Macular Degeneration: Improving your Vision

Macular Degeneration: Improving your Vision

Edited by Veronica Martin

hayle
medical

New York

Hayle Medical,
750 Third Avenue, 9th Floor,
New York, NY 10017, USA

Visit us on the World Wide Web at:
www.haylemedical.com

ISBN: 978-1-63241-709-1

Trademark Notice: Registered trademark of products or corporate names are used only for explanation and identification without intent to infringe.

Cataloging-in-Publication Data

    Macular degeneration : improving your vision / edited by Veronica Martin.
      p. cm.
Includes bibliographical references and index.
ISBN 978-1-63241-709-1
    1. Retinal degeneration. 2. Retina--Diseases. 3. Vision disorders--Treatment. I. Martin, Veronica.
RE661.D3 M33 2019
617.735--dc23

Table of Contents

Preface

The world is advancing at a fast pace like never before. Therefore, the need is to keep up with the latest developments. This book was an idea that came to fruition when the specialists in the area realized the need to coordinate together and document essential themes in the subject. That's when I was requested to be the editor. Editing this book has been an honour as it brings together diverse authors researching on different streams of the field. The book collates essential materials contributed by veterans in the area which can be utilized by students and researchers alike.

Macular degeneration is a condition of the eye, characterized by loss of central vision caused due to a damaged macula. Signs and symptoms generally occurring in people with macular degeneration are distorted or blurred vision, loss in contrast sensitivity, visual hallucinations and flashing lights, drastic decrease in visual acuity, etc. In macular degeneration, there arises a progressive accumulation of drusen in the various parts of retina, leading to its damage over time. It can be divided into early, intermediate and late stages, depending on its progression. A complete eye exam can establish a diagnosis of the condition. There are no treatments for reversing the effects of macular degeneration. Innovative interventions such as cell based therapies involving bone marrow stem cells, retinal pigment epithelial transplantation and use of associated genetic markers are being explored for the management and early prediction of macular degeneration. Some of the diverse topics covered in this book address the various clinical aspects of macular degeneration. The various studies that are constantly contributing towards advancing diagnosis and evolution of this field are examined in detail. It is a vital tool for all researching or studying macular degeneration as it gives incredible insights into emerging trends and concepts.

Each chapter is a sole-standing publication that reflects each author's interpretation. Thus, the book displays a multi-facetted picture of our current understanding of application, resources and aspects of the field. I would like to thank the contributors of this book and my family for their endless support.

Editor

Estimated Cases of Blindness and Visual Impairment from Neovascular Age-Related Macular Degeneration Avoided in Australia by Ranibizumab Treatment

Paul Mitchell[1]*, Neil Bressler[2], Quan V. Doan[3], Chantal Dolan[4], Alberto Ferreira[5], Aaron Osborne[¤5], Elena Rochtchina[1], Mark Danese[3], Shoshana Colman[6], Tien Y. Wong[7,8]

1 Department of Ophthalmology and Westmead Millennium Institute, University of Sydney, Westmead, New South Wales, Australia, 2 Wilmer Eye Institute, Johns Hopkins University, Baltimore, Maryland, United States of America, 3 Outcomes Insights, Inc., Westlake Village, California, United States of America, 4 CMD Consulting, Inc., Sandy, Utah, United States of America, 5 Novartis, Basel, Switzerland, 6 Genentech, Inc., South San Francisco, California, United States of America, 7 Singapore Eye Research Institute, National University of Singapore, Singapore, Singapore, 8 Centre for Eye Research Australia, University of Melbourne, Parkville, Victoria, Australia

Abstract

Intravitreal injections of anti-vascular endothelial growth factor agents, such as ranibizumab, have significantly improved the management of neovascular age-related macular degeneration. This study used patient-level simulation modelling to estimate the number of individuals in Australia who would have been likely to avoid legal blindness or visual impairment due to neovascular age-related macular degeneration over a 2-year period as a result of intravitreal ranibizumab injections. The modelling approach used existing data for the incidence of neovascular age-related macular degeneration in Australia and outcomes from ranibizumab trials. Blindness and visual impairment were defined as visual acuity in the better-seeing eye of worse than 6/60 or 6/12, respectively. In 2010, 14 634 individuals in Australia were estimated to develop neovascular age-related macular degeneration who would be eligible for ranibizumab therapy. Without treatment, 2246 individuals would become legally blind over 2 years. Monthly 0.5 mg intravitreal ranibizumab would reduce incident blindness by 72% (95% simulation interval, 70–74%). Ranibizumab given as needed would reduce incident blindness by 68% (64–71%). Without treatment, 4846 individuals would become visually impaired over 2 years; this proportion would be reduced by 37% (34–39%) with monthly intravitreal ranibizumab, and by 28% (23–33%) with ranibizumab given as needed. These data suggest that intravitreal injections of ranibizumab, given either monthly or as needed, can substantially lower the number of cases of blindness and visual impairment over 2 years after the diagnosis of neovascular age-related macular degeneration.

Editor: Keisuke Mori, Saitama Medical University, Japan

Funding: This study was funded by Novartis AG and Genentech, Inc. Novartis AG and Genentech, Inc. participated in the design and conduct of the study, in the distribution of the raw data to Outcomes Insights, in the analysis and interpretation of the data and in the preparation of the manuscript. Novartis AG and Genentech, Inc. reviewed the manuscript before submission. Third-party medical writing assistance, but not editorial content sufficient to meet International Committee of Medical Journal Editors (ICMJE) authorship criteria, was funded by Novartis AG.

Competing Interests: The authors have read the journal's policy and have the following conflicts: Dr. Bressler's employer, the Johns Hopkins University (JHU), but not Dr. Bressler himself, receives funding from Bayer, Genentech, Inc., Roche, Novartis and Regeneron, and Steba Pharmaceuticals for sponsored projects by the Department of Ophthalmology for the efforts of Dr. Bressler. Dr. Bressler receives salary support for these sponsored projects; the terms of these projects are negotiated and administered by JHU's Office of Research Administration. Under JHU's policy, support for the costs of research, administered by the institution, does not constitute a conflict of interest. Paul Mitchell has received consultancy fees, lecture fees and travel support from Novartis Pharma AG, Pfizer, Solvay (Abbott), Bayer, Alcon and Allergan. Novartis Pharma AG also funds a retina fellowship at Westmead Hospital, Sydney, which he supervises. Alberto Ferreira is an employee of Novartis Pharma AG. Aaron Osborne is currently with Alcon Research Ltd and is a former employee of Novartis Pharma AG. Shoshana Colman is an employee of Genentech, both Novartis Pharma AG and Genentech sponsored this study. Quan Doan and Mark Danese are employees of Outcomes Insights, Inc., and Chantal Dolan is an employee of CMD Consulting, Inc.; these companies were paid for analysis work. Genentech and Novartis market ranibizumab. No financial benefit is anticipated as a result of this study.

* Email: paul.mitchell@sydney.edu.au

¤Current address: Alcon Research Ltd., Fort Worth, Texas, United States of America

Introduction

Neovascular age-related macular degeneration (AMD) is the leading cause of blindness in many developed countries, including Australia [1,2]. Over the past 7 years, landmark clinical trials have shown that suppression of vascular endothelial growth factor (VEGF) with monthly or less frequent as-needed intravitreal injections of anti-VEGF agents prevented at least moderate visual acuity (VA) loss in nearly 95% of patients with neovascular AMD after 1 year and nearly 90% after 2 years, and at least moderate VA improvement has been noted in up to 40% of patients [3-5].

However, despite the clinical efficacy of this treatment and its widespread use in many countries, few studies have investigated the population-wide impact of anti-VEGF therapy on the incidence of blindness and visual impairment [6]. A Danish study recently showed that legal blindness attributable to AMD has halved since the introduction of anti-VEGF therapies and an Israeli study showed a reduction in overall blindness over time after anti-VEGF therapy [7,8].

In the USA, a recent model estimated that the number of cases of legal blindness caused by neovascular AMD would reduce dramatically if monthly ranibizumab (Lucentis, Genentech, Inc., South San Francisco, CA, USA/Novartis AG, Basel, Switzerland) was used when indicated compared with no treatment [9]. Treatment was expected to reduce cases of legal blindness (defined in the USA as best-corrected visual acuity [BCVA] of 20/200 or worse in the better-seeing eye) by approximately 72% (95% confidence interval [CI], 70–74%) and visual impairment (defined as BCVA worse than 20/40 in both eyes) by approximately 37% (95% CI, 35–39%). These data suggested that the impact of neovascular AMD on legal blindness and visual impairment is reduced dramatically when monthly ranibizumab is available.

Additionally, a retrospective US study confirmed that the prevalence of legal blindness and visual impairment 2 years after the diagnosis of neovascular AMD has decreased substantially since the introduction of anti-VEGF therapy [10]. Some patients in this retrospective study received dosing as needed instead of monthly.

In Australia, AMD is the leading cause of blindness and visual impairment in individuals aged 65 years or older and has been estimated to cost the country over $5 billion per year (2010 figures) [11,12]. The impact of ranibizumab therapy on the number of cases of legal blindness and visual impairment caused by neovascular AMD in Australia is unknown. Estimates from the recent model for the USA [9] are unlikely to be directly applicable to Australia due to potential differences in patient characteristics, incidence of neovascular AMD and treatment behaviours. In particular, the US model only considered patients receiving monthly ranibizumab treatment, which is only relevant to a subset of patients with neovascular AMD worldwide. In most other countries, including Australia, patients treated with ranibizumab for visual impairment due to neovascular AMD typically receive therapy on an as-needed basis. Thus, the aim of the present study was to estimate the proportion of cases of legal blindness and visual impairment due to neovascular AMD in Australia that were avoided by treatment with ranibizumab given monthly or as needed over 2 years. A model was constructed assuming that all eligible patients would receive treatment.

Materials and Methods

Subjects

The analysis was based on all Australians aged 60 years or over in 2010 (Table 1). Incident cases of neovascular AMD were derived from the estimated 10-year cumulative incidence of AMD in the Blue Mountains Eye Study (BMES) [13], extrapolated to the Australian population in 2010, and assuming that events occurred evenly over the observation period. Among individuals with neovascular AMD, it was assumed that 33% had existing neovascular AMD in the fellow eye at baseline using information from the Age-Related Eye Disease Study (AREDS), and ANCHOR and MARINA phase 3 ranibizumab trials [3,5,14]. Base-case distribution of lesion types was based on the population used in the recent US model [9]; 5% were predominantly haemorrhagic, 5% extrafoveal, 10% minimally classic, 20% predominantly classic and 60% occult. Patients were classified according to lesion type into three cohorts, which determined their eligibility for treatment (Figure 1). The 'PC lesion' cohort had predominantly classic lesions on fluorescein angiography; the 'OC/MC lesion' cohort had occult with no classic or minimally classic lesions; the 'treatment-ineligible' cohort had lesions that were considered, by the authors, as unlikely to receive ranibizumab treatment and this cohort was not included in the model.

Model structure

The 2-year rates of blindness and visual impairment were estimated using a patient-level simulation developed in TreeAge Pro 2009 Suite (TreeAge Software, Inc., Williamstown, MA, USA) that included three primary health states: 'active treatment', 'no treatment' and 'death' (Figure 1). Each patient began the model on a specific treatment and remained on active treatment until discontinuation or death. The model accounted for VA changes in each eye, treatment discontinuation, risk of AMD in the fellow eye and mortality risk over each monthly interval for 2 years. Separate simulations were run for the PC lesion cohort and the OC/MC lesion cohort to estimate the 2-year rates of outcomes. These rates were then applied to the size of each cohort to determine the magnitude of the outcomes at the population level using @Risk for Excel (version 5.5.1; Palisade Corporation, Ithaca, NY, USA). Change over 2 years in patients with incident neovascular AMD in year 1 was simulated in the model. Model parameters are specified in Table 2.

Treatments

The treatment alternatives were ranibizumab 0.5 mg, given monthly (specified as every 30 ± 7 days) [3,5], ranibizumab dosed as needed (i.e. according to signs of AMD as detected on 4-weekly optical coherence tomography [OCT], as used in the Comparison of AMD Treatment Trials [CATT] study) [4], and photodynamic therapy (PDT) with verteporfin (vPDT) or no treatment if vPDT was not indicated. Across these scenarios, all eligible patients in the model received only the specified treatment. The PC lesion cohort received treatment similar to patients in the ANCHOR trial (ranibizumab, vPDT or no treatment) and the OC/MC lesion cohort received treatment as received by patients in the MARINA trial (ranibizumab or no treatment).

Baseline visual acuity and visual acuity change

The baseline VA for the PC lesion and OC/MC lesion cohorts was based on BCVA distributions in the treated and fellow eyes for patients in ANCHOR and MARINA, respectively [3,5]. Because the results from a subgroup analysis of ANCHOR suggested that the extent of VA change is conditional on baseline VA, the Early Treatment Diabetic Retinopathy Study [ETDRS] chart letter score change over 2 years was sampled from the same patients selected at baseline to preserve the relationship between baseline VA and VA change [15]. For monthly ranibizumab treatment, the VA change from each study and each treatment was applied to the corresponding neovascular AMD lesion subtype and treatment group in the model. For ranibizumab dosed as needed, it was assumed that the gain in VA letter score achieved at 24 months was 2.1 (95% CI, −1.0–5.2) less than that achieved with monthly dosing, based on 2-year data from the CATT study [4]. This adjustment was applied to the patient-level ANCHOR and MARINA data. The model also accounted for the risk of treatment discontinuation each month using discontinuation rates from the ANCHOR and MARINA trials. While the patient was not receiving treatment, VA change was assumed to decline by 1.6% per month based on the 2-year sham-treatment results in MARINA (a loss of 14.9 letters over 24 months) [5]. Patients could not return to active treatment after discontinuation. The VA letter scores in each eye were tracked for each month up to month 24 or the time of death, whichever occurred first. A monthly risk of death was applied using Australian age- and gender-specific mortality data [16,17].

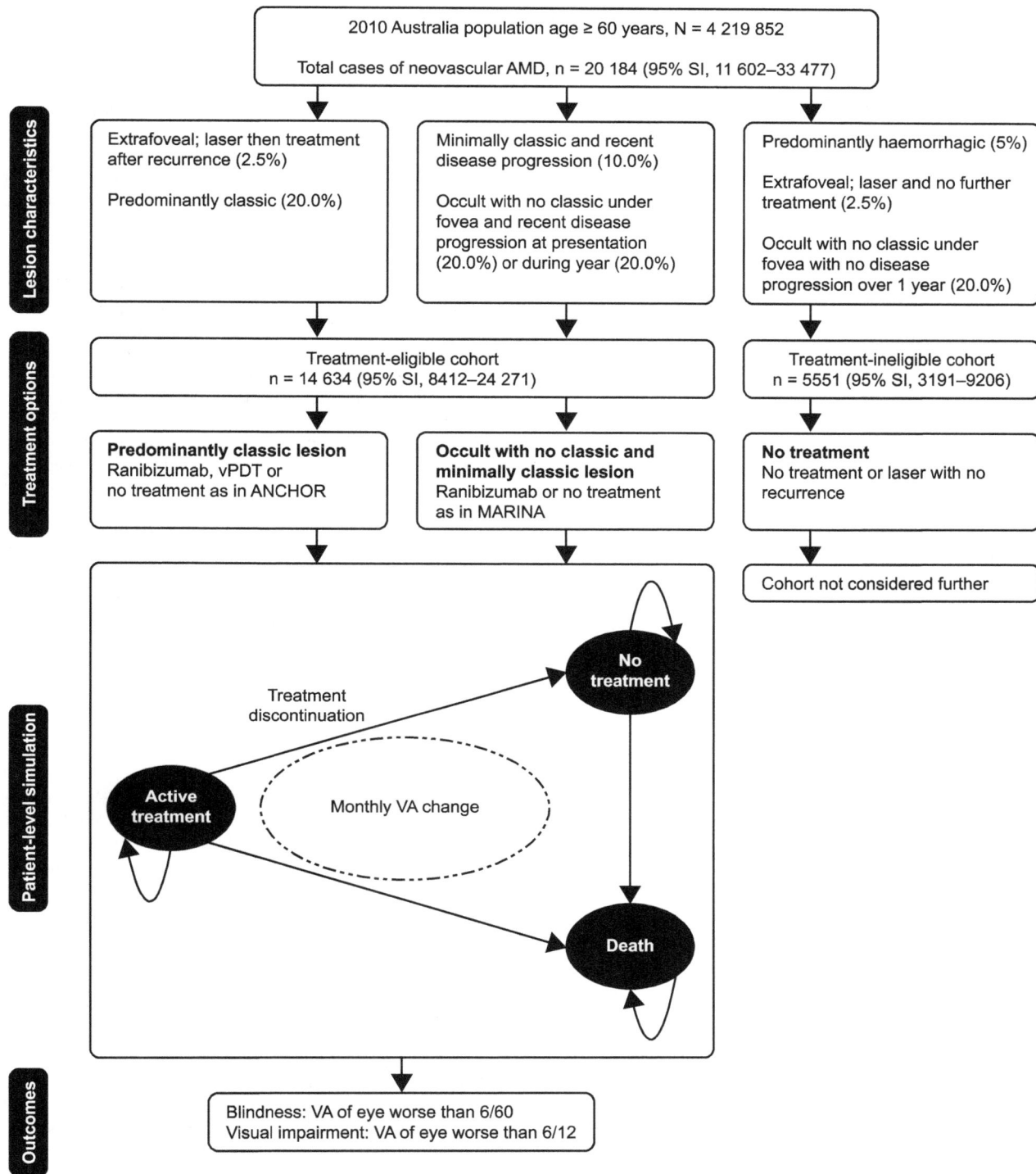

Figure 1. Model schematic. Incident cases of neovascular age-related macular degeneration (AMD) were derived by multiplying the number of individuals in each age group and gender by the respective incidences in the Blue Mountains Eye Study. Incident cases of neovascular AMD from 1 year were in the model for 2 years. Among individuals with AMD in one eye, 33% were estimated to have AMD in the fellow eye at baseline [3,5,14]. SI: simulation interval; VA: visual acuity; vPDT: photodynamic therapy with verteporfin.

Model outcomes

The key outputs from the model were the number of cases of legal blindness, defined as a VA score worse than 6/60 (approximated as a letter score of 38) in the better-seeing eye, and the number of cases of vision impairment, defined as a VA score of worse than 6/12 (approximated as a letter score of 68) in the better-seeing eye, over 2 years, including those patients already classified as having legal blindness [18]. For these outcomes,

Table 1. The Australian population aged 60 years or over in June 2010; distribution by age and gender.

Australian total population	60–69 years	70–79 years	≥ 80 years	Total
Male	1 053 685	599 729	326 947	**1 980 361**
Female	1 067 032	662 006	510 453	**2 239 491**
Total	**2 120 717**	**1 261 735**	**837 400**	**4 219 852**

Australian Bureau of Statistics (2011) 3101.0- Australian Demographic Statistics, Dec 2010. (Accessed September 2013 from http://www.abs.gov.au/AUSSTATS/abs@.nsf/mediareleasesbyCatalogue/251ECE081EC4B2EECA2579190013DCED).

ranibizumab was compared against no treatment, because PDT is now rarely used in Australia.

Sensitivity analyses

One-way sensitivity analyses were conducted on the proportions of neovascular AMD lesion types to assess the impact of these on blindness and visual impairment. Probabilistic sensitivity analysis was undertaken to account for various sources of patient variability and parameter uncertainty. Whenever possible, the distribution of patient-level characteristics was informed by the patient-level variability from trial data (e.g. baseline VA of each eye, VA change at 24 months in each eye). Parameter uncertainty was characterized as either a normal or gamma distribution. Patient-level variability was sampled in the first level, while parameter uncertainty was sampled in the second level, of a two-dimensional Monte Carlo simulation. To achieve stable rates, 300 averages of 10 000 iterations were sampled. Most of the key inputs into the model (Table 2) were evaluated. The confidence in the results is reported as an interval around the expected mean that captured 95% of all possible simulated values (95% simulation interval [SI]) for each outcome.

Results

Incidence of neovascular AMD

The model predicted that 20 184 (95% SI, 11 602–33 477) people would have developed neovascular AMD in Australia in 2010. Of these, 33% (6728) would have had pre-existing neovascular AMD in the fellow eye at the start of 2010.

Patients ineligible to receive ranibizumab

As shown in Figure 1, approximately 27.5% of incident cases of neovascular AMD (n = 5551) would have lesion types that would not be considered eligible for ranibizumab treatment. Assuming that all of the predominantly haemorrhagic cases progressed to a VA of worse than 6/60, and 33% of the extrafoveal and occult with no classic cases for which treatment was not judged to be indicated developed similar disease in the fellow eye, 2553 individuals would become legally blind over the following 2 years.

Patients eligible to receive ranibizumab

If none of the patients eligible to receive ranibizumab who were included in the model received treatment (n = 14 634; 95% SI, 8412–24 271), 2246 (95% SI, 1300–3695) patients would become legally blind over 2 years (Table 3). If they all received ranibizumab on a monthly basis, this number would drop to 624 patients (95% SI, 357–1031), a decrease of 72% (95% SI, 70–74%). If ranibizumab was dosed as needed, 724 patients (95% SI, 414–1211) would become blind, a decrease of 68% (95% SI, 64–71%). Treatment with PDT in those eligible to receive it would

result in a 12% (95% SI, 10–15%) reduction in cases of blindness (n = 1968; 95% SI, 1141–3220) compared with no treatment.

As summarized in Table 3, substantial reductions in the risk of bilateral visual impairment (BCVA worse than 6/60 in the incident eye) were predicted for ranibizumab dosed monthly or as needed. Bilateral visual impairment was predicted to develop over the 2-year period in 4846 patients with no treatment (95% SI, 2782–8027). Risk reductions of 37% and 28%, compared with no treatment, would be achieved with monthly ranibizumab and ranibizumab dosed as needed, respectively (Table 3). The corresponding reduction with PDT would be 1%. A BCVA worse than 6/60 in the incident eye would occur in 7865 patients (95% SI, 4534–13 120) with no treatment over the 2-year period; treatment with monthly or as-needed ranibizumab would achieve risk reductions of 68% and 65%, respectively, compared with no treatment, and the risk reduction for PDT would be 3%. A BCVA worse than 6/12 in the incident eye would occur in 8676 (95% SI, 4987–14 456) patients with no treatment, with risk reductions of 35%, 29% and 1% achieved with monthly ranibizumab, ranibizumab dosed as needed and PDT, respectively.

Sensitivity analyses

In the one-way sensitivity analyses, the proportions of patients with each neovascular AMD lesion type had the greatest impact on the cases of blindness and visual impairment avoided (Figure 2 and Figure 3, respectively). The SIs derived from the probabilistic sensitivity analyses showed moderate uncertainty around the estimates of legal blindness and visual impairment (Table 3).

Discussion

This study estimated the number of cases of blindness and visual impairment caused by neovascular AMD that can be avoided in Australia through the use of intravitreal ranibizumab injections. This model builds and expands on previous work by Bressler *et al.* [9] by accounting for characteristics specific to the Australian population, including Australian incidence data for neovascular AMD, Australian definitions for legal blindness and visual impairment, and Australian AMD incidence characteristics from population-level data. We modelled VA outcomes using 2-year, phase 3 ranibizumab trial data, which allowed us to use patient-level profiles following monthly treatment [3,5]. Results from the CATT study were used to estimate cases of blindness avoided with as-needed treatment [4]. The inclusion of as-needed therapy is a further important expansion of the previous model [9] because in many countries, including Australia, patients treated with ranibizumab for visual impairment due to neovascular AMD typically receive therapy on an as-needed basis. Furthermore, the inclusion of both monthly and as-needed regimens for the same population permits a comparison of predicted outcomes.

The model predicted that 20 184 people would develop AMD in Australia in 2010. Of these, about 5500 patients would not be

Table 2. Specification of the model parameters.

Model parameter		Value	Data source
Mortality		Overall death rate: 5.63/1000; age- and gender-specific rates used	Australian Bureau of Statistics[16,17]
Patients with health insurance/access problems		All residents of Australia are covered under Medicare plan and ranibizumab is fully covered for subfoveal neovascular AMD	Australian Health Service[a]
1-year incidence (SE) of neovascular AMD, women by age, years	< 60	0	BMES[13]
	60–69	0.0027 (0.0008)	
	70–79	0.0064 (0.0016)	
	≥ 80	0.0155 (0.0093)	
1-year incidence (SE) of neovascular AMD, men by age, years	< 60	0	BMES[13]
	60–69	0.0011 (0.0006)	
	70–79	0.0023 (0.0010)	
	≥ 80	0.0083 (0.0080)	
Patients with neovascular AMD in the fellow eye at baseline, %		33	Bressler et al. 2003[14]
Probability of developing neovascular AMD in the fellow eye, per month		0.0071	AREDS report number 8[b]
Baseline BCVA, LogMAR letter score, mean (SD) for the PC lesion cohort	Treated eye	46.5 (13.1)	ANCHOR trial data [3]; sampled from empirical trial data distribution
	Fellow eye without neovascular AMD at baseline	77.4 (13.7)	
	Fellow eye with neovascular AMD at baseline	34.5 (26.1)	
Baseline BCVA, LogMAR letter score, mean (SD) for the OC/MC lesion cohort	Treated eye	53.5 (13.2)	MARINA trial data;[5] sampled from empirical trial data distribution
	Fellow eye without neovascular AMD at baseline	76.1 (14.7)	
	Fellow eye with neovascular AMD at baseline	38.6 (26.2)	
Distribution of lesion subtypes, %	No treatment	27.5	Assumptions established in Bressler et al. 2011[9]
	PC lesion cohort	22.5	
	OC/MC lesion cohort	50.0	
Change in BCVA at 24 months		From empirical distributions	ANCHOR[3] and MARINA[5] trial data
Difference between monthly versus as-needed ranibizumab dosing in BCVA change at 24 months, letters (95% CI)		−2.1 (−5.2–1.0)	CATT study data[4]
Treatment discontinuation, monthly probability	Ranibizumab (PC lesions)	0.00178	ANCHOR (unpublished data, 2009)[9]
	Ranibizumab (OC/MC lesions)	0.00173	MARINA (unpublished data, 2006)[9]
	Photodynamic therapy	0.00407	ANCHOR (unpublished data, 2009)[9]
Patients, by BCVA letter score, after 2 years without treatment in PC lesion cohort, % (SD)	≤ 38 (worse than 6/60) in incident eye	67 (5.16)	TAP report number 3[c] (predominantly classic CNV)[d], SD reported in Bressler et al. 2011[9]
	≤ 38 (worse than 6/60) in better-seeing eye	22.3 (0.05)	TAP report number 3[d] and ANCHOR[3]
	≤ 68 (worse than 6/12) in incident eye	97.0 (1.86)	Assumption from Bressler et al. 2011[9]
	≤ 68 (worse than 6/12) in both eyes	52.6 (0.10)	Estimated based on TAP report number 3[c,d]
BCVA change per month after discontinuation from active treatment, %		1.6	Based on 2-year sham-treatment results in MARINA (−14.9 letters in 24 months)[5]

[a]Pharmaceutical Benefits Scheme. Ranibizumab. (Accessed September 2013 from www.pbs.gov.au). 2011.
[b]A randomized, placebo-controlled, clinical trial of high-dose supplementation with vitamins C and E, beta carotene, and zinc for age-related macular degeneration and vision loss: AREDS report no. 8. Arch Ophthalmol 2001; 119: 1417–1436.
[c]The mean baseline visual acuity of patients in TAP report number 3 is a 50-letter score.
[d]Bressler NM, Arnold J, Benchaboune M, Blumenkranz MS, Fish GE, Gragoudas ES et al. (2002) Verteporfin therapy of subfoveal choroidal neovascularization in patients with age-related macular degeneration: additional information regarding baseline lesion composition's impact on vision outcomes-TAP report No. 3. Arch Ophthalmol

120: 1443–1454.
AMD: age-related macular degeneration; BCVA: best-corrected visual acuity; CI: confidence interval; CNV: choroidal neovascularization; OC/MC lesion: occult with no classic lesions or minimally classic lesions; PC lesion: predominantly classic lesions; SD: standard deviation; SE: standard error.

eligible for ranibizumab treatment. Without treatment, 2246 of the remaining patients would become legally blind over a 2-year period. The results suggest that monthly ranibizumab would reduce the risk of legal blindness by 72% compared with no treatment, while the risk of visual impairment would be reduced by 37%. Dosing ranibizumab as needed with monthly monitoring provides a comparable reduction in the risk of blindness and visual impairment: 68% and 28%, respectively. Given the comparable VA outcomes between monthly and as-needed dosing regimens observed in the CATT study over 2 years [4], it is not surprising that there were only slightly fewer cases of blindness avoided with as-needed treatment than with monthly treatment, despite less frequent dosing. The extent to which these benefits can be extended beyond the 2-year period considered in this study is currently unknown.

The results of this modelling exercise confirm findings from a real-world database study in Denmark [7]. In that study, cases of blindness due to neovascular AMD were halved during the latter half of a 10-year period during which ranibizumab was introduced with a similar availability as in Australia. Since that study assessed

registered blindness and might not have used high-contrast charts to evaluate vision, it is difficult to compare the results with those of our study; however, the Danish study suggests that benefits can be extended beyond the 2-year window that we considered. Although comparison with real-world data was not the aim of this study, future validation of our findings with real-world data on the impact of anti-VEGF therapy in the Australian population is warranted. To date, no studies have been conducted to evaluate real-world reductions in blindness or visual impairment due to neovascular AMD in Australia following the introduction of anti-VEGF therapies. However, several ongoing studies may provide suitable real-world data for future validation in the Australian population [19,20] or for comparison with the UK [21].

Particularly in older populations, blindness and visual impairment have been shown to have substantial clinical, humanistic and economic impacts including increased risk of falls and fractures, reduced mobility and independence, earlier need for supportive care (e.g. entry into a nursing home), and increased risk of mortality [22-30]. Thus, our findings may be of value to healthcare policy experts, recognizing that our results are

Table 3. Blindness and visual impairment outcomes in patients with neovascular age-related macular degeneration with and without monthly treatment with ranibizumab.

Scenario	Number of patients (% of total cohort of 14 634)	95% SI, n (%)	Relative risk reduction compared with no treatment, % (95% SI)
Legal blindness (BCVA worse than 6/60 in better-seeing eye[a])			
No treatment	2246 (15)	1300–3695 (9–25)	–
Monthly ranibizumab	624 (4)	357–1031 (2–7)	72 (70–74)
Ranibizumab dosed as needed	724 (5)	414–1211 (3–8)	68 (64–71)
PDT scenario: PDT indicated and accessible; ranibizumab not accessible	1968 (13)	1141–3220 (8–22)	12 (10–15)
Visual impairment (BCVA worse than 6/12 in better-seeing eye[b])			
No treatment	4846 (33)	2782–8027 (19–55)	–
Monthly ranibizumab	3072 (21)	1763–5114 (12–35)	37 (34–39)
Ranibizumab dosed as needed	3504 (24)	1990–5833 (14–40)	28 (23–33)
PDT scenario: PDT indicated and accessible; ranibizumab not accessible	4773 (33)	2750–7884 (19–54)	1 (−1–4)
BCVA worse than 6/60 in the incident eye			
No treatment	7865 (54)	4534–13 120 (31–90)	–
Monthly ranibizumab	2538 (17)	1463–4197 (10–29)	68 (66–70)
Ranibizumab dosed as needed	2791 (19)	1604–4625 (11–32)	65 (61–68)
PDT scenario: PDT indicated and accessible; ranibizumab not accessible	7635 (52)	4433–12 616 (30–86)	3 (−3–8)
BCVA worse than 6/12 in the incident eye			
No treatment	8676 (59)	4987–14 456 (34–99)	–
Monthly ranibizumab	5632 (38)	3237–9336 (22–64)	35 (33–36)
Ranibizumab dosed as needed	6125 (42)	3513–10 166 (24–69)	29 (26–33)
PDT scenario: PDT indicated and accessible; ranibizumab not accessible	8606 (59)	4943–14 271 (34–98)	1 (−2–2)

[a]Legal blindness was defined as a BCVA letter score worse than 6/60 (approximate ETDRS letter score ≤ 38) in the better-seeing eye.
[b]Visual impairment was defined as a BCVA letter score worse than 6/12 (approximate ETDRS letter score ≤ 68) in the better-seeing eye.
BCVA: best-corrected visual acuity; ETDRS: Early Treatment Diabetic Retinopathy Study; PDT: photodynamic therapy; SI: simulation interval.

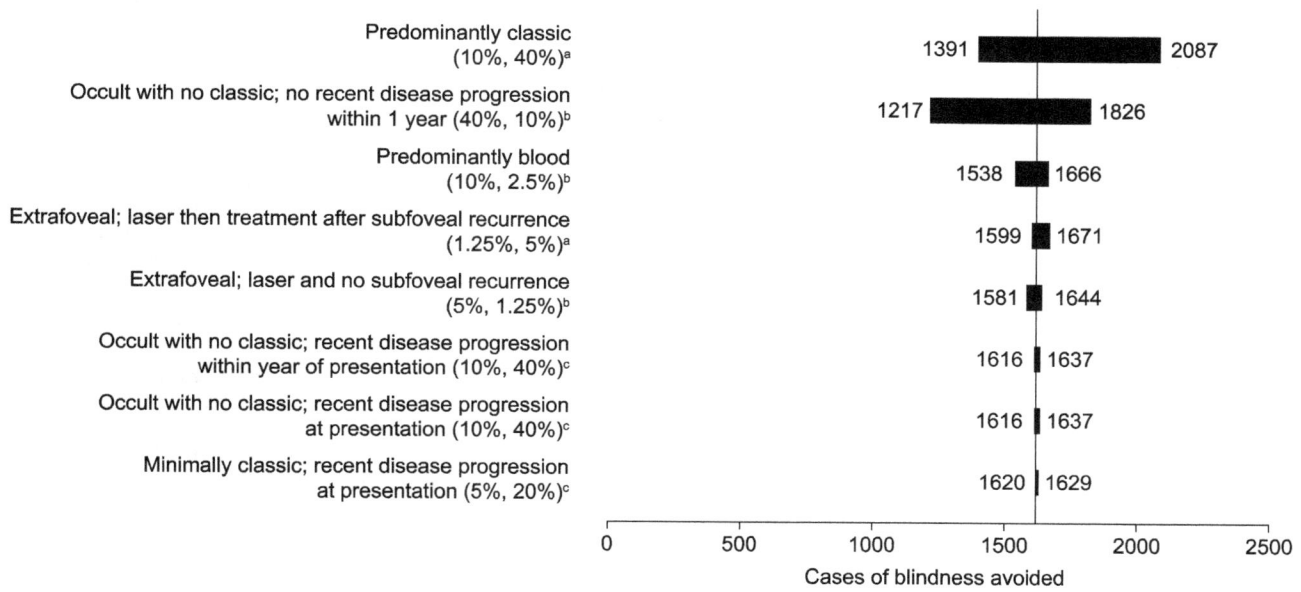

Figure 2. Sensitivity analyses. The impact of neovascular age-related macular degeneration lesion type on the cases of blindness (best-corrected visual acuity in better-seeing eye worse than 6/60) avoided using a monthly ranibizumab scenario compared with a no-treatment scenario. In the base analysis, 1622 cases of legal blindness were avoided with monthly ranibizumab, as indicated by the vertical line. [a]Eligible for PDT and ranibizumab. [b]Ineligible for any treatment. [c]Eligible for ranibizumab, but not for PDT. PDT: photodynamic therapy.

theoretical in nature and need to be considered in context along with factors such as patient preferences for therapy, treatment costs and healthcare resources. The information provided in this study may also be of value to health economists for incorporation in future cost-effectiveness models.

This study has some limitations that need to be considered. First, the incidence rates of neovascular AMD were based on the

BMES and there was no allowance for national variability; however, this study is considered representative of the portion of the Australian population that is affected by neovascular AMD (i.e. the Caucasian population), and applies to the older population of Australia in this study [31]. Secondly, there is a lack of patient-level data to estimate results for as-needed dosing. Nevertheless, since the VA profile found in the CATT study after treatment was

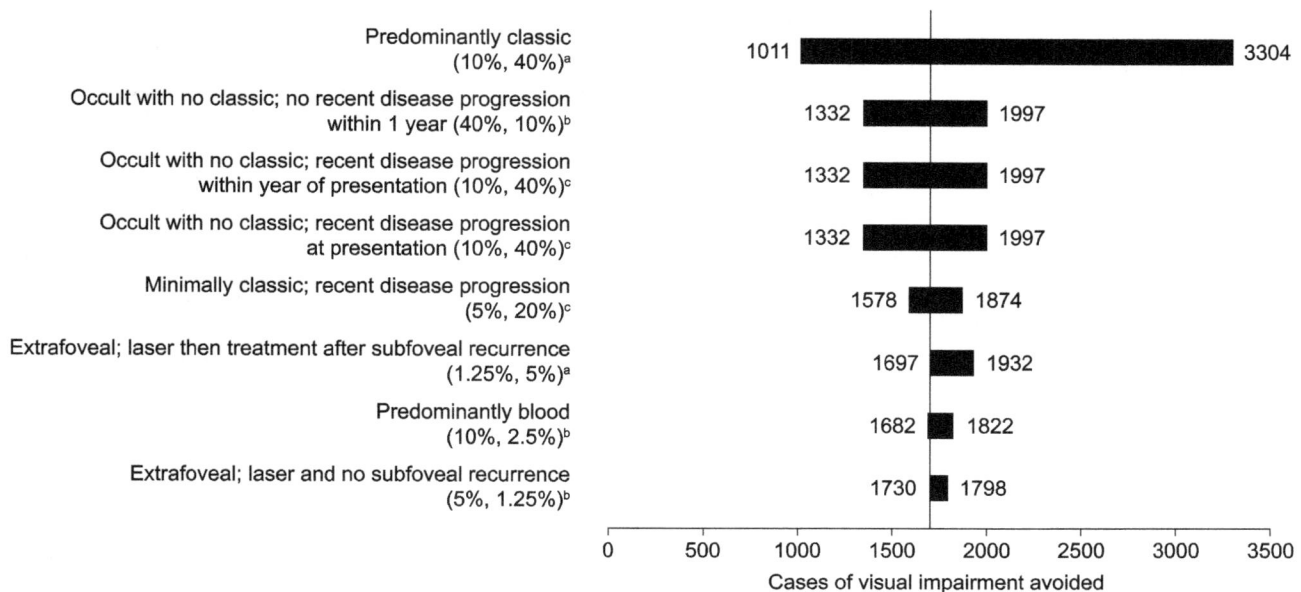

Figure 3. Sensitivity analyses. The impact of neovascular age-related macular degeneration lesion type on the cases of visual impairment (best-corrected visual acuity in better-seeing eye worse than 6/12) avoided using a monthly ranibizumab scenario compared with a no-treatment scenario. In the base analysis, 1774 cases of visual impairment were avoided with monthly ranibizumab, as indicated by the vertical line. [a]Eligible for PDT and ranibizumab. [b]Ineligible for any treatment. [c]Eligible for ranibizumab, but not for PDT. PDT: photodynamic therapy.

consistent across both groups (monthly and as-needed ranibizumab) [4], it was considered appropriate to also use the MARINA[5] and ANCHOR[3] profiles for as-needed dosing. Thirdly, there is limited evidence for the distribution of lesion types in patients in Australia. Since lesion type has an impact on avoidable blindness, according to the sensitivity analysis, it is important to know which types of lesions occur in the real world and how they respond to ranibizumab. Fourthly, the results might not be generalizable when the frequency of treatment is reduced below that used in the CATT study, or when monitoring of disease activity is limited to less than the monthly monitoring used in the CATT study. Also, further work is needed to understand the impact of 'treat-and-extend' regimens, as used in some countries, on the prevention of blindness.

To conclude, the results of this study suggest that, in Australia, ranibizumab given for neovascular AMD would reduce the number of cases of legal blindness over a 2-year period by 68% and 72%, and the number of cases of visual impairment by 28% and 37%, with as-needed and monthly treatment, respectively. These results are consistent with the known clinical benefits of anti-VEGF therapy for neovascular AMD, and extend the positive impacts of this treatment to the Australian population. In the future, neovascular AMD may no longer be the leading cause of blindness in older adults in Australia.

Acknowledgments

The authors would like to thank Jennifer Duryea of Outcomes Insights, Inc. for her work on the simulation model and technical report. In addition, Rowena Hughes and Polly Field from Oxford PharmaGenesis Ltd, Oxford, UK, provided editorial assistance in collating and addressing author comments.

Author Contributions

Conceived and designed the experiments: PM NB QVD CD AF AO ER MD SC TYW. Performed the experiments: PM NB QVD CD AF AO ER MD SC TYW. Analyzed the data: PM NB QVD CD AF AO ER MD SC TYW. Contributed reagents/materials/analysis tools: PM NB QVD CD AF AO ER MD SC TYW. Wrote the paper: PM NB QVD CD AF AO ER MD SC TYW.

References

1. Lim LS, Mitchell P, Seddon JM, Holz FG, Wong TY (2012) Age-related macular degeneration. Lancet 379: 1728–1738.

2. Resnikoff S, Pascolini D, Etya'ale D, Kocur I, Pararajasegaram R, et al. (2004) Global data on visual impairment in the year 2002. Bull World Health Organ 82: 844–851.

3. Brown DM, Michels M, Kaiser PK, Heier JS, Sy JP, et al. (2009) Ranibizumab versus verteporfin photodynamic therapy for neovascular age-related macular degeneration: two-year results of the ANCHOR study. Ophthalmology 116: 57–65.

4. Martin DF, Maguire MG, Fine SL, Ying GS, Jaffe GJ, et al. (2012) Ranibizumab and bevacizumab for treatment of neovascular age-related macular degeneration: two-year results. Ophthalmology 119: 1388–1398.

5. Rosenfeld PJ, Brown DM, Heier JS, Boyer DS, Kaiser PK, et al. (2006) Ranibizumab for neovascular age-related macular degeneration. N Eng J Med 355: 1419–1431.

6. Cheung N, Wong TY (2012) Changing trends of blindness: the initial harvest from translational public health and clinical research in ophthalmology. Am J Ophthalmol 153: 193–195.

7. Bloch SB, Larsen M, Munch IC (2012) Incidence of legal blindness from age-related macular degeneration in Denmark: year 2000 to 2010. Am J Ophthalmol 153: 209–213 e202.

8. Skaat A, Chetrit A, Belkin M, Kinori M, Kalter-Leibovici O (2012) Time trends in the incidence and causes of blindness in Israel. Am J Ophthalmol 153: 214–221 e211.

9. Bressler NM, Doan QV, Varma R, Lee PP, Suner IJ, et al. (2011) Estimated cases of legal blindness and visual impairment avoided using ranibizumab for choroidal neovascularization: non-Hispanic white population in the United States with age-related macular degeneration. Arch Ophthalmol 129: 709–717.

10. Campbell JP, Bressler SB, Bressler NM (2012) Impact of availability of anti-vascular endothelial growth factor therapy on visual impairment and blindness due to neovascular age-related macular degeneration. Arch Ophthalmol 130: 794–795.

11. Australian Institute of Health and Welfare (2005) *Vision problems among older Australians*. Bulletin no. 27. AIHW cat. No. AUS 60. Canberra. 2005. Accessed September 2013. Available: http://www.aihw.gov.au/WorkArea/DownloadAsset. aspx?id=6442453394.

12. Macular Degeneration Foundation (2011) *Eyes on the future*. Accessed September 2013. Available: http://www.mdfoundation.com.au/LatestNews/Deloitte_ Eyes_on_the_Future_Report_Exec_Summary%20web.pdf.

13. Wang JJ, Rochtchina E, Lee AJ, Chia EM, Smith W, et al. (2007) Ten-year incidence and progression of age-related maculopathy: the Blue Mountains Eye Study. Ophthalmology 114: 92–98.

14. Bressler NM, Bressler SB, Congdon NG, Ferris FL, 3rd, Friedman DS, et al. (2003) Potential public health impact of Age-Related Eye Disease Study results: AREDS report no. 11. Arch Ophthalmol 121: 1621–1624.

15. Kaiser PK, Brown DM, Zhang K, Hudson HL, Holz FG, et al. (2007) Ranibizumab for predominantly classic neovascular age-related macular degeneration: subgroup analysis of first-year ANCHOR results. Am J Ophthalmol 144: 850–857.

16. Australian Bureau of Statistics (2010) 3201.0 *Population by Age and Sex, Australian States and Territories*. Accessed September 2013. Available: http://www.abs.gov. au/ausstats/abs@.nsf/mf/3201.0/.

17. Australian Bureau of Statistics (2010) 3302.0 - Deaths, Australia, 2009; Table 2: Death rates, Summary, States and territories - 1999 to 2009. 2010. Accessed September 2013. Available: http://www.abs.gov.au/ausstats/abs@.nsf/ detailspage/3302.02009.

18. Commonwealth of Australia (2011) Guide to Social Security Law. 7 Jan 2011. Accessed September 2013. Available: http://www.facsia.gov.au/guides_acts/ ssg/ssguide-1/ssguide-1.1/ssguide-1.1.p/ssguide-1.1.p.210.html.

19. Abedi F, Wickremasinghe S, Islam AF, Inglis KM, Guymer RH (2014) Anti-VEGF treatment in neovascular age-related macular degeneration: a treat-and-extend protocol over 2 years. Retina Epub ahead of print.

20. Gillies MC, Walton RJ, Arnold JJ, McAllister IL, Simpson JM, et al. (2014) Comparison of outcomes from a phase 3 study of age-related macular degeneration with a matched, observational cohort. Ophthalmology 121: 676–681.

21. Writing Committee for the UK Age-Related Macular Degeneration EMR Users Group (2014) The Neovascular Age-Related Macular Degeneration Database: multicenter study of 92 976 ranibizumab injections: report 1: visual acuity. Ophthalmology 121: 1092–1101.

22. Cruess A, Zlateva G, Xu X, Rochon S (2007) Burden of illness of neovascular age-related macular degeneration in Canada. Can J Ophthalmol 42: 836–843.

23. Hochberg C, Maul E, Chan ES, Van Landingham S, Ferrucci L, et al. (2012) Association of vision loss in glaucoma and age-related macular degeneration with IADL disability. Invest Ophthalmol Vis Sci 53: 3201–3206.

24. Ivers RQ, Cumming RG, Mitchell P, Attebo K (1998) Visual impairment and falls in older adults: the Blue Mountains Eye Study. J Am Geriatr Soc 46: 58–64.

25. Klein BE, Moss SE, Klein R, Lee KE, Cruickshanks KJ (2003) Associations of visual function with physical outcomes and limitations 5 years later in an older population: the Beaver Dam eye study. Ophthalmology 110: 644–650.

26. Lotery A, Xu X, Zlateva G, Loftus J (2007) Burden of illness, visual impairment and health resource utilisation of patients with neovascular age-related macular degeneration: results from the UK cohort of a five-country cross-sectional study. Br J Ophthalmol 91: 1303–1307.

27. Popescu ML, Boisjoly H, Schmaltz H, Kergoat MJ, Rousseau J, et al. (2011) Age-related eye disease and mobility limitations in older adults. Invest Ophthalmol Vis Sci 52: 7168–7174.

28. Soubrane G, Cruess A, Lotery A, Pauleikhoff D, Mones J, et al. (2007) Burden and health care resource utilization in neovascular age-related macular degeneration: Findings of a multicountry study. Arch Ophthalmol 125: 1249–1254.

29. Szabo SM, Janssen PA, Khan K, Lord SR, Potter MJ (2010) Neovascular AMD: an overlooked risk factor for injurious falls. Osteoporos Int 21: 855–862.

30. Wood JM, Lacherez P, Black AA, Cole MH, Boon MY, et al. (2011) Risk of falls, injurious falls, and other injuries resulting from visual impairment among older adults with age-related macular degeneration. Invest Ophthalmol Vis Sci 52: 5088–5092.

31. Mitchell P, Wang JJ, Foran S, Smith W (2002) Five-year incidence of age-related maculopathy lesions: the Blue Mountains Eye Study. Ophthalmology 109: 1092–1097.

2

Mitochondrial DNA Variants Mediate Energy Production and Expression Levels for CFH, C3 and EFEMP1 Genes: Implications for Age-Related Macular Degeneration

M. Cristina Kenney[1]*, **Marilyn Chwa**[1], **Shari R. Atilano**[1], **Janelle M. Pavlis**[1], **Payam Falatoonzadeh**[1], **Claudio Ramirez**[1], **Deepika Malik**[1], **Tiffany Hsu**[1], **Grace Woo**[1], **Kyaw Soe**[1], **Anthony B. Nesburn**[1,2], **David S. Boyer**[3], **Baruch D. Kuppermann**[1], **S. Michal Jazwinski**[4], **Michael V. Miceli**[4], **Douglas C. Wallace**[5], **Nitin Udar**[1]

1 Gavin Herbert Eye Institute, University of California Irvine, Irvine, California, United States of America, 2 Cedars-Sinai Medical Center, Los Angeles, California, United States of America, 3 Retina-Vitreous Associates Medical Group, Beverly Hills, California, United States of America, 4 Tulane Center for Aging and Department of Medicine, Tulane University, New Orleans, Louisiana, United States of America, 5 Children's Hospital of Pittsburgh, Pittsburgh, Pennsylvania, United States of America

Abstract

Background: Mitochondrial dysfunction is associated with the development and progression of age-related macular degeneration (AMD). Recent studies using populations from the United States and Australia have demonstrated that AMD is associated with mitochondrial (mt) DNA haplogroups (as defined by combinations of mtDNA polymorphisms) that represent Northern European Caucasians. The aim of this study was to use the cytoplasmic hybrid (cybrid) model to investigate the molecular and biological functional consequences that occur when comparing the mtDNA H haplogroup (protective for AMD) versus J haplogroup (high risk for AMD).

Methodology/Principal Findings: Cybrids were created by introducing mitochondria from individuals with either H or J haplogroups into a human retinal epithelial cell line (ARPE-19) that was devoid of mitochondrial DNA (Rho0). In cybrid lines, all of the cells carry the same nuclear genes but vary in mtDNA content. The J cybrids had significantly lower levels of ATP and reactive oxygen/nitrogen species production, but increased lactate levels and rates of growth. Q-PCR analyses showed J cybrids had decreased expressions for CFH, C3, and EFEMP1 genes, high risk genes for AMD, and higher expression for MYO7A, a gene associated with retinal degeneration in Usher type IB syndrome. The H and J cybrids also have comparatively altered expression of nuclear genes involved in pathways for cell signaling, inflammation, and metabolism.

Conclusion/Significance: Our findings demonstrate that mtDNA haplogroup variants mediate not only energy production and cell growth, but also cell signaling for major molecular pathways. These data support the hypothesis that mtDNA variants play important roles in numerous cellular functions and disease processes, including AMD.

Editor: Walter Lukiw, Louisiana State University Health Sciences Center, United States of America

Funding: Funding provided by The Discovery Eye Foundation www.discoveryeye.org, Lincy Foundation lincyinstitute.unlv.edu/lincy.html, Beckman Macular Research Initiative www.beckmanmacular.org, The Henry Guenther Foundation, Polly and Michael Smith Foundation, Research to Prevent Blindness Foundation www.rpbusa.org, and the National Institute on Aging (AG006168). The funders had no role in study design, data collection and analysis, decision to publish, or preparation of the manuscript.

Competing Interests: The authors have declared that no competing interests exist.

* E-mail: mkenney@uci.edu

Introduction

Mitochondria provide critical cellular energy using the tricarboxylic acid (TCA) cycle, oxidative phosphorylation (OXPHOS), and beta-oxidation of fatty acids for metabolism, cell division, production of reactive oxygen species (ROS), and apoptosis. Human mitochondrial (mt) DNA forms a circle of double stranded DNA with 16,569 nucleotide pairs. The non-coding mtDNA Dloop contains 1121 nucleotides and is important for replication and transcription. The coding region of mtDNA encodes for 37 genes including 13 protein subunits essential for OXPHOS, 2 ribosomal RNAs, and 22 transfer RNAs [1–3]. The mtDNA can be categorized into haplogroups that are defined by a set of specific SNP variants that have accumulated over tens of thousands of years and correspond to different geographic populations of the world. The H haplogroup is the most common European haplogroup, while the J haplogroup originates from the Northern European region and is defined by SNP variants that are associated with heat production as an adaptation to colder climates [4].

The mtDNA plays an important role in aging and diseases [4–6]. Specific haplogroups are associated with a variety of eye diseases including age-related macular degeneration (AMD) [7–10], diabetic retinopathy [11], pseudoexfoliation glaucoma [12,13], primary open-angle glaucoma [14], keratoconus [15], multiple sclerosis-related optic neuritis [16,17], and Leber hereditary optic neuropathy [1,18]. In AMD, the J, T and U haplogroups are high risk while the H haplogroup is protective against developing the disease [7–10,19]. The actual cellular mechanisms or pathways by which mtDNA variants contribute to disease states have not been identified. One difficulty in studying the functional consequences of different mtDNA SNP variants is that the vast majority of proteins which contribute to energy biogenesis are encoded by nuclear DNA and imported into the mitochondria [4,20]. The contribution to energy production by the mtDNA is relatively small by comparison and experimental models have not been available to identify the nuclear-mitochondria interactions. In the present study, we have developed a human ARPE-19 cell cybrid (cytoplasmic hybrid) model, a system where individual cell lines have mitochondria representing H or J haplogroups from different individuals but contain identical nuclei. Using this model, we have taken a systematic approach to understand some of the basic mechanisms related to cellular functions that are potentially different within the H and J haplogroups. Our results show that the H and J haplogroups have different rates of energy production, cell growth, ROS production, and altered expression of nuclear genes involved in inflammation and human retinal diseases. Our findings are significant because they demonstrate that mtDNA mediates not only energy production but also cell signaling for major molecular pathways. These data support a paradigm shift in thinking about the role that mitochondria play in numerous cellular functions and disease processes.

Materials and Methods

Ethics Statement

All research involving human participants was approved by the Institutional review board of the University of California, Irvine (#2003-3131). Written informed consent was obtained and all clinical investigations were conducted according to the principles expressed in the Declaration of Helsinki.

Cybrid Cultures and Culture Conditions

For DNA analyses, 10 ml of peripheral blood was collected via venipuncture in tubes containing 10 mM EDTA. DNA was isolated with a DNA extraction kit (PUREGENE, Qiagen, Valencia, CA). Platelets were collected in tubes containing 3.2% sodium citrate, isolated by a series of centrifugation steps, and final pellets were suspended in Tris buffered saline. The ARPE-19 cells deficient in mtDNA (Rho0) were created by serial passages in low dose ethidium bromide [21]. Cybrids were produced by polyethylene glycol fusion of platelets with Rho0 ARPE-19 cells according to modified procedures of Chomyn [22]. Verification of transfer of the mitochondria into the Rho0 ARPE-19 cells was accomplished by using polymerase chain reaction (PCR), restriction enzyme digestion, and sequencing of the mtDNA to identify the mitochondrial haplogroup of each cybrid [9]. The SNPs defining the J haplogroup were G13708A, C16069T and T16126C. The H defining SNPs were T7028C and A73G. All experiments used passage 5 cybrid cells for the assays described below.

Identification of Cybrid Haplogroups

Cybrid DNA was extracted from cell pellets using a spin column kit (DNeasy Blood and Tissue Kit, Qiagen) and quantified using the Nanodrop 1000 (Thermo Scientific, Wilmington, DE). Restriction enzyme digests were performed as described in Udar and coworkers to determine mitochondrial haplogroups [9]. The digestion products were run on 3% agarose gels for the H cybrids and 1.2% agarose gels for the J cybrids. Allelic discrimination was

also performed to confirm the haplogroups. The primers for allelic discrimination were synthesized by ABI Assay-by-Design. The samples were run at GenoSeq, the UCLA Genoytyping and Sequencing Core, on an ABI 7900HT. The data was analyzed with Sequence Detection Systems software from ABI.

Reactive Oxygen/Nitrogen Species (ROS/RNS) Assay

The H haplogroup and J haplogroup cybrid cultures were incubated in 24 well plates (1×10^5 cells/well). After 24 hours, the cells were exposed to the reagent and ROS/RNS production measured with a scanning unit (FMBio III, Hitachi, San Francisco, CA) for the fluorescent dye 2′,7′-dichlorodihydrofluorescein diacetate (H_2DCFDA, Invitrogen-Molecular Probes, Carlsbad, CA) using 490 nm for the emission and 520 nm for the excitation wavelengths. The values represent combined results of experiments using three different H cybrids and three different J cybrids, each experiment repeated twice and the assays run in quadruplicate.

ATP Production Assay

Intracellular ATP levels were measured for H and J cybrids using the luminescence ATP detection assay (ATPlite Perkin Elmer Inc., Waltham, MA USA) as per the supplier's instructions. Cybrid lines (H cybrids n = 3, J cybrids n = 3) were cultured 24 hours on a 96 well plate at 3 different concentrations, 100K, 50K, and 10K cells per well with a final volume of 100 μl/well. Luminescence was measured using a Synergy HT Multi-Mode microplate reader and Gen5 Data Analysis software (BioTek instruments, Winooski, VT USA). All experiments were repeated twice and assayed in quadruplicate.

Lactate Assay

Lactate concentrations in the samples were measured by the Lactate Assay Kit (Eton Bioscience Inc, San Diego, CA). Cells were plated at 100K and 50K in 96-well plates and incubated overnight. Lactate levels were measured according to the manufacturer's protocol. Standards and samples were set up as duplicates and quadruplicates and experiments were repeated twice.

Growth Curve Assay

The growth curves of six different cybrids were assessed over six days under similar environmental conditions. Three different H cybrids and three J cybrids were grown to passage 5 using methods described above. For each time point, 300K cells per well were plated onto six-well plates and each cybrid cell line was assayed in duplicate. Cells were incubated in standard conditions and culture medium was changed every other day. The cell numbers were measured using a Cell Viability Analyzer (ViCell, Beckman Coulter, Miami, FL). The numbers of cells plated at timepoint 0 were designated as 100% and the percentage increase in growth for each cybrid at 2, 4, and 6 days were calculated. A mean percentage increase value of all three H cybrids and three J cybrids were compared by nonlinear regression analysis (Prism, version. 3.0; GraphPad Software Inc., San Diego, CA). Within each experiment, the assays were run in duplicate and the experiments repeated twice.

Isolation of RNA and Amplification of cDNA

Cells from cybrid cultures (H cybrids, n = 3, J cybrids, n = 3) were pelleted, and RNA isolated using the RNeasy Mini-Extraction kit (Qiagen, Inc.) following the manufacturer's protocol. The RNA was quantified using a NanoDrop 1000 (Thermo-

Scientific). For Q-PCR analyses, 100 ng of individual RNA samples were reverse transcribed into cDNA using the QuantiTect Reverse Transcription Kit (Qiagen).

Gene Expression Assay and Statistical Analyses

RNA was isolated as described above. For the gene expression analyses, the RNAs from the three H haplogroup cybrid cultures were combined (250 ng/µl per sample) into a single sample for analyses. Then three J haplogroup cybrid cultures were also combined into one sample. The H cybrid and J cybrid RNAs were sent to the UCLA Clinical MicroArray Core Lab for analyses with the Affymetrix Human U133 Plus 2.0 Array. The gene expression results were analyzed with pathway analysis software (INGENUITY Systems, Redwood City, CA).

Quantitative PCR (Q-PCR) Analyses

Q-PCR was performed using primers for genes associated with AMD and retinal disorders (CFH, C3, EFEMP1, ARMS2, MYO7A, BBS10), antioxidant enzymes (SOD1, SOD2, SOD3, PRDX6, GPX3), and genes related to metabolic homeostasis (FOXO1, ME3, GFM1) (QuantiTect Primer Assay, Qiagen). Total RNA was isolated from pellets of cultured cells of haplogroup J cybrids, n = 3 and haplogroup H cybrids, n = 3 as described above. The Q-PCR was performed using a QuantiFast SYBR Green PCR Kit (Qiagen) on a Bio-Rad iCycler iQ5 detection system and expression levels were standardized for all primers using TATA box binding protein (TBP) as the reference gene. The analyses were performed in triplicate. Statistical analyses of gene expression levels were performed to measure difference between haplogroups using Prism version 5.0 (Graph-Pad Software, Inc., San Diego, CA).

Statistical Analyses

Data were subjected to statistical analysis by ANOVA (Prism, version. 3.0; GraphPad Software Inc.). Newman-Keuls multiple-comparison test was done to compare the data within each experiment. $P < 0.05$ was considered statistically significant. The p values are designated as the following: *$p < 0.05$; **$p < 0.01$; ***< 0.001. Error bars in the graphs represent SEM (standard error mean). Experiments were performed two or three times and each treatment run in quadruplicate.

Results

Studies were designed to first confirm the identity of each of the cybrids created from the common Rho0 cell line. Figure 1a shows that after PCR amplification and digestion with AluI enzyme, the H cybrids have mtDNA with the C allele in the SNP 7028 representing the H haplogroup (156 bp+152 bp bands; lanes 3 and 4). The non-H haplogroup mtDNA, represented by the T allele, shows bands at 152 bp+126 bp (lanes 1 and 5). Figure 1b shows the restriction digest with BstNI enzyme and reveals a single band at 1210 bp representing the A allele of J haplogroup mtDNA (lanes 4 and 5). The non-J haplogroup is represented by the G allele (874 bp+336 bp, lanes 1 and 3). The mtDNA is absent in the Rho0 cells (lane 2). Each donor mitochondrial haplogroup matched up with the corresponding cybrid, confirming their identity.

Biochemical parameters related to mitochondrial function (production of ROS/RNS, ATP, and lactate) were measured for the different cybrids. It was shown that the H haplogroup cybrids produced 21% more ROS/RNS than the J haplogroups cybrids ($100 \pm 3.4\%$ versus $79 \pm 6.1\%$, p = 0.006, Figure 2). Next, the cybrids were plated in concentrations of 100K cells, 50K cells or

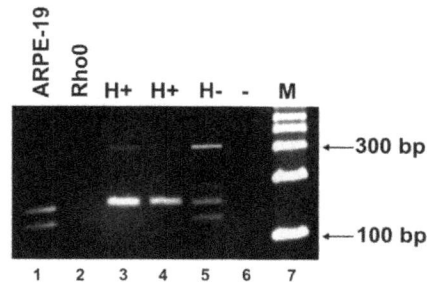

Haplogroup H - T7028C

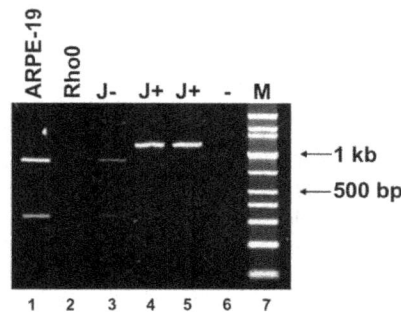

Haplogroup J - G13708A

Figure 1. Agarose gels showing bands obtained after PCR amplification and restriction enzyme digestion of the H haplogroup and J haplogroup cybrids. Figure 1a: Panel Upper – Digestion pattern of T7028C that defines the H haplogroup appears in lanes 3 and 4. The non-H haplogroup samples appear in lanes 1 and 5. Figure 1b: Panel Lower – Digestion pattern of G13708A that defines the J haplogroup is found in lanes 4 and 5. The non-J samples are in lanes 1 and 3. The Rho0 sample lacks mtDNA PCR amplification product (lane 2, upper and lower panels). M = marker; - indicates water only; bp, basepair.

10K cells and the relative amounts of ATP were measured (Figure 3a). The ATP production levels at all cell concentrations were significantly lower in the J cybrid samples compared to the H cybrids: 100K group, $100 \pm 3.4\%$ in H versus $62 \pm 3.9\%$ in J, $p < 0.001$; 50K group, $100 \pm 5.9\%$ in H versus $59 \pm 4.7\%$ in J, $p < 0.001$; 10K group, $100 \pm 6.2\%$ in H versus $40 \pm 4.9\%$ in J, $p < 0.0001$. In contrast, when the lactate levels were measured, the J haplogroup cybrids produced significantly higher levels compared to the H haplogroup (Figure 3b). When plated at a density of 100K cells, the J cultures showed a 1.8 fold increase in lactate production (3.57 ± 0.15) compared to H cybrids (1.98 ± 0.21, p = 0.0009). The J cultures plated with 50K cells showed 2.80 ± 0.23 mM lactate concentration levels versus 1.78 ± 0.13 in the H cybrid cultures, p = 0.008. Our findings indicate that the H haplogroup cybrids had lower levels of glycolysis than the J cybrids.

Cell growth was then compared for the cybrids. The H cybrids and J cybrids were plated with 30k cells per well, cultured over a 144 hour time period and then analyzed for cell viability at Days 0, 2, 4, and 6 (Figure 4). The Day 0 values were normalized to 100% in both H and J cultures. At each time point, the J cybrids

ROS/RNS Levels

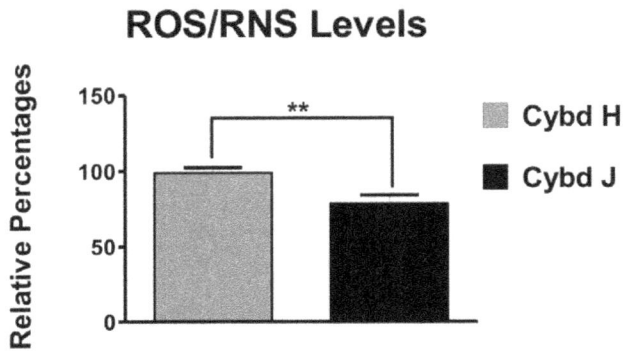

Figure 2. Differences in relative ROS/RNS levels are shown in H cybrid versus J cybrid cultures after 24 hours. Cybrids H produced increased levels of ROS/RNS compared to the J cybrids (**p<0.01). ROS/RNS, reactive oxygen/nitrogen species; Cybd, cybrid.

ATP Levels in Cybrids H and J

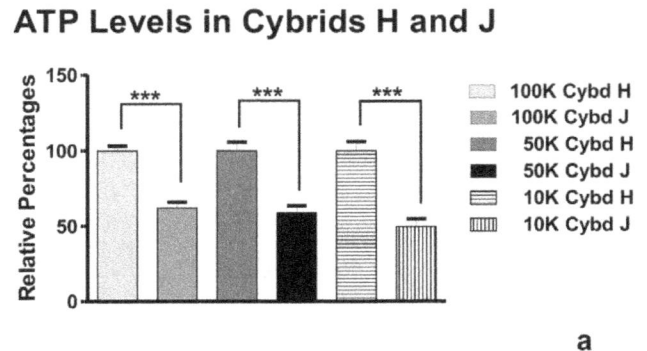

a

Lactate Assay

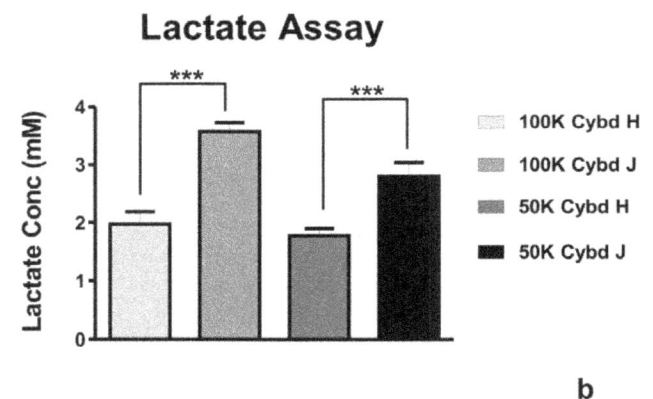

b

Figure 3. The H cybrid versus J cybrid cultures show differences in the ATP production and lactate levels. Figure 3a. Relative ATP levels in H versus J cybrid cultures at three different cell concentrations incubated for 24 hours. The H cybrids produced increased ATP levels compared to J cybrid cultures (***p<0.001). Figure 3b. Lactate levels in cybrid H versus cybrid J cultures at two different cell concentrations incubated for 24 hours. The H cybrids had decreased lactate production when compared to the J cybrids (**p<0.01, ***p<0.001) indicating lower glycolysis activity. Cybd, cybrid.

showed greater growth than the H cybrids (Day 2, 232% vs 159%; Day 4, 329% vs 234%) and by Day 6 the J cultures showed 420% growth while the H cultures had 284% growth. Regression analyses showed the J cybrid cultures had greater growth rates than the H cybrid cultures. It was an unexpected finding that the H cybrids were producing more ATP but had lower growth rates compared to J cybrid cultures.

Not only is the influence of haplogroup important for cellular mechanisms, the total number of mitochondria can also significantly influence various pathways. The mtDNA copy numbers in the H cybrids and J cybrids were determined by Q-PCR using 18S to represent nuclear DNA (nDNA) and MT-ND2 to represent mtDNA (TaqMan, Life Technologies). An average of 3 independent representatives was used for each haplogroup. We found that at Day 1 the mtDNA copy numbers (nDNA:mtDNA ratio) were similar in the H cybrid and J cybrid cultures (1.34 ± 0.0228 versus 1.36 ± 0.017, p = 0.59). At Day 7 the nDNA:mtDNA ratios in the H and J cybrid cultures were 1.3 ± 0.020 versus 1.26 ± 0.016, p = 0.14, indicating that the mtDNA copy numbers were similar after the longer incubation period. Therefore, our results showed that the H cybrids and J cybrids had similar mtDNA copy numbers.

Based upon differences found between H cybrids and J cybrids in the growth studies as well as the energy pathway assays, we hypothesized that the H and J cybrids would have different expression patterns of the nuclear genes. Therefore, we isolated the RNA of the cultured three H cybrids (Cybd 10.07, Cybd 10.04, Cybd 10.03) and three J cybrids (Cybd 10.05, Cybd 10.01, Cybd 11.32), and pooled equal quantities from each sample The H cybrid RNA and J cybrid RNA were then analyzed using the Affymetrix array that characterizes the gene expression for over 40K genes. Analyses of the data using the INGENUITY systems statistical program showed that the predominant pathways altered in the H cybrids versus J cybrids were Cell Death, Cell-to-Cell Signaling, Growth and Proliferation, Cellular Movement, and Morphology (Table 1). The program also reported that the diseases and disorders affected by varying the mitochondrial haplogroups but having cells with identical nuclei were Cancer, Genetic Disorders, Dermatologic Diseases, Developmental Disorders, and Connective Tissue Diseases (Table 2).

We then performed additional in-depth analyses for genes of interest associated with AMD, ROS/RNS production and mitochondrial functions. For these studies, Q-PCR analyses were performed on individual H or J cybrid samples (n = 3 each) in

triplicate. Figure 5 shows expression patterns for 14 different genes: (a) Six genes (CFH, C3, EFEMP1, MYO7A, BBS10, and ARMS2) that are reported to have high risk polymorphic associations with retinal diseases; (b) Five genes (SOD1, SOD2, SOD3, PRDX6, and GPX3) related to the production of ROS/RNS; and (c) Three nuclear encoded genes (FOXO1, GFM1, and ME3) that function in metabolic homeostasis. The Q-PCR showed that the J cybrids had decreased RNA expression levels for CFH (-1.0 ± 0.8 $\Delta\Delta C_T$; 0.5 fold, p = 0.0001), C3 (-1.8 ± 0.5 $\Delta\Delta C_T$; 0.29 fold, p = 0.0003), and EFEMP1 (-2.0 ± 0.4 $\Delta\Delta C_T$; 0.25 fold, p<0.0001), compared to the H cybrids. The MYO7A gene expression was higher in the J cybrids compared to the H cybrids (0.83 ± 0.29 $\Delta\Delta C_T$; 1.78 fold, p = 0.007). The BBS10 gene was expressed at similar levels in the H and J cybrids (p = 0.2). The ARMS2 expression levels were very low but similar in H and J cybrids (p = 0.89, data not shown). These Q-PCR findings were in agreement with the Affymetrix chip analyses which showed these genes to be elevated in the combined H haplogroup cybrid sample

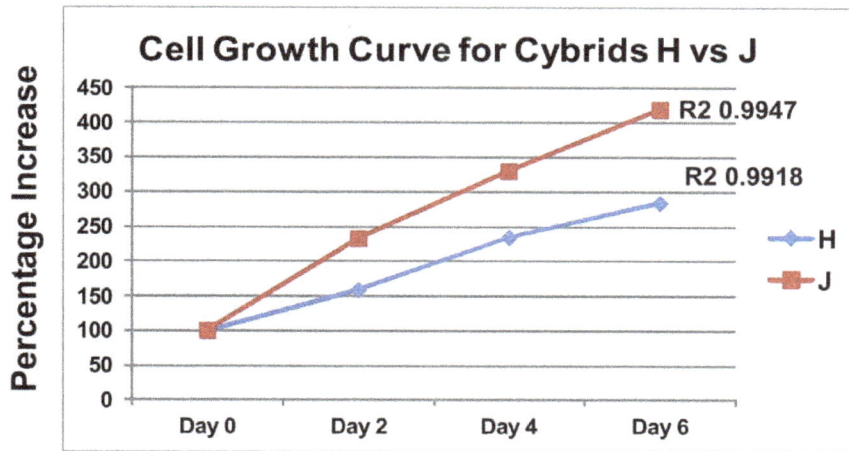

Figure 4. Six day growth curve shows a differential growth pattern for the H cybrids versus J cybrids. At Day 0, 30k cells per well were plated and the cell viabilities measured at Days 2, 4, and 6. The graph shows that the J cybrids grew at a faster rate than the H cybrids.

compared to the combined J cybrid sample. The antioxidant enzyme genes (SOD1 ($p = 0.6$), SOD2 ($p = 0.3$), SOD3 ($p = 0.6$), PRDX6 ($p = 0.1$), and GPX3 ($p = 0.2$) and nuclear encoded mitochondrial genes (FOXO1 ($p = 0.9$), ME3 ($p = 0.4$), and GFM1 ($p = 0.3$) showed no statistically significant differences by Q-PCR analyses between the H cybrid and J cybrid groups.

Discussion

This study was designed to provide insights into the different molecular and functional outcomes of having the J haplogroup mtDNA variants versus the H mtDNA variants within cells that had identical nuclei. We found that the H and J cybrids have different modes of energy production. The H cybrids have higher levels of ATP production regardless of the plating density, indicating they utilize OXPHOS more effectively than the J cybrids. Elevated production of ATP levels has been reported in Huntington's patients that have the H haplogroup compared to non-H individuals [23]. Our analyses also showed that the H cybrids produced significantly higher levels of ROS/RNS compared to the J cybrids. Endogenous production of ROS occurs as electrons leak from the electron transport chain (ETC) within the mitochondria [24]. Our findings suggest that the J cybrids may have lower efficiency of the ETC leading to lower ATP and ROS levels which is similar to that described in osteosarcoma cybrids with J haplogroups [25]. Similar relationships between the H and J haplogroups have been reported in human subjects. Marcuello studied 114 healthy males and showed

that those with the J haplogroup had lower maximum oxygen consumption (VO2max) rates than the non-J haplogroups [26], but that a steady state of exercise could eliminate this disparity [27]. Further analyses showed that this disparity was because the H haplogroup had significantly higher VO2max and oxidative damage than the J haplogroup individuals [28]. The inefficiency of the OXPHOS mitochondrial energy production found in J haplogroups may lead to lower ROS production and less oxidative damage, which in part may explain high correlations between centenarians and the J haplogroup population [29–31].

Using the cybrid model we found significantly higher lactate levels in the J cybrids indicating that these cells relied on glycolysis to a much greater degree than the OXPHOS-utilizing H cybrids. It has been shown in mitochondrial diseases (i.e., Leigh and MELAS syndromes) that diminished efficiency of the ETC is accompanied by higher lactate levels. Interestingly, when H cybrid and UK cybrid properties were compared, the UK cybrids had a 32% higher ATP production level and similar ROS levels compared to H cybrids [32]. This supports the idea that specific mtDNA SNPs that define the haplogroups can affect the cell energy function, pathway utilization and levels of oxidative stress.

In our study, comparison of the mtDNA to nDNA showed that the mtDNA copy numbers were similar in the H cybrids and J cybrids. We used 18S amplicon to represent the nDNA and MT-ND2 amplicon for the mtDNA. Suissa et al showed that cells with the J haplogroup backgrounds had increased mtDNA copy numbers compared to the H haplogroups [33]. The differences in the mtDNA copy numbers between Suissa and our studies may

Table 1. Molecular and Cellular Functions Associated with Gene Expression Differences Between H vs J Cybrids.

NAME	P-value	# Molecules
Cell Death	$3.77E^{-05} - 2.59E^{-02}$	107
Cell-to-Cell Signaling & Interactions	$6.86E^{-05} - 2.44E^{-02}$	55
Cellular Growth & Proliferation	$2.61E^{-05} - 2.66E^{-02}$	159
Cellular Movement	$6.56E^{-08} - 2.63E^{-02}$	117
Cell Morphology	$2.64E^{-05} - 2.68E^{-02}$	52

Table 2. Diseases and Disorders Associated with Gene Expression Differences Between H vs J Cybrids.

NAME	P-value	# Molecules
Cancer	$4.62E^{-06} - 2.63E^{-02}$	205
Genetic Disorders	$3.60E^{-05} - 2.17E^{-02}$	182
Dermatological Diseases & Conditions	$3.60E^{-05} - 2.03E^{-02}$	45
Developmental Disorders	$3.60E^{-05} - 2.64E^{-02}$	56
Connective Tissue Disorders	$3.60E^{-05} - 9.11E^{-04}$	13

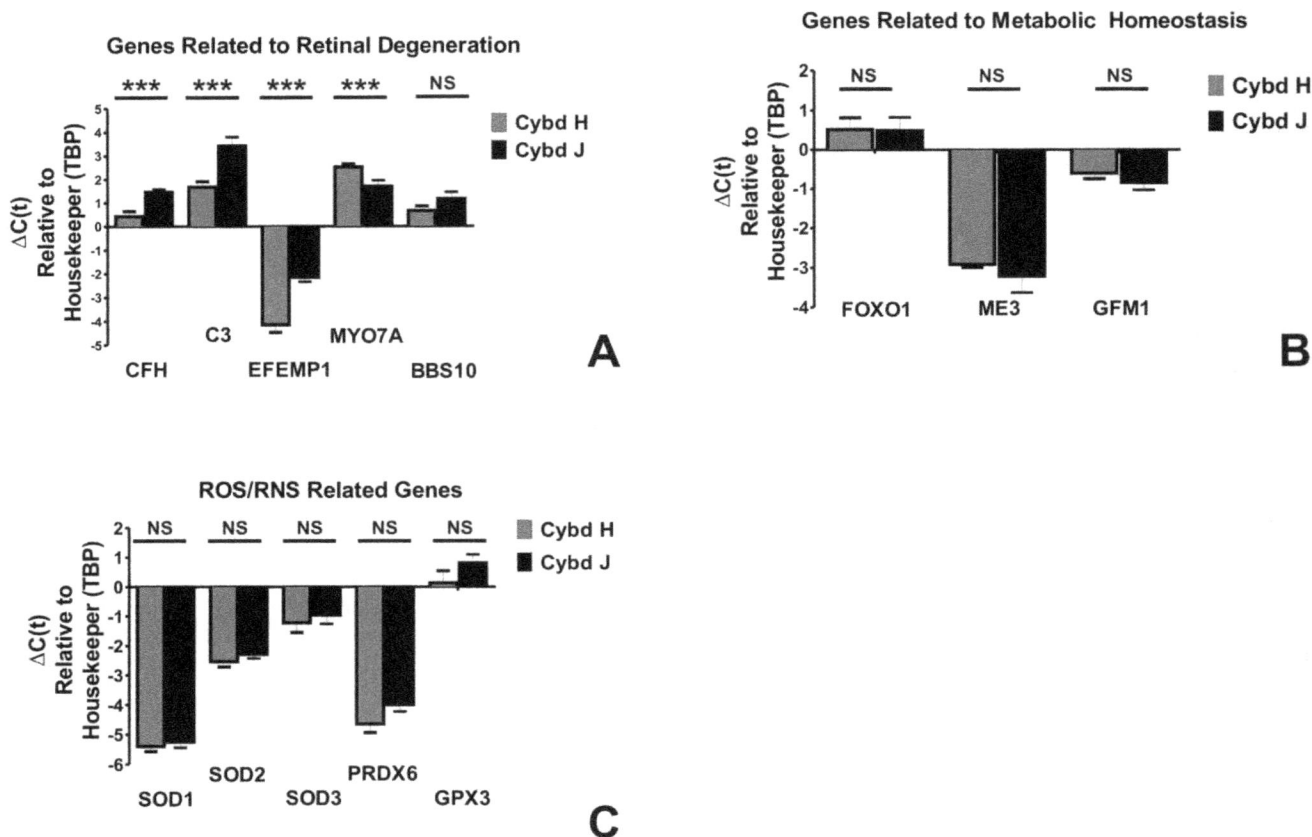

Figure 5. Q-PCR shows differential gene expression patterns for H cybrids versus the J cybrids. The relative delta C(t) values of the H cybrid cultures versus the J cybrid cultures are shown. Values are the average of three different H or J cybrids (originating from different individuals) run in six Q-PCR determinations. Error bars are SEM. *** p<0.001). The abbreviations for gene names are as follows: **Genes Related to Retinal Degeneration.** CFH, Complement Factor H; C3, Complement Component 3; EFEMP1, EGF-Containing Fibrilin-like Extracellular Matrix Protein 1; ARMS2, Age-Related Maculopathy Susceptibility 2; MYO7A, Myosin VIIA; BBS10, Chromosome 12, Open Reading Frame 58 for Bardet-Biedl syndrome. **Nuclear Encoded Genes.** FOXO1, Forkhead Box1; ME3, Malic Enzyme 3, NADP(+)-Dependent, Mitochondrial; GFM1, Mitochondrial Elongation Factor G1. **ROS/RNS Related Genes.** SOD1, Superoxide Dismutase 1; SOD2, Superoxide Dismutase 2; SOD3, Superoxide Dismutase 3; PRDX6, Peroxiredoxin 6; GPX3, Glutathione Peroxidase 3. NS, not significant; Cybd, cybrid; ROS/RNS, reactive oxygen/nitrogen species; TBP, TATA box binding protein.

be related to different cell types for the Rho0 cells and the source of mitochondria. Their study used a Wal2 Rho0 cell line suspension which was then fused with chemically enucleated lymphoblasts containing either H or J haplogroups. In our study we used ARPE-19 cells which attach to the plate and the source of mitochondria was from platelets that lack nuclei and therefore, did not have to undergo chemical enucleation. In our study, with the mtDNA copy numbers similar in H cybrids and J cybrids, it implies that the changes found in ATP production and ROS formation were not simply due to lower numbers of mitochondria within the cells but were properties of mitochondrial haplogroups.

The differences in mtDNA SNP variants between H and J haplogroups are considerable. The H defining 7028C allele is a synonymous SNP located in the MT-CO1 gene. Further subtyping of the J haplogroups used in our study showed two cybrids were J1c and one was J1d1a. The J1c mtDNA has 14 SNP variants with 4 of those being non-synonymous, leading to amino acid changes in the MT-CYB, MT-ND3, and MT-ND5 genes compared to H mtDNA. The J1d1a variant has 15 SNPs with 3 non-synonymous changes in the MT-CYB, MT-ND3 and MT-ND5 genes. We believe these SNP variants could affect protein functions leading to altered ATP, lactate, and ROS production

compared to the H cybrids. However, further work will be necessary to clarify the mechanisms.

The present study uses ARPE-19 cells, a cell line commonly used to analyze human RPE cell functions, as the background for cybrids to study mitochondrial function. Studies previously showed that removal of mtDNA in ARPE-19 cells caused significant changes in nuclear gene expression [21]. Moreover, osteosarcoma cells with depleted mtDNA are resistant to chemically induced apoptosis [34]. This suggests that the absence or alterations of mitochondria can affect the expression of some genes. One goal of the present study was to investigate the influence of mtDNA variants on expression of genes important to development of AMD and to this end we utilized the Affymetrix chip assay with its large number of genes. Analyses of the H and J cybrids showed differences of 107 genes within the Cell Death pathways and 55 genes within the Cell-to-Cell Signaling pathways (Table 1). In terms of diseases that might be affected, the INGENUITY system analyses showed 205 genes from the Cancer category while 182 genes were associated with the Genetic Disorder category. At this time the mechanisms for these differences are not known. However, the H and J cybrids have identical nuclei and one can speculate that the influences may be within the nuclear-mitochondrial interactions, or possibly based upon energy requirements within the cells that could mediate pathway regulation. In either case, our findings show that mtDNA can affect changes in numerous important pathways and can mediate cell signaling and molecular functions. Our results indicate that 1) subtle changes in mtDNA can lead to a set of changes at the molecular and cellular level that are similar to those that occur with complete loss of mtDNA [21,35], and 2) that these pathways changes are reminiscent of the retrograde response in yeast, C. elegans, Drosophila, mouse and human cells that is known to affect lifespan (in human cell population doubling levels; for review see [36,37]).

Based upon the delta Ct values obtained from the Affymetrix array, we targeted three groups of genes for further analyses by Q-PCR:

1) Genes Related to Retinal Degeneration

Recent studies have demonstrated a close relationship between mitochondria, oxidative stress and inflammation. Complement activation and inflammation play a role in AMD, diabetic retinopathy and uveitis. The CFH and C3 genes are known high risk genes associated with AMD. In our study, the J cybrids had significantly lower expression levels of CFH and C3 than the H cybrids. The CFH gene polymorphism (rs1061170, T1277C, Tyr402His) has been associated with the AMD in Caucasian populations [38–42] but not Asians [43–45]. The CFH protein is a major regulator for the alternative complement pathway as it blocks C3 activation to C3b and causes C3b degradation. Using animal models, it has been shown that CFH is critical for long-term retinal function [46]. The CFH protein with the high risk Tyr402His polymorphism has a reduced capacity to bind with malondialdehyde (MDA), a lipid peroxidation cytotoxin, which could possibly contribute to a defective innate immune response for AMD patients [47]. In our study, the higher expression of CFH in the H cybrids would mean higher levels of the CFH inhibitor protein and may be a mechanistic way that the H haplogroup could be protective for AMD [19]. If the H cybrids have higher expression levels for CFH, then the products of the complement cascade should be lower, resulting in less oxidative stress, reduced inflammatory-related debris, and more protection for RPE cells.

The C3 gene expression was also lower in J cybrids (0.29 fold, p = 0.0003) compared to H cybrids. In Caucasian English and Scottish populations, sequencing studies showed that within exon 3 of C3, the common functional R102G polymorphism (rs2230199; 120700.0001) was strongly associated with AMD [48–50]. Studies show that AMD individuals have significantly elevated levels of C3a des Arg in their plasma compared with the age-matched control group, irrespective of the CFH polymorphism status [51]. In AMD eyes, drusen have an accumulation of complement-associated proteins including C3 [52,53]. Cultured human RPE cells show a dramatically increased production of CFH and C3 after exposure to activated T cells [54] and oxidative stress induced by hydrogen peroxide [55]. It may be that the higher ROS production levels in the H cybrids stimulate upregulation of the complement components, including C3. Further studies will be needed to determine these interactions.

EFEMP1 is the third high risk AMD gene with lower expression in the J cybrids compared to H cybrids (0.25 fold, p = 0.0001). EFEMP1 is an extracellular matrix protein associated with drusen formation and complement activation in EFEMP1-R345W knock-in mice [56]. Histology of AMD eyes shows that EFEMP1 protein can be found between the RPE cell layer and drusen [57]. It has been suggested that misfolded EFEMP1 protein accumulates within RPE cells causing altered cellular function and inflamma-

tion. Higher EFEMP1 levels also play a role in tumor metastasis [58,59]. ARMS2 was the fourth AMD-associated gene investigated. It has been suggested that expression of the LOC387715/ARMS2 gene yields a 12 kDa protein that localizes to the outer mitochondrial membrane [60,61], although this has not been found by others [62]. In our study we found that the H cybrids and J cybrids have similar low levels of expression for ARMS2 (data not shown).

Our findings suggest that the mtDNA haplogroup defining variants mediate the expression of CFH, C3, and EFEMP1 genes and play a role in the inflammatory pathway of human RPE cells. The mechanism is not known at this time but one can speculate that the type of energy pathway, OXPHOS versus glycolysis, might feed back to the cell, influencing its innate immunity status. Studies using cybrids created from osteosarcoma cells have shown that mitochondrial haplogroups can influence the mRNA expression and intra-mitochondrial protein levels of HSP60 and HSP75, major elements in the stress responses for cells [63]. In addition, differences have been reported in expression for stress responsive nuclear genes interleukin-6, interleukin-1, and tumor necrosis factor receptor 2 [64]. Our findings suggest that cybrids with the H haplogroup mtDNA have different cellular homeostasis which may influence the response to oxidative stress, complement pathways, and degree of inflammation. This is significant because these responses are critical for the development of diseases, especially those related to the retina which has high metabolically active photoreceptor cells and is constantly exposed to UV light, both sources of oxidative stress. Another possible mechanism by which mtDNA variants may mediate cellular functions is through an as of yet unknown nuclear-mitochondrial DNA interaction(s) similar to that described for Saccharomyces cerevisiae cells grown under different metabolic conditions [65]. Studies show that mitochondrial dysfunction and damage can lead to a retrograde response that triggers many intracellular signaling pathways and nuclear genes [36]. The outcome is a compensatory adaptation that prolongs longevity (see excellent review [37]). No matter the mechanism occurring, our findings provide significant evidence that although the mtDNA is relatively small, in addition to energy production, it can mediate important cellular functions associated with inflammation which warrants further investigation.

Another gene investigated was MYO7A which was higher in J cybrids compared to H cybrids (1.78 fold, p = 0.006). This gene encodes an unconventional myosin that has structurally conserved heads but divergent tails to bind different macromolecules, allowing them to move along the actin filaments. Using this mechanism, the unconventional myosins can transport "cargo" within the cells [66]. The MYO7A gene is expressed in the RPE and photoreceptor cells, and has been associated with the retinal degeneration found in Usher syndrome type IB [67,68]. In shaker-1 mice a mutation of the MYO7a gene caused abnormalities in the melanosome distribution in the RPE cells [69]. The RPE and photoreceptor cells are highly metabolically active and the different utilization of the energy pathways (OXPHOS vs glycolysis) of the H versus the J cybrids may affect the efficiency of the MYO7A protein and lead to cell death. Further work needs to be performed to understand the relationship between the bioenergetics of the cells and MYO7A protein function.

The BBS10 gene is related to the Bardet-Biedl syndrome, a rare autosomal recessive disease characterized by systemic abnormalities including progressive rod-cone retinal dystrophy, cognitive impairment, postnatal obesity, renal dysplasia, and polydactyly. In our study the expression of the BBS10 gene was similar in the H cybrid and J cybrid samples.

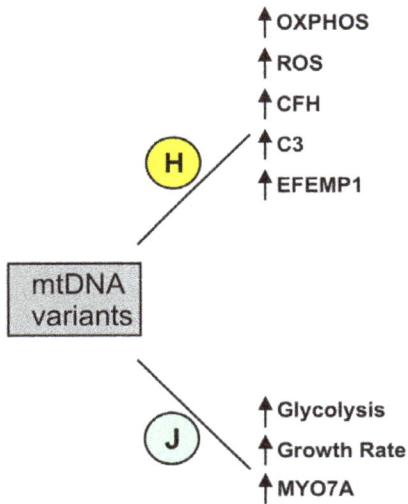

Figure 6. Schematic summary of the changes found in cybrids with H haplogroup mtDNA variants compared to cybrids with the H haplogroup mtDNA variants.

2) ROS/RNS Related Genes

Elevated ROS levels, such as seen in the H cybrid culture, can trigger activation or overexpression of various antioxidant genes. The SOD1, SOD2, SOD3 genes are important for conversion from superoxides into hydrogen peroxide, which is then converted by PRDX6 and GPX3 to water and oxygen. In our study, there were no differences in the expression levels for these antioxidant genes between the H and J cybrids. This is similar to results for H versus Uk cybrids which reported similar levels for MnSOD [32]. It may be that the levels of ROS produced by haplogroup-related SNPs are important for cell signaling but are not high enough to

cause overexpression of antioxidant enzymes associated with pathological mutations or disease processes. It should be noted that in patients with osteoarthritis, the J haplogroup population did have higher levels of catalase, an antioxidant enzyme involved in the removal of hydrogen peroxide [70]. Furthermore, combining the haplogroup types with specific biomarkers allowed for phenotypic identification of osteoarthritis patients [71].

3) Genes Related to Metabolic Homeostasis

We found that three genes important for maintaining metabolic functions (FOXO1, ME3, and GFM1) had similar expression levels present in the H and J cybrids. This finding suggests that the haplogroup SNP variants do not mediate a generalized increase of expression of all metabolically-related genes, but rather elevation of specific pathways, in this case the inflammatory, stress responsive, and alternative complement pathways. This may be important for the retina, which is very metabolically active, and AMD, which has been associated with both mitochondrial dysfunction and inflammation.

In summary, our findings demonstrate the valuable information that can be obtained using cybrid cell models. This study provides evidence that the mtDNA SNP variants associated with H versus J haplogroups can mediate differences in ROS, ATP and lactate production, influence cell growth rates, and modulate expression for genes involved in inflammation, oxidative stress, and apoptosis (Figure 6), which have been strongly associated with AMD. These findings are important because they provide possible mechanisms by which mitochondria-nuclear interactions can occur and they identify targets for possible drug interventions for AMD.

Author Contributions

Conceived and designed the experiments: MCK ABN DSB BDK DCW NU. Performed the experiments: MC SRA JMP CR DM KS PF TH GW. Analyzed the data: MCK MC SRA BDK DCW NU. Contributed reagents/materials/analysis tools: SMJ MVM. Wrote the paper: MCK.

References

1. Wallace DC (1992) Diseases of the mitochondrial DNA. Annu Rev Biochem 61: 1175–1212.
2. Wallace DC (1994) Mitochondrial DNA mutations in diseases of energy metabolism. J Bioenerg Biomembr 26: 241–250.
3. McFarland R, Turnbull DM (2009) Batteries not included: diagnosis and management of mitochondrial disease. J Intern Med 265: 210–228.
4. Wallace DC (2005) A mitochondrial paradigm of metabolic and degenerative diseases, aging, and cancer: a dawn for evolutionary medicine. Annu Rev Genet 39: 359–407.
5. Wallace DC, Lott MT, Procaccio V (2007) Mitochondrial genes in degenerative diseases, cancer and aging; Rimoin DL, Connor J.M., Pyeritz, R.E., Korf, B.R., editor. Philadelphis, PA: Churchill Livingstonr Elsevier. 194–298 (Chapter 113) p.
6. Czarnecka AM, Bartnik E (2011) The role of the mitochondrial genome in ageing and carcinogenesis. J Aging Res 2011: 136435.
7. Canter JA, Olson LM, Spencer K, Schnetz-Boutaud N, Anderson B, et al. (2008) Mitochondrial DNA polymorphism A4917G is independently associated with age-related macular degeneration. PLoS ONE 3: e2091.
8. Jones MM, Manwaring N, Wang JJ, Rochtchina E, Mitchell P, et al. (2007) Mitochondrial DNA haplogroups and age-related maculopathy. Arch Ophthalmol 125: 1235–1240.
9. Udar N, Atilano SR, Memarzadeh M, Boyer D, Chwa M, et al. (2009) Mitochondrial DNA haplogroups associated with Age-related macular degeneration. Invest Ophthalmol Vis Sci 50: 2966–2974.
10. SanGiovanni JP, Arking DE, Iyengar SK, Elashoff M, Clemons TE, et al. (2009) Mitochondrial DNA variants of respiratory complex I that uniquely characterize haplogroup T2 are associated with increased risk of age-related macular degeneration. PLoS One 4: e5508.
11. Kofler B, Mueller EE, Eder W, Stanger O, Maier R, et al. (2009) Mitochondrial DNA haplogroup T is associated with coronary artery disease and diabetic retinopathy: a case control study. BMC Med Genet 10: 35.
12. Wolf C, Gramer E, Muller-Myhsok B, Pasutto F, Wissinger B, et al. (2010) Mitochondrial haplogroup U is associated with a reduced risk to develop exfoliation glaucoma in the German population. BMC Genet 11: 8.

13. Abu-Amero KK, Cabrera VM, Larruga JM, Osman EA, Gonzalez AM, et al. (2011) Eurasian and Sub-Saharan African mitochondrial DNA haplogroup influences pseudoexfoliation glaucoma development in Saudi patients. Mol Vis 17: 543–547.
14. Abu-Amero KK, Gonzalez AM, Osman EA, Larruga JM, Cabrera VM, et al. (2011) Mitochondrial DNA lineages of African origin confer susceptibility to primary open-angle glaucoma in Saudi patients. Mol Vis 17: 1468–1472.
15. Pathak D, Nayak B, Singh M, Sharma N, Tandon R, et al. (2011) Mitochondrial complex 1 gene analysis in keratoconus. Mol Vis 17: 1514–1525.
16. Reynier P, Penisson-Besnier I, Moreau C, Savagner F, Vielle B, et al. (1999) mtDNA haplogroup J: a contributing factor of optic neuritis. Eur J Hum Genet 7: 404–406.
17. Penisson-Besnier I, Moreau C, Jacques C, Roger JC, Dubas F, et al. (2001) [Multiple sclerosis and Leber's hereditary optic neuropathy mitochondrial DNA mutations]. Rev Neurol (Paris) 157: 537–541.
18. Brown MD, Yang CC, Trounce I, Torroni A, Lott MT, et al. (1992) A mitochondrial DNA variant, identified in Leber hereditary optic neuropathy patients, which extends the amino acid sequence of cytochrome c oxidase subunit I. Am J Hum Genet 51: 378–385.
19. Mueller EE, Schaier E, Brunner SM, Eder W, Mayr JA, et al. (2012) Mitochondrial haplogroups and control region polymorphisms in age-related macular degeneration: a case-control study. PLoS ONE 7: e30874.
20. Yates JR, 3rd, Gilchrist A, Howell KE, Bergeron JJ (2005) Proteomics of organelles and large cellular structures. Nat Rev Mol Cell Biol 6: 702–714.
21. Miceli MV, Jazwinski SM (2005) Nuclear gene expression changes due to mitochondrial dysfunction in ARPE-19 cells: implications for age-related macular degeneration. Invest Ophthalmol Vis Sci 46: 1765–1773.
22. Chomyn A (1996) Platelet-mediated transformation of human mitochondrial DNA-less cells; Rubin. B, editor. Salt Lake City, UT: Academic Press, Inc.
23. Arning L, Haghikia A, Taherzadeh-Fard E, Saft C, Andrich J, et al. (2010) Mitochondrial haplogroup H correlates with ATP levels and age at onset in Huntington disease. J Mol Med (Berl) 88: 431–436.

24. Ruiz-Pesini E, Mishmar D, Brandon M, Procaccio V, Wallace DC (2004) Effects of purifying and adaptive selection on regional variation in human mtDNA. Science 303: 223–226.

25. Bellizzi D, D'Aquila P, Giordano M, Montesanto A, Passarino G (2012) Global DNA methylation levels are modulated by mitochondrial DNA variants. Epigenomics 4: 17–27.

26. Marcuello A, Martinez-Redondo D, Dahmani Y, Casajus JA, Ruiz-Pesini E, et al. (2009) Human mitochondrial variants influence on oxygen consumption. Mitochondrion 9: 27–30.

27. Marcuello A, Martinez-Redondo D, Dahmani Y, Terreros JL, Aragones T, et al. (2009) Steady exercise removes VO(2max) difference between mitochondrial genomic variants. Mitochondrion 9: 326–330.

28. Martinez-Redondo D, Marcuello A, Casajus JA, Ara I, Dahmani Y, et al. (2010) Human mitochondrial haplogroup H: the highest VO2max consumer–is it a paradox? Mitochondrion 10: 102–107.

29. De Benedictis G, Rose G, Carrieri G, De Luca M, Falcone E, et al. (1999) Mitochondrial DNA inherited variants are associated with successful aging and longevity in humans. Faseb J 13: 1532–1536.

30. Niemi AK, Hervonen A, Hurme M, Karhunen PJ, Jylha M, et al. (2003) Mitochondrial DNA polymorphisms associated with longevity in a Finnish population. Hum Genet 112: 29–33.

31. Ross OA, McCormack R, Curran MD, Duguid RA, Barnett YA, et al. (2001) Mitochondrial DNA polymorphism: its role in longevity of the Irish population. Exp Gerontol 36: 1161–1178.

32. Gomez-Duran A, Pacheu-Grau D, Lopez-Gallardo E, Diez-Sanchez C, Montoya J, et al. (2010) Unmasking the causes of multifactorial disorders: OXPHOS differences between mitochondrial haplogroups. Hum Mol Genet 19: 3343–3353.

33. Suissa S, Wang Z, Poole J, Wittkopp S, Feder J, et al. (2009) Ancient mtDNA genetic variants modulate mtDNA transcription and replication. PLoS Genet 5: e1000474.

34. Ferraresi R, Troiano L, Pinti M, Roat E, Lugli E, et al. (2008) Resistance of mtDNA-depleted cells to apoptosis. Cytometry A 73: 528–537.

35. Miceli MV, Jazwinski SM (2005) Common and cell type-specific responses of human cells to mitochondrial dysfunction. Exp Cell Res 302: 270–280.

36. Jazwinski SM (2012) The retrograde response: When mitochondrial quality control is not enough. Biochim Biophys Acta.

37. Jazwinski SM, Kriete A (2012) The yeast retrograde response as a model of intracellular signaling of mitochondrial dysfunction. Front Physiol 3: 139.

38. Edwards AO, Ritter R, 3rd, Abel KJ, Manning A, Panhuysen C, et al. (2005) Complement factor H polymorphism and age-related macular degeneration. Science 308: 421–424.

39. Klein RJ, Zeiss C, Chew EY, Tsai JY, Sackler RS, et al. (2005) Complement factor H polymorphism in age-related macular degeneration. Science 308: 385–389.

40. Haines JL, Hauser MA, Schmidt S, Scott WK, Olson LM, et al. (2005) Complement factor H variant increases the risk of age-related macular degeneration. Science 308: 419–421.

41. Conley YP, Thalamuthu A, Jakobsdottir J, Weeks DE, Mah T, et al. (2005) Candidate gene analysis suggests a role for fatty acid biosynthesis and regulation of the complement system in the etiology of age-related maculopathy. Hum Mol Genet 14: 1991–2002.

42. Narayanan R, Butani V, Boyer DS, Atilano SR, Resende GP, et al. (2007) Complement factor H polymorphism in age-related macular degeneration. Ophthalmology 114: 1327–1331.

43. Gotoh N, Yamada R, Hiratani H, Renault V, Kuroiwa S, et al. (2006) No association between complement factor H gene polymorphism and exudative age-related macular degeneration in Japanese. Hum Genet 120: 139–143.

44. Grassi MA, Fingert JH, Scheetz TE, Roos BR, Ritch R, et al. (2006) Ethnic variation in AMD-associated complement factor H polymorphism p.Tyr402His. Hum Mutat 27: 921–925.

45. Okamoto H, Umeda S, Obazawa M, Minami M, Noda T, et al. (2006) Complement factor H polymorphisms in Japanese population with age-related macular degeneration. Mol Vis 12: 156–158.

46. Coffey PJ, Gias C, McDermott CJ, Lundh P, Pickering MC, et al. (2007) Complement factor H deficiency in aged mice causes retinal abnormalities and visual dysfunction. Proc Natl Acad Sci U S A 104: 16651–16656.

47. Weismann D, Hartvigsen K, Lauer N, Bennett KL, Scholl HP, et al. (2011) Complement factor H binds malondialdehyde epitopes and protects from oxidative stress. Nature 478: 76–81.

48. Yates JR, Sepp T, Matharu BK, Khan JC, Thurlby DA, et al. (2007) Complement C3 variant and the risk of age-related macular degeneration. N Engl J Med 357: 553–561.

49. Maller JB, Fagerness JA, Reynolds RC, Neale BM, Daly MJ, et al. (2007) Variation in complement factor 3 is associated with risk of age-related macular degeneration. Nat Genet 39: 1200–1201.

50. Bergeron-Sawitzke J, Gold B, Olsh A, Schlotterbeck S, Lemon K, et al. (2009) Multilocus analysis of age-related macular degeneration. Eur J Hum Genet 17: 1190–1199.

51. Sivaprasad S, Adewoyin T, Bailey TA, Dandekar SS, Jenkins S, et al. (2007) Estimation of systemic complement C3 activity in age-related macular degeneration. Arch Ophthalmol 125: 515–519.

52. Johnson LV, Leitner WP, Staples MK, Anderson DH (2001) Complement activation and inflammatory processes in Drusen formation and age related macular degeneration. Exp Eye Res 73: 887–896.

53. Crabb JW, Miyagi M, Gu X, Shadrach K, West KA, et al. (2002) Drusen proteome analysis: an approach to the etiology of age-related macular degeneration. Proc Natl Acad Sci U S A 99: 14682–14687.

54. Juel HB, Kaestel C, Folkersen L, Faber C, Heegaard NH, et al. (2011) Retinal pigment epithelial cells upregulate expression of complement factors after co-culture with activated T cells. Exp Eye Res 92: 180–188.

55. Thurman JM, Renner B, Kunchithapautham K, Ferreira VP, Pangburn MK, et al. (2009) Oxidative stress renders retinal pigment epithelial cells susceptible to complement-mediated injury. J Biol Chem 284: 16939–16947.

56. Fu L, Garland D, Yang Z, Shukla D, Rajendran A, et al. (2007) The R345W mutation in EFEMP1 is pathogenic and causes AMD-like deposits in mice. Hum Mol Genet 16: 2411–2422.

57. Marmorstein LY, Munier FL, Arsenijevic Y, Schorderet DF, McLaughlin PJ, et al. (2002) Aberrant accumulation of EFEMP1 underlies drusen formation in Malattia Leventinese and age-related macular degeneration. Proc Natl Acad Sci U S A 99: 13067–13072.

58. Song EL, Hou YP, Yu SP, Chen SG, Huang JT, et al. (2011) EFEMP1 expression promotes angiogenesis and accelerates the growth of cervical cancer in vivo. Gynecol Oncol 121: 174–180.

59. En-lin S, Sheng-guo C, Hua-qiao W (2010) The expression of EFEMP1 in cervical carcinoma and its relationship with prognosis. Gynecol Oncol 117: 417–422.

60. Kaur I, Katta S, Hussain A, Hussain N, Mathai A, et al. (2008) Variants in the 10q26 gene cluster (LOC387715 and HTRA1) exhibit enhanced risk of age-related macular degeneration along with CFH in Indian patients. Invest Ophthalmol Vis Sci 49: 1771–1776.

61. Kanda A, Chen W, Othman M, Branham KE, Brooks M, et al. (2007) A variant of mitochondrial protein LOC387715/ARMS2, not HTRA1, is strongly associated with age-related macular degeneration. Proc Natl Acad Sci U S A 104: 16227–16232.

62. Wang G, Spencer KL, Court BL, Olson LM, Scott WK, et al. (2009) Localization of age-related macular degeneration-associated ARMS2 in cytosol, not mitochondria. Invest Ophthalmol Vis Sci 50: 3084–3090.

63. Bellizzi D, Taverna D, D'Aquila P, De Blasi S, De Benedictis G (2009) Mitochondrial DNA variability modulates mRNA and intra-mitochondrial protein levels of HSP60 and HSP75: experimental evidence from cybrid lines. Cell Stress Chaperones 14: 265–271.

64. Bellizzi D, Cavalcante P, Taverna D, Rose G, Passarino G, et al. (2006) Gene expression of cytokines and cytokine receptors is modulated by the common variability of the mitochondrial DNA in cybrid cell lines. Genes Cells 11: 883–891.

65. Rodley CD, Grand RS, Gehlen LR, Greyling G, Jones MB, et al. (2012) Mitochondrial-nuclear DNA interactions contribute to the regulation of nuclear transcript levels as part of the inter-organelle communication system. PLoS ONE 7: e30943.

66. Weil D, Blanchard S, Kaplan J, Guilford P, Gibson F, et al. (1995) Defective myosin VIIA gene responsible for Usher syndrome type 1B. Nature 374: 60–61.

67. Hasson T, Heintzelman MB, Santos-Sacchi J, Corey DP, Mooseker MS (1995) Expression in cochlea and retina of myosin VIIa, the gene product defective in Usher syndrome type 1B. Proc Natl Acad Sci U S A 92: 9815–9819.

68. Weil D, Levy G, Sahly I, Levi-Acobas F, Blanchard S, et al. (1996) Human myosin VIIA responsible for the Usher 1B syndrome: a predicted membrane-associated motor protein expressed in developing sensory epithelia. Proc Natl Acad Sci U S A 93: 3232–3237.

69. Liu X, Ondek B, Williams DS (1998) Mutant myosin VIIa causes defective melanosome distribution in the RPE of shaker-1 mice. Nat Genet 19: 117–118.

70. Fernandez-Moreno M, Soto-Hermida A, Pertega S, Oreiro N, Fernandez-Lopez C, et al. (2011) Mitochondrial DNA (mtDNA) haplogroups and serum levels of anti-oxidant enzymes in patients with osteoarthritis. BMC Musculoskelet Disord 12: 264.

71. Fernandez-Moreno M, Soto-Hermida A, Oreiro N, Pertega S, Fenandez-Lopez C, et al. (2012) Mitochondrial haplogroups define two phenotypes of osteoarthritis. Front Physiol 3: 129.

αA Crystallin May Protect against Geographic Atrophy—Meta-Analysis of Cataract vs. Cataract Surgery for Geographic Atrophy and Experimental Studies

Peng Zhou[1,9], Hong-Fei Ye[1,9], Yong-Xiang Jiang[1], Jin Yang[1], Xiang-Jia Zhu[1], Xing-Huai Sun[1], Yi Luo[1], Guo-Rui Dou[2], Yu-Sheng Wang[2], Yi Lu[1]*

1 Department of Ophthalmology, Eye and ENT Hospital of Fudan University, Shanghai, People's Republic of China, 2 Department of Ophthalmology, Xijing Hospital, Fourth Military Medical University, Xi'an, People's Republic of China

Abstract

Background: Cataract and geographic atrophy (GA, also called advanced "dry" age-related macular degeneration) are the two major causes of visual impairment in the developed world. The association between cataract surgery and the development of GA was controversial in previous studies.

Methods/Principal Findings: We performed a meta-analysis by pooling the current evidence in literature and found that cataract is associated with an increased risk of geographic atrophy with a summary odds ratio (OR) of 3.75 (95% CI: 95% CI: 1.84–7.62). However, cataract surgery is not associated with the risk of geographic atrophy (polled OR = 3.23, 95% CI: 0.63–16.47). Further experiments were performed to analyze how the αA-crystallin, the major component of the lens, influences the development of GA in a mouse model. We found that theαA-crystallin mRNA and protein expression increased after oxidative stress induced by NaIO$_3$ in immunohistochemistry of retinal section and western blot of posterior eyecups. Both functional and histopathological evidence confirmed that GA is more severe in αA-crystallin knockout mice compared to wild-type mice.

Conclusions: Therefore, αA-crystallin may protect against geographic atrophy. This study provides a better understanding of the relationship between cataract, cataract surgery, and GA.

Editor: Demetrios Vavvas, Massachusetts Eye & Ear Infirmary, Harvard Medical School, United States of America

Funding: This research was supported by grant from the National Basic Research Program of China (973 Program) No. 2011CB510200, National Natural Science Foundation of China (NSFC) No. 81070740 and No. 81070717. The funders had no role in study design, data collection and analysis, decision to publish, or preparation of the manuscript.

Competing Interests: The authors have declared that no competing interests exist.

* E-mail: luyi0705@yahoo.com.cn

9 These authors contributed equally to this work.

Introduction

Cataract and age-related macular degeneration (AMD) are the two major causes of visual impairment in the developed world [1]. Cataract is a clouding that develops in the crystalline lens of the eye. Cataract surgery is currently one of the most frequently performed and successful surgical procedures [2]. Advanced AMD has two major subtypes: geographic atrophy (GA, also called advanced "dry" AMD) and choroidal neovascularization (also called "wet" AMD) [3]. Geographic atrophy [4–6] is characterized by confluent areas of cell death in photoreceptors and retinal pigment epithelium, is bilateral in more than half of patients, and is responsible for 10% of the cases of legal blindness resulting from age-related macular degeneration. Both cataract and GA are strongly age related.

The association between cataract surgery and the development of GA was controversial in previous studies. In the Beaver Dam Eye Study (BDES) [7], a positive cross-sectional association was found between cataract surgery and GA. The association was consistent with findings in the Los Angeles Latino Eye Study (LALES) [8], but not with findings in the Blue Mountains Eye Study (BMES) [9] or the Age-related Eye Disease Study (AREDS) [10]. However, the positive association between cataracts and GA was consistent in the Beaver Dam Eye Study [7] and LALES [8].

The pathogenesis of the association between cataract surgery and GA is less clear. The previous hypothesis is that cataract removal results in increased risk because the cataract, a barrier to ultraviolet radiation, has been removed [11]. Based on this hypothesis, in theory, the prevalence of GA should be decreased in patients with cataract. However, the truth is that the prevalence of GA is higher in patients with cataract than the control. Therefore, this hypothesis is not sufficient to explain the clinical phenomenon.

One common change involving cataracts and cataract surgery has been neglected: the change of α-crystallins, which are the major protein of lens. The α-crystallins are small heat shock proteins which play central roles in maintaining lens transparency and refractive properties [12]. The discovery in 1992 that these proteins possess chaperone-like activity has led most researchers to focus on the ability of α-crystallins to prevent protein aggregation in vitro. While the ability of α-crystallins to efficiently trap aggregation-prone denatured proteins in vitro is thought to delay the development of age-related cataracts in vivo, α-crystallins have additional functions which may also contribute to cataract pathology. In addition to chaperone activity, α-crystallins are known to protect cells from stress-induced apoptosis, regulate cell growth, and enhance genomic stability [13]. They also physically and functionally interact with both the cell membrane and cytoskeleton. Functional changes in α-crystallin have been shown to modify membrane and cell-cell interactions and lead to lens cell pathology in vivo [14].

Because most studies on geographic atrophy and cataract surgery or cataracts had relatively small sample sizes, we combined pieces of evidence from the published literature for a meta-analysis. In this study, we preformed a meta-analysis focusing on the association between GA and cataracts or cataract surgery. Furthermore, the function of α-crystallins was studied in a GA animal model to investigate its role in the development of GA.

Materials and Methods

Meta-analysis

This meta-analysis followed the PISMA statement guidelines. [15] The meta-analysis of the association between GA and cataract or cataract surgery was performed as we have described previously [16]. In brief, relevant studies were selected by searching PubMed and Web of Science database (updated to December 5, 2011) using the following search terms: ("cataract" OR "cataract surgery") AND ("age-related macular degeneration" OR "geographic atrophy") with the limit "humans". All the resulting studies were retrieved, and their references were checked for other relevant publications. Review articles were also searched to find additional eligible studies. Only studies published in English with full-text articles were included in this meta-analysis. We did not define any minimum number of patients for a study to be included in the meta-analysis. For overlapping studies, only the one with the latest published was included. The identified articles were read carefully and assessed independently by two of the authors (Zhou, P and Lu, Y), and any discrepancies in their eligibility were adjudicated by Sun, XH.

The inclusion criteria were: (1) evaluating the association between the cataract and risk of geographic atrophy; (2) evaluating the association between the cataract surgery and risk of geographic atrophy; and (3) with sufficient available data to estimate an OR with its 95% CI. The included studies had to meet [(1)+(3)] or [(2)+(3)] of the above-mentioned criteria. Any study with internally inconsistent data was excluded. The following variables were extracted from each study, if available: first author's surname, publication year, numbers of cases and controls, and numbers of cases and controls in different groups whenever possible. Information was carefully and independently extracted from all the eligible publications by two of the authors (Zhou, P and Lu, Y). Disagreement was resolved by discussion between the authors. If they could not reach a consensus, another investigator (Sun, XH) adjudicated over the disagreements. (Figure S1, Table S1)

ORs and their 95% CIs were obtained directly or calculated from the data given in the articles. A random- or a fixed-effects model was used to calculate the pooled effect estimates in the presence (P<0.10) or absence (P>0.10) of heterogeneity, respectively. The potential publication bias was examined visually in a funnel plot of log [OR] against its standard error (SE), and the degree of asymmetry was tested using Egger's test (P<0.05 considered to be statistically significant). We conducted influence analysis by omitting each study to find potential outliers. All of the statistical analyses were performed using Stata/SE version 11.0 (Stata Corporation, College Station, TX).

Animals

The 129S6/SvEvTac wild-type mice were purchased from Chinese Scientific Academy (Shanghai, China), while the αA-crystallin knockout mice in 129S6/SvEvTac background [17] were obtained from the National Eye Institute. Mice between 6 and 8 weeks old were fed the standard laboratory chow in an air-conditioned room equipped with a 12-hour light/12-hour dark cycle. All procedures were performed in compliance with the Fudan University Institutional Animal Care and Use Committee's approved protocols and the ARVO Statement for the Use of Animals in Ophthalmic and Vision Research.

Chemical formulation and experimental procedure

Mice were briefly restrained. Sodium iodate ($NaIO_3$; Sigma, St. Louis, MO) was diluted with Phosphate buffered saline (PBS) solution and 20 mg/kg body weight of $NaIO_3$ was injected through the tail vein. [18] Animals injected with equivalent volumes of PBS solution served as controls. Electroretinography and fundus photographs were assessed at 21 days post injection. After the tests were made, mice were euthanized with CO_2 and their eyes processed for histology.

Experimental groups

The mice were divided into four groups: control wild type (PBS-treated WT), $NaIO_3$-treated wild type ($NaIO_3$-treated WT), control αA-crystallin knockout mice (PBS-treated αA−/−), and $NaIO_3$-treated αA-crystallin knockout mice ($NaIO_3$-treated αA−/−). Each group consisted of seven mice in the age range of 6–8 weeks.

Electroretinography (ERG)

Mice were dark-adapted overnight and anesthetized by intraperitoneal injection of ketamine (100 mg/kg body weight) and xylazine (10 mg/kg body weight). Pupils were dilated with topical administration of 2.5% phenylephrine containing 0.5% tropicamide, and the cornea was anesthetized with 0.5% proparacaine. Scotopic ERGs were measured from dark-adapted mice using a low-intensity stimulus, and mesopic ERGs were measured using a non-attenuated light stimulus. To measure cone responses, a 6 lux white background light was delivered through the other arm of the coaxial cable to suppress rod responses, and a non-attenuated light stimulus was applied. The a-wave amplitude was measured from the baseline to the trough of the a-wave, while b-wave amplitude was measured from the trough of the a-wave to the peak of the b-wave.

Histopathologic analysis

For histopathologic analysis, eyes were enucleated, and the anterior poles were removed. The remaining eyecups were snap-frozen in tissue-freezing medium (Triangle Biomedical Sciences, Durham, NC). Sections (8 μm) were stained with hematoxylin and eosin (H&E) to assess the histopathologic changes of retina.

Western blot analysis

The western blot was performed as described previously. [19,20] Lysed posterior eyecups, including retina and RPE, were centrifuged at 11,000 g for 20 minutes. Supernatants were collected, and proteins were resolved on Tris-HCl 10% polyacrylamide gels (Ready Gel; Bio-Rad, Hercules, CA) at 120 V. The proteins were transferred to PVDF blotting membrane (Millipore, Bedford, MA). The membranes were probed with antibody for αA-crystallin (Stressgen, San Diego, CA) and GAPDH (Millipore) at 1:1,000 dilution. Membranes were washed and incubated with a horseradish peroxidase (HRP)-conjugated secondary antibody (1:3,000, Vector Laboratories, Burlingame, CA) for 30 min at room temperature. Images were developed by adding ECL chemiluminescence detection solution (Amersham Pharmacia Biotech, Cleveland, OH).

Immunohistochemistry

Immunohistochemical stains were performed on freezing tissue sections. After blocking with 20% normal donkey serum for 30 minutes, slides were probed overnight at 4°C with primary αA-crystallin antibody (Stressgen, San Diego, CA) diluted into blocking solution. Slides were incubated with biotinylated goat anti-rabbit immunoglobulin Ig G (1:500) for 1 h at room temperature. The signal was detected using streptavidin-conjugated horseradish peroxidase and peroxidase activity was visualized with diaminobenzidine/H2O2 (Vector Laboratories, Burlingame, CA). After color development, slides were counterstained with hematoxylin.

Reverse transcription PCR and relative quantitative real-time PCR

The reverse transcription PCR (RT-PCRwas performed as described previously. [16] Total RNA was isolated using a TRIzol reagent (Invitrogen, Carlsbad, CA, USA). The first strand of cDNA was synthesized with 1 μg of total RNA, oligo(dT) primer and AMV reverse transcriptase (Promega, Madison, WI, USA). The primers used in RT-PCR were as follows: CRYAA forward: 5′- TTTTGAGTATGACCTGCTGCC - 3′, reverse: 5′-TGGAACTCACGGGAAATGTAG -3′; GAPDH, forward: 5′-GAAGGTGAAGGTCGGAGTC -3′, reverse: 5′- GAA-GATGGTGATGGGATTTC -3′. [21] The specificity of the PCR amplification products was checked by performing dissociation melting-curve analysis and by 1% agarose gel electrophoresis. Quantification analysis of CRYAA mRNA was normalized with a housekeeping gene, GAPDH, as an internal control.

Isolation of primary cultured RPE cells from mice

Primary cultured RPE cells were isolated from knockout mice as previously described. [22] The cornea, lens, vitreous, and retina were removed from eyes soaked in phosphate buffered saline (PBS) containing 5% penicillin/streptomycin (Sigma). The choroid/sclera tissue was then placed into a 2% dispase solution in PBS for 20 min at 37°C. After the incubation, the tissue was rapidly pipetted up and down for 30 s. The dispase solution containing the RPE cells was passed through a 70 μ filter followed by a 40 μ filter after which the cells were spun down and resuspended in Ham's F-12 Media (Cellgro, Herndon, VA) containing at least 25% fetal bovine serum (FBS; Irvine Scientific, Santa Ana, CA). The RPE were then grown on laminin coated plates (Becton Dickinson and Company, Franklin Lakes, NJ).

Detection of ROS Production

To determine the compartmentalized accumulation of reactive oxygen species (ROS), cells on an eight-well Lab-TekTM chamber were stained with carboxy-H2-DCFDA (Molecular Probes; 5 μM for 1 h at 37°C), and rapidly evaluated by confocal microscopy (LSM510, Zeiss, Thornwood, NY, USA). A green color is observed when ROS accumulated. Nucleus were stained with propidium Iodide (PI) as red fluorescence.

Statistics

All experiments were repeated at least three times. Values in the figures were expressed as means ± SE. Statistical analyses were performed with Student's t test. Values in the figures are expressed as means±SE. Values of P<0.05 were considered statistically significant.

Results

Meta-analysis shows that cataract, not cataract surgery, is associated with an increased risk of geographic atrophy

We performed a meta-analysis focusing on the relationship between geographic atrophy and cataract or cataract surgery. There were four published articles [7–10] investigating the association between cataract surgery and geographic atrophy risk (Figure S1). Two studies investigated the association between cataract and geographic atrophy risk [7,8] (Figure S1). Table 1 lists the main characteristics of relevant studies.

Positive association between cataract and risk of geographic atrophy was found (polled OR = 3.75, 95% CI: 1.84–7.62, $P=$ <0.001). However, no significant association between cataract

Table 1. Characteristics of studies included in meta-analysis.

No.	Year	First Author	Studies	Cataract surgery				Cataract			
				surgery		control		cataract		control	
				(n = 988)		(n = 21,918)		(n = 1,969)		(n = 12,924)	
				GA	No GA	GA	No GA	GA	No GA	GA	No GA
1	2002	Klein	BDES	3	94	17	3328	8	562	11	2718
2	2006	Cugati	BMES	4	128	51	2271	N.A.	N.A.	N.A.	N.A.
3	2008	Chew	AREDS	14	525	205	5383	N.A.	N.A.	N.A.	N.A.
4	2010	Fraser-Bell	LALES	4	216	9	10654	5	1394	8	9287

BDES = Beaver Dam Eye Study;
LALES = Los Angeles Latino Eye Study;
BMES = Blue Mountains Eye Study;
AREDS = Age-related Eye Disease Study;
N.A. = not available.

a. Cataract Surgery – Geographic Atrophy

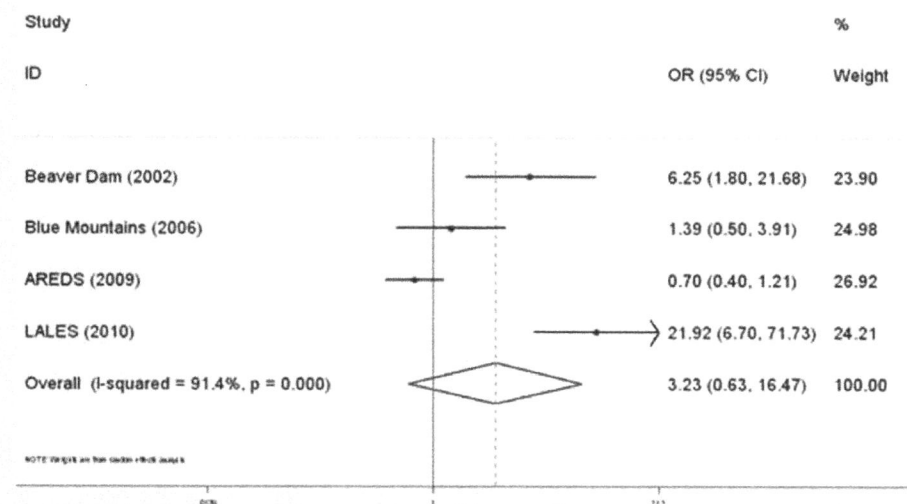

Study ID		OR (95% CI)	% Weight
Beaver Dam (2002)		6.25 (1.80, 21.68)	23.90
Blue Mountains (2006)		1.39 (0.50, 3.91)	24.98
AREDS (2009)		0.70 (0.40, 1.21)	26.92
LALES (2010)		21.92 (6.70, 71.73)	24.21
Overall (I-squared = 91.4%, p = 0.000)		3.23 (0.63, 16.47)	100.00

NOTE: Weights are from random effects analysis

b. Cataract – Geographic Atrophy

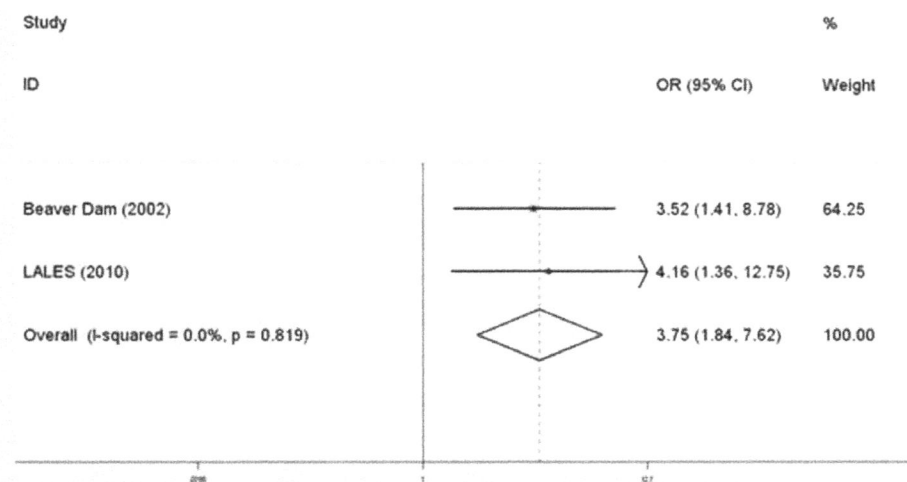

Study ID		OR (95% CI)	% Weight
Beaver Dam (2002)		3.52 (1.41, 8.78)	64.25
LALES (2010)		4.16 (1.36, 12.75)	35.75
Overall (I-squared = 0.0%, p = 0.819)		3.75 (1.84, 7.62)	100.00

Figure 1. The forest plot of meta-analysis. Each study is shown by the point estimate of the odds ratio (OR) (the size of the square is proportional to the weight of each study) and the 95% confidence interval (CI) for the OR (extending lines). a. the association of cataract surgery with geographic atrophy; b. the association of cataract with geographic atrophy. LALES = Los Angeles Latino Eye Study; BMES = Blue Mountains Eye Study; AREDS = Age-related Eye Disease Study.

surgery and risk of geographic atrophy was found (polled OR = 3.23, 95% CI: 0.63–16.47, $P = 0.159$). (Figure 1, Table 2).

Reduced ERG amplitudes in NaIO$_3$-treated αA-crystallin knockout mice

To determine whether the absence of αA-crystallin had an effect on the retinal function of NaIO$_3$-induced retinal degeneration, we compared mesopic (mixed rod and cone) ERG responses of the four groups of mice (PBS-treated WT, NaIO$_3$-treated WT, PBS-treated αA−/−, and NaIO$_3$-treated αA−/−) at the end of 3 weeks. Significant differences were observed in the ERGs of NaIO$_3$-treated αA−/− mice compared with the PBS-treated αA−/− mice (Figure 2). No significant differences were found between the ERGs of the NaIO$_3$-treated and control in wild-type mice.

The amplitudes of a-wave of the ERG of NaIO$_3$-treated αA−/− mice decreased by 78.11% of that of PBS-treated αA−/−

Table 2. Pooled ORs of TLR3 1234C>T in different genetic models.

	Ph	Polling Model	Polled OR (95%CI)	P
Cataract surgery - GA	<0.001	Random M-H	3.23 (0.63–16.47)	0.159
Cataract - GA	0.819	Fixed M-H	3.75 (1.84–7.62)	<0.001

Ph = P value of Q test for heterogeneity test;
OR = odds ratio;
CI = confidence interval.
M-H = Mantel-Haenszel.

mice. The amplitudes of b-wave of the ERG of NaIO$_3$-treated αA−/− mice decreased by 60.26%, compared with that of PBS-treated αA−/− mice. Generally speaking, a-wave of ERG demonstrates the function of the outer layer of the retina, while b-wave shows that of the inner layer. The ERG results suggested that the function of the outer layer of retina was more suppressed than that of the inner layer.

Histopathological evidence for accelerated NaIO$_3$-induced degeneration in αA-crystallin knockout mice

Retinas from αA-crystallin knockout mice revealed more severe degeneration from NaIO$_3$ injection as compared to wild-type retinas. An assessment of the extent of retinal damage by NaIO$_3$ was made by counting the number of nuclei in the inner nuclear layer, outer nuclear layer, and ganglion cell layer of wild type and

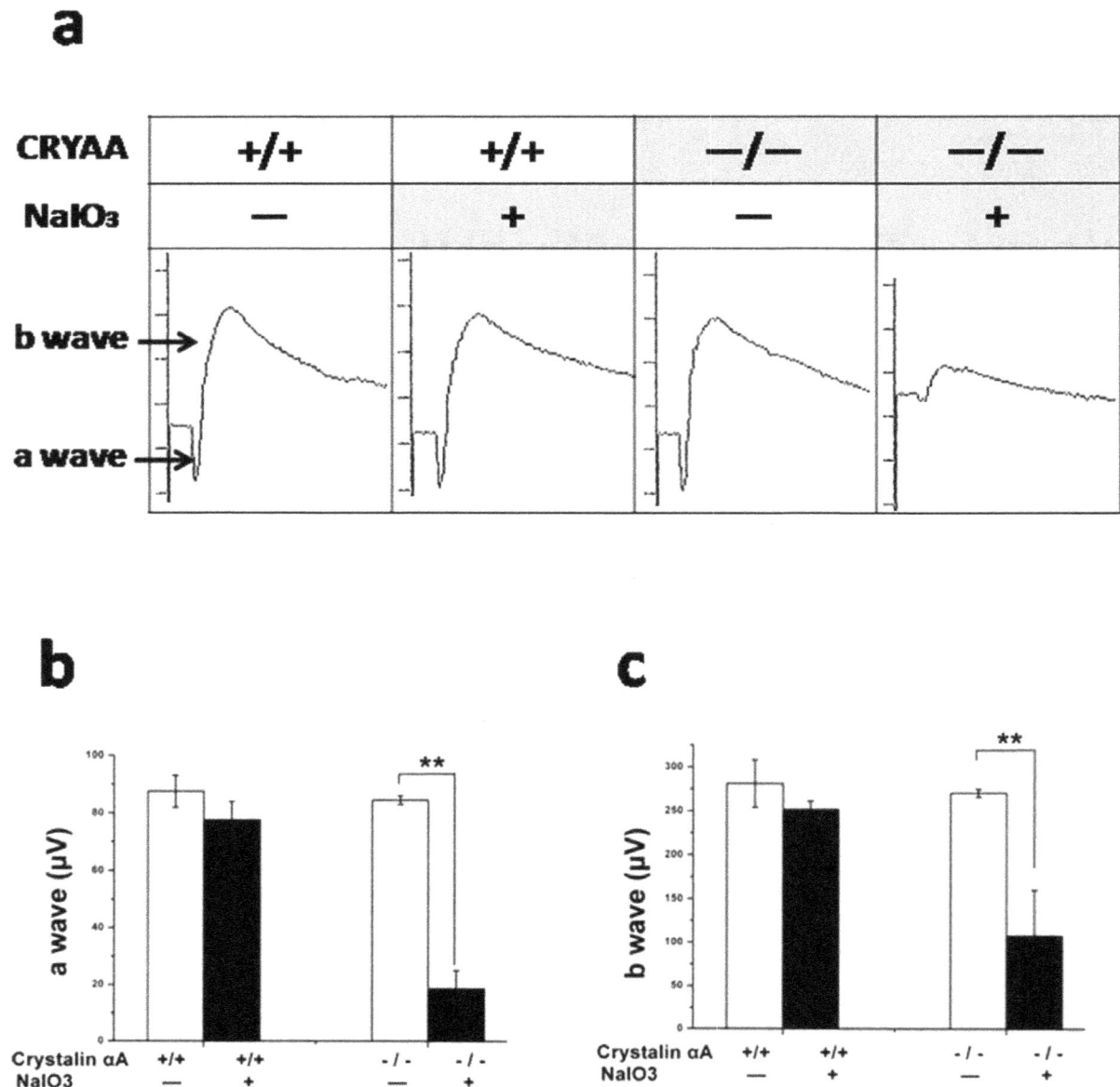

Figure 2. Reduced ERG amplitudes in NaIO$_3$-treated αA-crystallin knockout mice. The amplitudes of a-wave of the ERG of NaIO$_3$-treated αA−/− mice decreased to 21.89% of that of PBS-treated αA−/− mice. The amplitudes of b-wave of the ERG of NaIO$_3$-treated αA−/− mice decreased by 60.26%, compared with that of PBS-treated αA−/− mice. Data are mean ± SEM, n = 5/group, **P<0.01.

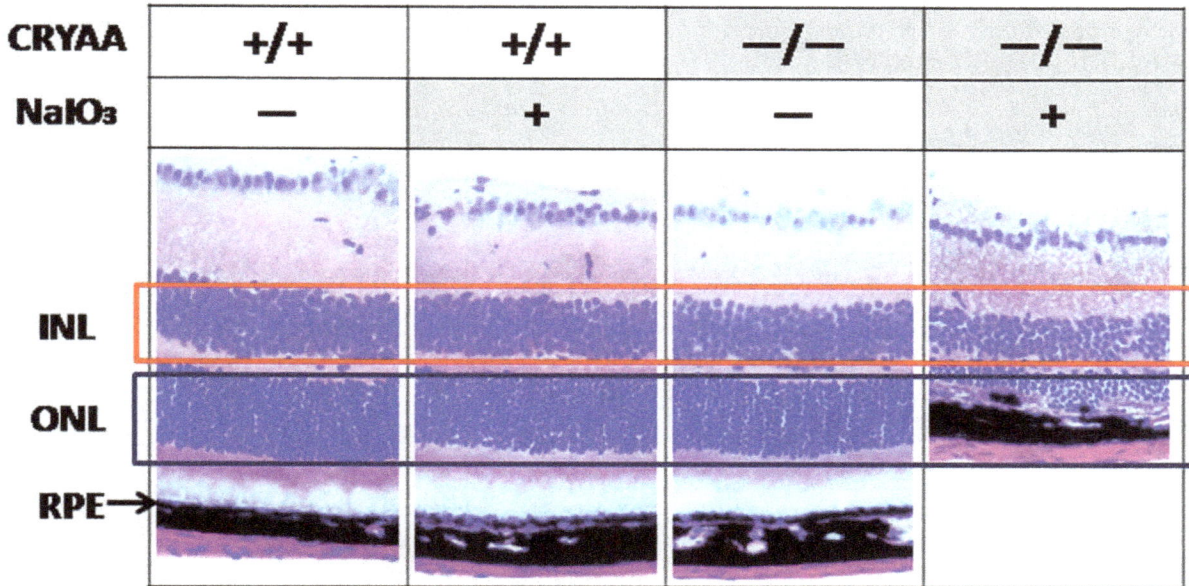

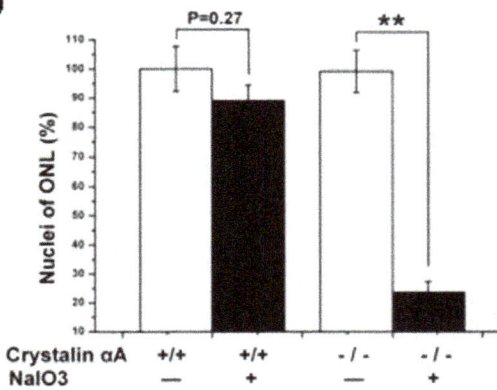

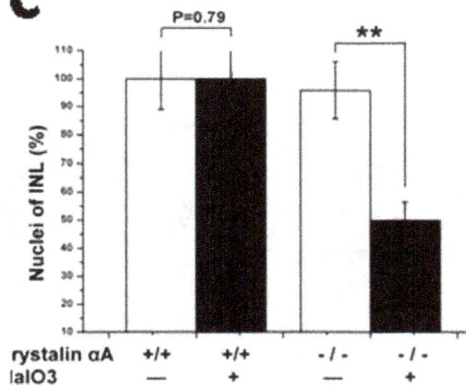

Figure 3. Histopathological evidence for accelerated NaIO₃-induced degeneration in αA-crystallin knockout mice. Retinas from αA-crystallin knockout mice revealed more severe degeneration from NaIO₃ injection as compared to wild-type retinas. The loss of nuclei was more prominent in αA-crystallin knockout retina vs. that of wild type. The decrease in the number of nuclei per unit area was statistically significant with NaIO₃ injection only in the outer nuclear layer of the crystallin knockout mice. No significant differences of nuclei numbers were found between the NaIO₃-injected and PBS-injected in wild-type mice. The RPE layers were discontinuous and damaged in αA-crystallin knockout mice with NaIO₃ injection, while they were continuous in wild-type mice. CRYAA = αA-crystallin; INL = inner nuclear layer; ONL = outer nuclear layer; RPE = retinal pigmental epithelium; **P<0.01.

αA-crystallin knockout retinas. This semi-quantitative analysis revealed that the loss of nuclei was more prominent at 3 weeks post injection of NaIO₃ in αA-crystallin knockout retina vs. that of wild type. The decrease in the number of nuclei per unit area was statistically significant (p<0.01) with NaIO₃ injection only in the outer nuclear layer of the crystallin knockout mice. No significant differences of nuclei numbers were found between the NaIO₃-injected and PBS-injected in wild-type mice (Figure 3).

The RPE layers were discontinuous and damaged in αA-crystallin knockout mice with NaIO₃ injection, while they were continuous in wild type mice.

Increased αA-crystallin expression after NaIO₃ treatment

Immunohistochemistry staining showed that αA-crystallin in retina increased after NaIO₃ treatment. (Figure 4a) Protein expression of αA-crystallin of mice eye cup after NaIO₃ treatment

a

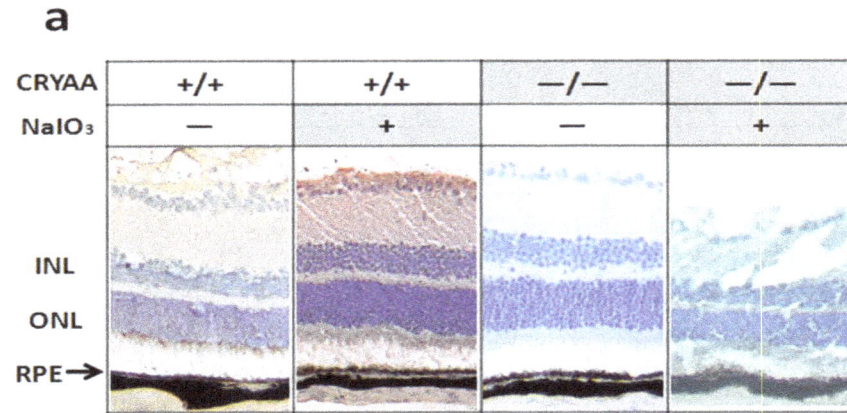

CRYAA	+/+	+/+	−/−	−/−
NaIO₃	−	+	−	+

INL
ONL
RPE→

b

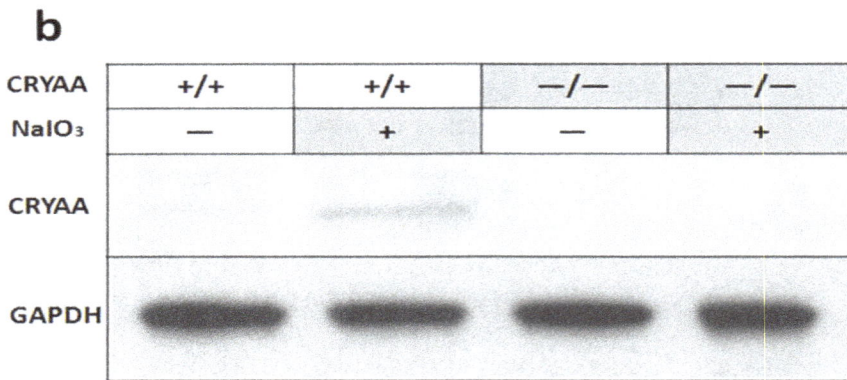

CRYAA	+/+	+/+	−/−	−/−
NaIO₃	−	+	−	+

CRYAA

GAPDH

c

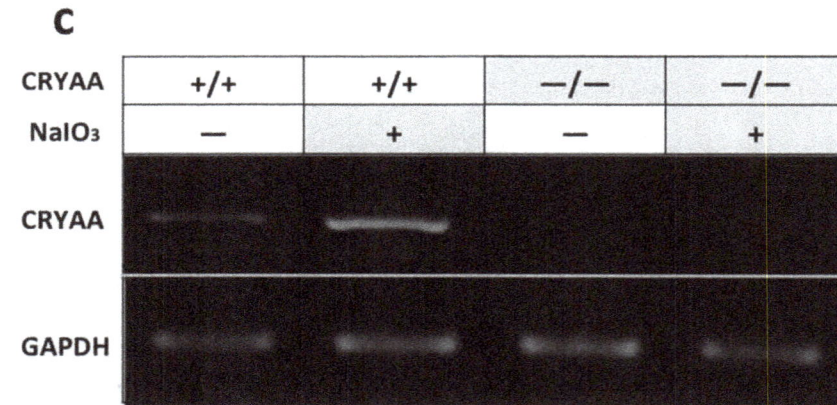

CRYAA	+/+	+/+	−/−	−/−
NaIO₃	−	+	−	+

CRYAA

GAPDH

d

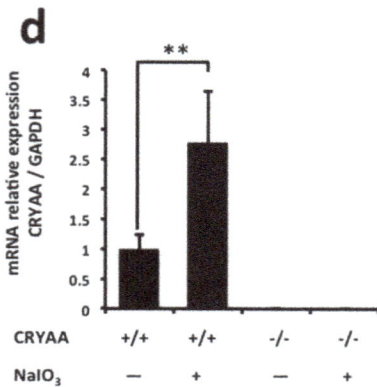

mRNA relative expression CRYAA / GAPDH

CRYAA	+/+	+/+	-/-	-/-
NaIO₃	−	+	−	+

e

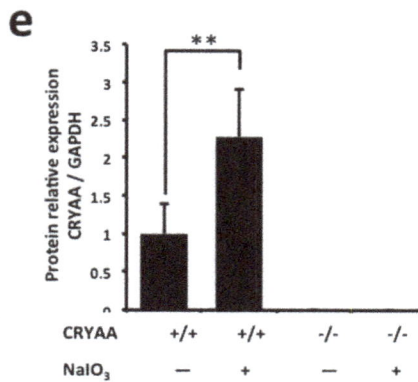

Protein relative expression CRYAA / GAPDH

CRYAA	+/+	+/+	-/-	-/-
NaIO₃	−	+	−	+

Figure 4. Increased αA-crystallin expression after NaIO₃ treatment. Immunohistochemistry staining showed that αA-crystallin in retina increased after NaIO₃ treatment. Protein expression of αA-crystallin of mice eye cup after NaIO₃ treatment was examined by Western blot analysis. αA-crystallin prtein increased to 2.28±0.62 times comparing to control (p<0.01), while mRNA increased 2.79±0.86 times comparing to control (p<0.01). No αA-crystallin was detected in αA-crystallin knockout mice. CRYAA = αA-crystallin, **P<0.01.

was examined by Western blot analysis. αA-crystallin increased to 2.28±0.62 times comparing to control (p<0.01). No αA-crystallin protein was detected in αA-crystallin knockout mice. (Figure 4b, d) mRNA expression of αA-crystallin of mice eye cup after NaIO₃ treatment was examined by RT-PCR analysis. αA-crystallin increased to 2.79±0.86 times comparing to control (p<0.01). No αA-crystallin mRNA was detected in αA-crystallin knockout mice. (Figure 4c, e) All experiments were repeated at least three times.

Increased accumulation of ROS in CRYAA −/− RPE cells

Primary cultured RPE cells was isolated from knockout mice and treated with NaIO₃. Figure 5 shows confocal images of ROS accumulation in RPE cells. The accumulation of ROS was much stronger in RPE cells from αA-crystallin knock our mice than that from wild type mice. These results show that knock out αA-crystallin results in increased accumulation of ROS in RPE cells treated with NaIO₃.

Discussion

The meta-analysis shows that cataract, not cataract surgery, is associated with an increased risk of geographic atrophy. Further experiments found that αA-crystallin may play an important role in this association.

Only a small number of publications could be included in the meta-analysis. The overall scientific level of evidence of these articles was not high. There were no trials at the highest level of evidence, which are randomized controlled trials (RCT). It needs to be mentioned that randomizing patients to not undergo cataract

surgery when their vision is poor enough to affect their daily life would neither be ethical nor practicable. Thus, observational cohort studies and non-randomized clinical trials are probably the best possible evidence. Both are rated as a level 2 on the five-step hierarchy of levels of evidence for medical studies [23].

The results of our meta-analysis is not consistent with previous theory that increased risk or progression of GA (dry age-related macular degeneration) after cataract surgery is related to the increased exposure of the retina to short-wavelength light [11,24,25]. However, the meta-analysis of 22,906 patients did not find significant association between cataract surgery and GA. Instead, we found that cataract is associated with an increased risk of geographic atrophy. That means that the risk of GA increased in cataract patients, although they had cataract as a barrier to short-wavelength light. Therefore, the short-wavelength light damage theory is not sufficient to explain our meta-analysis findings.

αA-Crystallin, which is a member of the small heat shock protein (sHSP also known as the HSP20) family, plays an important neuroprotection function in retina. [22,26–28] We analyzed cataracts and cataract surgery, and found that they have a common change: the crystallins in the lens. Cataracts cause crystallins to degenerate, and cataract surgery removes the lens, the largest bank of crystallins from the eyes. Furthermore, experiments were performed to analyze the effect of αA-crystallin on GA in a mouse model. We found that αA-crystallin expression increased after oxidative stress induced by NaIO3. Both functional and histopathological evidence confirmed that GA is more severe in αA-crystallin knockout mice compared with wild-type mice.

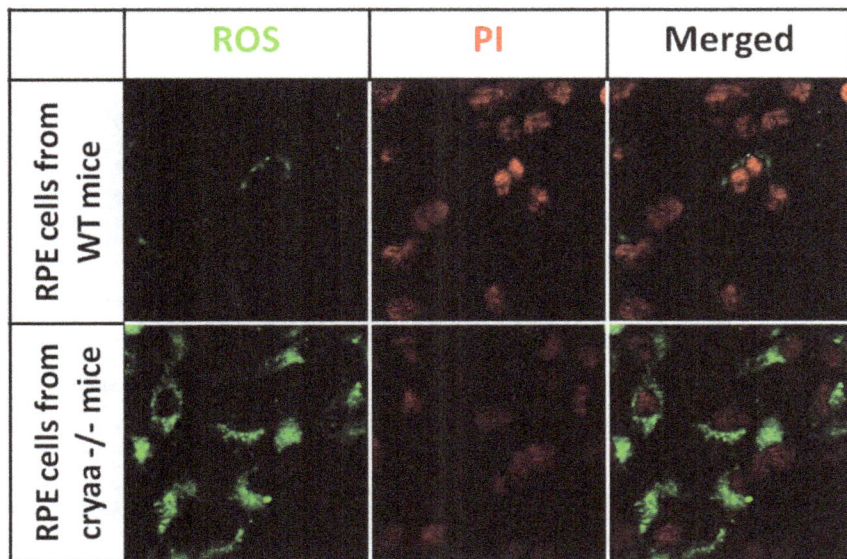

Figure 5. Increased accumulation of ROS in CRYAA −/− RPE cells. Primary cultured RPE cells was isolated from knockout mice and treated with NaIO3. Confocal images show ROS accumulation in RPE cells. The accumulation of ROS was much stronger in RPE cells from αA-crystallin knock our mice than that from wild type mice. These results show that knock out αA-crystallin results in increased accumulation of ROS in RPE cells treated with NaIO3.

Dry AMD is a challenging disease to study because of its complex genetics, late onset, and confounding environmental risk factors. As with other human diseases, finding a model system for AMD has been a demanding task. The pathology of dry AMD consists of degeneration of photoreceptors and the RPE, lipofuscin accumulation, and drusen formation. Genetically engineered mice have been used for generating models that simulate human AMD features. However, most mice develop retinal lesions at an older age (6–24 months). [29] Furthermore, there is no CRYAA −/− genetically engineered dry AMD mice. Therefore, we tried to find another way to mimic the dry AMD. Oxidative stress plays an important role in the pathogenesis of dry AMD. [30] NaIO3 can induce oxidative stress. NaIO3 damages mostly the central pole of the retina in low dose. Such a pathological phenomenon resembles those observed in dry AMD in their clinical course that initially involve the central part of the retina and spread gradually. Therefore, chemical damage induced by NaIO3 mimics dry AMD in humans and may serve as a model useful for studying retinal damage. [31] Therefore, we selected this model in our study.

The association of cataract with an increased risk of geographic atrophy can be explained by our findings. The pathogenesis of cataract is the degeneration of crystallins [32]. αA-crystallin is the major protein of the lens [17]. Neal's study showed that the concentration of alpha-A crystallins in vitreous is decreased in cataract patients. [33] After having cataract, the αA-crystallin degenerates. The total of active αA-crystallin decreases. Therefore, those people with cataract are more susceptible to have GA compared with people without cataract in the same dose of oxidative stress.

The phenomenon that cataract surgery is not associated with an increased risk of geographic atrophy can also be explained by our findings. Neal et. al reported that the concentration of αA-crystallin in vitreous is increased after cataract surgery [33]. Increased αA-crystallin may protect retina from GA. The protective αA-crystallins is produced by "after cataract". Over the year, many patients who have an uncomplicated routine cataract surgery will developed a clouding or a thickening of a natural membrane in the eye which sits just behind the lens implant, called the posterior lens capsule. This has been referred to as "after-cataract" or a secondary capsular opacification. The "after cataract" will produce new αA-crystallins and leak into vitreous.

In this study, ERG findings, the a-wave amplitude decreased more than that of b-wave in knockout mice exposed to oxidative stress. This suggests that the function of the outer retina was more suppressed than the inner, in relation to controls. However, only outer retinal atrophy was seen in histopathological findings. This phenomenon may because that the changes of function are earlier than that of anatomy. [34] ERG may be a better test to evaluate the retinal response to oxidative stress damage.

Some limitations of this meta-analysis should be acknowledged. First, this study involves two subjects, human patients with unknown genetic background and mice with clear genetic defects. However, there is not a sub-population of human subjects with congenital aA-Crystallin defects, which may share similarity to the aA-crystallin KO mice and contribute the correlations between lens and retina degenerating defects.

We put forward a hypothesis that the eye has an oxidation/anti-oxidation homeostasis. αA-crystallin is an important anti-oxidation factor. In young people, the αA-crystallin is sufficient to fend off oxidative stress damage, so their eyes do not have GA. When people have cataracts, the degenerative αA-crystallin cannot protect against oxidative stress damage, and they get GA. After cataract surgery, the concentration of αA-crystallin increases in the vitreous, and those eyes have more anti-oxidation factors. They are less likely to have GA than those who did not have cataract surgeries.

Author Contributions

Conceived and designed the experiments: YL PZ YSW. Performed the experiments: PZ HFY YXJ JY XJZ GRD. Analyzed the data: XHS YL. Contributed reagents/materials/analysis tools: PZ. Wrote the paper: PZ.

References

1. Chang JR, Koo E, Agron E, Hallak J, Clemons T, et al. (2011) Risk Factors Associated with Incident Cataracts and Cataract Surgery in the Age-Related Eye Disease Study (AREDS): AREDS Report Number 32. Ophthalmology 118: 2113–2119.

2. Meekins LC, Afshari NA (2011) Ever-evolving technological advances in cataract surgery: can perfection be achieved? Curr Opin Ophthalmol.

3. Yang Z, Stratton C, Francis PJ, Kleinman ME, Tan PL, et al. (2008) Toll-like receptor 3 and geographic atrophy in age-related macular degeneration. N Engl J Med 359: 1456–1463.

4. Ferris FL 3rd, Fine SL, Hyman L (1984) Age-related macular degeneration and blindness due to neovascular maculopathy. Arch Ophthalmol 102: 1640–1642.

5. Hyman LG, Lilienfeld AM, Ferris FL 3rd, Fine SL (1983) Senile macular degeneration: a case-control study. Am J Epidemiol 118: 213–227.

6. Sarks JP, Sarks SH, Killingsworth MC (1988) Evolution of geographic atrophy of the retinal pigment epithelium. Eye (Lond) 2 (Pt 5): 552–577.

7. Klein R, Klein BE, Wong TY, Tomany SC, Cruickshanks KJ (2002) The association of cataract and cataract surgery with the long-term incidence of age-related maculopathy: the Beaver Dam eye study. Arch Ophthalmol 120: 1551–1558.

8. Fraser-Bell S, Choudhury F, Klein R, Azen S, Varma R (2010) Ocular risk factors for age-related macular degeneration: the Los Angeles Latino Eye Study. Am J Ophthalmol 149: 735–740.

9. Cugati S, Mitchell P, Rochtchina E, Tan AG, Smith W, et al. (2006) Cataract surgery and the 10-year incidence of age-related maculopathy: the Blue Mountains Eye Study. Ophthalmology 113: 2020–2025.

10. Chew EY, Sperduto RD, Milton RC, Clemons TE, Gensler GR, et al. (2009) Risk of advanced age-related macular degeneration after cataract surgery in the Age-Related Eye Disease Study: AREDS report 25. Ophthalmology 116: 297–303.

11. Patel JI (2007) Is cataract surgery a risk factor for progression of macular degeneration? Curr Opin Ophthalmol 18: 9–12.

12. Maulucci G, Papi M, Arcovito G, De Spirito M (2011) The thermal structural transition of alpha-crystallin inhibits the heat induced self-aggregation. PLoS One 6: e18906.

13. Derham BK, Harding JJ (1999) Alpha-crystallin as a molecular chaperone. Prog Retin Eye Res 18: 463–509.

14. Andley UP (2009) Effects of alpha-crystallin on lens cell function and cataract pathology. Curr Mol Med 9: 887–892.

15. Liberati A, Altman DG, Tetzlaff J, Mulrow C, Gotzsche PC, et al. (2009) The PRISMA statement for reporting systematic reviews and meta-analyses of studies that evaluate health care interventions: explanation and elaboration. PLoS Med 6: e1000100.

16. Zhou P, Fan L, Yu KD, Zhao MW, Li XX (2011) Toll-like receptor 3 C1234T may protect against geographic atrophy through decreased dsRNA binding capacity. FASEB J 25: 3489–3495.

17. Brady JP, Garland D, Duglas-Tabor Y, Robison WG Jr, Groome A, et al. (1997) Targeted disruption of the mouse alpha A-crystallin gene induces cataract and cytoplasmic inclusion bodies containing the small heat shock protein alpha B-crystallin. Proc Natl Acad Sci U S A 94: 884–889.

18. Kiuchi K, Yoshizawa K, Shikata N, Moriguchi K, Tsubura A (2002) Morphologic characteristics of retinal degeneration induced by sodium iodate in mice. Curr Eye Res 25: 373–379.

19. Zhou P, Lu Y, Sun XH (2011) Zebularine suppresses TGF-beta-induced lens epithelial cell-myofibroblast transdifferentiation by inhibiting MeCP2. Mol Vis 17: 2717–2723.

20. Zhou P, Lu Y, Sun XH (2012) Effects of a novel DNA methyltransferase inhibitor Zebularine on human lens epithelial cells. Mol Vis 18: 22–28.

21. Zhou P, Zhao MW, Li XX, Yu WZ, Bian ZM (2007) siRNA targeting mammalian target of rapamycin (mTOR) attenuates experimental proliferative vitreoretinopathy. Curr Eye Res 32: 973–984.

22. Yaung J, Jin M, Barron E, Spee C, Wawrousek EF, et al. (2007) alpha-Crystallin distribution in retinal pigment epithelium and effect of gene knockouts on sensitivity to oxidative stress. Mol Vis 13: 566–577.

23. Bockelbrink A, Roll S, Ruether K, Rasch A, Greiner W, et al. (2008) Cataract surgery and the development or progression of age-related macular degeneration: a systematic review. Surv Ophthalmol 53: 359–367.

24. Nolan JM, O'Reilly P, Loughman J, Stack J, Loane E, et al. (2009) Augmentation of macular pigment following implantation of blue light-filtering intraocular lenses at the time of cataract surgery. Invest Ophthalmol Vis Sci 50: 4777–4785.

25. Algvere PV, Marshall J, Seregard S (2006) Age-related maculopathy and the impact of blue light hazard. Acta Ophthalmol Scand 84: 4–15.

26. Kase S, He S, Sonoda S, Kitamura M, Spee C, et al. (2010) alphaB-crystallin regulation of angiogenesis by modulation of VEGF. Blood 115: 3398–3406.

27. Rao NA, Saraswathy S, Wu GS, Katselis GS, Wawrousek EF, et al. (2008) Elevated retina-specific expression of the small heat shock protein, alphaA-crystallin, is associated with photoreceptor protection in experimental uveitis. Invest Ophthalmol Vis Sci 49: 1161–1171.

28. Yaung J, Kannan R, Wawrousek EF, Spee C, Sreekumar PG, et al. (2008) Exacerbation of retinal degeneration in the absence of alpha crystallins in an in vivo model of chemically induced hypoxia. Exp Eye Res 86: 355–365.

29. Ramkumar HL, Zhang J, Chan CC (2010) Retinal ultrastructure of murine models of dry age-related macular degeneration (AMD). Prog Retin Eye Res 29: 169–190.

30. Cai X, McGinnis JF (2012) Oxidative stress: the achilles' heel of neurodegenerative diseases of the retina. Front Biosci 17: 1976–1995.

31. Machalinska A, Lubinski W, Klos P, Kawa M, Baumert B, et al. (2010) Sodium iodate selectively injuries the posterior pole of the retina in a dose-dependent manner: morphological and electrophysiological study. Neurochem Res 35: 1819–1827.

32. Michael R, Bron AJ (2011) The ageing lens and cataract: a model of normal and pathological ageing. Philos Trans R Soc Lond B Biol Sci 366: 1278–1292.

33. Neal RE, Bettelheim FA, Lin C, Winn KC, Garland DL, et al. (2005) Alterations in human vitreous humour following cataract extraction. Exp Eye Res 80: 337–347.

34. Franco LM, Zulliger R, Wolf-Schnurrbusch UE, Katagiri Y, Kaplan HJ, et al. (2009) Decreased visual function after patchy loss of retinal pigment epithelium induced by low-dose sodium iodate. Invest Ophthalmol Vis Sci 50: 4004–4010.

4

A Pilot Study of Morphometric Analysis of Choroidal Vasculature *In Vivo*, Using En Face Optical Coherence Tomography

Mahsa Sohrab, Katherine Wu, Amani A. Fawzi*

Department of Ophthalmology, Northwestern University, Feinberg School of Medicine, Chicago, Illinois, United States of America

Abstract

Purpose: To study the ability of volumetric spectral domain optical coherence tomography (SD-OCT) to perform quantitative measurement of the choroidal vasculature *in vivo*.

Methods: Choroidal vascular density and vessel size were quantified using en face choroidal scans from various depths below the retinal pigment epithelium (RPE) in 58 eyes of 58 patients with either epiretinal membranes (ERM), early age-related macular degeneration (AMD), or reticular pseudo-drusen (RPD). For each patient, we used the macular volume scan (6×6 mm cube) for vessel quantification, while high-definition (HD) cross-section raster scans were used to qualitatively assess vascularity of the choroidal sub-layers, and measure choroidal thickness.

Results: Of the 58 patients, more were female (66% versus 34% male), of whom 14 (24%) had ERM, 11 (19%) early AMD, and 33 (57%) RPD. Compared to intact choriocapillaris in all ERM (100%), none of the RPD and only 5/11 (45%) early AMD eyes had visible choriocapillaris on either cross section or C-scans (p-value<0.001). When comparing select regions from the most superficial C-scans, early AMD group had lowest vascular density and RPD had highest (p-value 0.04). Qualitative evaluation of C-scans from all three groups revealed a more granular appearance of the choriocapillaris in ERM versus increased stroma and larger vessels in the RPD eyes.

Conclusions: SD-OCT can be used to qualitatively and quantitatively assess choroidal vascularity *in vivo*. Our findings correlate to previously reported histopathologic studies. Lack of choriocapillaris on HD cross-sections or C-scans in all RPD and about half of early AMD eyes suggests earlier choroidal involvement in AMD and specifically, RPD.

Editor: Andreas Wedrich, Medical University Graz, Austria

Funding: This work was supported by the National Eye Institute EY03040 and EY021470. The funders had no role in study design, data collection and analysis, decision to publish, or preparation of the manuscript.

Competing Interests: The authors have declared that no competing interests exist.

* E-mail: Afawzimd@gmail.com

Introduction

The role of choroidal vasculature in the pathogenesis of age-related macular degeneration (AMD) has been explored using various structural and functional approaches [1], [2], [3], [4], [5], [6], [7], [8]. Until recently, studies of the choroid have been limited to postmortem tissue. Histopathologic comparisons of eyes with early AMD to age-matched controls have shown correlations between choriocapillaris loss and drusen density [1], [2], [3], [5], [6], [7], [8]. Choroidal vascular flatmounts in late-stage AMD have shown loss of choriocapillaris underlying retinal pigment epithelium (RPE) atrophy in atrophic AMD with constriction of remaining choriocapillaris and loss of normal choroidal vasculature underlying areas of intact RPE surrounding choroidal neovascular membranes, suggesting diversity of interactions between the choroid and RPE in late AMD [4], [5].

Clinically, indocyanine green angiography has been used to study choroidal vasculature [9], though it does not allow three-dimensional visualization of the choriocapillaris. While many advances have been made in retinal imaging with spectral-domain

optical coherence tomography (SD-OCT), visualization of the choroid has remained a challenge. Recently, the sensitivity of choroidal imaging in SD-OCT was improved through enhanced depth imaging [10], [11], [12], [13], [14], [15], [16], revealing that about one-third of patients with advanced AMD have thin choroid significantly below the mean thickness of age-matched controls [10], [11], [12], [13]. Additionally, choroidal thickness was found to be highly correlated with age, axial length, and refraction, emphasizing the importance of controlling for these variables when studying any patient population [16]. More interestingly, choroidal thickness varies on a diurnal basis by as much as 29+/−16 microns in one study, suggesting that it can be an highly variable measure of choroidal vasculature and further emphasizing the need to develop novel approaches to reliably assess choroidal vascular health *in vivo* [16], [17], [18].

Our understanding of the role played by the choroid *in vivo* can be significantly enhanced by detailed choroidal vascular reconstructions. In a previous study, we used multimodal imaging and registered OCT volume scans of reticular pseudodrusen (RPD)

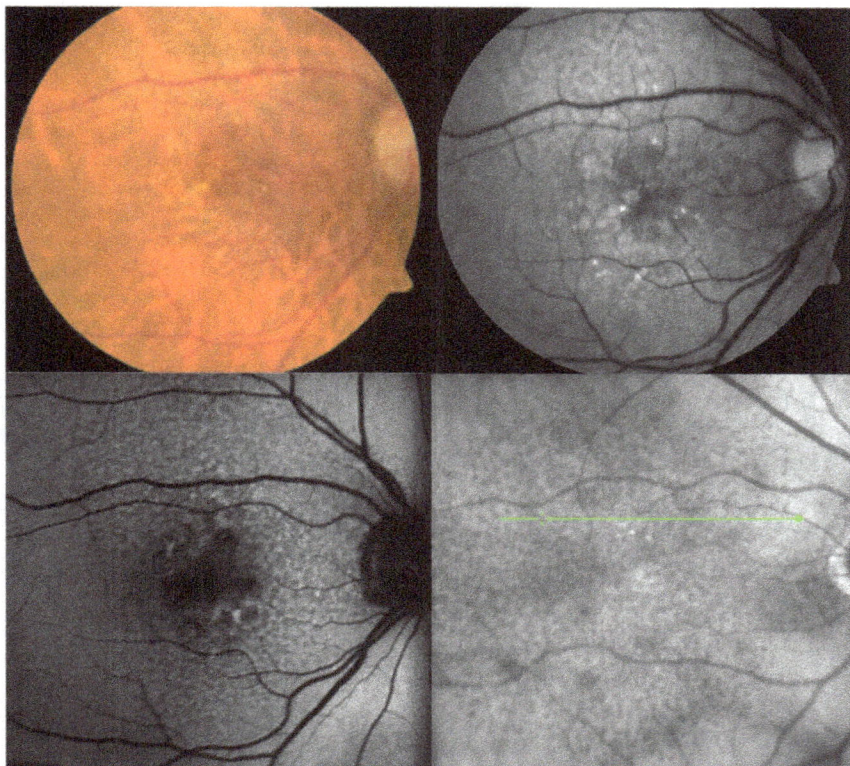

Figure 1. Imaging Characteristics of Reticular Pseudodrusen. Reticular pseudodrusen appear as faint, yellowish, interlacing networks along the arcades on color fundus images (top left) and as light interlacing networks on red-free imaging (top right). Imaging with autofluorescence (bottom left) and infrared (bottom right) improves visualization of reticular pseudodrusen as hypoautofluorescent or hyporeflectant lesions, respectively, extending along the arcades and through the fovea.

lesions and showed the lesions overlapped with the choroidal stroma [19], illustrating that reconstructed high-density volume OCT scans can be used to study the choroidal vascular patterns. In the current study we wanted to explore the use of reconstructed OCT scans to quantify choroidal vasculature in patients with early AMD and various stages of RPD, with the goal of using SD-OCT to obtain quantitative maps of the choroidal vasculature *in vivo*, similar to histopathologic sections and vascular flat-mounts of the choroid. Our results are the first to demonstrate the utility of this approach through comparison to results of prior histopathologic studies of the choroidal vasculature.

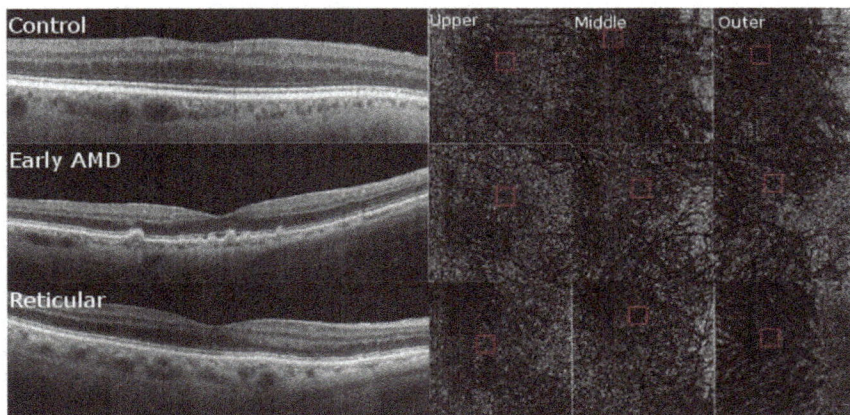

Figure 2. En Face Optical Coherence Tomography (OCT) Choroidal Sub-Layer C-Scans. Examples of 2 micron-thick C-scans obtained from control (top panel), early age-related macular degeneration (AMD, middle panel) and reticular groups (bottom panel). C-scans were obtained from the choriocapillaris or most representative layer below the RPE in the reticular group (center left column), Sattler's or the middle choroidal layer (center right column), and Haller's or the outermost layer (far right column) for further analysis.

Methods

Study Population

The study was approved by the Institutional Review Board at the Doheny Eye Institute and adhered to the tenets set forth by the Declaration of Helsinki. A retrospective review of all patients diagnosed with AMD between June 2008 and July 2011 identified 58 patients between the ages of 41 and 97 who had undergone infrared (IR), fundus autofluorescence (FAF) and SD-OCT imaging. Patients scanned with the Cirrus high-definition SD-OCT device (HD-OCT, Carl Zeiss Meditec Inc, Dublin, CA USA) were included. Some patients had red-free (RF) images with the Spectralis HRA+OCT (Heidelberg Engineering Inc, Dossenheim, Germany), though the majority had RF images obtained as part of the standard fluorescein angiography protocol using the Topcon TRC-50IX (Topcon Medical Systems Inc, Paramus, NJ, USA).

The strict criteria for the presence of RPD as described in the Definitions section below was applied to the entire portfolio of imaging studies for each patient. We enrolled patients with epiretinal membranes (ERM) without evidence of AMD to serve as the control group. The eye with the best image quality or most obvious display of the characteristic of interest was selected for each patient in the study. Eyes that were eligible for more than one category (early AMD, RPD, and/or ERM) were excluded. Only one eye per patient was included in the study.

Image Acquisition

All 58 patients underwent scanning with the Cirrus HD-OCT Model 4000 device, using super-luminescent diode at 840 nm, which achieves 5 microns of axial and 15 microns of transverse tissue resolution. The device captures 27,000 A-scans per second at 2 mm of depth, and the images were viewed with the latest Cirrus HD-OCT software (Version 5.0; Carl Zeiss Meditec Inc, Dublin, CA, USA). As part of the standard Cirrus imaging protocol, all eyes undergo two scanning protocols, a 5-line raster consisting of 4,096 A-scans for each of the 5 B-scans, and a 512×128 Macular Cube volume scan consisting of 128 equally-spaced horizontal B-scans (each composed of 512 A-scans) over a 6 mm square grid. The line scanning laser ophthalmoscope (LSLO) feature also obtained a registered OCT fundus image for each data cube. The Cirrus OCT imaging protocol further requires photographers to repeat OCT volume scans if the summed OCT projection image suggests that significant motion artifact is present.

Definitions

Identification of patients with evidence of early AMD, RPD, or ERM was based on recognition of characteristic features as seen in the Cirrus OCT and fundus imaging.

Patients with early AMD were identified on the basis of the presence of soft and hard drusen (dry AMD) on imaging. Patients with RPD were identified on the basis of characteristic features on various imaging modalities as defined in previous reports (Figure 1) [19]. Evidence of RPD on RF imaging was defined by the presence of light, interlacing networks ranging from 125 to 250 microns in width. RPD on FAF was defined by the presence of clusters of ill-defined, hypo-autofluorescent lesions interspersed against a background of mildly increased AF occurring in regular and well-defined array. RPD on IR was defined as groups of hyporeflective lesions interspersed against a background of mild hyperreflectance. Advanced RPD was defined as RPD lesions in eyes with evidence of atrophic or neovascular AMD.

Analysis Protocol

En face OCT choroidal sub-layer C-scans. The following analysis was performed on each of the 58 patients. OCT volume scans (512×128 macular cubes) obtained on Cirrus HD-OCT were reviewed on the Cirrus version 5.0 software using the advanced visualization feature. As previously described [19], the RPE feature was used to obtain en face slices that were contoured based on each patient's RPE curvature. The slice feature was selected to ensure that the RPE band or sclera were not included in any of the sections. We obtained 2 micron-thick C-scans for each eye at three levels of the choroid, the choriocapillaris, Sattler's layer (middle), and Haller's layer (outermost) to undergo further analysis (Figure 2).

The slice location within each choroidal layer was placed with guidance from the HD OCT scan. In patients in whom choriocapillaris was not visible or difficult to visualize in the en face slice, we confirmed the absence of choriocapillaris using the HD scan and selected the most representative C-scan immediately beneath the RPE.

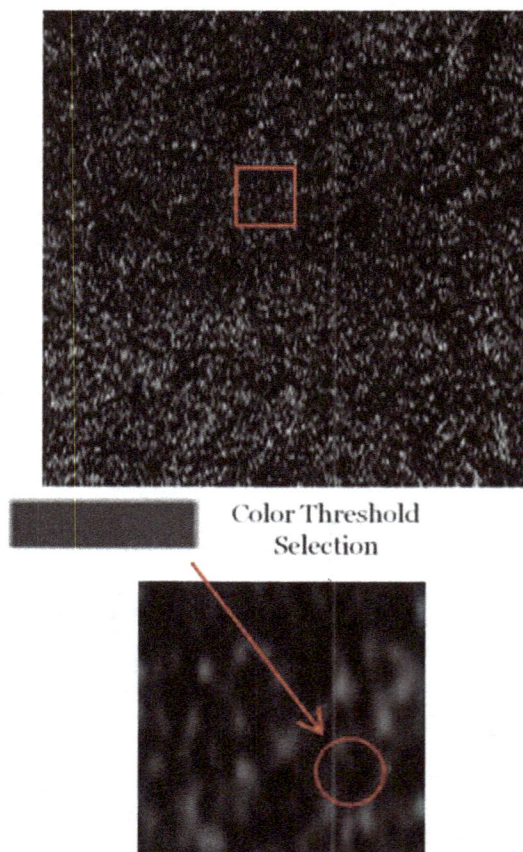

Figure 3. Selecting Pixel Intensity Threshold for Choroidal Vessel Density Analysis. Choroidal C-scans (top image) were obtained using the advanced visualization feature of macular cubes consisting of 512×128 optical coherence tomography volume scans over a 6 mm square grid. Each C-scan was a 2 micron-thick scan from each of the three choroidal layers. A customized image analysis program was used for both full C-scans (top image) and a selected region of each scan (inset) for all patients. A strict threshold of R=65, G=65, and B=65 pixel intensity combination was selected for vessel versus stroma (center).

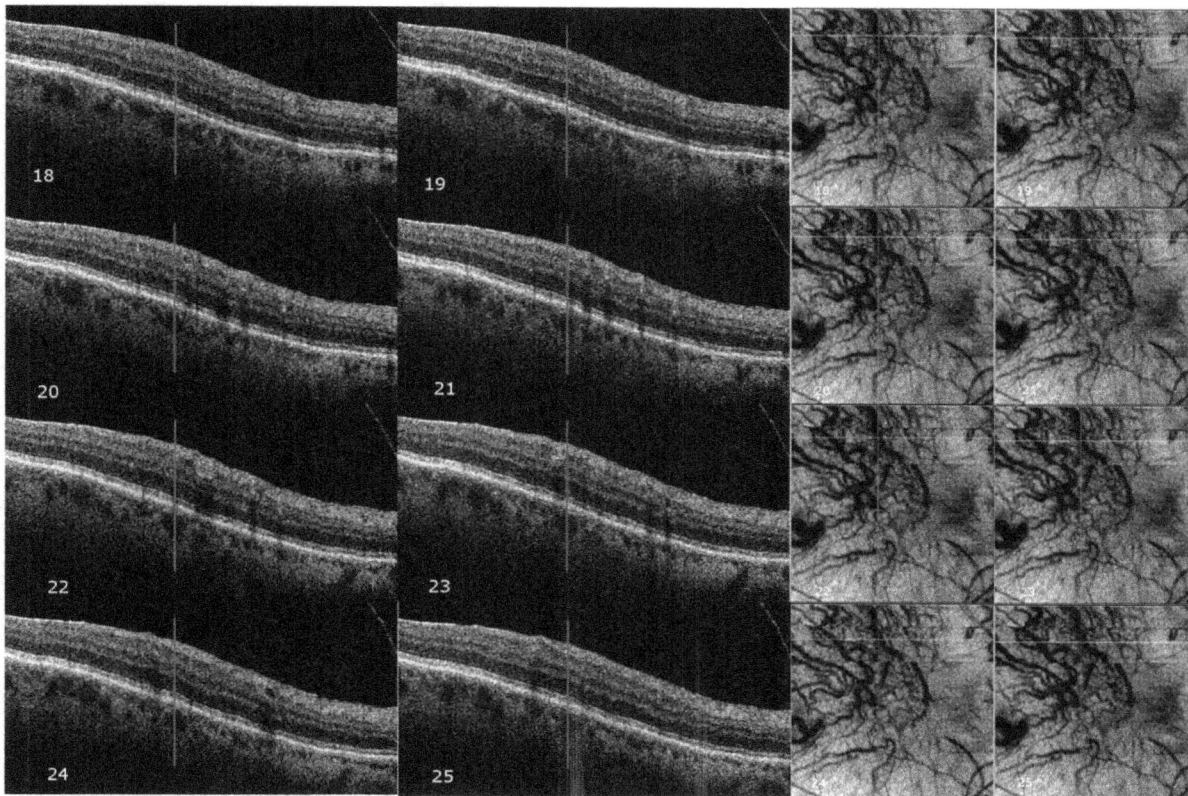

Figure 4. Cross-Correlation of Choroidal Vascular Appearance on Optical Coherence Tomography (OCT) Comparing B- and C-Scans. A large choroidal vessel is identified as a well-defined round hypo-reflective structure in cross-section on individual B-Scans (purple line). Sequential B-scan slices (18–25) are shown with the purple line centered on the same choroidal vessel. On the C-scans shown, the blue horizontal lines correspond to the location of the respective B-scan, while the purple line follows the vertical axis of the corresponding choroidal vessel on C-scan.

Vessel density on choroidal C-scans (Figure 3). We developed a custom image analysis program to compare the vessel density present in each choroidal sub-layer for each patient. Since every image is composed of a certain number of pixels, the image analysis program analyses the entire array of pixels, each coded with a specific red, green and blue (RGB) intensity, where the combination of RGB intensities code a specific gray-scale.

Each pixel intensity ranges from 0 to 255, and pixels that are a similar shade of black or white, have the same R, G, and B values. For example, the combination for pure white is R = 255, G = 255, B = 255 while the combination for pure black is R = 0, G = 0, B = 0. We selected a threshold RGB combination from the

spectrum of black to white and all pixel combinations with RGB values at or below this threshold were classified as vessel (black) while those above the threshold were considered stroma. In order to confirm that the round hypo-reflective structures seen on individual B-scans correspond to the choroidal vessel lumen, we tracked one of these structures in eight consecutive raster B-scans and cofirmed that the circular lumen coincided with the course of the corresponding choroidal vessel seen on the en face OCT slice (Figure 4). We ran two analyses for all the images, one with a loose cutoff at a gray shade of R = 110, G = 110, B = 110 and one with a stricter cutoff at an almost black shade of R = 65, G = 65, B = 65,

Table 1. Patient Demographics.

	Control n = 14	Early AMD n = 11	Reticular n = 23	Advanced Reticular n = 10	Overall n = 58	p-value
Gender						
Female	7 (50%)	4 (36.4%)	19 (82.6%)	8 (80%)	38 (66%)	0.02
Male, n(%)	7 (50%)	7 (63.6%)	4 (17.4%)	2 (20%)	20 (34%)	0.02
Mean Age (+/− SD)	61(10.7)	76.7(9)	82.6(7)	84.3(7.6)	76.6	<0.001[*]

AMD = age-related macular degeneration; Control = epiretinal membranes; early AMD = drusen, advanced reticular patients = reticular pseudodrusen with advanced atrophic or neovascular AMD.
*Age Comparisons were statistically significant (p<0.001) between each of the AMD subgroups and control, but not significant between the individual AMD groups.

selecting the latter cutoff for the vascular analyses of the entire database.

In calculating vessel density, we initially analyzed the full 6×6 mm en-face scans for each patient, which provided an averaged vascular density for the entire macula. We then manually selected representative areas (0.5×0.5 mm) within each en face slice, where the choroidal vasculature was visible to calculate select area vessel density.

Measurement of Vessel Diameter in Choroidal C-scans. The customized image analysis tool allowed us to measure the diameter of the individual vessels in each choroidal slice by calculating the distance between the coordinates of the edges of the vessels. Using Cartesian mathematics with the horizontal base as the x-axis and the vertical edge as the y axis, and selecting two coordinates directly across from each other on the border in the x-axis (horizontal dimension), the software calculated the horizontal diameter of the vessels in pixels.

Since some of the vessels in the choriocapillaris were extremely narrow, it was difficult to accurately pinpoint the coordinates of the edges of the vessels. To eliminate error, we programmed the image analysis software to magnify the images from its original size of 644 by 644 pixels to approximately 760 by 760 pixels so we could more easily select the coordinates located on the diameter of the vessels. This discrepancy created by magnification was rectified by modifying the image analysis software to directly proportion the size of the magnified image to the size of its corresponding original image and subsequently correlate the coordinates on the magnified

image with the actual coordinates in the original image. Using these adjusted coordinates, the program calculated the diameter of vessels in pixels.

Each C-scan image contained numerous vessels with varying diameters, so to obtain the measurements for the average vessel sizes we took the average of two measurements from the diameter of the largest and smallest visible vessels per image. For the most superficial choroidal layer in eyes with RPD (without visible choriocapillaris), the values were obtained from 5 averaged measurements of the large, medium, and small vessels.

Choroidal Thickness. The linear measurement tool was used to measure the choroidal thickness from the base of the RPE to the junction of the sclera and the choroid on the foveal HD raster scans (6 mm lines of 4096 A-scans) obtained on the Cirrus HD-OCT device.

Statistical Analysis

The analysis of variance (ANOVA) test was used to compare parameters including age, gender and choroidal thickness as well as vessel density (in percentage) and vessel diameter (pixels) for each layer. Analysis of covariance (ANCOVA) was performed for choroidal thickness, vessel diameter and vessel density after adjusting for choroidal thickness and for age and gender. When the ANOVA and ANCOVA were statistically significant ($p < 0.05$), Bonferroni adjusted p-values were calculated for the comparisons.

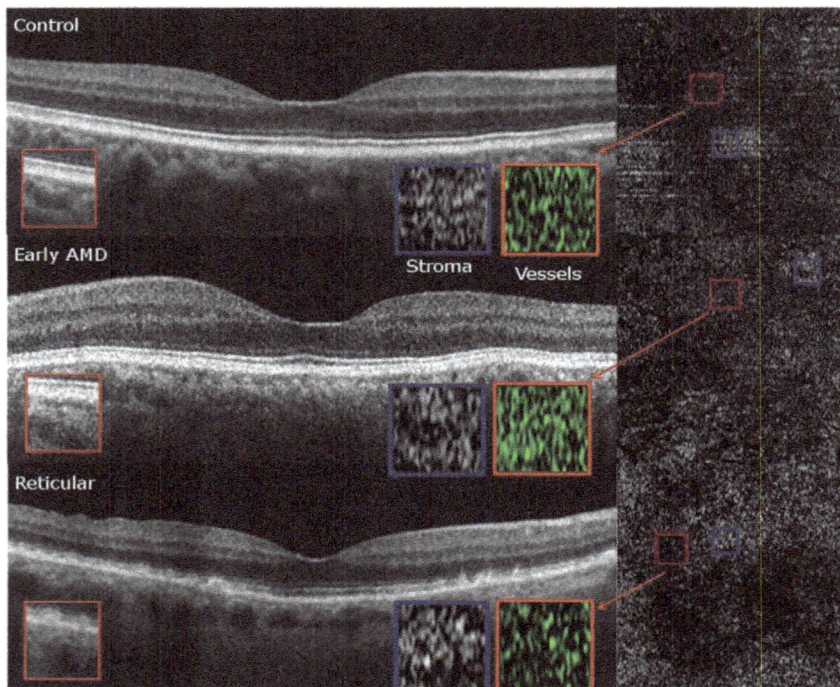

Figure 5. Qualitative Choriocapillaris Assessment Comparing C-Scans and B-Scans (Example 1). When comparing control (top panel), early age-related macular degeneration (AMD, middle panel) and reticular (bottom panel) patients, the appearance of representative C-scans obtained just below the retinal pigment epithelium in reticular groups (bottom right) was qualitatively different from the choriocapillaris scans obtained in the control and AMD groups (top right and center right, respectively). Red boxes on the B-Scans (left) show magnified and colorized selected areas of choroidal vasculature from the regions contained by the smaller red boxes on the C-Scans (right) for each group. Blue boxes on the B-Scans (left) show magnified areas of selected stroma from the regions contained by the smaller blue boxes on the C-Scans (right). Stromal sections demonstrate more patchy whitish regions in the RPD group (bottom panel) as compared to the control and AMD groups (top and middle panels) but similar vessel density due to the presence of larger vessels.

Results

Study Population (Table 1)

Of the 58 patients selected for inclusion in the study, there was a twofold preponderance of females, higher in the reticular groups where the ratio of female to male was 4:1 (p = 0.02). Of all eyes examined, 14 (24%) were classified as controls, 11 (19%) as early AMD, and 33 (57%) as RPD, of whom 10/33 (30%) were classified as advanced RPD (defined in the methods). The control group had the lowest average age while the reticular groups had the highest (p<0.001).

Qualitative Choriocapillaris Assessment on HD-OCT B-scans and Choroidal slice C-scans (Figures 5, 6, 7, 8)

None of the RPD eyes and only 5 (45%) of the early AMD eyes had visible choriocapillaris in the HD-OCT scans, compared to all control eyes (p<0.001, Fisher's exact test).

C-scans of the choriocapillaris layer in control eyes showed a regular, honeycomb-like pattern of alternating vessels and stroma that was distinguishable from the deeper choroidal layers which showed well-defined interlacing vascular channels separated by stromal regions in the middle and outer layers. In contrast, C-scans taken just beneath the RPE in patients without evident choriocapillaris (100% of RPD eyes and 55% of early AMD eyes), showed larger sized vascular channels more closely resembling the middle layer of control eyes (Figures 5, 6, 7). Given the qualitative differences noted on comparing sections from different groups, it is unlikely that the layer immediately external to the RPE in the early AMD and reticular eyes without visible choriocapillaris is analogous to the normal choriocapillaris seen in controls.

Choroidal vessel density on C-scans (Tables 2 and 3)

In order to understand the relationship between choroidal thickness and vascular density, we explored the average vessel density in each full 6×6 mm choroidal slice as a function of choroidal thickness. The deepest choroidal layers had the highest vascular density, regardless of the range of choroidal thickness (Graph S1). Overall, eyes with thicker choroids were found to have higher vascular densities in each choroidal sublayer (Graph S1). Based on this finding, we decided to control for choroidal thickness when evaluating vascular densities.

In Table 2 we tested two models of analyzing the data for covariance, with the first adjusting for choroidal thickness and the second adjusting for age and gender. Comparing the choroidal vascular density between groups using an entire 6×6 mm slice (full scan) versus a smaller selected region (500×500 micons) for each choroidal sublayer, we did not find statistically significant sublayer vessel density differences in the full slice group between groups but did find statistically significant differences in the smaller selected regions, with the lowest vascular density in the early AMD group and the highest density in the reticular group (p-value = 0.0003). Controlling for age and gender, superficial choroidal thickness in the small region remained statistically significant (p = 0.04). Detailed raw values of vessel density data in each group are shown in Table 3.

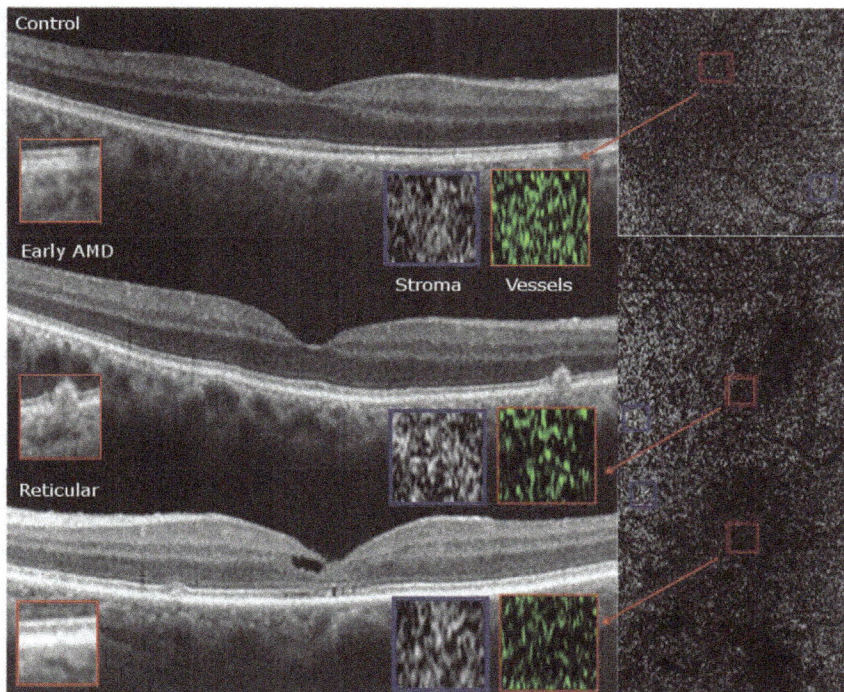

Figure 6. Qualitative Choriocapillaris Assessment Comparing C-Scans and B-Scans (Example 2). Comparing another example of control (top panel), early age-related macular degeneration (AMD, middle panel) and reticular (bottom panel) patients, reveals qualitatively different appearance of representative C-scans obtained just below the retinal pigment epithelium in reticular groups (bottom right) than in the control and AMD groups (top right and center right, respectively). Red boxes on the B-Scans (left) show magnified and colorized selected areas of choroidal vasculature from the regions contained by the smaller red boxes on the C-Scans (right) for each group. Blue boxes on the B-Scans (left) show magnified areas of selected stroma from the regions contained by the smaller blue boxes on the C-Scans (right). Stromal sections demonstrate more patchy whitish regions in the RPD group (bottom panel) as compared to the control and AMD groups (top and middle panels) but similar vessel density due to the presence of larger vessels.

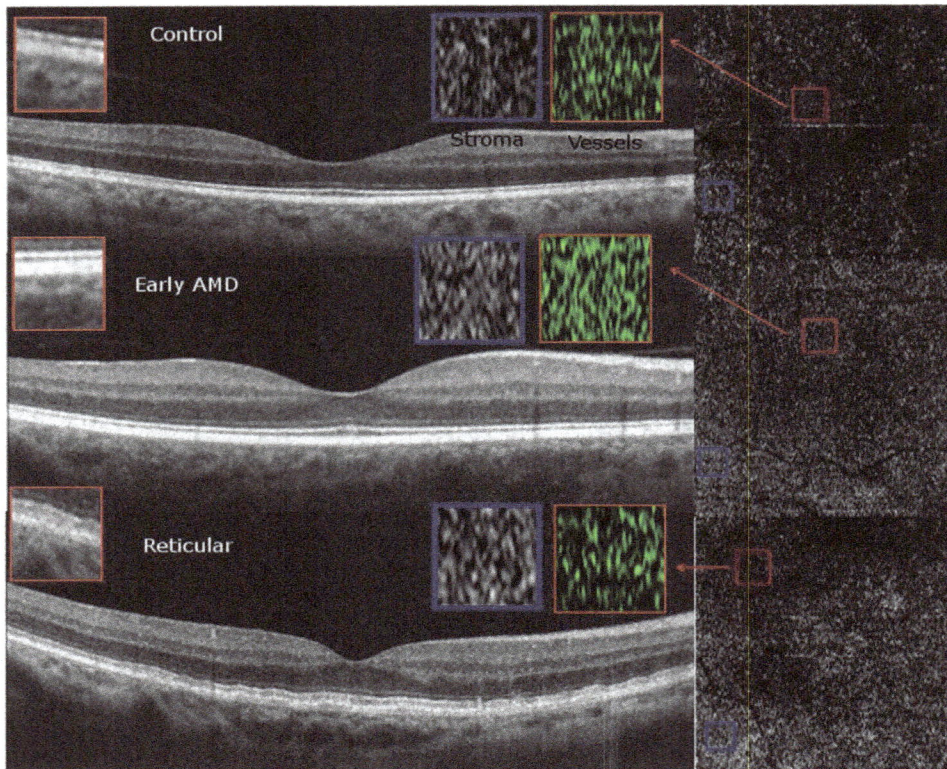

Figure 7. Qualitative Choriocapillaris Assessment Comparing C-Scans and B-Scans (Example 3). Comparisons of control (top panel), early age-related macular degeneration (AMD, middle panel) and reticular (bottom panel) patients reveals qualitatively different appearance of representative C-scans obtained just below the retinal pigment epithelium in reticular groups (bottom right) than in the control and AMD groups (top right and center right, respectively). Red boxes on the B-Scans (left) show magnified and colorized selected areas of choroidal vasculature from the regions contained by the smaller red boxes on the C-Scans (right) for each group. Blue boxes on the B-Scans (left) show magnified areas of selected stroma from the regions contained by the smaller blue boxes on the C-Scans (right). Stromal sections demonstrate more patchy whitish regions in the RPD group (bottom panel) as compared to the control and AMD groups (top and middle panels) but similar vessel density due to the presence of larger vessels.

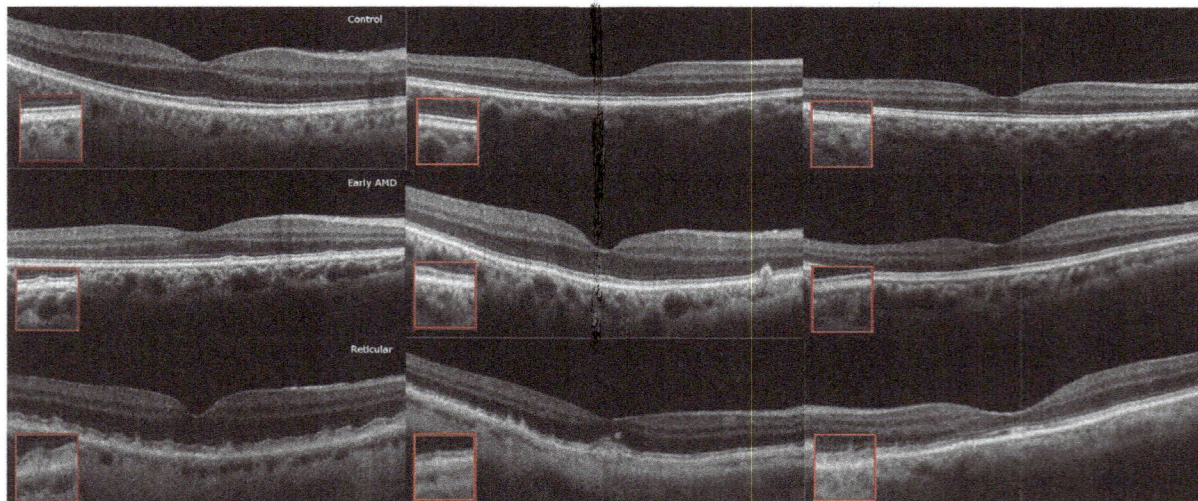

Figure 8. Qualitative High Density (HD) Raster Scan Assessment of Choriocapillaris. HD-raster scans of the control group (top) had a distinct granular-appearing choriocapillaris layer, in contrast to only 45% of the early age-related macular degeneration group (center) and none of the reticular group (bottom), in whom this layer was lacking.

Table 2. Choroidal Vascular Density on C-Scans: Macular (6×6 mm) versus Regional (500×500 microns).

	Control n = 14	Early AMD n = 11	Reticular n = 23	Advanced Reticular n = 10	p-value[Ac]
6×6 mm C-scan Vascular Density (%)					
Inner					
Model 1	75.4±2.3	71.7±3.6	74.5±1.9	74.4±2.8	0.86
Model 2	78.5±3.2	72.7±4.0	72.1±2.5	72.7±3.5	0.53
Middle					
Model 1	83.2±1.4	80.1±1.6	80.4±1.1	84.2±2.1	0.18
Model 2	83.3±1.9	80.1±1.7	80.5±1.4	84.4±2.3	0.22
Outer					
Model 1	86.4±1.5	86.8±1.6	86.4±1.1	86.5±1.6	1.00
Model 2	85.5±2.0	87.3±1.6	86.1±1.3	86.9±1.9	0.89
500×500 micron Regional Vascular Density (%)					
Inner					
Model 1	85.2±1.8	79.5±2.8	91.6±1.5	86.5±2.2	0.003*
Model 2	86.7±2.5	79.7±3.1	90.7±1.9	86.4±2.8	0.04^
Middle					
Model 1	89.6±1.4	90.5±1.5	91.3±1.1	90.3±2.0	0.81
Model 2	87.8±1.8	90.3±1.5	92.2±1.3	91.7±2.2	0.36
Outer					
Model 1	95.7±0.9	95.6±1.0	95.6±0.7	97.2±1.0	0.59
Model 2	94.8±1.2	95.7±0.9	95.7±0.8	97.4±1.1	0.41

AMD = age-related macular degeneration; Control = epiretinal membranes; early AMD patients = drusen, advanced reticular patients = reticular pseudodrusen with advanced atrophic or neovascular AMD.
[Ac] = Analysis of covariance (ANCOVA) p-value. Model 1. Adjusting for choroidal thickness. Model 2. Adjusting for age and gender. When the ANCOVA was statistically significant (p<0.05), Bonferroni adjusted p-values were calculated for the pairwise comparisons. NS = non-significant (p>0.05).
*When comparing Drusen vs early reticulars, p = 0.004, while all other comparisons were non-significant.
^When comparing Drusen vs early reticulars, p = 0.04, while all other comparisons were non-significant.

Measurement of Vessel Diameter in choroidal C-scans (Table 4)

Choriocapillaris vessel diameter measured in the horizontal axis in controls ranged from 2.8 to 6.5 pixels (average 4.42), middle choroidal vessels 7.0 to 10.8 pixels (average 8.31), and deeper choroidal vessels 15.6 to 22.1 pixels (average 18.38). Vessel diameters were similar in the early AMD and RPD groups (in layers in which they were present), without statistically significant differences. Given the cube is 6×6 mm, with 512× 128 A-scans, the pixel separation in the horizontal direction is 6000/512 or 11.7 microns (and 6000/128 in the vertical direction or 47 microns), hence the choriocapillaris horizontal dimensions were on average 50 microns, the middle vessels ~100 microns, and the large vessels ~215 microns.

Choroidal Thickness (Table 5)

Overall, choroid was thicker in the control and early AMD groups and thinner in the RPD and advanced RPD groups (p = 0.04), though the differences were not statistically significant after controlling for age and gender (p = 0.5). We examined the effect of age and gender on choroidal thickness, and found a trend for females to have thinner choroids up to age 80, after which there was reversal of the pattern, though differences were not statistically significant (Graph S2).

Discussion

To our knowledge, this is the first study to evaluate choroidal vascular patterns and density using reconstructed SD-OCT volume imaging. While histopathologic studies have documented a range of choroidal vascular changes in normal aging and in

Table 3. Choroidal Vessel Density by Choroidal Sublayer.

Vessel Density (%)	Control	Early AMD	Reticular
Inner	63.8%–91.2% (76.5%)	67.2%–78.7% (72.2%)	54.8%–91.0% (73.8%)
Middle	75.9%–88.4% (83.6%)	74.9%–84.5% (80.3%)	69.7%–89.9% (80.%)
Outer	79.3%–93.9% (87.2%)	72.4%–94.4% (87.2%)	76.9%–91.6% (85.9%)

Full slices (6×6 mm) data; Control = epiretinal membranes; early AMD patients = drusen, reticular patients = reticular pseudodrusen with or without advanced atrophic or neovascular AMD, average densities in parentheses.

Table 4. Choroidal Vessel Diameter.

	Control n = 14	Early AMD n = 11	Reticular n = 23	Advanced Reticular n = 10	p-value	Early AMD vs Reticular
Diameter (pixels)						
Inner						
Crude	4.43±0.98	4.18±0.36	–	–	0.60	
Adjusted	4.49±0.38	4.19±0.45	–	–	0.54	
Middle						
Crude	8.31±1.22	7.51±2.22	7.36±2.47	7.52±1.47	0.61[A]	0.87[A]
Adjusted	8.30±0.78	7.51±0.66	7.36±0.51	7.52±0.93	0.83[Ac]	0.87[Ac]
Outer						
Crude	19.49±0.07	18.38±2.07	17.61±4.22	18.02±3.21	0.61[A]	0.26[A]
Adjusted	19.45±1.16	17.36±1.44	17.98±0.88	18.51±1.30	0.63[Ac]	0.84[Ac]

AMD = age-related macular degeneration; crude versus adjusted for age and gender; Control = epiretinal membranes; early AMD patients = drusen, advanced reticular patients = reticular pseudodrusen with advanced atrophic or neovascular AMD.
[A] = Analysis of variance (ANOVA) p-value.
[Ac] = Analysis of covariance (ANCOVA) p-value, adjusting for age and gender. When the ANOVA or ANCOVA was statistically significant (p<0.05), Bonferroni adjusted p-values were calculated for the pairwise comparisons.

AMD [1], [2], [3], [4], [5], [6], [7], [8], the exact sequence of events remains a subject of considerable debate. The ability to perform quantitative choroidal vascular analysis *in vivo* as shown in our study opens avenues for longitudinal detailed study of the choroid in aging eyes and an opportunity to address these controversies definitively.

In evaluating choroidal vessel density, we utilized two different approaches. Vessel density in the 6×6 mm *en-face* C-scan provided an averaged macular vascular density and found similar densities among the different groups. We found that approach suffered from segmentation artifact, especially when evaluating the choriocapillaris, which might be related to RPE curvature especially in eyes with thin choroid (Figure 9). Qualitative evaluation of the entire C-scans in these eyes showed non-uniform appearance of the vascular patterns suggesting patchy vascular loss (Figures 5, 6, 7). We therefore performed an additional quantitative analysis on manually selected regions (500×500 microns) with visible vasculature (Figures 5, 6, 7). Using these select areas, we found that early RPD eyes had statistically significant increased superficial choroidal vascular density compared to early AMD, after adjusting for age and gender (p = 0.04) and choroidal thickness (p = 0.004). Taken together with absent choriocapillaris

on HD-OCT cross sections in 100% of RPD eyes, we believe that the most superficial C-scan analyzed in these eyes included larger choroidal vessels interspersed with atrophic choriocapillaris. It is further possible that residual "ghost" or non-perfused choriocapillaris, which are likely less than a horizontal pixel (11 microns), are under-estimated by this approach due to lack of adequate resolution.

Qualitatively, the regular "honeycomb" pattern of the most superficial C-scan in control eyes was distinctly absent in reticular eyes, further validating our conclusions (Figures 5, 6, 7, 8). Instead, RPD eyes show interlacing larger diameter choroidal vessels in the most superficial vascular layer of the choroid (Figures 5, 6, 7, 8). Qualitative evaluation of HD-raster B-scans further confirmed the lack of a "granular appearing" choriocapillaris in the immediate sub-RPE region of RPD eyes (Figure 8). The lack of statistically significant differences in superficial vascular density of the full slices reflects a combination of the patchy distribution of the larger vasculature and dense stroma noted on C-scans in RPD eyes. In contrast, analysis of selected areas with visible vascular patterns demonstrated focally increased vascular density in RPD.

HD cross-section OCT scans showed that less than half of eyes with early AMD had visible choriocapillaris. This is similar to

Table 5. Choroidal Thickness.

	Control n = 14	Early AMD n = 11	Reticular n = 23	Advanced Reticular n = 10	p-value
Thickness (Average +/− SD, microns)					
Crude	207.0+/−42.5	228.6+/−58.4	163.4+/−68.5	179.0+/−99.4	0.04*
Adjusted	209.7+/−20.6	198.1+/−24.7	169.4+/−16.7	188.8+/−23.6	0.50[Ac]

AMD = age-related macular degeneration; crude versus adjusted for age and gender; Control = epiretinal membranes; early AMD patients = drusen, advanced reticular patients = reticular pseudodrusen with advanced atrophic or neovascular lesions.
*Analysis of variance (ANOVA) p-values. Pairwise comparisons were statistically significant between Drusen and early reticulars (p = 0.04), but not significant when comparing other subtypes of AMD (p>0.05).
[Ac]: Analysis of covariance (ANCOVA) p-value, adjusting for age and gender. When the ANOVA or ANCOVA were statistically significant (p<0.05), Bonferroni adjusted p-values were calculated for the pairwise comparisons.

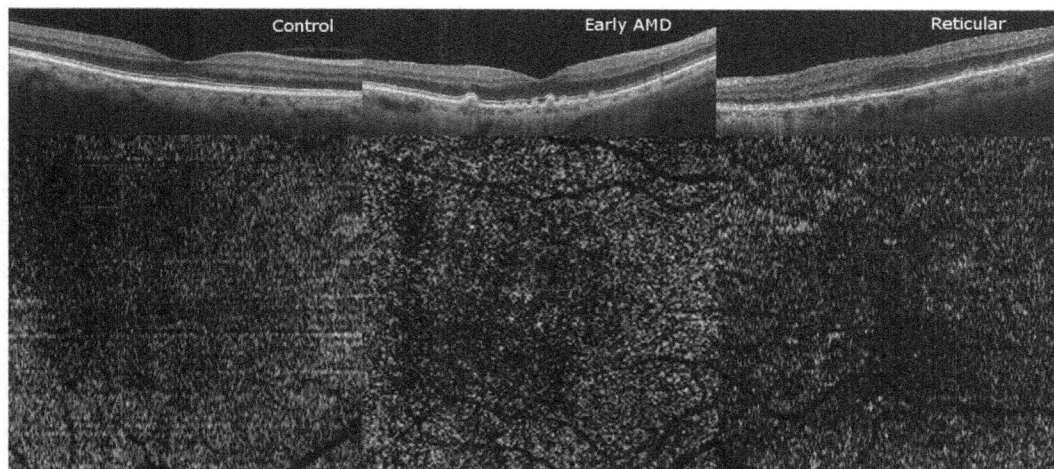

Figure 9. Altered Curvature of the Retinal Pigment Epithelium (RPE). Analyzing 6×6 mm C- scans obtained in the most superficial choroidal layers for all groups were affected by the variance in curvature of the RPE, especially in eyes with thin choroid (middle panel). Examples of high density (HD) raster scans and 6×6 mm C-scans from the control (left), early age-related macular degeneration (AMD, center) and reticular (right) groups are shown. In order to overcome these differences, selected 1×1 mm representative areas from the full C-scans were used for further analysis (red squares, bottom panel).

histopathologic findings of choriocapillaris atrophy and vascular dropout in areas of basal laminar and basal linear deposits [1], [2], [4]. Furthermore, we found statistically significantly decreased choroidal vessel density in the superficial choroid in early AMD eyes versus controls (79.7% versus 86.7%, p = 0.04). Choriocapillaris diameter in early AMD eyes was slightly reduced compared to control eyes, though this was not statistically significant (4.19 versus 4.49 pixels, respectively). In control eyes, we found an overall choriocapillaris vessel density (6×6 mm) of 78.5%, closely paralleling 79.6% reported in histopathologic studies, supporting the utility of OCT scans as a reliable tool for quantitative choroidal vascular mapping *in vivo*.

The vessel diameters found in this study are consistent among eyes, averaging 40–50 microns for the choriocapillaris compared to 100 and 200 microns for medium and large choroidal vessels, respectively. These measurements are consistent with histopathologic evidence in the posterior pole, though our approach probably leads to overestimation of the choriocapillaris size. The average macular choriocapillaris size on histopathology is ~20 microns as compared to the lateral resolution of the OCT system, which is 15 microns, making it inadequate for accurate choriocapillaris size assessment [20]. This problem could potentially be solved by incorporating the axial dimension of the choriocapillaris (from cross-sectional b-scans) into the calculation of choriocapilaris diameter. By assuming the choriocapillaris are round *in vivo*, and then further correcting for anisometric pixel resolution of this OCT, the accuracy of choriocapillaris size assessment with current OCT could be improved.

Three-dimensional high-density OCT volume data allowed us to study the relationship between choroidal thickness and the choroidal sublayer vascular structures. We found that patients with severely thin choroids (0 to 100 microns) had a lower average vessel density in the innermost choroidal layers as compared to thicker choroids (300 to 400 microns), in whom vessel density was similar between the layers (Graph S1). This is consistent with previous histopathologic evidence of decreased choroidal vessel density and diameter with decreased choroidal thickness [1], [2], [3], [4], [5]. In contrast, previous histopathologic reports did not compare vessel density or size in the different choroidal layers.

Our data suggests that with choroidal thinning, vessel density decreases most in the inner layer of the choroid, with less effect on the outer vasculature. The proximity of the choriocapillaris to the RPE allows a high oxygen supply to the highly metabolic outer retina, and the effect of decreased density of choriocapillaris in the setting of early AMD can have important implications on disease progression.

Comparing choroidal thickness among the patient groups, we found RPD eyes had thinner choroids compared to those with AMD without RPD, though these differences were not statistically significant after adjusting for age and gender. Previous studies found that the choroid becomes thinner with increasing age, regardless of disease status [11], [12], [13], [14], [15], [16]. Further analysis of our results demonstrated that, while overall choroidal thickness decreases in both men and women with age, choroid tends to be relatively thinner in younger women and older men (Graph S2). A recent cross-sectional study of young healthy subjects similarly found that women had thinner choroids compared to men for the same axial length [21]. Although the underlying reason for this difference is unclear, future population-based studies are indicated to further explore gender differences in the choroid. Our results suggest that age and gender may play a more important role in determining choroidal thickness than the underlying disease processes.

Limitations of the present study include the use of arbitrary cut-offs for distinguishing between vessel and stroma, compared to histopathology where more specific vascular labeling is possible. However, the pixel intensity cut-offs were standardized and applied to all groups allowing these comparisons. Furthermore, whereas histopathology can differentiate between healthy and ghost choriocapillaris, structural imaging cannot reveal these distinctions. Imaging approaches that are currently in development, such as phase-resolved OCT [22], may allow visualization of choroidal vascular flow to answer this question in the future. Finally, our study selected the layer immediately external to the RPE in patients who did not show evidence of choriocapillaris with the assumption that this layer would be analogous to the choriocapillaris, though this is likely not the case given the qualitative differences noted on our comparisons of sections obtained from each of the groups. Finally, our groups were not balanced with regards to age and gender, but we have controlled for these differences in our statistical analyses to avoid any bias.

In summary, this study is a first step towards using SD-OCT to quantify choroidal vasculature in the aging population *in vivo*. We found distinct differences in the macular choroid between the three groups studied, which were in agreement to previous histopathologic findings. Larger populations, longitudinal studies and the use of phase-resolved approaches will help elucidate the particular sequence of RPE and choroidal changes in the pathogenesis of various AMD subtypes. Further studies are needed to examine these findings in a larger population and to explore whether choriocapillaris atrophy topographically correlates with the location of RPD lesions.

Author Contributions

Conceived and designed the experiments: MAS AAF KW. Performed the experiments: AAF KW. Analyzed the data: MAS AAF KW. Contributed reagents/materials/analysis tools: MAS AAF KW. Wrote the paper: MAS AAF.

References

1. Mullins RF, Johnson MN, Faidley EA, Skeie JM, Huang J (2011) Choriocapillaris vascular dropout related to density of drusen in human eyes with early age-related macular degeneration. Invest Ophthalmol Vis Sci ;52: 1606–12.
2. Lengyel I, Tufail A, Hosaini HA, Luthert P, Bird AC, et al. (2004) Association of drusen deposition with choroidal intercapillary pillars in the aging human eye. Invest Ophthalmol Vis Sci 45: 2886–92.
3. Ramrattan RS, van der Schaft TL, Mooy CM, de Bruijn WC, Mulder PG, et al. (1994) Morphometric analysis of Bruch's membrane, the choriocapillaris, and the choroid in aging. Invest Ophthalmol Vis Sci 35: 2857–64.
4. McLeod DS, Taomoto M, Otsuji T, Green WR, Sunness JS, et al. (2002) Quantifying changes in RPE and choroidal vasculature in eyes with age-related macular degeneration. Invest Ophthalmol Vis Sci 43: 1986–93.
5. McLeod DS, Grebe R, Bhutto I, Merges C, Baba T, et al. (2009) Relationship between RPE and choriocapillaris in age-related macular degeneration. Invest Ophthalmol Vis Sci 50: 4982–91.
6. Spraul CW, Lang GE, Grossniklaus HE, Lang GK (1999) Histologic and morphometric analysis of the choroid, Bruch's membrane, and retinal pigment epithelium in postmortem eyes with age-related macular degeneration and histologic examination of surgically excised choroidal neovascular membranes. Surv Ophthalmol 44 Suppl 1: S10–32.
7. McLeod DS, Lutty GA (1994) High-resolution histologic analysis of the human choroidal vasculature. Invest Ophthalmol Vis Sci 35: 3799–3811.
8. Lutty G, Grunwald J, Majji AB, Uyama M, Yoneya S (1999) Changes in choriocapillaris and retinal pigment epithelium in age-related macular degeneration. Mol Vis 5: 35.
9. Stanga PE, Lim JI, Hamilton P (2003) Indocyanine green angiography in chorioretinal diseases: indications and interpretation: an evidence-based update. Ophthalmology 110: 15–21; quiz 22–13.
10. Margolis R, Spaide RF (2009) A pilot study of enhanced depth imaging optical coherence tomography of the choroid in normal eyes. Am J Ophthalmol 147: 811–5.
11. Spaide RF (2009) Age-related choroidal atrophy. Am J Ophthalmol 147: 801–10.
12. Manjunath V, Goren J, Fujimoto JG, Duker JS (2011) Analysis of choroidal thickness in age-related macular degeneration using spectral-domain optical coherence tomography. Am J Ophthalmol 152: 663–8.
13. Koizumi H, Yamagishi T, Yamazaki T, Kawasaki R, Kinoshita S (2011) Subfoveal choroidal thickness in typical age-related macular degeneration and polypoidal choroidal vasculopathy. Graefes Arch Clin Exp Ophthalmol 249: 1123–8.
14. Kim SW, Oh J, Kwon SS, Yoo J, Huh K (2011) Comparison of choroidal thickness among patients with healthy eyes, early age-related maculopathy, neovascular age-related macular degeneration, central serous chorioretinopathy, and polypoidal choroidal vasculopathy. Retina 31: 1904–11.
15. Chung SE, Kang SW, Lee JH, Kim YT (2011) Choroidal thickness in polypoidal choroidal vasculopathy and exudative age-related macular degeneration. Ophthalmology 118: 840–5.
16. Ikuno Y, Kawaguchi K, Nouchi T, Yasuno Y (2010) Choroidal Thickness in Healthy Japanese Subjects. Invest Ophthalmol Vis Sci 51: 2173–6.
17. Brown JS, Flitcroft DI, Ying GS, Francis EL, Schmid GF, et al. (2009) In Vivo Human Choroidal Thickness Measurements: Evidence for Diurnal Fluctuations. Invest Ophthalmol Vis Sci 50: 5–12.
18. Chakraborty R, Read SA, Collins MJ (2011) Diurnal Variations in Axial Length, Choroidal Thickness, Intraocular Pressure, and Ocular Biometrics. Invest Ophthalmol Vis Sci 52: 5121–9.
19. Sohrab MA, Smith RT, Salehi-Had H, Sadda SR, Fawzi AA (2011) Image registration and multimodal imaging of reticular pseudodrusen. Invest Ophthalmol Vis Sci 52: 5743–8.
20. Choroid (1971) In:Hogan MJ, Alvarado JA, Weddell JE, editors. Histology of the Human Eye. Philadelphia: W.B. Saunders pp.320–392.
21. Li XQ, Larsen M, Munch IC (2011) Subfoveal choroidal thickness in relation to sex and axial length in 93 Danish university students. Invest Ophthalmol Vis Sci 52: 8438–41.
22. Wang RK, An L (2011) Multifunctional imaging of human retina and choroid with 1050-nm spectral domain optical coherence tomography at 92-kHz line scan rate. J Biomed Opt 16: 050503.

5

DNA Sequence Variants in *PPARGC1A*, a Gene Encoding a Coactivator of the ω-3 LCPUFA Sensing PPAR-RXR Transcription Complex, Are Associated with NV AMD and AMD-Associated Loci in Genes of Complement and VEGF Signaling Pathways

John Paul SanGiovanni[1]*, Jing Chen[2], Przemyslaw Sapieha[3], Christopher M. Aderman[2], Andreas Stahl[4], Traci E. Clemons[5], Emily Y. Chew[1], Lois E. H. Smith[2]

1 Clinical Trials Branch, National Eye Institute, National Institutes of Health, Bethesda, Maryland, United States of America, 2 Department of Ophthalmology, Harvard Medical School, The Children's Hospital, Boston, Massachusetts, United States of America, 3 Department of Ophthalmology, Maisonneuve-Rosemont Hospital Research Centre, University of Montreal, Montreal, Quebec, Canada, 4 Department of Ophthalmology, University Eye Hospital Freiburg, Freiburg, Germany, 5 The EMMES Corp., Rockville, Maryland, United States of America

Abstract

Background: Increased intake of ω-3 long-chain polyunsaturated fatty acids (LCPUFAs) and use of peroxisome proliferator activator receptor (PPAR)-activating drugs are associated with attenuation of pathologic retinal angiogenesis. ω-3 LCPUFAs are endogenous agonists of PPARs. We postulated that DNA sequence variation in PPAR gamma (PPARG) co-activator 1 alpha (*PPARGC1A*), a gene encoding a co-activator of the LCPUFA-sensing PPARG-retinoid X receptor (RXR) transcription complex, may influence neovascularization (NV) in age-related macular degeneration (AMD).

Methods: We applied exact testing methods to examine distributions of DNA sequence variants in *PPARGC1A* for association with NV AMD and interaction of AMD-associated loci in genes of complement, lipid metabolism, and VEGF signaling systems. Our sample contained 1858 people from 3 elderly cohorts of western European ancestry. We concurrently investigated retinal gene expression profiles in 17-day-old neonatal mice on a 2% LCPUFA feeding paradigm to identify LCPUFA-regulated genes both associated with pathologic retinal angiogenesis and known to interact with PPARs or *PPARGC1A*.

Results: A DNA coding variant (rs3736265) and a 3'UTR-resident regulatory variant (rs3774923) in *PPARGC1A* were independently associated with NV AMD (exact $P = 0.003$, both SNPs). SNP-SNP interactions existed for NV AMD ($P < 0.005$) with rs3736265 and a AMD-associated variant in complement factor B (CFB, rs512559). PPARGC1A influences activation of the AMD-associated complement component 3 (*C3*) promoter fragment and CFB influences activation and proteolysis of C3. We observed interaction ($P \leq 0.003$) of rs3736265 with a variant in vascular endothelial growth factor A (*VEGFA*, rs3025033), a key molecule in retinal angiogenesis. Another *PPARGC1A* coding variant (rs8192678) showed statistical interaction with a SNP in the VEGFA receptor fms-related tyrosine kinase 1 (*FLT1*, rs10507386; $P \leq 0.003$). C3 expression was down-regulated 2-fold in retinas of ω-3 LCPUFA-fed mice – these animals also showed 70% reduction in retinal NV ($P \leq 0.001$).

Conclusion: Ligands and co-activators of the ω-3 LCPUFA sensing PPAR-RXR axis may influence retinal angiogenesis in NV AMD via the complement and VEGF signaling systems. We have linked the co-activator of a lipid-sensing transcription factor (PPARG co-activator 1 alpha, PPARGC1A) to age-related macular degeneration (AMD) and AMD-associated genes.

Editor: Lynette Kay Rogers, The Ohio State Unversity, United States of America

Funding: Funding support for NEI-AMD was provided by the National Eye Institute (JPSG); EY017017 and Research to Prevent Blindness (RPB) Senior Investigator Award (LEHS). Additional support was provided by Children's Hospital Ophthalmology Foundation and Charles H. Hood Foundation (JC), the Canadian Institues of Health Research (Institute of Nutrition, Metabolism and Diabetes) (PS) and the Deutsche Forschungsgemeinschaft, Freifrau von Nauendorf Stiftung and Deutsche Ophthalmologische Gesellschaft (AS). Mouse microarray studies were performed by the Molecular Genetics Core Facility at Children's Hospital Boston supported by National Institutes of Health NIH-P50-NS40828, and NIH-P30-HD18655. The funders had no role in study design, data collection and analysis, decision to publish, or preparation of the manuscript.

* E-mail: jpsangio@post.harvard.edu

Introduction

Neovascular (NV) age-related macular degeneration (AMD) is a common sight-threatening disease in the elderly, accounting for more than 80% of all AMD-related vision loss in people of western European ancestry. [1] The cardinal lesions of NV AMD are proliferative growth of and exudation from vessels in the choriocapillaris, the major vascular network of the outer retina. [2,3,4] More than 2 million U.S. residents have advanced AMD. [5] Current treatments (intraocular injections with anti-angiogenic drugs) are a substantial financial burden on society, with direct annual medical costs reaching ~570 million dollars. AMD-related outpatient services are incurred annually by ~1.4 million people aged 65-and-older and contribute to ~0.5 billion dollars in Medicare claims per year. [6] Less expensive and non-invasive treatment options for AMD are needed.

Nutrient-based approaches to AMD treatment have been focused on compounds demonstrating: 1) intake-dependent and –modifiable accretion to retinal cell types affected in AMD; and 2) biophysical and biochemical capacity to act on processes implicated in pathogenesis and pathophysiology. Large-scale human studies on AMD suggest a reduced likelihood of having or progressing to NV AMD among people reporting highest dietary intakes of omega-3 (ω-3) long-chain polyunsaturated fatty acids (LCPUFAs). [7,8,9,10] ω-3 LCPUFAs act as key structural and signaling molecules in the retina. [11] Findings from work on *in vivo* model systems support the idea that increasing retinal tissue status of these nutrients protects against pathologic intraretinal [12,13,14] and choroidal [15,16] neovascularization. The role of ω-3 LCPUFAs in cell survival and rescue is an emerging area of research, as these nutrients are precursors to families of potent neuroprotective autacoids. [17,18,19] Biosynthetic and cleavage enzymes, transporters, receptors, and transcriptional regulators that interact with ω-3 LCPUFAs, their precursors, metabolites, and targets are expressed in retinal areas manifesting neurode-generative and angiogenic lesions of AMD (Institute of Human Genetics, University of Regensburg, http://www.retinacentral.org/. Accessed 2012 Nov 30). Among these are cognate lipid-sensing nuclear receptors of the peroxisome proliferator-activated receptor (PPAR) family. ω-3 LCPUFAs are endogenous PPAR agonists. [20].

PPARs act as master regulators of gene transcription and have been studied in the context of retinal vascular disease. In 2005 we first discussed the putative role of LCPUFA-PPAR relationships in the retina [11] and have recently demonstrated direct PPAR-gamma (PPARG)-mediated effects of dietary ω-3 LCPUFAs on retinal vessel formation in a oxygen-induced retinopathy (OIR) model of pathologic retinal angiogenesis. [13,14] Use of synthetic PPAR agonists has been associated with lower likelihood and severity of pathologic retinal neovascularization. Troglitazone, a PPARG agonist, inhibited laser-induced choroidal neovascular-ization (a hallmark of NV AMD) in cynomoglus monkeys. [21] Fenofibrate, a PPAR activator, reduced the need for laser treatment for proliferative (neovascular) retinopathy in a large phase III clinical trial of 9795 people with type 2 diabetes. [22] The rationale for using PPAR ligands as therapeutic agents for NV AMD has been raised elsewhere. [23].

The PPARG-retinoid X receptor (PPAR-RXR) transcription complex is involved in ligand-activated transcription; this complex typically binds the *AGGTCANAGGTCA* DNA consensus sequence in peroxisome proliferator hormone response elements (PPREs) within the promoter region of target genes – when the PPAR is bound by a ligand (e.g. LCPUFAs or drugs), transcription is altered. The activity of PPARs is dependent on the shape of their ligand-binding domains and the physical interaction with co-activator and co-repressor proteins. PPAR agonists bind the PPARG-RXR transcription complex, causing a conformational shift that permits displacement of co-repressor proteins and a subsequent docking of co-activator proteins. We examined the possible influence of DNA variation in the PPARG co-activator 1 alpha gene (*PPARGC1A*), as an extension of the work on endogenous and pharmacologic PPAR agonists in pathologic retinal angiogenesis (discussed in the previous paragraph). *PPARGC1A* encodes a transcriptional regulator protein involved in constitutive activation of ω-3 LCPUFA-sensing PPARG-RXR complex target genes. PPARGC1A is a major PPARG co-activator. Our results suggest that multiple constituents (ligands and transcriptional co-activators) of the PPAR-RXR system may influence pathogenic processes implicated in NV AMD and offer promise for efficiently examining combined therapies for this blinding disease of public health significance.

Results

We examined DNA sequence variants in *PPARGC1A* for association with NV AMD in three independent U.S.-based cohorts of western European ancestry. All data are from large-scale projects designed to investigate the molecular genetics of AMD. The panel of 20 sequence variants we tested were taken from the ILLUMINA HumanCNV370v1 microarray and included 2 single nucleotide polymorphisms (SNPs) resident in exonic *PPARGC1A* regions and one resident in the 3′ untranslated region (UTR) of this gene. We applied a 4-phase approach to testing, first using our largest independent cohort as a 'discovery' sample, then examining the magnitude and direction of measures of NV AMD-*PPARGC1A* relationships in two other large-scale genotyping projects on AMD, and then combining measures of association with meta-analytic techniques – finally, testing these combined estimates with exact methods. After observing relationships of NV AMD with SNPs in exonic and regulatory regions of *PPARGC1A* from the meta-analysis, we examined interactions of these variants with established genetic loci for NV AMD resident in systems: 1) associated with AMD in other studies (complement, lipid metabolism, and vascular endothelial growth factor (VEGF) signaling systems); and, 2) responsive to ω-3 LCPUFA feeding in our animal models (complement cascade). **Figure 1** is a schematic of putative relationships between PPARGC1A, an ω-3 LCPUFA activator of PPARs (docosahexaenoic acid, DHA), PPARs, and genes containing AMD-associated variants (symbols for these genes are colored red).

In summary, we applied age-, sex-, and smoking-adjusted logistic regression models to analyze 843 people with NV AMD and 1032 of their elderly peers who were both AMD-free and ≥65 years-of-age. A cohort of 506 cases and 512 controls from a major university-based clinical center served as the discovery sample in phase 1. Our phase 2 replication samples consisted of 123+205 cases and 198+314 AMD-free elderly peers from 2 independent and geographically distinct university based research centers. **Table 1** contains demographic characteristics of our cohorts. After examining single locus tests for between-cohort concordance, we computed combined age-, sex-, and smoking-adjusted estimates of NV AMD-SNP relationships with meta-regression, applying random effects models to account for sample heterogeneity (phase 3). We then used max(T) permutation (10,000 iterations) on the combined samples to derive exact P-values for sequence variants significant at $P<0.005$ in covariate-adjusted meta-analysis (phase 4). Two-locus epistatic (SNP-SNP) interactions of AMD-associated PPARGC1A variants were then

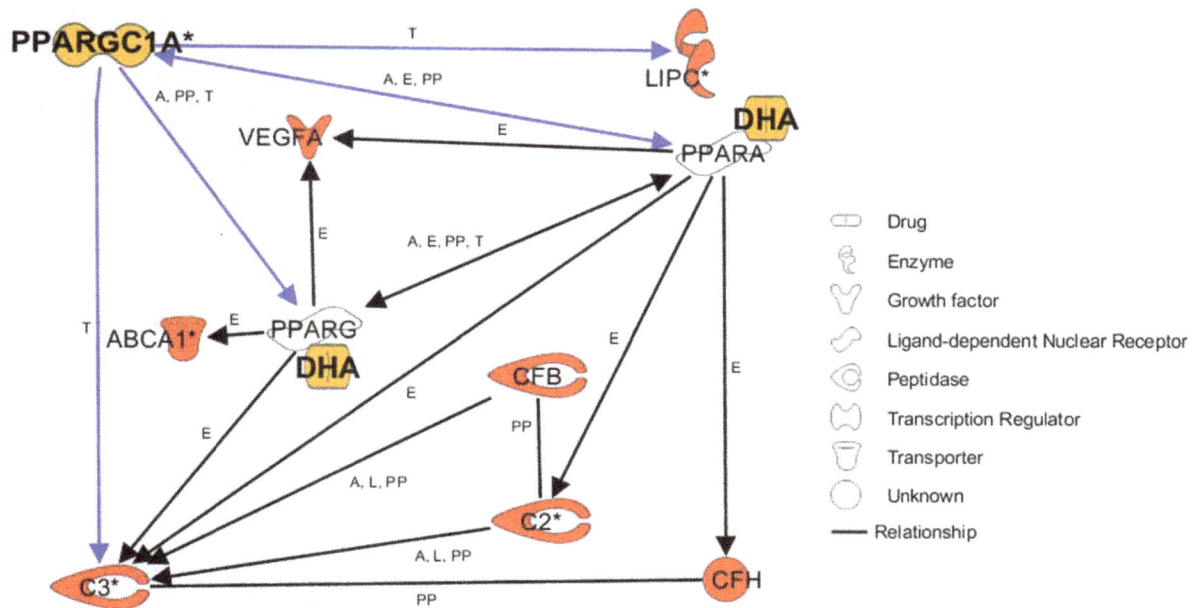

Figure 1. Relationships of PPARG co-activator 1 alpha (PPARGC1A) with AMD-associated genes or their products. Genes associated with AMD in extant studies are shaded in red. DHA = docosahexaenoic acid (a PPAR agonist). Diagram was generated with Ingenuity Pathway Analysis® software. Full names for genes represented by symbols exist at http://www.ncbi.nlm.nih.gov/gene/. Direct effects of PPARGC1A are represented by blue arrows. Letters on the arrows represent the nature of evidence and are defined as follows: A = activation, E = expression, L = proteolysis, PP = protein-protein interaction, T = transcription.

conducted with established AMD risk loci of genes in the complement, lipoprotein metabolism, and VEGF signaling systems. These genes included complement factor H (*CFH*), complement component 3 (*C3*), complement factor B (*CFB*) complement component 2 (*C2*), LIPC hepatic lipase (*LIPC*), ATP-binding cassette transporter A1 (*ABCA1*), vascular endothelial growth factor A (*VEGFA*) and its receptors fms-related tyrosine kinase 1 (*FLT1*, *VEGFR1*) and kinase insert domain receptor (*KDR*, *VEGFR2*, *FLK1*)).

Single Locus Tests of *PPARGC1A* Variants for NV AMD

Findings from single locus tests on *PPARGC1A* are presented in **Table 2**. A relationship emerged for rs3736265 (odds ratio (OR) = 0.63, exact P = 0.005), a variant in exon 9 yielding a deleterious peptide transition (SIFT score 0.01) from threonine to methionine or lysine at amino acid 612. People carrying the minor allele (AA or AG) were ~40% less likely than their peers (GG) to have NV AMD. This variant allele was predicted with HaploReg (Broad Institute. www.broadinstitute.org/mammals/haploreg/. Accessed 2012 Nov 30) to enhance affinity to consensus sequence in hypoxia inducible factor 1 beta (aryl hydrocarbon receptor nuclear translocator, ARNT) a heterodimeric transcription factor involved with in hypoxia-induced angiogenesis. rs3736265 is in proximity to a highly conserved RNA binding domain (RNA recognition motif overlapping amino acids 678–738) involved in post-transcriptional gene expression processes (e.g. mRNA and rRNA processing, RNA stability, and RNA export). We observed relationships of the PPARGC1A intronic variant rs3755862 with NV AMD (OR = 0.61, exact P = 0.002); this SNP is in nearly complete linkage disequilibrium (r^2 = 0.96) with the rs3736265 coding variant. Our inferences on a PPARGC1A-NV AMD relationship were strengthened by the observation that the 3′UTR

in *PPARGC1A* also contains a NV AMD-associated variant (rs3774923, OR = 0.58, exact P = 0.003). As with SNP rs3736265, people carrying one or two copies of the minor allele showed a 40% reduced likelihood of having NV AMD, relative to their peers who were homozygous for the major allele. We do not have reason to believe that the rs3736265 coding SNP and the rs3774923 UTR SNP are co-inherited, based on measures of linkage disequilibrium (r^2 = 0.64 in our analytic sample and r^2 = 0.55 within the CEU+TSI cohorts from the International HAPMAP Project). It is important to acknowledge that the 300K SNP chip used for genotyping did not permit dense mapping of *PPARGC1A*, and thus constrained our range of inferences. Our conclusion from single-locus tests on *PPARGC1A* variants is that co-activators of PPAR-mediated processes may be reasonably implicated in pathogenesis of NV AMD.

Interaction Testing of NV AMD-associated *PPARGC1A* SNPs with AMD-associated Variants

Extant relationships depicted in Figure 1 justified our decision to examine statistical interactions of AMD-associated *PPARGC1A* variants discussed in the section above with those in genes of complement, lipid metabolism, and VEGF signaling systems. In model systems, PPARGC1A has been shown to directly activate promoter elements of *C3* [24] and *LIPC*. [25] *C3* and *LIPC* carry AMD-associated sequence variants. [26,27] *Via* co-activation of PPARG [28], PPARGC1A may alter expression of *ABCA1* [29,30,31] and *VEGFA*. [32,33] *ABCA1* and *VEGFA* carry AMD-associated sequence variants. [26,34,35,36] *Via* co-activation of PPARA [37,38,39,40], PPARGC1A may alter expression of CFH [41], and C2. [42] These genes carry AMD-associated sequence variants. [43,44] In our cohorts, *PPARGC1A* SNPs showed

Table 1. Description of Cohorts.

	Outcome	
Cohort	No AMD	NV AMD
Discovery Cohort (Michigan)		
Total, N	514	506
Mean age at exam (SE)	76.6 (0.23)	80.4 (0.30)
Female (% of cohort)	58	63
Current smoker (% of cohort)	4	7
Replication 1 (Pennsylvania)		
Total, N	198	123
Mean age at exam (SE)	76.2 (0.34)	77.5 (0.64)
Female (% of cohort)	55	58
Current smoker (% of cohort)	7	6
Replication 2 (Mayo Clinic)		
Total, N	318	205
Mean age at exam (SE)	73.7(0.34)	79.7 (0.55)
Female (% of cohort)	53	65
Current smoker (% of cohort)	6	8

Abbreviations: SE, standard error; NV AMD, neovascular AMD.

statistical interactions with *CFB*, *C3*, *C2*, *VEGFA*, *FLT1*, and *KDR* variants. *FLT1* and *KDR* encode VEGFA receptors.

In examining interactions, we first considered single variant findings for AMD-associated SNPs in *CFH*, *C3*, *CFB*, *C2*, *LIPC*, and *ABCA1* reported in independent studies. [26,43,45] In our cohorts, AMD-associated loci in the complement system genes, LIPC, and ABCA1 also existed (**Table S1**). VEGF is a key molecule implicated in pathologic retinal angiogenesis variants in VEGFA have been implicated in AMD [46,47,48] – although, relationships have not always been replicated. [49,50,51,52] While NV AMD-VEGF relationships did not exist in our cohorts for the SNPs on our microarray feature set (this may have been due to sparse coverage of the gene on the testing panel), we saw value in examining possible interactions with *PPARGC1A* SNPs.

Table 3 contains results for NV AMD-related interactions of *PPARGC1A* SNPs significant at $P<0.005$. Most notable are findings for the *PPARGC1A* coding variant (rs3736265) with *CFB* (rs512559, $P≤0.0046$) and VEGFA (rs3025033, $P≤0.0037$). CFB influences activation and proteolysis of C3. Commentary exists in the *Discussion* on a *PPARGC1A-VEGF* interaction ($P≤0.003$) for another coding SNP in *PPARGC1A* (Gly482Ser, rs8192678) with a variant in VEGFA receptor *FLT1* (rs10507386) that changes the binding motif of the RXR consensus sequence. Inferences on the interactions of ω-3 LCPUFA-sensing PPARG-RXR complex constituents with complement and angiogenesis pathway genes in NV AMD are further strengthened by findings from: 1) large-scale population-based studies demonstrating interactions of fish (a primary source of ω-3 LCPUFAs) intake with CFH gene variants in early [53,54] and late AMD [54]; and 2) ω-3 LCPUFA related alterations in C3 expression and attenuation of pathologic retinal neovascularization in *in vivo* systems (discussed in the section below). Our conclusion from interaction tests on *PPARGC1A* variants is that PPAR-mediated processes may be reasonably implicated to influence complement and VEGF signaling systems in the pathogenesis of NV AMD. Additional work on this concept is necessary to make conclusive inferences.

Genome-wide Expression Profiling of Murine Retinal Response to LCPUFAs

To consider the role of LCPUFA-regulated genes both associated with pathologic retinal angiogenesis and known to interact with PPARs or *PPARGC1A* we compared retinal gene expression profiles from an Illumina Mouse-ref 6 microarray in 17-day-old (P17) mice on a diet of 2.0% total fatty acids from ω-6 LCPUFAs (arachidonic acid, C20:4 ω-6) to those P17 mice on a 2.0% ω-3 LCPUFA diet (1% EPA +1% DHA). Both diets were fed from time of birth. We found a 2.0-fold reduction in retinal expression of the AMD-associated *C3* gene among animals fed the 2.0% ω-3 LCPUFA diet (FDR (false discovery rate) ∼ 0.8%). Notably, identical LCPUFA exposures led to retinal tissue LCPUFA status changes and subsequent alterations in the severity of pathologic retinal angiogenesis within the OIR model. Animals receiving ω-3 LCPUFAs showed a ∼20% reduction in retinal vessel loss ($P≤0.05$) and a ∼70% reduction in pathologic retinal angiogenesis ($P≤0.001$) (**Figure 2**). [12] These findings strengthen inferences from work in humans supporting links on the influences of dietary (ω-3 LCPUFAs), pharmacologic (trolitazone, fenofibrate), and constitutive (PPARGC1A) PPAR activators as they may relate to the complement and VEGF signaling systems, and development of neovascular pathology of the retina.

Discussion

We tested two highly conserved DNA sequence variants that code for changes in the peptide structure (rs3736265 and rs8192678) and one highly conserved SNP (rs3774923) in the regulatory 3'UTR of *PPARGC1A*; all were associated with NV AMD. An association of NV AMD with rs3736265 emerged from exact tests in age-, sex-, and smoking-adjusted models. Statistical interactions existed between rs3736265 and SNPs resident in AMD-associated loci of genes encoding key factors in complement and VEGF signaling systems. rs8192678 was associated with NV AMD through an interaction with a SNP in the VEGFA receptor FLT1. rs3774923 was related with NV AMD in single locus analyses.

Our findings extend evidence implicating endogenous (ω-3 LCPUFAs) and pharmacologic (troglitazone, fenofibrate) PPAR agonists/activators as protective agents against pathologic retinal angiogenesis to support the action of a constitutive PPAR co-activator protein (PPARGC1A) in a similar capacity. PPARGC1A may serve as a hub molecule influencing AMD pathogenesis and pathophysiology as it activates the glitazone target PPARG [28,55], the fenofibrate target PPARA [37,55], and C3 [24], LIPC [25], and VEGF [33] promoter fragments. Glitazones have been tested in model systems for their protective effects on retinal cell survival. [56] Troglitazone inhibited choroidal neovascularization in a *in vivo* primate model of NV AMD. [21] Fenofibrate, a synthetic PPAR activator, reduced the need for laser treatment for proliferative diabetic retinopathy. [22] Chemical structures for PPAR agonists exist at (Kanehisa Laboratories, www.genome.jp/kegg/pathway/map/map07222.html. Accessed 2012 Nov 30); those for RXR agonists and antagonists are presented at (Kanehisa Laboratories, www.genome.jp/kegg/pathway/map/map07223.html. Accessed 2012 Nov 30).

We did not observe single locus associations of NV AMD with the *VEGFA*, *FLT1*, or *KDR* variants present on our microarray test panel. However, interaction of *PPARGC1A* SNPs with those in each of these genes existed at *P*-values ≤0.005. Notable PPARGC1A-VEGF interactions emerged for coding SNPs in *PPARGC1A*: rs8192678 with a variant in *FLT1* (rs10507386, $P≤0.003$); and rs3736265 with a variant in *VEGFA* (rs3025033,

Table 2. Association results of *PPARGC1A* SNPs for NV AMD in three cohorts and in meta-analysis using multivariable models.

SNP	Feature	Alleles	Model	Discovery Michigan OR (95% CI)	P	Replication Pennsylvania OR (95% CI)	P	Mayo OR (95% CI)	P	OR$_{meta}$	P$_{exact}$
rs3774923	**3'UTR**	**A/G**	**DOM**	**0.52 (0.33–0.83)**	**0.006**	**0.69 (0.31–1.53)**	**0.181**	**0.66 (0.30–1.42)**	**0.142**	**0.580**	**0.003**
rs12650562	INTRON	T/C	ADD	1.07 (0.89–1.30)	0.459	1.16 (0.85–1.59)	0.181	1.02 (0.77–1.33)	0.453	1.074	0.380
rs7682765	INTRON	C/T	DOM	1.52 (1.02–2.28)	0.041	0.49 (0.23–1.06)	0.035	1.48 (0.84–2.60)	0.088	1.306	0.206
rs2932965	INTRON	A/G	ADD	0.97 (0.71–1.34)	0.856	0.99 (0.52–1.86)	0.486	0.99 (0.65–1.52)	0.480	0.910	0.831
rs3774921	INTRON	G/A	ADD	1.07 (0.89–1.28)	0.494	1.01 (0.74–1.38)	0.479	1.13 (0.86–1.48)	0.195	1.070	0.316
rs3736265[a]	**EXON**	**A/G**	**DOM**	**0.63 (0.42–0.94)**	**0.022**	**0.70 (0.34–1.46)**	**0.171**	**0.58 (0.30–1.13)**	**0.055**	**0.630**	**0.005**
rs8192678	EXON	A/G	ADD	1.02 (0.82–1.27)	0.830	1.27 (0.88–1.82)	0.101	0.88 (0.63–1.23)	0.226	1.032	0.847
rs3755862[a]	**INTRON**	**A/G**	**DOM**	**0.62 (0.42–0.92)**	**0.018**	**0.58 (0.28–1.23)**	**0.079**	**0.60 (0.32–1.14)**	**0.059**	**0.611**	**0.002**
rs2970848	INTRON	G/A	ADD	1.07 (0.86–1.32)	0.568	0.65 (0.41–1.02)	0.030	0.99 (0.71–1.37)	0.465	0.975	0.673
rs2932976	INTRON	A/G	ADD	1.26 (0.96–1.64)	0.097	0.78 (0.47–1.30)	0.170	1.07 (0.73–1.57)	0.367	1.114	0.387
rs2970853	INTRON	A/G	ADD	0.98 (0.75–1.29)	0.906	0.99 (0.62–1.56)	0.476	0.82 (0.54–1.23)	0.165	0.939	0.489
rs6448226	INTRON	G/A	DOM	0.74 (0.57–0.97)	0.029	0.91 (0.57–1.45)	0.341	1.01 (0.68–1.50)	0.486	0.832	0.127
rs7665116	INTRON	C/T	DOM	0.86 (0.64–1.16)	0.325	0.79 (0.47–1.32)	0.184	0.88 (0.56–1.38)	0.288	0.850	0.160
rs6850464	INTRON	G/A	ADD	1.01 (0.67–1.51)	0.967	0.75 (0.24–2.37)	0.310	0.69 (0.22–2.14)	0.260	0.943	0.908
rs4235308	INTRON	C/T	ADD	1.17 (0.96–1.43)	0.113	0.75 (0.51–1.10)	0.073	1.03 (0.77–1.37)	0.428	1.057	0.490
rs4550905	INTRON	G/A	ADD	0.83 (0.66–1.05)	0.115	1.07 (0.75–1.51)	0.364	1.10 (0.77–1.55)	0.303	0.939	0.391
rs4361373	INTRON	C/T	ADD	0.79 (0.52–1.20)	0.267	1.45 (0.85–2.50)	0.088	1.09 (0.61–1.94)	0.387	1.014	0.917
rs17637318	INTRON	C/T	ADD	1.06 (0.84–1.32)	0.644	1.30 (0.88–1.92)	0.093	1.02 (0.73–1.43)	0.454	1.088	0.383
rs4469064	INTRON	G/A	DOM	1.28 (0.91–1.82)	0.154	1.16(0.50–2.27)	0.329	1.27 (0.72–2.19)	0.210	1.260	0.056
rs2946385	INTRON	T/G	ADD	1.03 (0.85–1.25)	0.752	0.72 (0.50–1.04)	0.041	1.06 (0.81–1.41)	0.331	0.984	0.965

Abbreviations: 3'UTR, 3' untranslated region; SNP, single-nucleotide polymorphism. a, SNPs in nearly complete linkage disequilibrium ($r^2 = 0.96$) – no other SNPs were in linkage disequilibrium; ADD, additive model (minor allele count –2|1|0); DOM, dominant model (grouping minor allele homozygotes with heterozygotes). SNPs were tested from the panel of the ILLUMINA HumanCNV370v1 chip (SNP batch IDs at http://www.ncbi.nlm.nih.gov/SNP/snp_viewBatch.cgi?sbid = 1047132). People in the reference groups (controls) were AMD-free and at least 65-years-of-age at the time of phenotype classification. We computed odds ratios (ORs) and 95% confidence intervals (95% CI) from age-, sex-, and smoking-adjusted logistic regression analyses on 506 cases and 512 controls in the Discovery Cohort (University of Michigan), 123 cases and 198 controls in Replication Cohort 1 (University of Pennsylvania), and 205 cases and 314 controls in Replication Cohort 2 (Mayo Clinic, Rochester). Combined estimates (OR$_{meta}$) were computed with age-, sex-, and smoking-adjusted meta-regression – random effects models were applied in instances indicated by Cochrane's Q statistic. All P values are 2-sided, with the exception of those for the replication cohorts. Exact (empirical) P values are from max(T) permutation with 10000 iterations on the full sample.

$P \leq 0.004$). *PPARGC1A* rs8192678 is resident in the conserved consensus sequence for the EVI1 transcription factor binding site. The *FLT1* rs10507386 variant with which it shows statistical interaction also changes the binding motif of the RXR consensus sequence.

There is a link between PPARGC1A, VEGF, and the estrogen signaling system. Arany *et al.* demonstrated a PPARGC1A-dependent regulation of VEGF *via* coactivation by estrogen related receptor alpha (ESRRA) and binding to the VEGF promoter sequence. [33] Our microarray feature set did not contain ESRRA variants. We have conducted preliminary work on a network of genes encoding constituents of a signaling system with the capacity to impact VEGFA *via* PPARGC1A- and ESRRA-mediated processes. Variants in estrogen receptor 1 (ESR1, rs1999805, $P_{meta} \leq 0.002$), estrogen related receptor beta (ESRRB, rs2361290, $P_{meta} \leq 0.009$), and estrogen related receptor gamma (ESRRG, rs1984137 and 2820879, respective $P_{meta} \leq 0.01$, 0.007) showed weak relationships with NV AMD. These genes encode proteins that interact with PPARGC1 and ESRRA and may impact VEGF signaling directly (ESR1) or via PPARs (ESRRB/ESRRG). PPARGC1A-VEGF relationships are germane to the present study since a number of drugs acting on VEGF or VEGF signaling have been tested in large-scale trials for

treatment of advanced AMD [57,58]; these include: the anti-VEGF monoclonal antibody bevacizumab [59] (Avastin), the VEGFA antibody ranibizumab [59,60] (Lucentis), and the anti-VEGF165 aptamer pegaptanib [60] (Macugen).

We observed single locus relationships of *ABCA1* and *LIPC* SNPs on NV AMD, but no interactions with the *PPARGC1A* SNPs on our test panel. Because PPARGC1A has both the capacity to alter ABCA1 expression through its interaction with PPARG [30,61] and to activate the LIPC promoter fragment [25], we believe this is a promising area for future work.

In conclusion, we propose that constituents of the ω-3 LCPUFA sensing PPAR-RXR axis have the capacity to act on processes impacting pathologic retinal angiogenesis *via* complement and VEGF signaling systems. A number of FDA-approved drugs targeting constituents of the axis now exist. Testing combinations of endogenous and pharmacologic PPAR agonists/activators ligands and compounds that influence PPAR co-activator proteins in pre-clinical studies on NV AMD may elucidate promising therapies for this complex blinding disease of public health significance.

Table 3. Summary of interaction analysis of *PPARGC1A* SNPs and SNPs in complement and VEGF genes for NV AMD in combined cohorts.

PPARGC1A	Interaction SNP			
SNP (Allele)	Gene Symbol	SNP (Allele)	OR	P
rs3736265[a] (A)	**CFB**	**rs512559 (C)**	**4.33**	**0.0046**
rs3755862[a] (A)	CFB	rs512559 (C)	4.40	0.0042
rs4235308 (C)	C3	rs2230205 (A)	0.61	0.0004
rs6448226 (G)	C2	rs638383 (A)	2.24	0.0041
rs6448226 (G)	CFB	rs512559 (C)	2.32	0.0025
rs7665116 (C)	C2	rs1042663 (A)	2.24	0.0041
rs7665116 (C)	C2	rs638383 (A)	3.21	0.0032
rs7665116 (C)	CFB	rs512559 (C)	3.37	0.0021
rs7682765 (C)	CFB	rs4151657 (C)	1.74	0.0048
rs12650562 (T)	FLT1	rs10507386 (T)	1.65	0.0049
rs2970848 (G)	FLT1	rs10507384 (G)	0.51	0.0014
rs8192678 (A)	**FLT1**	**rs10507386 (T)**	**1.76**	**0.0033**
rs4550905 (G)	KDR	rs2125489 (T)	1.59	0.0046
rs7682765 (C)	VEGFA	rs833069 (G)	1.80	0.0037
rs3736265[a] (A)	**VEGFA**	**rs3025033 (G)**	**0.41**	**0.0037**
rs3755862[a] (A)	VEGFA	rs3025033 (G)	0.41	0.0035

Abbreviations: SNP, single-nucleotide polymorphism. *PPARGC1A*, PPAR gamma co-activator 1 alpha gene. Tests of SNP x SNP interactions (allelic by allelic epistasis) were conducted for *PPARGC1A* with AMD-related SNPs in complement, lipid metabolism, and, VEGF signaling genes. Text in bold type represents interactions of *PPARGC1A* SNPs in exonic regions leading to changes in protein structure. Models were based on allele dosage. Only* relationships significant at P≤0.005 are reported in this table. a, SNPs in nearly complete linkage disequilibrium (r^2 = 0.96) – no other SNPs were in linkage disequilibrium. Full names for the genes listed in the 'Gene Symbol' column exist at: http://www.ncbi.nlm.nih.gov/gene.

Materials and Methods

Large-scale Genotyping Study in Elderly Humans

Data used for human genetic analyses in this report were obtained from the NEI Study of Age-Related Macular Degeneration (NEI-AMD) Database at the U.S. National Center for Biotechnology Information (NCBI) database of Genotypes and Phenotypes (dbGaP). NEI-AMD is a collaborative of researchers from the University of Michigan (Ann Arbor, MI), Mayo Clinic (Rochester, MN), University of Pennsylvania (Philadelphia, PA), and the Age-related Eye Disease Study (AREDS) group including National Eye Institute intramural investigators. Institutional review boards at each NEI-AMD study site reviewed and approved the study protocols. Each participant provided written informed consent in accordance with the *Declaration of Helsinki*.

Subjects and Study Design. Our analytic sample contained, respectively 506, 123, 205 people with NV AMD, and 514, 198, 318 AMD-free people (age ≥65 years) from the University of Michigan, University of Pennsylvania, and The Mayo Clinic. Details on the NEI-AMD genome-wide association (GWA) study and links to peer-reviewed publications from the project exist at: http://www.ncbi.nlm.nih.gov/gap/?term = MMAP.

Outcome Ascertainment. Experienced graders (ophthalmologists) classified outcomes according to AMD diagnosis in the worse eye. All participants had negative history of: 1) severe macular disease or vision loss onset prior to 40-years-of-age; 2)

juvenile retinal degeneration, macular damage resulting from ocular trauma, retinal detachment, high myopia, chorioretinal infection/inflammatory disease, or choroidal dystrophy; and, 3) retinal insult that would render the fundus ungradable. Existence of neovascularization in at least one eye, according to diagnostic criteria established by the International Age-Related Maculopathy Epidemiological Study and the Modified Wisconsin Age-Related Maculopathy Grading System, was the basis for classifying people with NV AMD. In all cases of unilateral NV AMD, drusen or pigment changes also existed in the fellow eye. The likelihood of developing AMD increases 2-to-6 fold after age 75 and it was therefore essential to select our oldest AMD-free participants to minimize the potential for non-random misclassification (false negatives) in the youngest members of the control group. Our AMD-free comparison group was composed of people ≥65-years-of-age who had no large or intermediate drusen in either eye; these participants received examinations and gradings by the NEI-AMD study ophthalmologists. If small drusen or pigment changes were present in the AMD-free group, they were neither bilateral nor extensive (≤5).

Array-Based SNP Genotyping. All NEI-AMD specimens were genotyped with DNA microarrays at the Johns Hopkins University Center for Inherited Disease Research (CIDR, Baltimore, MD, USA) using the ILLUMINA HumanCNV370v1 chip (SNP batch IDs at http://www.ncbi.nlm.nih.gov/SNP/snp_viewBatch.cgi?sbid = 1047132) with the Illumina Infinium II assay protocol. The Illumina BeadStudio Genotyping module (version 3.2.32) was used with the combined intensity of 99% of the samples to assign allele cluster definitions. The threshold for genotype calls was a gencall score ≥0.25. Reproducibility of blind duplicate samples was 99.992%. All sequence variants analyzed for the current study passed process quality and analytic filters for missingness (<5%), minor allele frequency (>1%) and Hardy-Weinberg equilibrium (HWE $P < 1 \times 10^{-6}$ in the AMD-free group).

Bioinformatics. We used positional coordinates (±1000 base pairs) to analyze *PPARGC1A*, and AMD-associated variants in genes of the complement, lipid metabolism, and VEGF signaling systems. To permit a deeper inference on our findings, we used public-access databases to annotate AMD-associated variants for residence within exons, consensus sequences of highly conserved transcription factor binding sites, epigenetic marks in histone protein H3 (mono- and tri-methylation and acetylation), DNase I hypersensitivity regions, and CpG islands.

Statistical Analyses. We used Plink (version 1.07, http://pngu.mgh.harvard.edu/purcell/plink/) and SAS (version 9.1, Cary, NC) software for data analysis, first examining the allelic distributions of SNPs in people with NV AMD (relative to the AMD-free comparison group) with age-, sex-, and smoking-adjusted logistic regression analyses. Genotype was coded using additive, dominant (grouping minor allele homozygotes with heterozygotes), and recessive (grouping major allele homozygotes with heterozygotes) models of inheritance to obtain odds ratios (ORs) for variants within the discovery cohort (University of Michigan). Additive, dominant, and recessive models were run in the two replication cohorts. Combined ORs for single locus tests were computed across cohorts with results from each of the three models using age-, sex-, and smoking-adjusted meta-regression. Combined estimates were only computed within a given model (e.g. results from the additive model in the discovery cohort were only combined with results from the additive models run on the replication cohort). Sample heterogeneity was assessed with Cochrane's Q statistic and random effects models were applied when indicated.

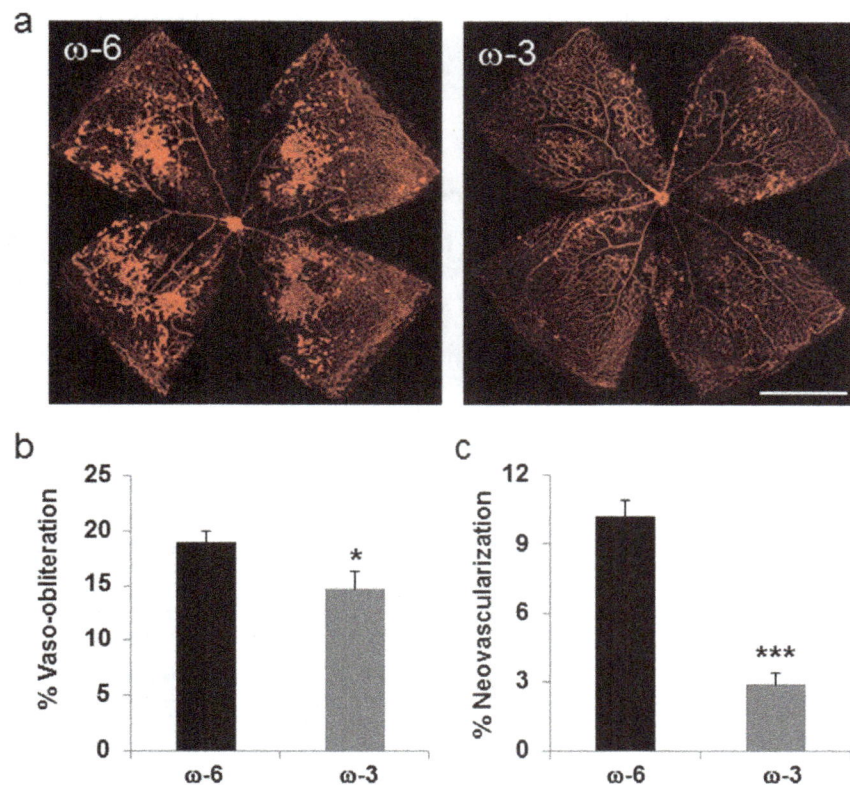

Figure 2. Dietary treatment of ω-3 PUFA protects against pathologic retinal neovascularization. C57 BL/6 mouse pups fed with ω-3 or ω-6 PUFA enhanced diet were exposed to oxygen-induced retinopathy. Retinas were flat mounted at postnatal day (P) 17 to visualize vasculature with contralateral retinas from the same mice isolated for gene array analysis. (**a**). Representative retina vasculature stained with isolectin B_4 shows vaso-obliteration and pathologic neovascularization in ω-6 or ω-3 fed mice. (ω-6, n = 7 and ω-3, n = 8). Scale bar: 1mm. Quantification of (**b**) vaso-obliteration and (**c**) neovascularization in ω-6 or ω-3 fed mice. * $P \leq 0.05$, *** $P \leq 0.001$.

For variants attaining significance in the meta-analysis, we applied exact tests on empirical distributions of P-values generated with a max(T) permutation procedure set to 10000 iterations. Permutation procedures permit the computation of significance levels from empirically derived distributions. Exact P-values yielded by the procedure have tractable properties in obviating constraints of small sample sizes, while providing a framework for correction for multiple testing, and controlling for population substructure. In our cohorts of unrelated individuals, we swapped data values with the assumption that individuals are interchangeable under the null – this permitted construction of a new dataset sampled under the null hypothesis. Through the permutation approach only the phenotype-genotype relationship is destroyed (patterns of linkage disequilibrium between sequence variants will be preserved under the observed and permuted samples). As permutation methods sustain the correlational structure between SNPs, the approach provides a less stringent correction for multiple testing than the Bonferroni test (which assumes all tests are independent). As such, the corrected P-value is the relevant construct, so it is usually sufficient to apply a much smaller number of tests; resulting P-values ≥ 0.05 were considered significant.

Tests of SNP × SNP interactions (allelic by allelic epistasis) were conducted for PPARGC1A with AMD-related SNPs in complement, lipid metabolism, and, VEGF signaling genes using Plink. The analytic models were based on allele dosage. For each SNP (e.g. SNP A and B) the model took the form of $Y \simeq \beta_0 + \beta_1 A + \beta_2 B + \beta_3 AB + e$. The test for interaction was based on the coefficient β_3.

LCPUFA Intake and Retinal Gene Expression in Mice

Our animal study adhered to the Association for Research in Vision and Ophthalmology (ARVO) Statement for the Use of Animals in Ophthalmic and Vision Research and was approved by the Children's Hospital Boston Animal Care and Use Committee. C57BL/6J mice (stock number 000664, the Jackson Laboratory) were used for the study. Beginning at postnatal day 0 (P0), nursing mothers were fed diets enriched with either 2% ω-3 (eicosapentaenoate+docosahexaenoate) to or 2% ω-6 (arachidonate) LCPUFAs [12]. To induce vessel loss, and subsequent pathological neovascularization, nursing mothers and pups were exposed to 75% oxygen from P7 to P12 and returned to room air and sacrificed at P17. Retinas from each group were isolated and flash frozen using RNase-free techniques. Total RNA was extracted and prepared for Illumina microarray analysis using the Mouse-ref 6 chip (n = 3 biological replicates for each diet group). The chip contained ~45,000 probe sets representing ~34,000 genes. Microarray studies, from cDNA synthesis to raw data normalization were performed by the Molecular Genetics Core Facility at Children's Hospital Boston. Briefly, total RNA (1 μg each) were reverse transcribed, followed by a single *in vitro* transcription amplification to incorporate biotin-labeled nucleotide, and subsequent hybridization and staining with strepatavidin-Cy3 according to the manufacturer's instructions. Data were acquired using the Illumina BeadStudio software and analyzed for quality control, background analysis and normalization with rank invariant algorithm. Further analysis was performed using Significance Analysis of Microarray (SAM), Gene Set Enrichment

Analysis (GSEA), and J-Express Pro 2.7 software. We profiled retinal gene expression with the 2% LCPUFA feeding paradigm identify LCPUFA-regulated genes both associated with pathologic NV and involved in PPAR-mediated processes.

Acknowledgments

We thank the NEI-AMD participants and the NEI-AMD Research Groups for their valuable contributions to this research. The data used for the genetic analyses were obtained from the NEI Study of Age-Related Macular Degeneration (NEI-AMD) Database found at: http://www.ncbi.nlm.nih.gov/projects/gap/cgi-bin/study.cgi?study_id = phs000182.v2.p1. Accessed 2012 Nov 30.

Author Contributions

Conceived and designed the experiments: JPSG JC PS LEHS. Performed the experiments: JPSG JC PS CMA. Analyzed the data: JPSG JC CMA. Contributed reagents/materials/analysis tools: TEC EYC LEHS. Wrote the paper: JPSG JC PS CMA AS TEC EYC LEHS.

References

1. Congdon N, O'Colmain B, Klaver CC, Klein R, Munoz B, et al. (2004) Causes and prevalence of visual impairment among adults in the United States. Arch Ophthalmol 122: 477–485.

2. Hageman GS, Gehrs K, Johnson LV, Anderson D (2008) Age-Related Macular Degeneration (AMD). In: Kolb H, editor. Webvision: The Organization of the Retina and Visual System. 2011/03/18 ed. Salt Lake City (UT). Available: http://www.ncbi.nlm.nih.gov/books/NBK27323/. Accessed 2012 Nov 30.

3. Bird AC (2010) Therapeutic targets in age-related macular disease. J Clin Invest 120: 3033–3041.

4. Ambati J, Ambati BK, Yoo SH, Ianchulev S, Adamis AP (2003) Age-related macular degeneration: etiology, pathogenesis, and therapeutic strategies. Surv Ophthalmol 48: 257–293.

5. Friedman DS, O'Colmain BJ, Munoz B, Tomany SC, McCarty C, et al. (2004) Prevalence of age-related macular degeneration in the United States. Arch Ophthalmol 122: 564–572.

6. (2007) Prevent Blindness America. The economic impact of vision problems. Available: http://www.preventblindness.net/site/DocServer/Impact_of_Vision_Problems.pdf?docID = 1321. Accessed 2012 Nov 30.

7. Chong EW, Kreis AJ, Wong TY, Simpson JA, Guymer RH (2008) Dietary omega-3 fatty acid and fish intake in the primary prevention of age-related macular degeneration: a systematic review and meta-analysis. Arch Ophthalmol 126: 826–833.

8. Weikel KA, Chiu CJ, Taylor A (2012) Nutritional modulation of age-related macular degeneration. Mol Aspects Med 33: 318–375.

9. SanGiovanni JP, Agron E, Clemons TE, Chew EY (2009) Omega-3 long-chain polyunsaturated fatty acid intake inversely associated with 12-year progression to advanced age-related macular degeneration. Arch Ophthalmol 127: 110–112.

10. SanGiovanni JP, Agron E, Meleth AD, Reed GF, Sperduto RD, et al. (2009) {omega}-3 Long-chain polyunsaturated fatty acid intake and 12-y incidence of neovascular age-related macular degeneration and central geographic atrophy: AREDS report 30, a prospective cohort study from the Age-Related Eye Disease Study. Am J Clin Nutr 90: 1601–1607.

11. SanGiovanni JP, Chew EY (2005) The role of omega-3 long-chain polyunsaturated fatty acids in health and disease of the retina. Prog Retin Eye Res 24: 87–138.

12. Connor KM, SanGiovanni JP, Lofqvist C, Aderman CM, Chen J, et al. (2007) Increased dietary intake of omega-3-polyunsaturated fatty acids reduces pathological retinal angiogenesis. Nat Med 13: 868–873.

13. Sapieha P, Stahl A, Chen J, Seaward MR, Willett KL, et al. (2011) 5-Lipoxygenase Metabolite 4-HDHA Is a Mediator of the Antiangiogenic Effect of I‰-3 Polyunsaturated Fatty Acids. Science Translational Medicine 3: 69ra12.

14. Stahl A, Sapieha P, Connor KM, Sangiovanni JP, Chen J, et al. (2010) Short communication: PPAR gamma mediates a direct antiangiogenic effect of omega 3-PUFAs in proliferative retinopathy. Circ Res 107: 495–500.

15. Koto T, Nagai N, Mochimaru H, Kurihara T, Izumi-Nagai K, et al. (2007) Eicosapentaenoic acid is anti-inflammatory in preventing choroidal neovascularization in mice. Invest Ophthalmol Vis Sci 48: 4328–4334.

16. Sheets KG, Zhou Y, Ertel MK, Knott EJ, Regan CE Jr, et al. (2010) Neuroprotectin D1 attenuates laser-induced choroidal neovascularization in mouse. Mol Vis 16: 320–329.

17. Mukherjee PK, Marcheselli VL, Serhan CN, Bazan NG (2004) Neuroprotectin D1: a docosahexaenoic acid-derived docosatriene protects human retinal pigment epithelial cells from oxidative stress. Proc Natl Acad Sci U S A 101: 8491–8496.

18. Halapin NA, Bazan NG (2010) NPD1 induction of retinal pigment epithelial cell survival involves PI3K/Akt phosphorylation signaling. Neurochem Res 35: 1944–1947.

19. Bazan NG, Calandria JM, Serhan CN (2010) Rescue and repair during photoreceptor cell renewal mediated by docosahexaenoic acid-derived neuroprotectin D1. J Lipid Res 51: 2018–2031.

20. Vanden Heuvel JP (2012) Nutrigenomics and nutrigenetics of omega3 polyunsaturated fatty acids. Prog Mol Biol Transl Sci 108: 75–112.

21. Murata T, He S, Hangai M, Ishibashi T, Xi XP, et al. (2000) Peroxisome proliferator-activated receptor-gamma ligands inhibit choroidal neovascularization. Invest Ophthalmol Vis Sci 41: 2309–2317.

22. Keech AC, Mitchell P, Summanen PA, O'Day J, Davis TME, et al. (2007) Effect of fenofibrate on the need for laser treatment for diabetic retinopathy (FIELD study): a randomised controlled trial. The Lancet 370: 1687–1697.

23. Del V Cano M, Gehlbach PL (2008) PPAR-alpha Ligands as Potential Therapeutic Agents for Wet Age-Related Macular Degeneration. PPAR Res 2008: 821592.

24. Kressler D, Schreiber SN, Knutti D, Kralli A (2002) The PGC-1-related protein PERC is a selective coactivator of estrogen receptor alpha. J Biol Chem 277: 13918–13925.

25. Rufibach LE, Duncan SA, Battle M, Deeb SS (2006) Transcriptional regulation of the human hepatic lipase (LIPC) gene promoter. J Lipid Res 47: 1463–1477.

26. Neale BM, Fagerness J, Reynolds R, Sobrin L, Parker M, et al. (2010) Genome-wide association study of advanced age-related macular degeneration identifies a role of the hepatic lipase gene (LIPC). Proc Natl Acad Sci U S A 107: 7395–7400.

27. Maller JB, Fagerness JA, Reynolds RC, Neale BM, Daly MJ, et al. (2007) Variation in complement factor 3 is associated with risk of age-related macular degeneration. Nat Genet 39: 1200–1201.

28. Puigserver P, Adelmant G, Wu Z, Fan M, Xu J, et al. (1999) Activation of PPARgamma coactivator-1 through transcription factor docking. Science 286: 1368–1371.

29. Glass CK, Witztum JL (2001) Atherosclerosis. the road ahead. Cell 104: 503–516.

30. Son NH, Park TS, Yamashita H, Yokoyama M, Huggins LA, et al. (2007) Cardiomyocyte expression of PPARgamma leads to cardiac dysfunction in mice. J Clin Invest 117: 2791–2801.

31. Yano M, Matsumura T, Senokuchi T, Ishii N, Murata Y, et al. (2007) Statins activate peroxisome proliferator-activated receptor gamma through extracellular signal-regulated kinase 1/2 and p38 mitogen-activated protein kinase-dependent cyclooxygenase-2 expression in macrophages. Circ Res 100: 1442–1451.

32. Fauconnet S, Lascombe I, Chabannes E, Adessi GL, Desvergne B, et al. (2002) Differential regulation of vascular endothelial growth factor expression by peroxisome proliferator-activated receptors in bladder cancer cells. J Biol Chem 277: 23534–23543.

33. Arany Z, Foo SY, Ma Y, Ruas JL, Bommi-Reddy A, et al. (2008) HIF-independent regulation of VEGF and angiogenesis by the transcriptional coactivator PGC-1alpha. Nature 451: 1008–1012.

34. Cipriani V, Leung HT, Plagnol V, Bunce C, Khan JC, et al. (2012) Genome-wide association study of age-related macular degeneration identifies associated variants in the TNXB-FKBPL-NOTCH4 region of chromosome 6p21.3. Hum Mol Genet 21: 4138–4150.

35. Smailhodzic D, Muether PS, Chen J, Kwestro A, Zhang AY, et al. (2012) Cumulative Effect of Risk Alleles in CFH, ARMS2, and VEGFA on the Response to Ranibizumab Treatment in Age-Related Macular Degeneration. Ophthalmology.

36. Yu Y, Reynolds R, Fagerness J, Rosner B, Daly MJ, et al. (2011) Association of variants in the LIPC and ABCA1 genes with intermediate and large drusen and advanced age-related macular degeneration. Invest Ophthalmol Vis Sci 52: 4663–4670.

37. Barger PM, Browning AC, Garner AN, Kelly DP (2001) p38 mitogen-activated protein kinase activates peroxisome proliferator-activated receptor alpha: a potential role in the cardiac metabolic stress response. J Biol Chem 276: 44495–44501.

38. Lee Y, Yu X, Gonzales F, Mangelsdorf DJ, Wang MY, et al. (2002) PPAR alpha is necessary for the lipopenic action of hyperleptinemia on white adipose and liver tissue. Proc Natl Acad Sci U S A 99: 11848–11853.

39. McGill JK, Beal MF (2006) PGC-1alpha, a new therapeutic target in Huntington's disease. Cell 127: 465–468.

40. Miura S, Kai Y, Ono M, Ezaki O (2003) Overexpression of peroxisome proliferator-activated receptor gamma coactivator-1alpha down-regulates GLUT4 mRNA in skeletal muscles. J Biol Chem 278: 31385–31390.

41. Anderson SP, Dunn C, Laughter A, Yoon L, Swanson C, et al. (2004) Overlapping transcriptional programs regulated by the nuclear receptors peroxisome proliferator-activated receptor alpha, retinoid X receptor, and liver X receptor in mouse liver. Mol Pharmacol 66: 1440–1452.

42. Leuenberger N, Pradervand S, Wahli W (2009) Sumoylated PPARalpha mediates sex-specific gene repression and protects the liver from estrogen-induced toxicity in mice. J Clin Invest 119: 3138–3148.

43. Chen W, Stambolian D, Edwards AO, Branham KE, Othman M, et al. (2010) Genetic variants near TIMP3 and high-density lipoprotein-associated loci influence susceptibility to age-related macular degeneration. Proc Natl Acad Sci U S A 107: 7401–7406.

44. Klein RJ, Zeiss C, Chew EY, Tsai JY, Sackler RS, et al. (2005) Complement factor H polymorphism in age-related macular degeneration. Science 308: 385–389.

45. Kopplin LJ, Igo RP Jr, Wang Y, Sivakumaran TA, Hagstrom SA, et al. (2010) Genome-wide association identifies SKIV2L and MYRIP as protective factors for age-related macular degeneration. Genes Immun 11: 609–621.

46. Churchill AJ, Carter JG, Lovell HC, Ramsden C, Turner SJ, et al. (2006) VEGF polymorphisms are associated with neovascular age-related macular degeneration. Hum Mol Genet 15: 2955–2961.

47. Almeida LN, Melilo-Carolino R, Veloso CE, Pereira PA, Miranda DM, et al. (2012) Homozygosity for the +674C>T polymorphism on VEGF gene is associated with age-related macular degeneration in a Brazilian cohort. Graefes Arch Clin Exp Ophthalmol 250: 185–189.

48. Galan A, Ferlin A, Caretti L, Buson G, Sato G, et al. (2010) Association of age-related macular degeneration with polymorphisms in vascular endothelial growth factor and its receptor. Ophthalmology 117: 1769–1774.

49. Brion M, Sanchez-Salorio M, Corton M, de la Fuente M, Pazos B, et al. (2011) Genetic association study of age-related macular degeneration in the Spanish population. Acta Ophthalmol 89: e12–22.

50. Qu Y, Dai H, Zhou F, Zhang X, Xu X, et al. (2011) Vascular endothelial growth factor gene polymorphisms and risk of neovascular age-related macular degeneration in a Chinese cohort. Ophthalmic Res 45: 142–148.

51. Mori K, Horie-Inoue K, Gehlbach PL, Takita H, Kabasawa S, et al. (2010) Phenotype and genotype characteristics of age-related macular degeneration in a Japanese population. Ophthalmology 117: 928–938.

52. Richardson AJ, Islam FM, Guymer RH, Cain M, Baird PN (2007) A tag-single nucleotide polymorphisms approach to the vascular endothelial growth factor-A gene in age-related macular degeneration. Mol Vis 13: 2148–2152.

53. Ho L, van Leeuwen R, Witteman JC, van Duijn CM, Uitterlinden AG, et al. (2011) Reducing the genetic risk of age-related macular degeneration with dietary antioxidants, zinc, and omega-3 fatty acids: the Rotterdam study. Arch Ophthalmol 129: 758–766.

54. Wang JJ, Rochtchina E, Smith W, Klein R, Klein BE, et al. (2009) Combined effects of complement factor H genotypes, fish consumption, and inflammatory markers on long-term risk for age-related macular degeneration in a cohort. Am J Epidemiol 169: 633–641.

55. Miura S, Kai Y, Kamei Y, Ezaki O (2008) Isoform-specific increases in murine skeletal muscle peroxisome proliferator-activated receptor-gamma coactivator-1alpha (PGC-1alpha) mRNA in response to beta2-adrenergic receptor activation and exercise. Endocrinology 149: 4527–4533.

56. Pershadsingh HA, Moore DM (2008) PPARgamma Agonists: Potential as Therapeutics for Neovascular Retinopathies. PPAR Res 2008: 164273.

57. Menon G, Walters G (2009) New paradigms in the treatment of wet AMD: the impact of anti-VEGF therapy. Eye (Lond) 23 Suppl 1: S1–7.

58. Vedula SS, Krzystolik MG (2008) Antiangiogenic therapy with anti-vascular endothelial growth factor modalities for neovascular age-related macular degeneration. Cochrane Database Syst Rev: CD005139.

59. Subramanian ML, Ness S, Abedi G, Ahmed E, Daly M, et al. (2009) Bevacizumab vs ranibizumab for age-related macular degeneration: early results of a prospective double-masked, randomized clinical trial. Am J Ophthalmol 148: 875–882 e871.

60. Takeda AL, Colquitt J, Clegg AJ, Jones J (2007) Pegaptanib and ranibizumab for neovascular age-related macular degeneration: a systematic review. Br J Ophthalmol 91: 1177–1182.

61. Chawla A, Boisvert WA, Lee CH, Laffitte BA, Barak Y, et al. (2001) A PPAR gamma-LXR-ABCA1 pathway in macrophages is involved in cholesterol efflux and atherogenesis. Mol Cell 7: 161–171.

6

Comprehensive Analysis of Copy Number Variation of Genes at Chromosome 1 and 10 Loci Associated with Late Age Related Macular Degeneration

Stuart Cantsilieris[1,2], Stefan J. White[2], Andrea J. Richardson[1], Robyn H. Guymer[1], Paul N. Baird[1]*

1 Centre for Eye Research Australia, University of Melbourne, Royal Victorian Eye and Ear Hospital, East Melbourne, Victoria, Australia, **2** Centre for Reproduction and Development, Monash Institute of Medical Research, Melbourne, Victoria, Australia

Abstract

Copy Number Variants (CNVs) are now recognized as playing a significant role in complex disease etiology. Age-related macular degeneration (AMD) is the most common cause of irreversible vision loss in the western world. While a number of genes and environmental factors have been associated with both risk and protection in AMD, the role of CNVs has remained largely unexplored. We analyzed the two major AMD risk-associated regions on chromosome 1q32 and 10q26 for CNVs using Multiplex Ligation-dependant Probe Amplification. The analysis targeted nine genes in these two key regions, including the Complement Factor H (*CFH*) gene, the 5 CFH-related (*CFHR*) genes representing a known copy number "hotspot", the *F13B* gene as well as the *ARMS2* and *HTRA1* genes in 387 cases of late AMD and 327 controls. No copy number variation was detected at the *ARMS2* and *HTRA1* genes in the chromosome 10 region, nor for the *CFH* and *F13B* genes at the chromosome 1 region. However, significant association was identified for the *CFHR3-1* deletion in AMD cases (p = 2.38×10^{-12}) OR = 0.31, CI-0.95 (0.23–0.44), for both neovascular disease (nAMD) (p = 8.3×10^{-9}) OR = 0.36 CI-0.95 (0.25–0.52) and geographic atrophy (GA) (p = 1.5×10^{-6}) OR = 0.36 CI-0.95 (0.25–0.52) compared to controls. In addition, a significant association with deletion of *CFHR1-4* was identified only in patients who presented with bilateral GA (p = 0.02) (OR = 7.6 CI-0.95 1.38–41.8). This is the first report of a phenotype specific association of a CNV for a major subtype of AMD and potentially allows for pre-diagnostic identification of individuals most likely to proceed to this end stage of disease.

Editor: Anneke I. den Hollander, Radboud University Nijmegen Medical Centre, The Netherlands

Funding: This study was supported by the National Health and Medical Research Council (NHMRC) Centre for Clinical Research Excellence #529923-Translational Clinical Research in Major Eye Diseases and NHMRC Project Grant #1008979 and NHMRC practitioner fellowship (RHG). CERA and MIMR receives Operational Infrastructure Support from the Victorian Government. The information contained in this manuscript has not been published before. The authors have no financial interests or involvements with companies regarding this work. The funders had no role in study design, data collection and analysis, decision to publish, or preparation of the manuscript.

* E-mail: pnb@unimelb.edu.au

Introduction

Age-related Macular Degeneration (AMD) is a complex disease associated with multiple gene and environment interactions [1]. It is also the leading cause of vision loss in the western world and ranks third among global causes of visual impairment [2]. Rapid progress in identifying genetic risk factors for AMD susceptibility has been made over the last few years including the identification of two major loci at chromosome 1q32 and 10q26. Whilst these two loci appear to account for the majority of genetic susceptibility in Caucasian populations with AMD, the mechanisms behind their involvement in AMD development and progression are still incompletely understood [3].

Copy Number Variations (CNVs) (deletions and duplications >1000 bp) have recently been shown to have an important role in complex disease phenotypes, most notably in autoimmune related disorders such as Psoriasis [4], Rheumatoid Arthritis [5], Systemic Lupus Erythematosus (SLE) [6] and Atypical Hemolytic Uremic Syndrome (aHUS) [7]. A great proportion of CNVs are enriched towards secreted, olfactory and immunity proteins [8] and it is well known that regions flanked by duplicons (regions of high sequence similarity >95% and a at least 10kb in length) are "hotspots" for CNV and thus more likely to undergo recurrent rearrangements due to non-allelic homologous recombination (NAHR) [9].

Analysis of the Regulators of Complement Activation (RCA) alpha block located on chromosome 1q32 that contain the *CFH*, *CFH* related 1–5 and *F13B* genes and analysis of the chromosome 10q26 region containing the *ARMS2* and *HTRA1* genes has identified a series of single nucleotide polymorphisms (SNPs) associated with both risk of, and protection against, AMD [10,11]. It has previously been shown that an 84 kb deletion encompassing the entire *CFHR3* and *CFHR1* genes is associated with protection in AMD [12,13]. This same deletion is inversely associated with aHUS, thus representing a significant genetic risk factor [14]. Of the five ancestrally related *CFHR* genes, *CFHR3*, *CFHR1* and *CFHR4* are flanked by segmental duplicons and re-arrangements between these duplicons are common but vary in frequency between ethnicities [15]. At the chromosome 10 locus, the two genes, *ARMS2* and *HTRA1* have been extensively screened using SNPs and inferred SNP haplotypes [11,16], but these genes have yet to be analyzed for larger structural variation which may impact on disease pathogenesis. Direct sequencing of this region in a small number of individuals has already revealed an insertion/deletion (indel) polymorphism in the 3'UTR (del443ins54) of *AMRS2*, showing significant association with increased risk of AMD [17].

On the basis of the genomic architecture of the RCA block and the as yet unexplored chromosome 10 regions for CNV, we hypothesized that, in addition to the common *CFHR3-1* deletion, other potential rearrangements encompassing the *CFH, CFHR4, CFHR2, CFHR5, F13B, ARMS2 and HTRA1* genes may contribute to AMD pathogenesis. Two recent reports of a rare *CFHR1-4* deletion further support this notion that other CNVs exist in these regions [18,19]. To assess this region in more detail we have applied Two-colour Multiplex Ligation-dependant Probe Amplification (MLPA), a well established method for detecting quantitative changes in DNA [20,21] and quantitative polymerase chain reaction (qPCR) to validate our findings in a cohort of AMD cases and controls from Australia.

Materials and Methods

Study Design

The study was conducted in accordance with the Declaration of Helsinki and according to the National Health and Medical Research Council of Australia's statement on ethical conduct in research involving humans, revised in 2000. Written informed consent was obtained from all individuals, and ethics approval for the project was provided by the Human Research and Ethics Committee of the Royal Victorian Eye and Ear Hospital (RVEEH), Melbourne. The detailed methods of clinical diagnosis of late AMD as well as control samples has been previously reported [22]. In brief, this was a prospective study with all patients recruited from the RVEEH upon attendance at the clinic. All individuals included in this study were Caucasian of Anglo-Celtic ethnic background. At the time of recruitment, a standard risk factor and disease history questionnaire was undertaken, a clinical examination was performed, a fundus photograph obtained, and a blood sample collected for DNA analysis. Cases had a diagnosis of late AMD which consisted of either neovascular disease (nAMD) or geographic atrophy (GA) whereas control individuals were included if they had a normal fundus (<10 hard drusen <63 µm in size) and no altered macular pigmentation in either eyes. 268 cases on nAMD, 86 Bilateral GA, 33 unilateral GA and 327 normal controls were utilized for this study (Table 1). Cases of nAMD were verified in the clinic on angiography or in clinical notes from the treating clinician. Cases and controls were graded using the modified International Classification System for AMD by two independent graders.

Multiplex Ligation-dependant Probe Amplification (MLPA)

Probe Design. Two-colour MLPA as described by White *et al.* [21] was used to assess CNVs. Probes were designed to each coding exon of *HTRA1* (9 exons) and *ARMS2* (2 exons), 17 of the

23 coding exons of *CFH* and 3 coding exons contained within *F13B*. To analyze the *CFHR1-5* region 5 probes were positioned within the 2 flanking segmental duplicons extending from *CFHR3* to *CFHR4*, while another 4 probes were designed within the remaining *CFHR2* and *CFHR5* genes (Table S1). To allow for simultaneous probe amplification, the common ends of each probe corresponded to the MLPA primers described by Schouten *et al.* [20] and the Multiplex Amplifiable Probe Hybridization (MAPH) primers described by White *et al.* [23]. The specificity of the probes was analyzed using the BLAT program at the University of California Santa Cruz (http://genome.ucsc.edu). Probes were designed to produce PCR products ranging from 80 base pairs (bp) to 130 bp. Oligonucleotides were ordered from Sigma Genosys (www.sigma.genosys.com) with the 5' end of the right hand half-probe phosphorylated to allow ligation to occur. Probe mixes were prepared by combining each oligonucleotide so that they were all present to a final concentration of 4 fmol/µl.

MLPA Reaction. Reagents for the MLPA reaction were purchased from Fisher Biotec (Australia) with the exception of MAPH primers that were purchased from Sigma Genosys. The MLPA reactions were performed according to the method published by Schouten *et al.* [20]. Briefly, 250 ng of DNA in a final volume of 5 µl was denatured at 98°C for 5 minutes, after cooling at room temperature, 1.5 µl of probe mix and 1.5 µl of Hybridization buffer was added to the sample, heat denatured at 95°C for 1 minute followed by hybridization at 60°C for 16 hours.

Ligation was performed at 54°C by adding 32 µl of ligation reaction, after 15 minutes the enzyme was inactivated by heating at 95°C for 5 minutes.

Polymerase Chain Reaction (PCR) amplification was carried out under the following conditions: 1 cycle of 98°C for 1 minute; 35 cycles of 95°C 30 seconds, 57°C 1 minute, 72°C 1 minute; and 1 cycle of 72°C 20 minutes. The PCR reaction was performed in 25 µl.

From each PCR reaction, 1 µl was mixed with 8.8 µl of HIDI formamide and 0.2 µl of LIZ500 size standard (Applied Biosystems). Product separation was performed on the ABI 3130 Electrophoresis 16 capillary sequencer (Applied Biosystems).

Data Analysis. Data Analysis was performed using the GeneMapper Software (Applied Biosystems) and the peak heights were exported to Microsoft Excel. A "global" or "population based" analysis was implemented whereby normalization was performed by calculating the sum of all peak heights from each sample and dividing by the individual peak heights of each probe [24]. The median was calculated for each probe which was then divided by each individual probe to calculate the number of copies of each exon. Thresholds for deletions and duplications were set at below 0.75 and above 1.25 respectively. All samples were tested at least twice.

Quantitative PCR (qPCR)

To verify the results of MLPA, a qPCR assay was designed for the *CFHR3* and *CFHR4* genes using *FOXP2* as the control gene

Table 1. Characteristics of the study population: Age and Gender Distribution of AMD Cases and Controls.

	Unilateral GA (n = 33)	nAMD (n = 268)	Bilateral Geographic Atrophy (n = 86)	Total Cases (n = 387)	Controls (n = 327)
Female n (%)	15 (45)	173 (64)	59 (68)	248 (64)	182 (47)
Age (SD)	69±(10.2)	76±(7.7)	71±(9.6)	74±(8.6)	71±(7)

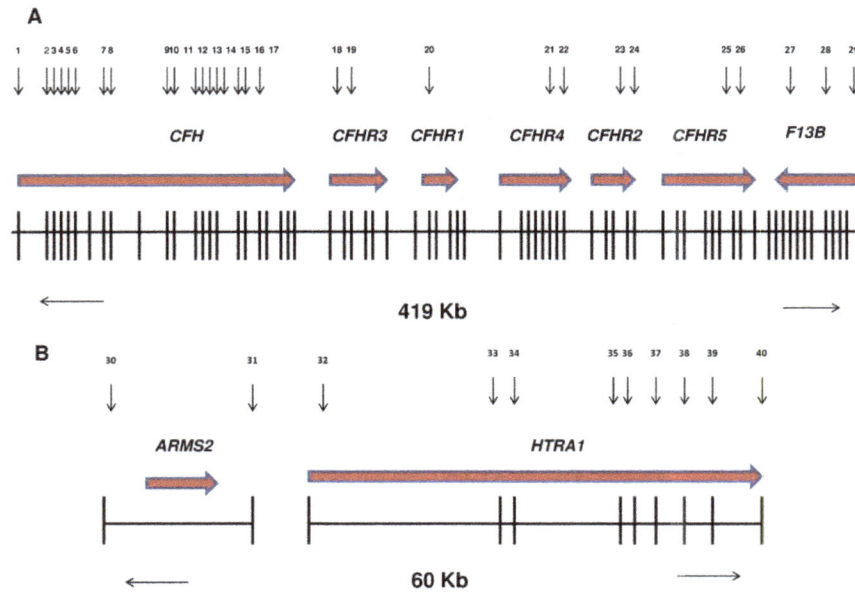

Figure 1. Schematic Representation of Chromosome 1q32 and Chromosome 10q26. (A) Chromosome 1q32 showing a 419 kb region containing the *CFH, CFHR1-5* and *F13B* genes. The vertical lines represent exons in each of the genes. The horizontal arrows at the top represent the direction of transcription. The numbers (top) represent the MLPA probe positions across each of the genes. (B) Chromosome 10q26 show a 60 kb region containing the *ARMS2* and *HTRA1* genes. The horizontal arrows at the top represent the direction of transcription. The numbers represent the MLPA probe positioning in each of the coding exons (vertical bars) across these genes.

[25]. The PCR primers for qPCR are listed in Table S2. qPCR was conducted in triplicate using 25 ng of DNA, PCR reactions were performed using 7.5 µl of 2× Bioline Syber Green Master Mix (www.bioline.com), 0.5 µl of 10 pmol/µl primers and 5 µl of DNA in a 15 µl reaction. qPCR cycling protocol consisted of 95°C for 3 minutes; 40 cycles of 95°C for 5 seconds, 63°C for 5 seconds, 72°C for 10 seconds. Copy number calculations were performed using the Delta-Delta CT method and average copy number was set at 2 [25].

Quantitative Multiplex PCR of Short Fluorescent Fragments (QMPSF)

To verify results of *CFH* exon 18 we employed QMPSF analysis as described by Casili *et al.* [26]. Briefly, primers were designed to flank *CFH* exon 18. The primers used were chimeric and had 5′ extensions of CGTTAGATAG on the forward primer or GATAGGGTTA on the reverse primer. All forward primers were 5′ labeled with 6-FAM. An additional primer pair amplifying the HMBS gene located on chromosome 11 was used as an internal control as described by Saugier-Veber *et al.* [27]. Primer Pairs are listed in the Table S4, PCR reactions were performed as previously described using a modified PCR protocol to allow for quantitative conditions [27].

Statistics

Chi Square analysis, Fisher's exact test and deviations from Hardy-Weinberg Equilibrium (HWE) was performed using PLINK software v1.07 [28]. All genotypes were in HWE (p = >0.001). Logistic regression models were constructed to determine the odds ratio (OR) and 95% confidence intervals (CI 0.95) for AMD cases while conditioning on the rs1061170 SNP in the *CFH* gene, the rs10490924 SNP in the *LOC387715* gene and the rs11200638 SNP in the *HTRA1* gene after adjustment for age,

gender and smoking. Logistic regression and conditional analysis was performed using PLINK v1.07.

Results

Patient Samples

A total of 714 individuals consisting of 387 late stage AMD cases with either nAMD (n = 268) or bilateral GA (n = 86) or unilateral GA (n = 33) and controls (n = 327) without AMD were included in the CNV analysis. The average age of all cases at examination was 74 years with those having nAMD having a mean age of 75 years and those having GA a mean age of 71 years. The average age of control participants was 71.4 years. Male to female ratios were 247/136 (64% vs 36%) in cases and 182/145 (53% vs 47%) in controls.

Probe Design

Copy number analysis was performed on genes from two well established AMD associated genomic loci, targeting seven genes on chromosome 1q32 (*CFH, CFHR1, CFHR2, CFHR3, CFHR4, CFHR5, F13B*) and two genes on chromosome 10q26 (*ARMS2 and HTRA1*) (Figure 1). The probe coverage on chromosome 1 extended almost 0.5 mega base (Mb) from exon 1 of the *CFH* gene to the final exon of the *F13B* gene, while on chromosome 10 the genomic coverage was 60 kilo bases (kb) extending from the first exon of the *ARMS2* gene to the final exon of the *HTRA1* gene. Not all coding exons within the *CFH* gene were amenable to MLPA probe design due to the extensive homology existing between the *CFH* and the *CFHR1-5* genes. Reliable MLPA probe designs could not be achieved for exon 7 and exons 20–23 of the *CFH* gene, but nevertheless we were able to design probes for the majority of the *CFH* gene covering 17/22 its exons. Reliability of probe designs was calculated by assessing the standard deviation (SD) of the normalized probe ratio (1.0 indicating CN of 2) for all 43 probes in

50 samples. The SD for all 43 probes was <10% indicating reliable performance of all probe designs (Table S1).

Detection of re-arrangements on 1q32 and 10q26

MLPA analysis did not reveal the presence of any large re-arrangements encompassing either the *ARMS2* or *HTRA1* genes at chromosome 10q26 in either cases or controls. Similarly the *CFH*, *CFHR2*, *CFHR5* and *F13B* genes did not show evidence of CNVs. Analysis of *CFH* exon 18, appeared to indicate the presence of a heterozygous deletion. Further analysis of the ligation site used to detect this deletion revealed a SNP (rs35292876) identified from recent 1000 genomes data (http://genome.ucsc.edu) likely leading to disturbance of the ligation site and thus giving the appearance of a heterozygous deletion. Confirmation that the exon was indeed only present as two copies was made using Quantitative Multiplex PCR of Short Fluorescent fragments (QMPSF) where primers were designed that flanked the exon (Table S4). Within the remaining *CFHR3*, *CFHR1* and *CFHR4* genes, we detected 6 different combinations of re-arrangements, the common *CFHR3-1* deletion (homozygous and heterozygous), the *CFHR1-4* deletion, deletion of *CFHR1* with reciprocal duplication as well as deletion of *CFHR3* (Figure 2).

Analysis of CNV's and late AMD

Analysis of the common *CFHR3-1* deletion demonstrated its association with protection in AMD being present in a total of 32.8% of controls compared to 13.75% of cases ($p = 2.38 \times 10^{-12}$) OR = 0.31, CI-0.95 (0.23–0.44) (Table 2). The homozygous deletion was almost 10 fold more frequent in controls (5.8%) compared to cases (0.75%), whereas in the heterozygous state it was 2 fold more frequent in controls (27%) compared to cases (13%). Subtype analysis in both end stage nAMD and GA showed that the deletion was protective in both subtypes at ($p = 8.3 \times 10^{-9}$) OR = 0.36 CI-0.95 (0.25–0.52) and ($p = 1.5 \times 10^{-6}$) OR = 0.36 CI-0.95 (0.25–0.52) (Table 2). We performed logistic regression analysis adjusting for gender, age, smoking and conditioning on the Y402H (rs1061170) polymorphism of the *CFH* gene. A statistically significant association remained after adjusting for these confounders (1.34×10^{-5}) OR = 0.40 CI-0.95 (0.27–0.60) (Table 3), consistent with previous reports [19,29,30]. We also conditioned on other *CFH* SNPs rs800292 and rs1061147 and found the same result (data not shown). Conditional analysis on two of the high risk SNPs in the chromosome 10 region rs10490924 and rs11200638 also showed a statistically significant association with protection from AMD (3.2×10^{-9}) OR = 0.28 CI 0.95 (0.19–0.43) (Table 3). Analysis of the rare *CFHR1-4* deletion showed that while the deletion was not associated with risk or protection in late AMD cases as a whole ($p = 0.46$), stratification by subtype revealed a statistically significant association with risk of cases with bilateral GA ($p = 0.02$) OR = 7.6 CI 0.95 (1.38–41.8). Analysis in 327 controls showed that the frequency of the deletion was below <1% compared to 4.7% in bilateral GA. We observed no significant difference in the nAMD subtype ($p = 1.0$). The other three re-arrangements detected in the *CFHR* genes were too rare to infer any statistical significance, consistent with previous reports [31].

Discussion

We have carried out a comprehensive analysis of copy number variation in nine genes from the two most significantly AMD risk associated loci. Identification of the rare heterozygous *CFHR1-4* deletion appears significantly associated with risk of bilateral GA, being 6 times more frequent in this late phenotype compared to

that of nAMD. Interestingly this deletion is present in only 0.74% of nAMD cases, but 4.7% in bilateral GA, suggesting that the deletion may contribute to a different pathophysiological process associated with the bilateral GA phenotype ($p = 0.03$). We also provide further evidence for the protective role of the *CFHR3-1* deletion in AMD, with the homozygous deletion being present in 5.4% of control samples compared to only 0.75% of cases. Three other rare re-arrangements in *CFHR1* and *CFHR3* were also identified in two control samples and one case including a heterozygous deletion of *CFHR3* and a heterozygous deletion and a duplication of *CFHR1*. Analysis of the coding exons of the *CFH* gene, did not reveal any contiguous or non-contiguous CNVs extending from the *CFHR* region. Similarly, analysis of the *F13B* gene in a subset of 100 cases and 100 controls did not show evidence of CNVs. The *ARMS2* and *HTRA1* genes also showed no evidence of CNVs, suggesting that the *ARMS2* indel (del443ins54) located in the promoter region may represent the only major and relatively large structural variant at this locus.

Population based frequencies of the *CFHR3-1* and *CFHR1-4* deletions show evidence of population stratification across multiple ethnicities [12,32]. A study by Hageman et al. showed that the frequency of the homozygous *CFHR3-1* deletion in Africans was as high as 16% compared to 7% in Hispanics, 5% in Caucasians, and only 2% in Asians [12]. Data from the 1000 genomes project [32] also supports this finding indicating that combined analysis of heterozygous and homozygous *CFHR3-1* deletions are present in approximately 50% of Africans compared to 25% in Europeans and less that 10% in Asians [32]. The European frequency is comparable to the combined analysis of homozygous and heterozygous deletions at 32.8% reported here [12,18]. The *CFHR3-1* deletion frequency within African populations may also account for the reduced prevalence of AMD within this population compared to Europeans [33] although it cannot be ruled out that this invariably reflects an earlier age of mortality in this group. Nevertheless it cannot be discounted that the presence of this CNV is positively selected given that these genes have recently been identified as functionally important in complement regulation [29]. Analysis of the rare *CFHR1-4* deletion in our Caucasian control population showed the frequency to be <1%. This frequency was similar to data from the 1000 genomes project which showed no evidence of this CNV in Caucasians and below 5% frequency in Africans and Asians (n = 159) [32].

Analysis of the *CFHR3-1* deletion in our study found similar frequencies to those described previously of homozygous deletions in cases (0.8%–1.2%) and controls (4.9%–5.2%), similarly heterozygous deletions between cases (17%–18%) and controls (22%–27%) [12,31]. Like others [12,13], we also identified a clear gene dosage effect between *CFHR3-1* heterozygous and homozygous deletion samples where individuals with homozygote deletions conferred higher protection from AMD. A study by Fritsche et al. demonstrated that homeostatic balance between *CFHR1*, *CFHR3* and *CFH* determines complement activity and influences inflammation [29]. *CFHR3* and *CFHR1* compete with *CFH* for C3b binding, the loss of two complement regulators from the homozygous deletion of *CFHR3/1* results in increased binding of *CFH to C3b* thereby regulating *CFH* mediated complement activity [29]. They also showed this affect was independent of the Y402H and A473A polymorphism of the *CFH* gene further confirming that this CNV is functionally relevant in AMD pathogenesis. Consistent with these findings and others [19,29,30], we also showed that this effect is independent of Y402H. Studies attempting to verify the independent effects of this deletion have shown that while the statistical strength is mitigated upon conditioning of several highly associated SNPs within *CFH*,

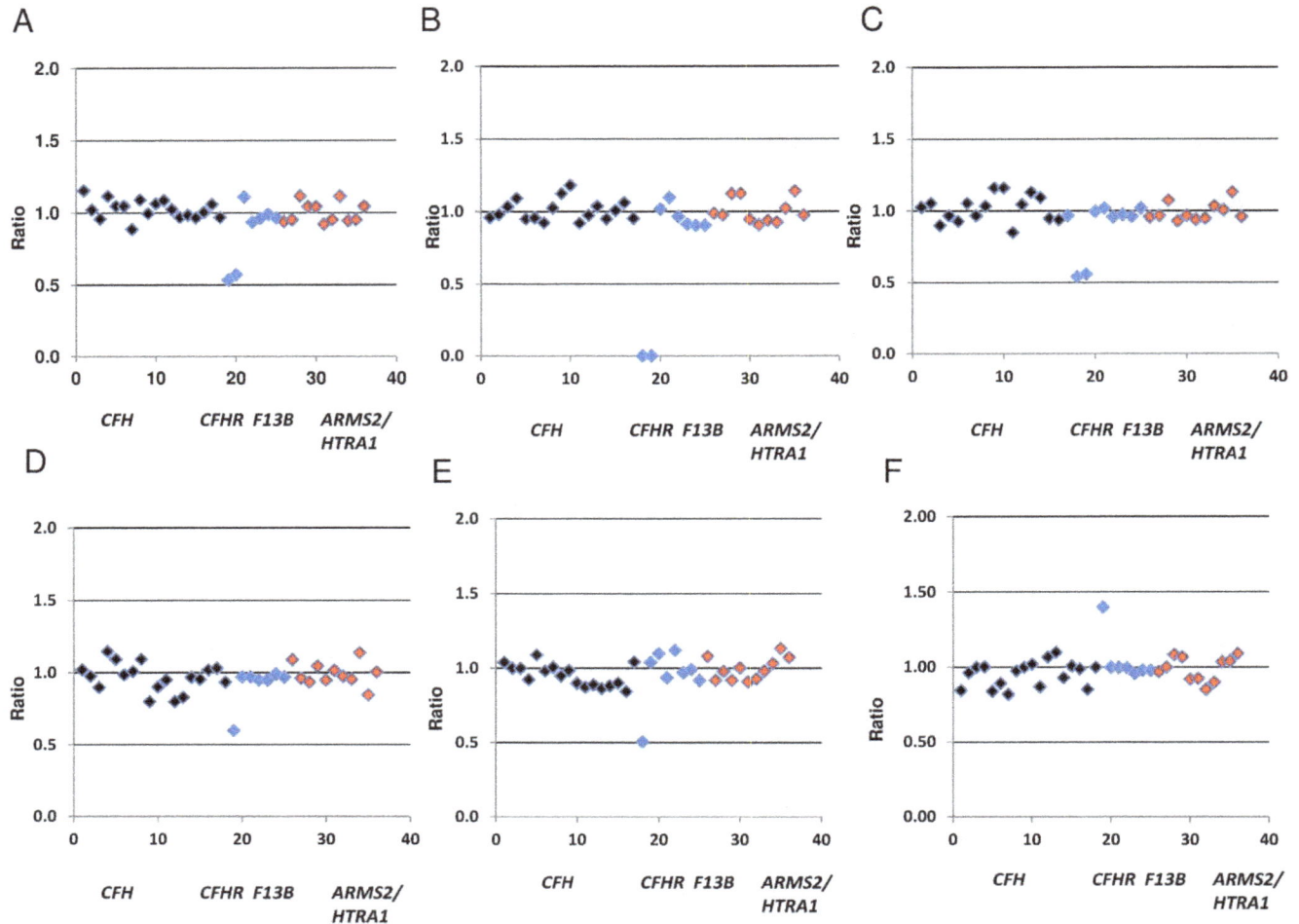

Figure 2. Peak Patterns and Scatter Plots. Scatter plots representing 5 different CNV re-arrangements detected in the *CFHR3*, *CFHR1* and *CFHR4* genes in our sample cohort. Probes targeting the *CFH* gene are represented in black, probes targeting the *CFHR1-5* and *F13B* genes are represented in blue and probes corresponding to the *ARMS2* and *HTRA1* genes are represented in red. The x axis describes each probe number which corresponds to the numbered probe list in Table S1. The y axis represents normalized probe ratios relative to a two copy locus (Normal range 0.75–1.25). The scatter plots describe (A) a heterozygous deletion of *CFHR3-1*, (B) a homozygous deletion of *CFHR3-1*, (C) a heterozygous deletion of *CFHR1-4*, (D) a heterozygous deletion of *CFHR3*, (E) heterozygous deletion of *CFHR1* (F) heterozygous duplication of *CFHR1*.

the statistical significance is not entirely removed [29,30]. A recent report by Hughes *et al.* suggested that the reduction in P value, was a reflection on allele frequency, rather than affect size, as the OR's between rs2274700 and rs10737680 confer almost equal effects to that of the *CFHR3-1* deletion (0.37–0.39) [34].

While this manuscript was in preparation three other studies reported on CNVs in the *CFHR1-5* region with AMD [18,19,35]. Sivakumaran *et al.* [35] reported that an increase *CFHR3-1* CN showed trends towards risk, before conditioning on the most significant SNPs in *CFH*. Interestingly, we and others [12,13,18,29,31] have not detected enrichment of increased *CFHR3-1* copy numbers in AMD cohorts, in fact this appears to be a rare event. In contrast to our data, and others, Sivakumaran *et al.* also reported that additional copies of *CFHR1-4* appeared to confer risk to AMD, suggesting that the deletion conferred protection [35]. The reciprocal duplication of *CFHR1-4* appears to also be a rare event in Africans, Asians and European control populations [32], and was not detected in two subsequent studies of AMD cases and controls [18,19]. This may be a reflection of ethnic differences between the cohorts or the methods used to

genotype the re-arrangements at the *CFHR1-5* region. Several rare re-arrangements, the majority of which, residing in intergenic regions between the *CFHR1-5* genes has been reported [35]. *De-novo* events affecting several exons within *CFH* were detected within samples from African ancestry. In support of our data, these changes were not detected among Caucasian samples suggesting that re-arrangements within *CFH* are rare events, unlikely to have an impact on AMD pathogenesis in individuals of European origin [35].

While there appears to be overwhelming consensus in relation to the association of the *CFHR3-1* deletion and protection from AMD, the same cannot be said for the rare CNV of *CFHR1-4*. Two recent studies found no significant association with this variant and AMD [18,19]. The frequency of this deletion appears to fluctuate depending on the cohort and methodologies used for genotyping. In addition, the deletion and or reciprocal duplication have not been found to be in linkage disequilibrium (LD) with flanking SNP markers [18,35], thus must be genotyped directly. Both studies by Sawitzke *et al.* and Sivakumaran *et al.* used samples from the Age Related Eye Disease Study (AREDS) but appeared

Table 2. Frequencies of Copy Number Rearrangements and Association with end stage AMD.

| | End stage AMD | | | | | | | | Unadjusted Analysis | | | | | |
| | Controls (n=327) | | Unilateral GA (n=33) | | Bilateral GA (n=86) | | nAMD(n=268) | | Bilateral GA | | nAMD | | ALL AMD | |
	n	%	n	%	n	%	n	%	OR (95% CI)	P Value	OR (95% CI)	P Value	OR (95% CI)	P Value
CFHR3-1 Deletion														
2 Copies	220	67.3	27	82	80	93	229	85.45	0.36 (0.25–0.52)	1.5×10^{-6}	0.36 (0.25–0.52)	8.3×10^{-9}	0.31 (0.23–0.44)	2.38×10^{-12}
1 Copy	88	26.9	6	18	6	7	37	13.8						
0 Copies	19	5.8	0	0	0	0	2	0.75						
CFHR1-4 Deletion														
2 Copies	325	99.4	33	100	82	95.3	266	99.26	7.6 (1.38–41.8)	0.02	0.6 (0.05–6.8)	1	2.1 (0.40–10.91)	0.46
1 Copy	2	0.006	0	0	4	4.7	2	0.74						
0 Copies	0	0	0	0	0	0	0	0						

to yield different frequencies of *CFHR1-4* copy numbers [19,35]. These findings of differing copy number changes in two sub populations of AREDS individuals cannot be easily explained. One explanation is the potential for admixture in the population and it would be interesting if the two sub cohorts were assessed for this effect. Ethnicity information was not reported in either of the Sawitzke or Sivakumaran studies. Another potential explanation is that two differing methodologies used to analyze this region (qPCR and array CGH) may have led to some methodological biases between the two studies [19,35].

Interestingly, several studies of CNVs in other diseases have shown similar conflicting data. Lower copy number of the FC Gamma Receptor 3B (*FCGR3B*) gene has been shown to be associated with Rheumatoid Arthritis (RA) [5], while other studies have failed to replicate this association [25,36]. Similarly, analysis of CC Chemokine Ligand 3-like 1 (*CCL3L1*) in HIV AIDS susceptibility has found evidence of lower copy number and HIV susceptibility [37], while others have found no association [38,39]. It remains unclear as to whether accurate assessment of CNVs, population sub structure, admixture, or whether small changes in detected frequencies of rare CNVs in cases and controls affected by sample size are the main contributing factors to the reproducibility of these associations.

Functionally the *CFHR4* gene has been shown to be important in complement regulation [40]. *CFHR4* protein binds to a pentameric form of C-reactive protein (pCRP) (different from the monomeric *CRP* bound by *CFH*) and recruits pCRP to the surface of necrotic cells enhancing removal of necrotic cells directly or facilitating C1q binding and complement activation [41]. In addition, it has been proposed that *CFHR4* limits inflammation by enhancing the co-factor activity of *CFH* and enhancing complement deposition by CRP binding which helps phagocytic clearance of microbes and necrotic cells in inflamed tissues [40]. If *CFHR4* regulates complement activation and opsonization on biological surfaces via interaction with pCRP [40], then potentially a deletion of this gene would lead to reduced pCRP binding and thus limit its capacity to inhibit inflammation leading to enhanced disease. A similar hypothesis has also been suggested for the *CFH* gene by Laine *et al.* [42] whereby binding affinity of CRP for *CFH* was influenced by the Y402H polymorphism. It was suggested that impaired binding of CRP to *CFH* reduced the ability for *CFH* to modulate inflammation [42]. Furthermore, no individuals in the current study presented with both the *CFHR3-1* and *CFHR1-4* deletions on both alleles as described previously [14]. As these genes represent a functionally different component to complement regulation, it suggests that homeostatic balance between *CFH*, *CFHR3*, *CFHR1* and *CFHR4* is necessary to maintain regulation of complement activation.

Typically, studies analyzing the *CFHR1-5* gene cluster have incorporated an MLPA based approach [13,14,18,29,31]. MLPA utilizes a ligation step to join two adjacent oligonucleotide probe sequences together after hybridization [20]. This step provides increased sensitivity to distinguish between two highly homologous sequences [43]. However, an unsuspected polymorphism near the ligation site of the two MLPA oligonucleotides can hamper accurate determination of CNV regions [44]. In most primer probe based assays, a polymorphism can disturb primer binding enough to give the appearance of a deletion [45]. In this case a deletion detected with a single probe should always be confirmed via an alternative method. With this in mind we implemented three methods of CNV detection through the use of MLPA, QMPSF and qPCR.

Data from Kubista *et al.* previously identified a heterozygous deletion of *CFHR2* at a frequency of less than 1% [18]. We and others [19,35] did not detect this deletion in our respective

Table 3. Logistic regression analysis of rs1061170, rs10490924, rs11200638 and CFHR3-1 deletion in AMD Cases and Controls.

CFHR3-1 Deletion	Bilateral GA		nAMD		ALL AMD	
	OR (95% CI)	P Value	OR (95% CI)	P Value	OR (95% CI)	P Value
Adjusted for Age, Gender, Smoking	0.16 (0.07–0.37)	2.2×10^{-5}	0.32 (0.21–0.48)	5.1×10^{-8}	0.30 (0.20–0.43)	3.04×10^{-10}
Adjusted for Age, Gender, smoking and conditioned on rs1061170	0.24 (0.09–0.62)	0.003	0.42 (0.27–0.64)	8.4×10^{-5}	0.40 (0.27–0.60)	1.37×10^{-5}
Adjusted for Age, Gender, smoking and conditioned on rs10490924, rs11200638	0.17 (0.07–0.40)	6.6×10^{-5}	0.32 (0.21–0.50)	4.4×10^{-7}	0.28 (0.19–0.43)	3.2×10^{-9}

Caucasian cohorts. One possible explanation is a potential polymorphism on the ligation site for the *CFHR2* MLPA probe used by Kubista *et al.* [18]. Sequence analysis revealed a polymorphism C>T (rs72736421) directly on the ligation site which is likely to disturb the probe binding sufficiently to give the appearance of a heterozygous deletion. We identified similar polymorphisms for probes used to analyze *CFH* exon 18 (rs115722139) and *CFH* intron 1 (rs77837548), although these polymorphisms were further away from the ligation site, 8 bp and 3 bp respectively [18]. In the case of the *CFH* exon 18 MLPA probe used in this study, analysis of the ligation site showed a polymorphism C>T (rs35292876) directly on the ligation site which would explain the presence of an apparent deletion that was initially detected using this technique but yet could not be detected in confirmatory studies using QMPSF (Table S3). The polymorphism was not identified during the original probe design and was only identified following release of the first draft of the 1000 genomes data.

Our understanding of CNVs and the role that they play in complex disease is likely to increase substantially in the next few years, especially with recent advancements in next generation sequencing and array based Comparative Genome Hybridization [46,47]. Of continuing interest is the apparent reversal of associations seen in seemingly unrelated complex diseases to what are essentially identical copy number variants. For example, studies of the RCA alpha block encompassing *CFH* and *CFHR1-5* genes have shown associations with AMD, aHUS, Membranoproliferative Glomerulonephritis [48] and SLE. Curiously, the *CFHR3-1* deletion has now been shown to be associated with risk in aHUS [14] and SLE [49] but protection in AMD [12]. The same study in aHUS individuals also showed that combined deletion of *CFHR3-1* and *CFHR1-4* on both alleles is associated with risk of aHUS [14]. Similarly studies analyzing the beta defensin gene cluster have shown that while increased beta defensin copy number (>5 copies) is associated with psoriasis, low copy numbers (<4 copies) are associated with Crohn's Disease [50,51]. Further investigation into the functionality of these CNV regions is required to assess their impact on complex disease pathogenesis. These findings may indicate a dosage response mechanism or differing action depending on the tissue type.

Our finding that the rare *CFHR1-4* deletion is associated with risk of bilateral GA may have important research and clinical implications, particularly as our current knowledge regarding how progression of AMD occurs towards the two late stage phenotypes of GA and nAMD is currently limited. While this is an interesting finding, we are cautious about reporting associations of rare variants especially given the conflicting data from three other reports. Replication in larger populations would strengthen the argument that the findings reported here are reproducible before any definitive conclusions can be drawn concerning a clinically relevant association between this variant and AMD.

Our data represents a comprehensive study of copy number variation in genes associated with AMD. Our cohort was collected from a single centre with all cases being seen by a small number of retinal specialists. The phenotype information was well characterized with ethnicity information collected. In summary we demonstrate that the relevant copy number "hotspot" in AMD lies in the region encompassing the *CFHR3*, *CFHR1* and *CFHR4* genes. These findings support the idea that CNVs do impart a likely functional role in AMD pathogenesis through gene dosage effects on genes regulating the complement cascade. Given that many copy number polymorphisms (CNPs) are poorly tagged by SNPs, and are likely to exert their own independent effects, a combined effort analyzing all classes of genetic variation such as SNPs, Indels and CNVs is likely to lead to a greater understanding of AMD pathogenesis. Given the substantial number of people affected by AMD this finding if replicated would greatly enhance our ability to predict which patients are most likely to go on to develop GA and thereby offer specific treatments targeted to such a group.

Author Contributions

Conceived and designed the experiments: SC SJW PNB. Performed the experiments: SC. Analyzed the data: SC SJW. Contributed reagents/materials/analysis tools: SC SJW AR RHG PNB. Wrote the paper: SC SJW RHG PNB.

References

1. Guymer RH, Chong EWT (2006) Modifiable risk factors for age-related macular degeneration. Med J Aust 184.

2. Resnikoff S, Pascolini D, Mariotti SP, Pokharel GP (2008) Global magnitude of visual impairment caused by uncorrected refractive errors in 2004. Bull World Health Organ 86: 63–70.

3. Robman L, Baird PN, Dimitrov PN, Richardson AJ, Guymer RH (2010) C-Reactive Protein Levels and Complement Factor H Polymorphism Interaction in Age-related Macular Degeneration and Its Progression. Ophthalmology 117: 1982–1988.

4. de Cid R, Riveira-Munoz E, Zeeuwen P, Robarge J, Liao W, et al. (2009) Deletion of the late cornified envelope LCE3B and LCE3C genes as a susceptibility factor for psoriasis. Nat Genet 41: 211–215.

5. McKinney C, Fanciulli M, Merriman ME, Phipps-Green A, Alizadeh BZ, et al. (2010) Association of variation in Fc gamma receptor 3B gene copy number with rheumatoid arthritis in Caucasian samples. Ann Rheum Dis 69: 1711–1716.

6. Fanciulli M, Norsworthy PJ, Petretto E, Dong R, Harper L, et al. (2007) FCGR3B copy number variation is associated with susceptibility to systemic, but not organ-specific, autoimmunity. Nat Genet 39: 721–723.

7. Zipfel PF, Edey M, Heinen S, Jozsi M, Richter H, et al. (2007) Deletion of Complement Factor Related Genes *CFHR1* and *CFHR3* Is Associated with Atypical Hemolytic Uremic Syndrome. PLoS Genet 3: e41.

8. Nguyen D-Q, Webber C, Ponting CP (2006) Bias of selection on human copy-number variants. PLoS Genet 2.

9. Sharp AJ, Locke DP, McGrath SD, Cheng Z, Bailey JA, et al. (2005) Segmental duplications and copy-number variation in the human genome. Am J Hum Genet 77: 78–88.

10. Hageman GS, Anderson DH, Johnson LV, Hancox LS, Taiber AJ, et al. (2005) A common haplotype in the complement regulatory gene factor H (HF1/CFH) predisposes individuals to age-related macular degeneration. Proc Natl Acad Sci U S A 102: 7227–7232.

11. DeWan A, Liu M, Hartman S, Zhang SS, Liu DT, et al. (2006) HTRA1 Promoter Polymorphism in Wet Age-Related Macular Degeneration. Science 314: 989–992.

12. Hageman GS, Hancox LS, Taiber AJ, Gehrs KM, Anderson DH, et al. (2006) Extended haplotypes in the complement factor H (CFH) and CFH-related (CFHR) family of genes protect against age-related macular degeneration: Characterization, ethnic distribution and evolutionary implications. Ann Med 38: 592–604.

13. Hughes AE, Orr N, Esfandiary H, Diaz-Torres M, Goodship T, et al. (2006) A common CFH haplotype, with deletion of CFHR1 and CFHR3, is associated with lower risk of age-related macular degeneration. Nat Genet 38: 1173–1177.

14. Moore I, Strain L, Pappworth I, Kavanagh D, Barlow PN, et al. (2010) Association of factor H autoantibodies with deletions of CFHR1, CFHR3, CFHR4, and with mutations in CFH, CFI, CD46, and C3 in patients with atypical hemolytic uremic syndrome. Blood 115: 379–387.

15. Campbell CD, Sampas N, Tsalenko A, Sudmant PH, Kidd JM, et al. (2011) Population-Genetic Properties of Differentiated Human Copy-Number Polymorphisms. Am J Hum Genet 88: 317–332.

16. Atsuhiro K, Wei C, Othman M, Branham KEH, Brooks M, et al. (2007) A variant of mitochondrial protein LOC387715/ARMS2, not HTRA1, is strongly associated with age-related macular degeneration. Proc Nat Acad Sci USA 104: 16227–16232.

17. Fritsche LG, Loenhardt T, Janssen A, Fisher SA, Rivera A, et al. (2008) Age-related macular degeneration is associated with an unstable ARMS2 (LOC387715) mRNA. Nat Genet 40: 892–896.

18. Kubista KE, Tosakulwong N, Wu Y, Ryu E, Roeder JL, et al. (2011) Copy number variation in the complement factor H-related genes and age-related macular degeneration. Mol Vis 17: 2080–2092.

19. Sawitzke J, Im KM, Kostiha B, Dean M, Gold B (2011) Association Assessment of Copy Number Polymorphism and Risk of Age-Related Macular Degeneration. Ophthalmology In Press, Corrected Proof.

20. Schouten JP, McElgunn CJ, Waaijer R, Zwijnenburg D, Diepvens F, et al. (2002) Relative quantification of 40 nucleic acid sequences by multiplex ligation-dependent probe amplification. Nucleic Acids Res 30: 1–13.

21. White SJ, Vink GR, Kriek M, Wuyts W, Schouten J, et al. (2004) Two-color multiplex ligation-dependent probe amplification: Detecting genomic rearrangements in hereditary multiple exostoses. Hum Mutat 24: 86–92.

22. Richardson AJ, Islam FMA, Aung KZ, Guymer RH, Baird PN (2010) An Intergenic Region between the tagSNP rs3793917 and rs11200638 in the HTRA1 Gene Indicates Association with Age-Related Macular Degeneration. Invest Ophthalmol Vis Sci 51: 4932–4936.

23. White S, Kalf M, Liu Q, Villerius M, Engelsma D, et al. (2002) Comprehensive Detection of Genomic Duplications and Deletions in the DMD Gene, by Use of Multiplex Amplifiable Probe Hybridization. Am J Hum Genet 71: 365–374.

24. White SJ, Breuning MH, den Dunnen JT (2004) Detecting Copy Number Changes in Genomic DNA: MLPA and MAPH. Methods Cell Biol 75: 751.

25. Marques RB, Thabet MM, White SJ, Houwing-Duistermaat JJ, Bakker AM, et al. (2010) Genetic Variation of the Fc Gamma Receptor 3B Gene and Association with Rheumatoid Arthritis. PloS One 5.

26. Casilli F, Di Rocco ZC, Gad S, Tournier I, Stoppa-Lyonnet D, et al. (2002) Rapid detection of novel BRCA1 rearrangements in high-risk breast-ovarian cancer families using multiplex PCR of short fluorescent fragments. Hum Mutat 20: 218–226.

27. Saugier-Veber P, Goldenberg A, Drouin-Garraud V, de la Rochebrochard C, Layet V, et al. (2006) Simple detection of genomic microdeletions and microduplications using QMPSF in patients with idiopathic mental retardation. Eur J Hum Genet 14: 1009–1017.

28. Purcell S, Neale B, Todd-Brown K, Thomas L, Ferreira MAR, et al. (2007) PLINK: A Tool Set for Whole-Genome Association and Population-Based Linkage Analyses. The American Journal of Human Genetics 81: 559–575.

29. Fritsche LG, Lauer N, Hartmann A, Stippa S, Keilhauer CN, et al. (2010) An imbalance of human complement regulatory proteins CFHR1, CFHR3 and factor H influences risk for age-related macular degeneration (AMD). Hum Mol Genet 19: 4694–4704.

30. Raychaudhuri S, Ripke S, Li M, Neale BM, Fagerness J, et al. (2010) Associations of CFHR1-CFHR3 deletion and a CFH SNP to age-related macular degeneration are not independent. Nat Genet 42: 553–555.

31. Schmid-Kubista KE, Tosakulwong N, Wu Y, Ryu E, Hecker LA, et al. (2009) Contribution of Copy Number Variation in the Regulation of Complement Activation Locus to Development of Age-Related Macular Degeneration. Invest Ophthalmol Vis Sci 50: 5070–5079.

32. Sudmant PH, Kitzman JO, Antonacci F, Alkan C, Malig M, et al. (2010) Diversity of Human Copy Number Variation and Multicopy Genes. Science 330: 641–646.

33. Klein R, Chou C-F, Klein BEK, Zhang X, Meuer SM, et al. (2011) Prevalence of Age-Related Macular Degeneration in the US Population. Arch Ophthalmol 129: 75–80.

34. Hughes AE, Orr N, Cordell HJ, Goodship T (2010) Reply to Associations of CFHR1-CFHR3 deletion and a CFH SNP to age-related macular degeneration are not independent. Nat Genet 42: 555–556.

35. Sivakumaran TA, Igo RP, Jr., Kidd JM, Itsara A, Kopplin LJ, et al. (2011) A 32 kb Critical Region Excluding Y402H in CFH Mediates Risk for Age-Related Macular Degeneration. Plos One 6: e25598.

36. Mamtani M, Anaya JM, He W, Ahuja SK (2010) Association of Copy Number Variation in the FCGR3B gene with risk of autoimmune diseases. Genes Immun 11: 155–160.

37. Gonzalez E, Kulkarni H, Bolivar H, Mangano A, Sanchez R, et al. (2005) The Influence of CCL3L1 Gene-Containing Segmental Duplications on HIV-1/AIDS Susceptibility. Science 307: 1434–1440.

38. Field SF, Howson JMM, Maier LM, Walker S, Walker NM, et al. (2009) Experimental aspects of copy number variant assays at CCL3L1. Nat Med 15: 1115–1117.

39. Bhattacharya T, Stanton J, Kim E-Y, Kunstman KJ, Phair JP, et al. (2009) CCL3L1 and HIV/AIDS susceptibility. Nat Med 15: 1112–1115.

40. Hebecker M, Okemefuna AI, Perkins SJ, Mihlan M, Huber-Lang M, et al. (2011) Molecular basis of C-reactive protein binding and modulation of complement activation by factor H-related protein 4. Mol Immunol 47: 1347–1355.

41. Mihlan M, Hebecker M, Dahse H-M, Halbich S, Huber-Lang M, et al. (2009) Human complement factor H-related protein 4 binds and recruits native pentameric C-reactive protein to necrotic cells. Mol Immunol 46: 335–344.

42. Laine M, Jarva H, Seitsonen S, Haapasalo K, Lehtinen MJ, et al. (2007) Y402H Polymorphism of Complement Factor H Affects Binding Affinity to C-Reactive Protein. J Immunol 178: 3831–3836.

43. White S, Vissers L, Geurts Van Kessel A, De Menezes R, Kalay E, et al. (2007) Variation of CNV distribution in five different ethnic populations. Cytogenet Genome Res 118: 19.

44. Notini AJ, Craig JM, White SJ (2008) Copy number variation and mosaicism. Cytogenetic And Genome Research 123: 270–277.

45. Janssen B, Hartmann C, Scholz V, Jauch A, Zschocke J (2005) MLPA analysis for the detection of deletions, duplications and complex rearrangements in the dystrophin gene: potential and pitfalls. Neurogenetics 6: 29–35.

46. Alkan C, Kidd JM, Marques-Bonet T, Aksay G, Antonacci F, et al. (2009) Personalized copy number and segmental duplication maps using next-generation sequencing. Nat Genet 41: 1061–1067.

47. Cooper GM, Coe BP, Girirajan S, Rosenfeld JA, Vu TH, et al. (2011) A copy number variation morbidity map of developmental delay. Nat Genet 43: 838–846.

48. Abrera-Abeleda MA, Nishimura C, Smith JLH, Sethi S, McRae JL, et al. (2006) Variations in the complement regulatory genes factor H (CFH) and factor H related 5 (CFHR5) are associated with membranoproliferative glomerulonephritis type II (dense deposit disease). J Med Gen 43: 582–589.

49. Zhao J, Wu H, Khosravi M, Cui H, Qian X, et al. (2011) Association of Genetic Variants in Complement Factor H and Factor H-Related Genes with Systemic Lupus Erythematosus Susceptibility. PLoS Genet 7: e1002079.

50. Fellermann K, Stange DE, Schaeffeler E, Schmalzl H, Wehkamp J, et al. (2006) A Chromosome 8 Gene-Cluster Polymorphism with Low Human Beta-Defensin 2 Gene Copy Number Predisposes to Crohn Disease of the Colon. Am J Hum Genet 79: 439–448.

51. Hollox EJ, Huffmeier U, Zeeuwen P, Palla R, Lascorz J, et al. (2008) Psoriasis is associated with increased beta-defensin genomic copy number. Nat Genet 40: 23–25.

7

Three New Genetic Loci (R1210C in *CFH*, Variants in *COL8A1* and *RAD51B*) Are Independently Related to Progression to Advanced Macular Degeneration

Johanna M. Seddon[1,2*], **Robyn Reynolds**[1], **Yi Yu**[1], **Bernard Rosner**[3]

1 Ophthalmic Epidemiology and Genetics Service, Tufts University School of Medicine and Tufts Medical Center, New England Eye Center, Boston, Massachusetts, United States of America, **2** Department of Ophthalmology, Tufts University School of Medicine, Boston, Massachusetts, United States of America, **3** Channing Laboratory, Brigham and Women's Hospital and Harvard School of Public Health, Harvard University, Boston, Massachusetts, United States of America

Abstract

Objectives: To assess the independent impact of new genetic variants on conversion to advanced stages of AMD, controlling for established risk factors, and to determine the contribution of genes in predictive models.

Methods: In this prospective longitudinal study of 2765 individuals, 777 subjects progressed to neovascular disease (NV) or geographic atrophy (GA) in either eye over 12 years. Recently reported genetic loci were assessed for their independent effects on incident advanced AMD after controlling for 6 established loci in 5 genes, and demographic, behavioral, and macular characteristics. New variants which remained significantly related to progression were then added to a final multivariate model to assess their independent effects. The contribution of genes to risk models was assessed using reclassification tables by determining risk within cross-classified quintiles for alternative models.

Results: Three new genetic variants were significantly related to progression: rare variant R1210C in *CFH* (hazard ratio (HR) 2.5, 95% confidence interval [CI] 1.2–5.3, P = 0.01), and common variants in genes *COL8A1* (HR 2.0, 95% CI 1.1–3.5, P = 0.02) and *RAD51B* (HR 0.8, 95% CI 0.60–0.97, P = 0.03). The area under the curve statistic (AUC) was significantly higher for the 9 gene model (.884) vs the 0 gene model (.873), P = .01. AUC's for the 9 vs 6 gene models were not significantly different, but reclassification analyses indicated significant added information for more genes, with adjusted odds ratios (OR) for progression within 5 years per one quintile increase in risk score of 2.7, P<0.001 for the 9 vs 6 loci model, and OR 3.5, P<0.001 for the 9 vs. 0 gene model. Similar results were seen for NV and GA.

Conclusions: Rare variant *CFH* R1210C and common variants in *COL8A1* and *RAD51B* plus six genes in previous models contribute additional predictive information for advanced AMD beyond macular and behavioral phenotypes.

Editor: Olaf Strauß, Eye Hospital, Charité, Germany

Funding: Supported by grant RO1-EY11309 from the National Institutes of Health; Massachusetts Lions Eye Research Fund; Foundation Fighting Blindness; unrestricted grants from Research to Prevent Blindness; American Macular Degeneration Foundation; Macula Vision Research Foundation; and the Macular Degeneration Research Fund, Ophthalmic Epidemiology and Genetics Service, Tufts Medical Center, Tufts University School of Medicine, Boston, MA, USA. The funders had no role in study design, data collection and analysis, decision to publish, or preparation of the manuscript.

Competing Interests: Tufts Medical Center has patents pending that are not in the public domain in relation to the prediction model and some genes analyzed in this study. There are no further patents, products in development or marketed products related to this study to declare.

* E-mail: jseddon@tuftsmedicalcenter.org

Introduction

There is a strong genetic component and an important environmental influence on the development of age-related macular degeneration (AMD) [1,2]. Common loci in genes in the complement and lipid pathways have been confirmed in several studies. Since 2011, associations with AMD have been shown for a novel rare variant (R1210C) in *CFH* [3] common variants in *COL10A1*[4–6], *COL8A1*[4–6], *VEGFA* [5], and *TNFRSF10A* [6,7] Additional common variants were also identified in our international consortium effort based on meta-analyses of several genome-wide case-control association studies. [6] All of these recently reported genes have been shown to be related to advanced AMD when compared with controls. However, the relative impact of most of these new genes on AMD progression has not been reported, and their independent effects, while controlling for all established genetic and non-genetic risk factors for progression, are unknown.

In this study we, therefore, determined: 1) the independent effect of each new genetic locus on AMD progression after controlling for the known genetic, demographic, behavioral and ocular risk factors related to progression, when each new locus was considered separately, 2) whether the new genetic loci related to AMD progression based on this initial analyses remained significant predictors of progression when combined with variables in our previous risk models, and 3) if genes and number of genes significantly add to risk models for AMD progression.

Table 1. Multivariate Associations between Baseline Demographic, Environmental, Macular Variables and Incidence of Advanced AMD.

		Progressors	Non-progressors	HR 95% CI*	p - value
Total patients:		**(N = 777)**	**(N = 1988)**		
Age (years)		N (%)	N (%)		
	<65	197 (25)	242 (12)	1.0 ref	
	65–74	476 (61)	1322 (66)	0.7 (0.6–0.9)	0.0007
	55–64	104 (13)	424 (21)	0.6 (0.5–0.7)	<0.0001
Sex					
	Female	425 (55)	1135 (57)	1.0 ref	
	Male	352 (45)	853 (43)	1.1 (0.9–1.2)	0.42
Education					
	≤ High School	309 (40)	624 (31)	1.0 ref	
	> High School	468 (60)	1364 (69)	0.9 (0.8–1.0)	0.07
Smoking					
	Never	300 (39)	1008 (51)	1.0 ref	
	Past	410 (53)	880 (44)	1.1 (1.0–1.3)	0.09
	Current	67 (9)	100 (5)	1.9 (1.4–2.4)	<0.0001
BMI					
	<25	227 (29)	672 (34)	1.0 ref	
	25–29	328 (42)	848 (43)	1.1 (0.9–1.3)	0.52
	30+	222 (29)	468 (24)	1.2 (1.0–1.5)	0.05
Advanced AMD in One Eye at Baseline					
	Neither Eye	522 (67)	1833 (92)	1.0 ref	
	Grade 4	49 (6)	6 (0.3)	7.1 (2.6–18.9)	<0.0001
	Grade 5	206 (27)	149 (7)	5.0 (1.9–12.6)	0.0008
Individuals with Advanced AMD in One Eye at Baseline: Largest Drusen Size in Non-advanced Eye (microns)					
	<63	6 (2)	46 (30)	1.0 ref	
	63–124	41 (16)	57 (37)	4.4 (1.9–10.4)	0.0007
	125–249	86 (34)	37 (24)	9.6 (4.2–22.0)	<0.0001
	≥250	122 (48)	15 (10)	16.6 (7.3–37.8)	<0.0001
Individuals Without Advanced AMD at Baseline: Size of Drusen (microns) in Each Eye					
	<63, <63	17 (3)	807 (44)	1.0 ref	
	63–124, <63	27 (5)	388 (21)	3.2 (1.8–6.0)	0.0002
	63–124, 63–124	35 (7)	171 (9)	8.4 (4.7–15.1)	<0.0001
	125–249, <63	21 (4)	127 (7)	7.3 (3.8–13.9)	<0.0001
	125–249, 63–124	64 (12)	155 (9)	15.3 (8.9–26.3)	<0.0001
	125–249, 125–249	88 (17)	93 (5)	30.1 (18.2–52.0)	<0.0001
	≥250, ≤124	24 (5)	25 (1)	29.6 (15.8–55.4)	<0.0001
	≥250, 125–249	92 (18)	41 (2)	49.7 (29.4–84.1)	<0.0001
	≥250, ≥250	154 (30)	26 (1)	75.0 (45.2–124.5)	<0.0001

HR = hazard ratio; CI = confidence interval.
*Controlling for all variables in the table.

Methods

The Age-Related Eye Disease Study included a randomized clinical trial to assess the effect of antioxidant and mineral supplements on risk of AMD and cataract and a longitudinal study of AMD that ended in December 2005 [8] Research adhered to the tenets of the Declaration of Helsinki. The research protocol was approved by institutional review boards and all participants signed consent statements. Follow-up time ranged from 0.5 to 13.0

years (mean 8.8 years). Phenotype data were accessed through the Database of Genotypes and Phenotypes (dbGaP). Participants were classified using the Clinical Age-Related Maculopathy Staging System (CARMS) [9], based on ocular examination and grading of fundus photographs at baseline, into 5 stages: normal or stage 1 in both eyes (essentially free of age-related macular abnormalities or a few small drusen), early AMD or stage 2 in the worse eye (mild changes including multiple small drusen, nonextensive intermediate drusen, and/or pigment abnormalities),

Table 2. Distribution of Age-Related Macular Degeneration Genetic Variants Among Progressors and Non-Progressors.

Gene/Genotype		Progression Yes	No	p-value*	Gene/Genotype		Progression Yes	No	p-value*
Total patients N (%)		777 (28.1)	1988 (71.9)				777 (28.1)	1988 (71.9)	
CFH(Y402H)	TT	123 (16)	723 (36)	<0.0001	LIPC	CC	420 (54)	1036 (52)	0.25
	CT	343 (44)	922 (46)			CT	308 (40)	805 (40)	
	CC	311 (40)	343 (17)			TT	49 (6)	147 (7)	
CFH	TT	29 (4)	329 (17)	<0.0001	ABCA1	CC	443 (57)	1094 (55)	0.28
	CT	231 (30)	903 (45)			CT	290 (37)	765 (38)	
	CC	517 (66)	756 (38)			TT	44 (6)	129 (6)	
ARMS2/HTRA1(A69S)	GG	244 (31)	1164 (59)	<0.0001	FRK/COL10A1	CC	401 (52)	1046 (53)	0.73
	GT	368 (47)	701 (35)			CT	315 (41)	784 (40)	
	TT	165 (21)	123 (6)			TT	60 (8)	155 (8)	
C2 (E318D)	GG	748 (96)	1827 (92)	<0.0001	APOC1/APOE	AA	568 (73)	1422 (72)	0.41
	CG/CC	29 (4)	161 (8)			AG/GG	209 (27)	566 (28)	
CFB (R32Q)	CC	715 (93)	1615 (84)	<0.0001	TIMP3	AA	712 (92)	1774 (89)	0.06
	CT/TT	56 (7)	318 (16)			AC/CC	65 (8)	214 (11)	
C3 (R102G)	CC	386 (50)	1234 (62)	<0.0001	TNFRSF10A	TT	222 (29)	540 (27)	0.87
	CG	318 (41)	669 (34)			GT	373 (48)	1020 (51)	
	GG	73 (9)	84 (4)			GG	182 (23)	428 (22)	
CFI	CC	181 (23)	526 (26)	0.01	ADAMTS9/AS2**	CC	241 (31)	581 (29)	0.27
	CT	373 (48)	983 (50)			CT	375 (48)	964 (48)	
	TT	223 (29)	479 (24)			TT	161 (21)	443 (22)	
CETP	CC	310 (40)	880 (44)	0.003	SLC16A8	CC	493 (64)	1267 (64)	0.46
	AC	356 (46)	902 (45)			CT	241 (31)	641 (32)	
	AA	111 (14)	205 (10)			TT	43 (6)	80 (4)	
COL8A1	TT	594 (76)	1636 (82)	0.0004	DDR1	CC	546 (70)	1394 (70)	0.59
	CT	170 (22)	332 (17)			CT	218 (28)	540 (27)	
	CC	13 (2)	20 (1)			TT	13 (2)	54 (3)	
COL10A1	AA	292 (38)	715 (36)	0.06	TGFBR1	TT	463 (60)	1137 (57)	0.20
	AG	379 (49)	921 (46)			GT	271 (35)	722 (36)	
	GG	106 (14)	351 (18)			GG	43 (6)	129 (6)	
CFH R1210C	CC	769 (99)	1982 (99.7)	0.02	VEGFA	CC	150 (19)	451 (23)	0.06
	CT	8 (1)	6 (0.3)			CT	399 (51)	996 (50)	
RAD51B	AA	331 (43)	791 (40)	0.02		TT	228 (29)	540 (27)	
	AG	367 (47)	914 (46)		HSPH1/B3GALTL	TT	232 (30)	666 (34)	0.006
	GG	79 (10)	283 (14)			CT	369 (47)	963 (48)	
HSPH1/B3GALTL	TT	232 (30)	666 (34)	0.006		CC	176 (23)	359 (18)	
	CT	369 (47)	963 (48)						
	CC	176 (23)	359 (18)						

*Mantel-Haenszel Chi-Square.
**ADAMTS9/ADAMTS9-AS2.

intermediate AMD or stage 3 in the worse eye (drusen 125 microns or greater diameter, extensive intermediate drusen), stage 4 in one eye (advanced dry AMD with central or non-central geographic atrophy (GA), and stage 5 with advanced neovascular (NV) AMD in one eye at baseline. Both cohorts were classified using this system. Since category 3 patients in the original AREDS classification included non-central geographic atrophy and category 4 included both advanced forms of AMD as well as visual loss regardless of phenotype [8], we reclassified these groups independent of visual acuity level into CARMS grades 4 (GA) and 5 (NV) as described above.

Maximum drusen size within the grid (a 3000 micron radius centered on the fovea) at baseline was used to assess drusen phenotypes for eyes without advanced AMD. Drusen size was based on standard circles with diameters corresponding to 63 µm, 125 µm, and 250 µm. Drusen size was divided into the following categories: <63 µm, 63–124 µm, 125–249 µm, and ≥250 µm. AMD status and drusen size in eyes without AMD at baseline were evaluated.

Table 3. Associations between New Age-Related Macular Degeneration Genetic Loci and Incidence of Advanced Age-Related Macular Degeneration, Controlling for Demographic, Environmental, Ocular and Genetic Factors.

Gene: SNP (Reference Genotype)/Genotype		Model A*			Model B‡		
		HR 95% CI	p-value	p-trend	HR 95% CI	p-value	p-trend
CFI:rs10033900 (CC)	CT	1.0 (0.9–1.2)	0.78		1.1 (0.9–1.3)	0.45	
	TT	1.1 (0.9–1.3)	0.48	0.47	1.1 (0.9–1.3)	0.38	0.39
LIPC:rs10468017 (CC)	CT	1.1 (0.9–1.2)	0.51		1.0 (0.9–1.2)	0.65	
	TT	1.1 (0.8–1.3)	0.42	0.35	1.1 (0.8–1.5)	0.40	0.41
CETP: rs3764261 (CC)	AC	1.1 (0.9–1.2)	0.48		1.0 (0.9–1.2)	0.56	
	AA	1.1 (0.9–1.4)	0.29	0.27	1.2 (0.9–1.4)	0.19	0.21
ABCA1: rs1883025 (CC)	CT	1.1 (0.9–1.2)	0.46		1.1 (0.9–1.2)	0.35	
	TT	1.0 (0.7–1.3)	0.75	0.78	0.9 (0.6–1.2)	0.32	0.95
TIMP3: rs9621532 (AA)	AC/CC	0.8 (0.6–1.0)	0.07	–	0.8 (0.6–1.0)	0.11	-
COL8A1:rs13095226 (TT)	CT	1.2 (1.0–1.4)	0.09		1.1 (0.9–1.3)	0.21	
	CC	1.9 (1.1–3.3)	0.02	0.02	1.9 (1.1–3.3)	0.02	0.04
FRK/COL10A1: rs1999930 (CC)	CT	1.1 (0.9–1.2)	0.45		1.0 (0.9–1.2)	0.93	
	TT	1.0 (0.7–1.3)	0.83	0.78	0.9 (0.7–1.2)	0.71	0.83
COL10A1: rs1064583 (AA)	AG	1.1 (0.9–1.3)	0.29		1.1 (0.9–1.3)	0.35	
	GG	0.8 (0.7–1.0)	0.13	0.36	0.8 (0.7–1.0)	0.10	0.28
VEGFA: rs943080 (CC)	CT	1.1 (0.9–1.3)	0.30		1.1 (0.9–1.3)	0.38	
	TT	1.0 (0.8–1.2)	0.72	0.54	1.0 (0.8–1.2)	0.96	0.82
TNFRSF10A: rs13278062 (TT)	GT	1.0 (0.8–1.2)	0.91		1.0 (0.8–1.2)	0.74	
	GG	1.2 (1.0–1.4)	0.11	0.14	1.1 (0.9–1.4)	0.22	0.27
CFH R1210C:rs121913059 (CC)	CT	1.4 (0.7–2.9)	0.31	–	2.4 (1.2–4.9)	0.02	–
APOC1/APOE: rs4420638 (AA)	AG/GG	1.0 (0.9–1.2)	0.80	–	1.0 (0.8–1.2)	0.94	–
DDR1:rs3094111 (CC)	CT	1.1 (0.9–1.3)	0.40		1.1 (0.9–1.3)	0.31	
	TT	0.9 (0.5–1.6)	0.82	0.54	1.1 (0.6–1.9)	0.77	0.32
SLC16A8: rs8135665 (CC)	CT	1.0 (0.9–1.2)	0.58		1.1 (0.9–1.2)	0.51	
	TT	1.2 (0.9–1.7)	0.23	0.25	1.2 (0.9–1.6)	0.29	0.27
TGFBR1: rs334353 (TT)	GT	1.0 (0.9–1.2)	0.85		1.0 (0.9–1.2)	0.98	
	GG	1.0 (0.8–1.4)	0.86	0.81	1.0 (0.7–1.4)	0.93	0.94
RAD51B: rs8017304 (AA)	AG	0.9 (0.7–0.99)	0.04		0.9 (0.7–0.99)	0.04	
	GG	0.7 (0.6–0.96)	0.02	0.007	0.8 (0.6–0.98)	0.04	0.01
ADAMTS9/AS2**: rs6795735 (CC)	CT	1.0 (0.8–1.1)	0.89		1.0 (0.8–1.1)	0.73	
	TT	0.9 (0.8–1.3)	0.51	0.70	0.9 (0.8–1.1)	0.49	0.83
HSPH1/B3GALTL: rs9542236 (TT)	CT	1.2 (1.0–1.4)	0.03		1.1 (1.0–1.3)	0.17	
	CC	1.2 (1.0–1.5)	0.06	0.04	1.1 (0.9–1.3)	0.40	0.33

*Model A = Controlling for: age, gender, education, body mass index, smoking, 4 treatment groups, baseline macular grade and drusen status.
‡Model B = Controlling for: age, gender, education, body mass index, smoking, 4 treatment groups, baseline macular grade, drusen status, CFHrs1410996, CFH Y402H, ARMS2/HTRA1, C3, C2 and CFB.
**ADAMTS9/ADAMTS9-AS2.

Progression was defined as either eye progressing from a stage 1, 2 or 3 to either stage 4 or stage 5 at any follow-up visit to the end of the study within each individual. In a subgroup analysis we classified progressors to each advanced stage of AMD separately as progression to GA and progression to NV. Time to progression was recorded for the first eye to progress if both eyes were at risk, and for the fellow eye if one eye was at risk. Individuals were considered progressors if a) there was no advanced AMD in either eye at baseline and they developed advanced AMD in at least one eye during follow-up, or b) they had advanced AMD in one eye at baseline and progressed to advanced AMD in the fellow eye

during follow-up. For subjects in group "a" above, we controlled for baseline grade in each eye and evaluated the time to progression in each eye and used the earlier of the two progression times if both eyes progressed at different times. For subjects in group "b" above, we controlled for AMD category in the affected eye at baseline (i.e., CARMS grades 4 and 5), AMD grade in the non-advanced eye at baseline, and evaluated the time to progress in the fellow eye. Demographic and risk factor data, including education, smoking history, and body mass index (BMI), were obtained at the baseline visit from questionnaires and height and weight measurements.

Table 4. Multivariate Associations Between Genes and Progression to Advanced Age-Related Macular Degeneration.

Gene: SNP/Genotype		6 Gene Model*			9 Gene Model‡		
		HR 95% CI	p-value	p-trend	HR 95% CI	p-value	p-trend
CFH:rs1061170 (Y402H)	TT	1.0 (ref.)			1.0 (ref.)		
	CT	1.1 (0.9–1.3)	0.63		1.1 (0.9–1.4)	0.40	
	CC	1.2 (0.9–1.5)	0.31	0.29	1.2 (0.9–1.5)	0.25	0.26
CFH:rs1410996	TT	1.0 (ref.)			1.0 (ref.)		
	CT	2.0 (1.3–3.0)	0.002		1.9 (1.2–2.9)	0.004	
	CC	2.4 (1.6–3.8)	<0.0001	0.0002	2.4 (1.5–3.7)	0.0001	0.0001
ARMS2/HTRA1:rs10490924(A69S)	GG	1.0 (ref.)			1.0 (ref.)		
	GT	1.3 (1.1–1.6)	0.001		1.3 (1.1–1.6)	0.0008	
	TT	1.8 (1.5–2.3)	<0.0001	<0.0001	1.9 (1.5–2.3)	<0.0001	<0.0001
C2:rs9332739(E318D)	GG	1.0 (ref.)			1.0 (ref.)		
	CG/CC	0.7 (0.5–1.0)	0.05	–	0.7 (0.5–1.0)	0.06	–
CFB:rs641153(R32Q)	CC	1.0 (ref.)			1.0 (ref.)		
	CT/TT	0.7 (0.5–0.9)	0.004	–	0.7 (0.5–0.9)	0.006	–
C3:rs2230199(R102G)	CC	1.0 (ref.)			1.0 (ref.)		
	CG	1.1 (1.0–1.3)	0.19		1.1 (1.0–1.3)	0.13	
	GG	1.4 (1.1–1.8)	0.01	0.01	1.4 (1.1–1.8)	0.009	0.006
COL8A1:rs13095226	TT	–	–		1.0 (ref.)		
	CT	–	–		1.1 (0.9–1.3)	0.21	
	CC	–	–		2.0 (1.1–3.5)	0.02	0.04
CFH R1210C:rs121913059	CC	–	–		1.0 (ref.)		
	CT	–	–		2.5 (1.2–5.3)	0.01	–
RAD51B: rs8017304	AA	–	–		1.0 (ref.)		
	AG	–	–		0.9 (0.7–1.0)	0.05	
	GG	–	–		0.8(0.6–0.97)	0.03	0.01

*6 Gene Model = Controlling for: age, gender, education, body mass index, smoking, baseline macular grade, drusen status, 4 treatment groups, CFH rs1410996, CFHY402H, ARMS2/HTRA1, C2,C3 and CFB genes.
‡9 Gene Model = Controlling for: age, gender, education, body mass index, smoking, baseline macular grade, drusen status, 4 treatment groups and all genes in the table.

Genotype Data

Common single nucleotide polymorphisms (SNPs) associated with AMD were evaluated 1) Complement Factor H (CFH) Y402H (rs1061170) [10], 2) CFH rs1410996, an independently associated single nucleotide polymorphism (SNP) variant within intron 14 of CFH [11], 3) ARMS2/HTRA1 (rs10490924) [12–14], 4) Complement component 2 or C2 E318D (rs9332739) [11,15], 5) Complement Factor B or CFB R32Q (rs641153) [11,15], 6) Complement component 3 or C3 R102G (rs2230199) [16,17], 7) complement factor I, or CFI (rs10033900), an independently associated SNP located in the linkage peak region of chromosome 4, 2781 base pairs upstream of the 3′ untranslated region of CFI [18], and 8) hepatic lipase C, or LIPC (rs10468017), a promoter variant on chromosome 15q22 [4], 9) Cholesteryl ester transfer protein, or CETP (rs3764261) [4,19], 10) ATP-binding cassette subfamily A member 1, or ABCA1 (rs1883025) [4,19] 11) TIMP metalloproteinase inhibitor 3, or TIMP3 (rs9621532) [4,19], 12) Collagen type VIII, alpha1 or COL8A1(rs13095226) [4,5], 13) FRK/COL10A1 rs199930 [4,5], 14) Collagen, type X, alpha 1 or COL10A1 (rs1064583) [5,6], 15) Vascular endothelial growth factor A, or VEGFA (rs943080) [5], 16) Tumor necrosis factor receptor superfamily, member 10a or TNFRSF10A (rs13278062 [6,7], 17) Apolipoprotein E and Apolipoprotein C- I or APOE/

APOC1 rs4420638 [6,20,21], 18) Discodin domain receptor tyrosine kinase 1, or DDR1 (rs3094111) [6], 19) Solute carrier family 16, member 8 (monocarboxylic acid transporter 3or SLC16A8 (rs8135665) [6], 20) Transforming growth factor, beta receptor 1 or TGFBR1 (rs334353) [6], 21) RAD51 homolog B (S. cerevisiae) or RAD51B (rs8017304) [6], 22) ADAM metallopeptidase with thrombospondin type 1 motif [6]; ADAMTS9 antisense RNA 2 (non-protein coding) or ADAMTS9/ADAMTS9-AS2 (rs6795735) [6] 23) Beta 1,3- galactosyltransferase -like or B3GALTL (rs9542236) [6]. The rare variant in CFH, R1210C rs121913059 was also evaluated [3].

Statistical Analyses

Analyses were performed using the Cox proportional hazards model to evaluate relationships between progression of AMD and the following variables: genotypes, age (<65, 65–74, 75+), gender, education (high school or less, more than high school), cigarette smoking (never, past, current), and BMI, which was calculated as the weight in kilograms divided by the square of the height in meters (<25, 25–29.9, and 30+), baseline stage of AMD and drusen characteristics in both eyes. Hazard ratios (HRs) and 95% confidence intervals (CI) were calculated for demographic, behavioral, ocular and genetic factors. The method for calculating

Table 5. 9 Gene Model for Geographic Atrophy and Neovascular Disease.

Gene: SNP/Genotype		Geographic Atrophy (N = 416)**			Neovascular Disease (N = 527)**		
		HR 95% CI*	p-value	p-trend	HR 95% CI*	p-value	p-trend
CFH:rs1061170 (Y402H)	TT	1.0 (ref)			1.0 (ref)		
	CT	1.08(0.78–1.5)	0.63		1.31(0.97–1.76)	0.08	
	CC	1.27(0.87–1.84)	0.22	0.19	1.26(0.9–1.76)	0.17	0.33
CFH:rs1410996	TT	1.0 (ref)			1.0 (ref)		
	CT	1.52(0.89–2.6)	0.13		1.77(1.01–3.1)	0.047	
	CC	1.69(0.96–2.99)	0.07	0.11	2.45(1.37–4.38)	0.002	<0.001
ARMS2/HTRA1:rs10490924(A69S)	GG	1.0 (ref)			1.0 (ref)		
	GT	1.39(1.1–1.75)	0.005		1.43(1.16–1.76)	<0.001	
	TT	1.74(1.3–2.32)	<0.001	<0.001	1.94(1.5–2.49)	<0.0001	<0.0001
C2:rs9332739(E318D)	GG	1.0 (ref)			1.0 (ref)		
	CG/CC	0.61(0.33–1.11)	0.11	0.10	0.78(0.5–1.21)	0.26	0.21
CFB:rs641153(R32Q)	CC	1.0 (ref)			1.0 (ref)		
	CT/TT	0.68(0.46–1.0)	0.050	0.06	0.62(0.44–0.88)	0.008	0.009
C3:rs2230199(R102G)	CC	1.0 (ref)			1.0 (ref)		
	CG	1.1(0.89–1.35)	0.39		1.13(0.94–1.36)	0.20	
	GG	1.26(0.87–1.83)	0.23	0.16	1.42(1.05–1.93)	0.026	0.021
COL8A1:rs13095226	TT	1.0 (ref)			1.0 (ref)		
	CT	1.05(0.83–1.34)	0.67		1.27(1.03–1.56)	0.025	
	CC	2.02(0.99–4.15)	0.055	0.24	1.61(0.79–3.24)	0.19	0.016
CFH R1210C:rs121913059	CC	1.0 (ref)			1.0 (ref)		
	CT	3.12(1.33–7.29)	0.009	0.006	3.09(1.33–7.19)	0.008	0.001
RAD51B: rs8017304	AA	1.0 (ref)			1.0 (ref)		
	AG	0.91(0.73–1.12)	0.36		0.90(0.76–1.08)	0.28	
	GG	0.96(0.68–1.34)	0.79	0.49	0.67(0.49–0.92)	0.013	0.016

*Controlling for: Age, gender, education, body mass index, smoking, baseline macular grade, drusen status, 4 treatment groups and all genes in the table.
**Some individuals progressed to Geographic Atrophy in one eye and Neovascular Disease in the fellow eye.

the AMD progression risk score and gene risk score based on regression coefficients of all demographic, environmental, genetic and ocular factors, has been reported previously [22–24].

Survival analysis was used to determine 5-year and 10-year cumulative incidence rates of AMD and the advanced AMD subtypes for individual subjects according to various risk factor levels at baseline. To assess discrimination, the AUC (area under the ROC, or receiver operating curve) was obtained for progression within 5 years and progression within 10 years. In addition, an age-adjusted concordance or "C" statistic based on

Table 6. Area Under the Curve Statistics for Progression to Advanced Age-Related Macular Degeneration, Geographic Atrophy and Neovascular Disease at 5 and 10 Years After Baseline.

	AUC (SE)	AUC (SE)	AUC (SE)	p-value	p-value
	0 Gene Model	6 Gene Model	9 Gene Model	6 vs 9 Gene Model	0 vs 9 Gene Model
5 Year					
All advanced AMD	0.873 (0.009)	0.883 (0.008)	0.884 (0.008)	0.24	0.01
Geographic Atrophy	0.886 (0.012)	0.892 (0.012)	0.893 (0.012)	0.64	0.12
Neovascular Disease	0.860 (0.012)	0.875 (0.011)	0.876 (0.011)	0.30	0.02
10 Year					
All advanced AMD	0.898 (0.007)	0.910 (0.006)	0.911 (0.006)	0.56	0.001
Geographic Atrophy	0.914 (0.009)	0.921 (0.008)	0.920 (0.008)	0.90	0.02
Neovascular Disease	0.879 (0.009)	0.896 (0.009)	0.897(0.009)	0.43	0.001

SE = Standard Error.

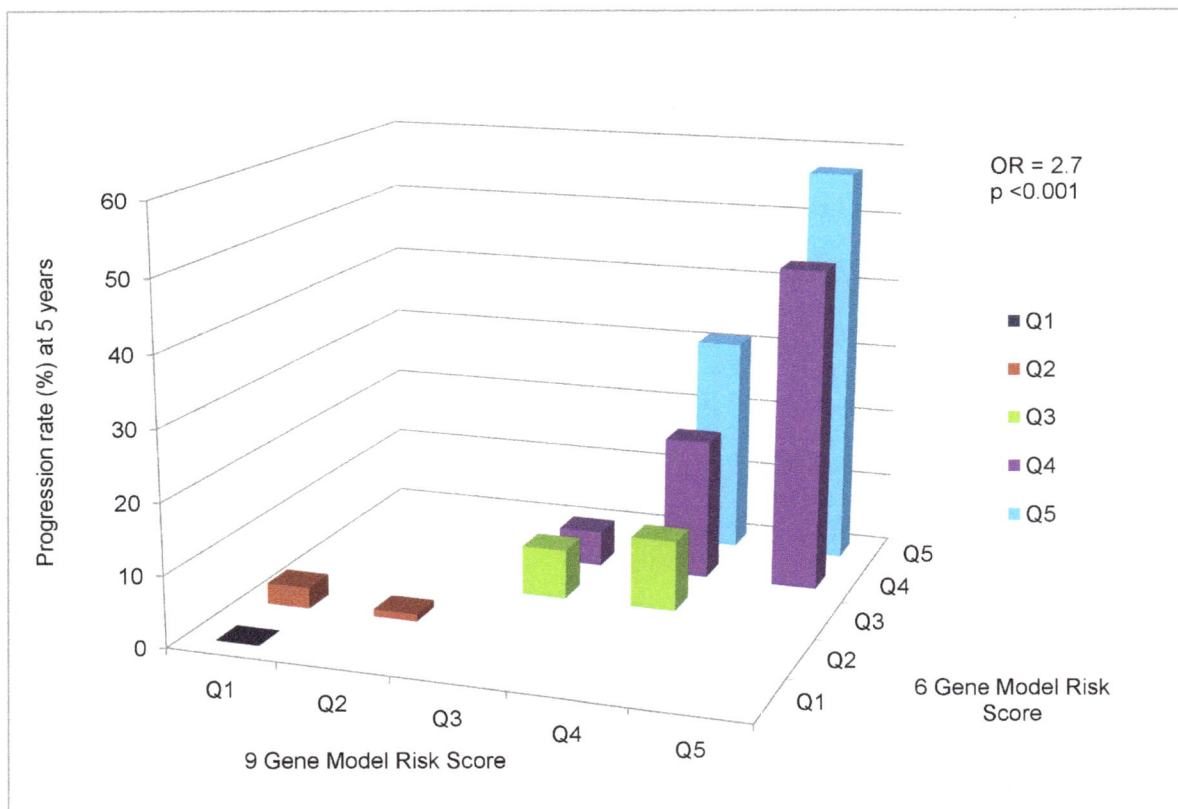

Figure 1. Cross-Classification of Progression Rates to Advanced AMD: 9 Gene Model vs 6 Gene Model. Cross-classification of subjects by risk score quintile for 9 and 6 gene models, with estimated progression rates for each combination of a 9 gene quintile by 6 gene quintile. OR = odds ratio of progression per one quintile increase in 9 gene model, holding 6 gene model quintile constant.

the curve was calculated to assess the probability that the risk score based on the group of risk factors in that model from a random progressor was higher than the corresponding risk score from a random non-progressor within the same 10-year age group [25]. Confidence limits were obtained and C statistics were compared between competing models [26].

To assess the added value of a model with genes vs. models with fewer or no genes, we calculated quintiles of risk score according to each model and cross-classified the quintile of risk score derived from one model by quintile of risk score derived from the other. We then ran a logistic regression of progression within 5 years (yes/no) on risk score quintile of the zero gene model (treated as a categorical variable with regression coefficients β_1, β_2, β_3, β_4) and the 9 gene model risk score quintile, expressed as an ordinal variable with values 1 to 5 with regression coefficient γ. The odds ratio (OR) of progression to advanced AMD per one unit increase in quintile of the 9 gene model risk score, holding the risk score quintile of the zero gene model constant, was measured by exp (γ). A similar approach was used to assess the added value of the 9 gene model vs the 6 gene model.

Results

Among 2765 individuals, there were 777 progressors to advanced stages of AMD in either eye, and 1988 non-progressors. Among the progressors, 416 progressed to GA in at least one eye and 527 progressed to NV in at least one eye. The mean ages (±

SD) of progressors and non-progressors at baseline were 70.2 (±5.2) and 68.2 (±4.7).

Table 1 displays the multivariate associations between baseline demographic, environmental and macular variables and incident advanced AMD. Increasing age, current smoking and higher BMI were related to progression. Advanced AMD in one eye and larger drusen size in the fellow eye, as well as larger drusen size in both eyes among individuals without advanced AMD at baseline were strongly related to higher rates of conversion from early and intermediate to advanced stages of AMD.

The distributions of genetic variants among progressors and non-progressors are shown in **Table 2**. There were significant and positive associations between progression and the number of risk alleles for *CFH Y402H*, *CFH* rs1410996, *ARMS2/HTRA1* and *C3*. In addition there were protective effects for the minor alleles of *C2* and *CFB*. We found significant positive associations with risk alleles for *CFI*, *CETP*, and *HSPH1/B3GALTL*, and a significant protective association for the minor allele of *RAD51B*. Furthermore, there were borderline positive associations with *VEGFA* (P = .06) and borderline protective associations for *COL10A1* and *TIMP3* (P = .06). No significant associations with progression to advanced AMD were found for *LIPC*, *ABCA1*, *TNFRSF10A*, *APOC1/APOE*, *DDR1*, *SLC16A8*, *TGFBR1*, and *ADAMTS9* in these analyses.

Table 3 displays the multivariate associations between incident AMD and the novel gene variants in two models: A) adjusted for demographic, environmental and macular variables, and B) controlling for the 6 genetic variants in 5 genes (referred to herein

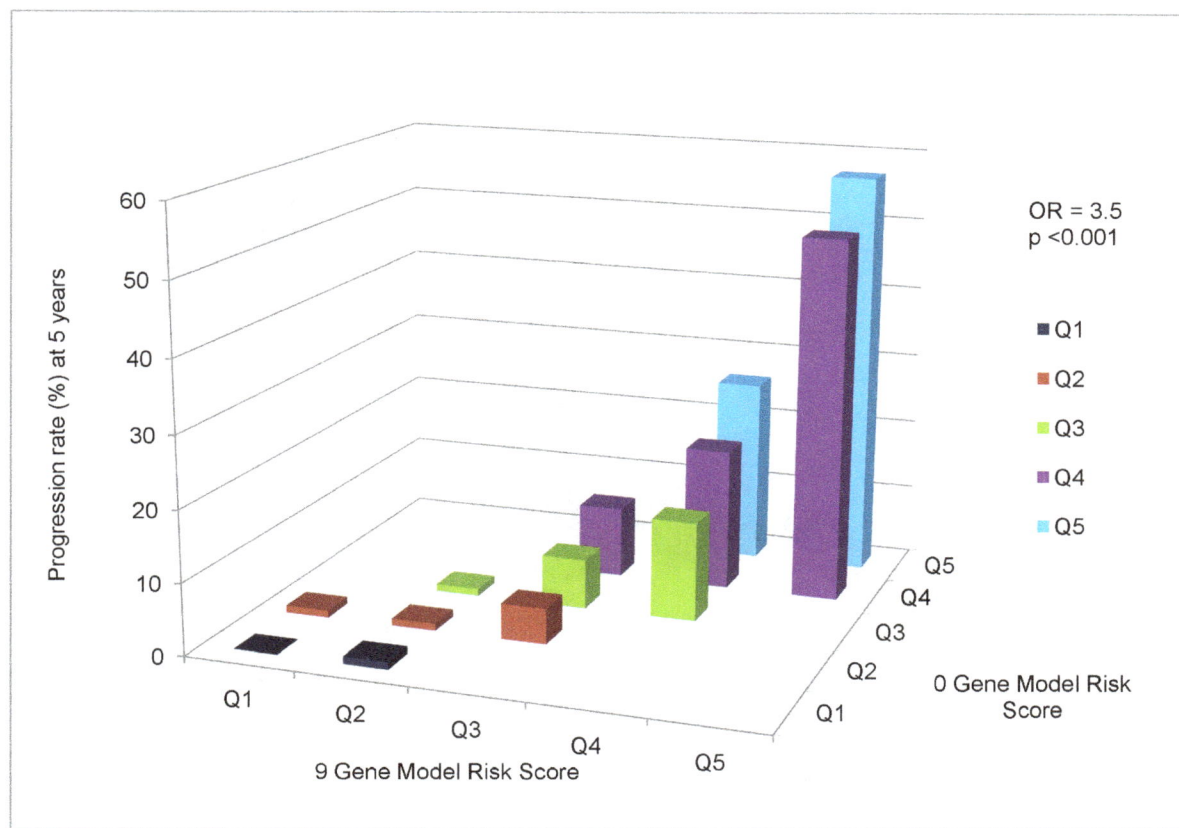

Figure 2. Cross-Classification of Progression Rates to Advanced AMD: 9 Gene Model vs 0 Gene Model. Cross-classification of subjects by risk score quintile for 9 and 0 gene models, with estimated progression rates for each combination of a 9 gene quintile by 0 gene quintile. OR = odds ratio of progression per one quintile increase in 9 gene model, holding 0 gene model quintile constant.

as the "6 gene model"), in addition to the non-genetic variables in Model A. In Model B, *COL8A1* (CC vs TT, HR = 1.9, P = .02, P trend = 0.04), *CFH R1210C* (HR 2.4, P = .02) and *RAD51B* (GG vs AA, HR 0.80, P = .04, P trend = 0.01), were significantly related to AMD progression to advanced stages independent of the other variables.

Table 4 shows two models: 1) the 6 gene model in our previous prediction paper [22–24], with multivariate associations between incident advanced AMD and the genetic variants adjusted for demographic, environmental, and macular phenotypes, and 2) the 9 gene model (9 genetic loci in 7 genes, herein referred to as the "9 gene model") with the addition of the 3 significant genetic loci identified in Table 3, mutually adjusted for each other as well as the other 6 genetic loci. We found independent effects of the variants in *COL8A1* (CC vs TT, HR = 2.0, P = .02, P trend = 0.04), *CFH R1210C* (CT vs CC, HR = 2.5, P = .01), and *RAD51B* (GG vs AA, HR = 0.80, P = .03, P trend = 0.01).

Table 5 depicts similar analyses for progression to GA and NV separately. Associations with some genetic variants were somewhat stronger for NV than GA, although HR's were in the same direction generally for both phenotypes, except for *RAD51B* which was not related to GA.

In **Table 6**, we estimated the AUC's corrected for age for gene models predicting progression at 5 years and 10 years. For 5 year progression, the AUC's were as follows: 0 gene model 0.873, 6 gene model 0.883, 9 gene model 0.884; P = 0.01 for 0 gene vs 9 gene model and P = 0.24 for 9 gene vs 6 gene model. Similarly, for 10 year progression, AUC's were 0.898, 0.910, and 0.911 for the

0, 6, and 9 gene models, respectively, with P = 0.001 for the 9 vs 0 gene model comparison of the AUC's but no significant difference in AUC's for the 9 vs 6 gene model. Changes in AUC's for the 9 gene vs 0 gene models were somewhat larger for NV than GA for both 5 and 10 year progression.

Previous studies in a variety of settings have revealed that the AUC is a relatively insensitive statistic for identifying improvement in model fit [27]. An alternative approach is provided by reclassification models where risk is cross-classified simultaneously for level of risk predicted by 2 different competing models. For this purpose we cross-classified subjects by risk score derived from the models and divided into quintiles (Q) and estimated rates of progression for each combination of a 6 gene risk score quintile by a 9 gene risk score quintile. The results are displayed in **Figure 1**. Qualitatively it appears, especially for high risk individuals (risk score Q4 and Q5), while holding the 6 gene model risk score quintile constant, there is an increasing progression rate as the 9 gene risk score quintile increases. Little additional information is provided for low risk individuals (Q1 and Q2). Overall, the OR per risk score quintile increase in the 9 gene model controlling for the 6 gene model risk score quintile was 2.7 (95% CI 1.7–4.4) P<0.001, indicating that significant additional information regarding progression is provided by the 9 gene model compared to the 6 gene model.

Given the ongoing discussion of the value in adding genetic information to predictive models, we also compared the model with 9 genetic loci to the model without genes (0 gene model) as shown in **Figure 2**. There are larger differences between the 9

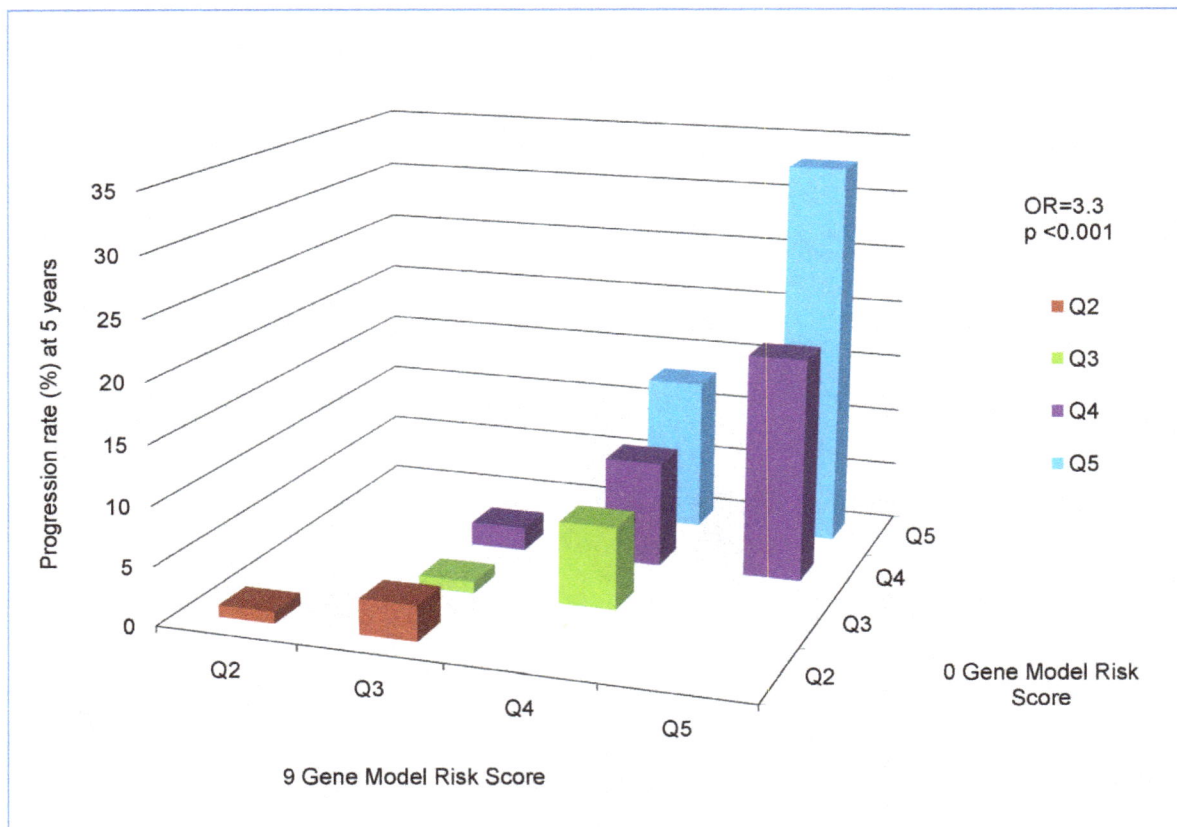

Figure 3. Cross-Classification of Progression Rates to Geographic Atrophy: 9 Gene Model vs 0 Gene Model. Cross-classification of subjects progressing to Geographic Atrophy by risk score quintile for 9 and 0 gene models, with estimated progression rates for each combination of a 9 gene quintile by 0 gene quintile. OR = odds ratio of progression per one quintile increase in 9 gene model, holding 0 gene model quintile constant.

gene vs the 0 gene model than between the 9 gene vs 6 gene models. There are large differences in progression rate as the 9 gene model risk score quintile increases, when holding the 0 gene model risk score quintile constant, for the highest risk individuals (i.e. Q4 and Q5 in the 0 gene model). For intermediate risk individuals (Q2 and Q3) for the 0 gene model, there are also discernible increases in progression rates as the 9 gene model risk score quintile increases. However, little added value is apparent for the lowest risk quintile (Q1) for the 9 gene loci vs 0 gene model. The OR per quintile increase in the 9 gene model controlling for the 0 gene model was 3.5 (95% CI 2.6–4.6), P<0.001, indicating that significant additional information is obtained by including genes in the predictive model.

In **Figures 3 and 4**, we depict the comparison of the 9 gene vs 0 gene models for progression at 5 years to GA and NV separately. The major incremental precision obtained from including 9 genes in the prediction model is obtained from subjects at high risk in the 0 gene model (i.e. Q4 and Q5), with smaller increments for intermediate risk subjects (Q3) and little benefit for low risk individuals (Q1 and Q2). The OR's are 3.3, P<0.001 for GA (**Figure 3**), and 3.1, P<0.001 for NV (**Figure 4**).

Discussion

To our knowledge this is the first report on the independent associations between R1210C in *CFH*, *COL8A1* and *RAD51B* and progression to advanced AMD, controlling for all known AMD

genetic loci. The AUC's for the 9 gene vs 0 gene models were significantly different but were similar for the 9 and 6 gene models. To further discriminate between the two models which included genes, we used a re-classification approach, which is novel for AMD risk models, but has been used in other settings [27]. Cross classifying quintile of risk in the 9 gene by 6 gene models, holding the 6 gene model constant, demonstrated an increased risk of progression in the 4th and 5th quintiles of the risk score, indicating that incorporating a larger number of independent AMD genetic loci enhanced predictive power. Using a similar approach, larger increases in predictive accuracy were apparent for the model with 9 genes compared to none.

Our first prediction models for advanced AMD beginning in 2006 included only genes [11], a model with environmental and demographic variables only (AUC 0.62), and a model that included *CFHY402H* genotype (AUC 0.74) [28]. These early models demonstrated the importance of genetic variants in predicting AMD risk. When *ARMS2/HTRA1* was added to the genetic model with *CFHY402H* along with demographic and environmental factors, the AUC increased moderately to 0.78 [29]. The first multi-gene prediction model with 6 loci in 5 genes in addition to demographic and environmental factors, increased the C statistic to 0.83, adding to the evidence that genetic susceptibility plays a large role in predicting AMD risk [22]. The addition of macular phenotype and baseline AMD grade to the genetic and environmental models increased the AUC to 0.89 [23]. Other prediction models include our Markov model of

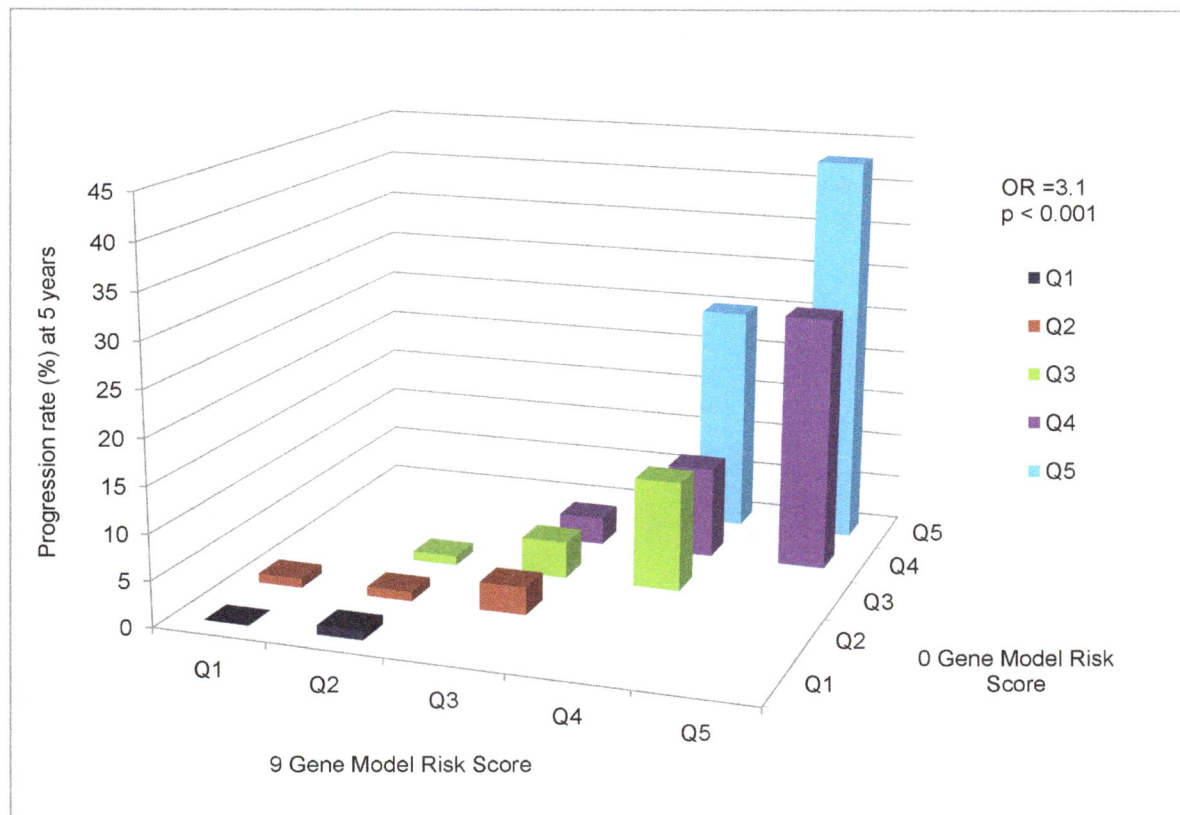

Figure 4. Cross-Classification of Progression Rates to Neovascular Disease: 9 Gene Model vs 0 Gene Model. Cross-classification of subjects progressing to Neovascular Disease by risk score quintile for 9 and 0 gene models, with estimated progression rates for each combination of a 9 gene quintile by 0 gene quintile. OR = odds ratio of progression per one quintile increase in 9 gene model, holding 0 gene model quintile constant.

transitions within different stages of AMD and inclusion of plasma complement levels in the model [30,31]. The Markov model included *CFH, ARMS2, C2, CFB, C3, CFI* and genes in the cholesterol and collagen pathways (*LIPC, CETP, COL8A1*) in addition to drusen phenotypes, demographic, and environmental characteristics. The 5 year AUC in that model was 0.88 [30]. The addition of complement plasma markers to a model in a case-control study, together with 6 complement pathway loci, *ARMS2/HTRA1*, demographic and environmental characteristics increased the C-statistic to 0.94 [31].

AUC is a reasonable measure of discrimination for a risk prediction rule and by definition is based on the relative order of risk between progressors and non-progressors. However, it does not take into account the magnitude of the differences in risk. Thus, it does not provide all the information in determination of risk. In populations dominated by low risk individuals, there are ways to re-classify higher risk subjects to obtain a more accurate risk profile. Cook et al. demonstrated this in the Women's Health Study population assessing cardiovascular risk in models with and without hsCRP [27]. In that study, hsCRP had little effect on the C-statistic. However, if one cross-classifies subjects by risk level with and without hsCRP, individuals in the low and medium risk groups (5–10% and 10–20% 10 year Framingham risk) were reclassified (21% and 19% of the time, respectively) into different risk groups [27]. Rosner et al. used a similar approach for cross-classifying breast cancer risk scores with and without estradiol [32]. Similar to the hsCRP study, the AUC did not increase

substantially with the addition of estradiol. However, when risk deciles in the estradiol and non-estradiol models were cross-classified, there was an estimated 67% increase in breast cancer incidence for an increase of one decile of risk for the estradiol model holding the non-estradiol model decile constant [32]. In our study of macular degeneration, 5–10% of subjects were reclassified into a different quintile for the 9 gene vs 6 gene models, and 15–30% of subjects were reclassified for the 9 vs 0 gene models, indicating an improvement in model accuracy with the addition of genetic variants.

The mechanisms by which *CFH* R1210C, *COL8A1*, and *RAD51B* genes are related to the development and progression of advanced AMD are being explored. The R1210C mutation has been shown to compromise portions of the complement cascade resulting in defective binding to C3d, C3b, heparin and endothelial cells [3]. The *COL8A1* gene, encodes one of the two alpha chains of type VIII collagen, a major component of the multiple basement membranes in the eye, including Bruch's membrane and the choroidal stroma [4,33]. The protein encoded by *RAD51B* is a member of the RAD51 protein family, and is essential for DNA repair mechanisms. This gene is also involved in cell cycle delay and apoptosis [34].

Conclusions

We have presented a model with 9 common and rare predictive genetic loci for progression to advanced stages of AMD that adds more predictive power than either a model with 6 common genetic loci or a model without any genetic information. New rare and highly penetrant loci in addition to the rare variant *CFH* R1210C [3,35] and several common loci included here, may further improve the accuracy of AMD risk models. Our models can be used for clinical research such as selecting individuals at high risk for increased surveillance and for inclusion in clinical trials of new therapies [23], and for assessing different responses to AMD treatments based on the risk score.

Acknowledgments

Presented at Association for Research in Vision and Ophthalmology, Seattle, WA, May 9, 2013, and American Academy of Ophthalmology, New Orleans, LA, November 17, 2013.

Author Contributions

Conceived and designed the experiments: JS BR. Performed the experiments: JS BR. Analyzed the data: JS BR. Contributed reagents/materials/analysis tools: JS BR. Wrote the paper: JS BR YY RR.

References

1. Seddon JM, Cote J, Page WF, Aggen SH, Neale MC (2005) The US twin study of age-related macular degeneration: relative roles of genetic and environmental influences. Arch Ophthalmol 123: 321–327.
2. Lim LS, Mitchell P, Seddon JM, Holz FG, Wong TY (2012) Age-related macular degeneration. Lancet 379: 1728–1738.
3. Raychaudhuri S, Iartchouk O, Chin K, Tan PL, Tai AK, et al. (2011) A rare penetrant mutation in CFH confers high risk of age-related macular degeneration. Nat Genet 43: 1232–1236.
4. Neale BM, Fagerness J, Reynolds R, Sobrin L, Parker M, et al. (2010) Genome-wide association study of advanced age-related macular degeneration identifies a role of the hepatic lipase gene (LIPC). Proc Natl Acad Sci U S A 107: 7395–7400.
5. Yu Y, Bhangale TR, Fagerness J, Ripke S, Thorleifsson G, et al. (2011) Common variants near FRK/COL10A1 and VEGFA are associated with advanced age-related macular degeneration. Hum Mol Genet 20: 3699–3709.
6. Fritsche LG, Chen W, Schu M, Yaspan BL, Yu Y, et al. (2013) Seven new loci associated with age-related macular degeneration. Nat Genet 45: 433–439, 439e431–432.
7. Arakawa S, Takahashi A, Ashikawa K, Hosono N, Aoi T, et al. (2011) Genome-wide association study identifies two susceptibility loci for exudative age-related macular degeneration in the Japanese population. Nat Genet 43: 1001–1004.
8. (2001) A randomized, placebo-controlled, clinical trial of high-dose supplementation with vitamins C and E, beta carotene, and zinc for age-related macular degeneration and vision loss: AREDS report no. 8. Arch Ophthalmol 119: 1417–1436.
9. Seddon JM, Sharma S, Adelman RA (2006) Evaluation of the clinical age-related maculopathy staging system. Ophthalmology 113: 260–266.
10. Klein RJ, Zeiss C, Chew EY, Tsai J-Y, Sackler RS, et al. (2005) Complement factor H polymorphism in age-related macular degeneration. Science 308: 385–389.
11. Maller J, George S, Purcell S, Fagerness J, Altshuler D, et al. (2006) Common variation in three genes, including a noncoding variant in CFH, strongly influences risk of age-related macular degeneration. Nat Genet 38: 1055–1059.
12. Jakobsdottir J, Conley YP, Weeks DE, Mah TS, Ferrell RE, et al. (2005) Susceptibility genes for age-related maculopathy on chromosome 10q26. Am J Hum Genet 77: 389–407.
13. Rivera A, Fisher SA, Fritsche LG, Keilhauer CN, Lichtner P, et al. (2005) Hypothetical LOC387715 is a second major susceptibility gene for age-related macular degeneration, contributing independently of complement factor H to disease risk. Hum Mol Genet 14: 3227–3236.
14. DeWan A, Liu M, Hartman S, Zhang SS-M, Liu DT, et al. (2006) HTRA1 promoter polymorphism in wet age-related macular degeneration. Science 314: 989–992.
15. Gold B, Merriam JE, Zernant J, Hancox LS, Taiber AJ, et al. (2006) Variation in factor B (BF) and complement component 2 (C2) genes is associated with age-related macular degeneration. Nat Genet 38: 458–462.
16. Maller JB, Fagerness JA, Reynolds RC, Neale BM, Daly MJ, et al. (2007) Variation in complement factor 3 is associated with risk of age-related macular degeneration. Nat Genet 39: 1200–1201.
17. Yates JR, Sepp T, Matharu BK, Khan JC, Thurlby DA, et al. (2007) Complement C3 variant and the risk of age-related macular degeneration. N Engl J Med 357: 553–561.
18. Fagerness JA, Maller JB, Neale BM, Reynolds RC, Daly MJ, et al. (2009) Variation near complement factor I is associated with risk of advanced AMD. Eur J Hum Genet 17: 100–104.
19. Chen W, Stambolian D, Edwards AO, Branham KE, Othman M, et al. (2010) Genetic variants near TIMP3 and high-density lipoprotein-associated loci influence susceptibility to age-related macular degeneration. Proc Natl Acad Sci U S A 107: 7401–7406.
20. Klaver CC, Kliffen M, van Duijn CM, Hofman A, Cruts M, et al. (1998) Genetic association of apolipoprotein E with age-related macular degeneration. Am J Hum Genet 63: 200–206.
21. Souied EH, Benlian P, Amouyel P, Feingold J, Lagarde J-P, et al. (1998) The γ e4 allele of the apolipoprotein E gene as a potential protective factor for exudative age-related macular degeneration. Am J Ophthalmol 125: 353–359.
22. Seddon JM, Reynolds R, Maller J, Fagerness JA, Daly MJ, et al. (2009) Prediction model for prevalence and incidence of advanced age-related macular degeneration based on genetic, demographic, and environmental variables. Invest Ophthalmol Vis Sci 50: 2044–2053.
23. Seddon JM, Reynolds R, Yu Y, Daly MJ, Rosner B (2011) Risk models for progression to advanced age-related macular degeneration using demographic, environmental, genetic, and ocular factors. Ophthalmology 118: 2203–2211.
24. Seddon JM, Reynolds R, Yu Y, Rosner B (2013) Validation of a prediction algorithm for progression to advanced macular degeneration subtypes. JAMA Ophthalmol 131: 448–455.
25. Hanely J, McNeil B (1982) The meaning and use of the area under a receiver operating characteristic (ROC) curve. Radiology 143: 29–36.
26. Rosner B, Glynn R (2009) Power and sample size estimation for the Wilcoxon rank sum test with application to comparisons of C statistics from alternative prediction models. Biometrics 65: 188–197.
27. Cook NR, Buring JE, Ridker PM (2006) The effect of including C-reactive protein in cardiovascular risk prediction models for women. Annals of Internal Medicine 145: 21–29.
28. Seddon JM, George S, Rosner B, Klein ML (2006) CFH gene variant, Y402H, and smoking, body mass index, environmental associations with advanced age-related macular degeneration. Hum Hered 61: 157–165.
29. Seddon JM, Francis PJ, George S, Schultz DW, Rosner B, et al. (2007) Association of CFH Y402H and LOC387715 A69S with progression of age-related macular degeneration. JAMA 297: 1793–1800.
30. Yu Y, Reynolds R, Rosner B, Daly MJ, Seddon JM (2012) Prospective assessment of genetic effects on progression to different stages of age-related macular degeneration using multistate Markov models. Invest Ophthalmol Vis Sci 53: 1548–1556.
31. Reynolds R, Hartnett ME, Atkinson JP, Giclas PC, Rosner B, et al. (2009) Plasma complement components and activation fragments: associations with age-related macular degeneration genotypes and phenotypes. Invest Ophthalmol Vis Sci 50: 5818–5827.
32. Rosner B, Colditz GA, Iglehart JD, Hankinson SE (2008) Risk prediction models with incomplete data with application to prediction of estrogen receptor-positive breast cancer: prospective data from the Nurses' Health Study. Breast Cancer Res 10: R55.
33. Tamura Y, Konomi H, Sawada H, Takashima S, Nakajima A (1991) Tissue distribution of type VIII collagen in human adult and fetal eyes. Invest Ophthalmol Vis Sci 32: 2636–2644.
34. Suwaki N, Klare K, Tarsounas M. RAD51 paralogs: roles in DNA damage signalling, recombinational repair and tumorigenesis; 2011. Elsevier. 898–905.
35. Seddon JM, Yu Y, Miller EC, Reynolds R, Tan PL, et al. (2013) Rare variants in CFI, C3 and C9 are associated with high risk of advanced age-related macular degeneration. Nat Genet 45: 1366–1370.

8

Single Nucleotide Polymorphisms in MCP-1 and Its Receptor Are Associated with the Risk of Age Related Macular Degeneration

Akshay Anand[1][*][9], **Neel Kamal Sharma**[1][9], **Amod Gupta**[2], **Sudesh Prabhakar**[1], **Suresh Kumar Sharma**[3], **Ramandeep Singh**[2], **Pawan Kumar Gupta**[1]

1 Department of Neurology, Post Graduate Institute of Medical Education and Research (PGIMER), Chandigarh, India, 2 Department of Ophthalmology, Post Graduate Institute of Medical Education and Research (PGIMER), Chandigarh, India, 3 Department of Statistics, Panjab University, Chandigarh, India

Abstract

Background: Age-related macular degeneration (AMD) is the leading cause of blindness in the elderly population. We have shown previously that mice deficient in monocyte chemoattractant protein-1 (MCP1/CCL2) or its receptor (CCR2) develop the features of AMD in senescent mice, however, the human genetic evidence so far is contradictory. We hypothesized that any dysfunction in the CCL2 and its receptor result could be the contributing factor in pathogenesis of AMD.

Methods and Findings: 133 AMD patients and 80 healthy controls were enrolled for this study. Single neucleotid Polymorphism for CCL2 and CCR2 was analyzed by real time PCR. CCL2 levels were determined by enzyme-linked immunosorbent assay (ELISA) after normalization to total serum protein and percentage (%) of CCR2 expressing peripheral blood mononuclear cells (PBMCs) was evaluated using Flow Cytometry. The genotype and allele frequency for both CCL2 and CCR2 was found to be significantly different between AMD and normal controls. The CCL2 ELISA levels were significantly higher in AMD patients and flow Cytometry analysis revealed significantly reduced CCR2 expressing PBMCs in AMD patients as compared to normal controls.

Conclusions: We analyzed the association between single neucleotide polymorphisms (SNPs) of CCL2 (rs4586) and CCR2 (rs1799865) with their respective protein levels. Our results revealed that individuals possessing both SNPs are at a higher risk of development of AMD.

Editor: Giuseppe Novelli, Tor Vergata University of Rome, Italy

Funding: The funding of study was from Department of Science and Technology(F.No. SR/SO/HS-109/205 dated 1-05-2007). The funders had no role in study design, data collection and analysis, decision to publish, or preparation of the manuscript.

Competing Interests: The authors have declared that no competing interests exist.

* E-mail: akshay1anand@rediffmail.com

9 These authors contributed equally to this work.

Introduction

Age related macular degeneration is the leading cause of irreversible blindness in the elderly population [1,2]. AMD is of two types: early and late. In the early stage of disease there is presence of drusen with pigmented and hyperpigmented area. After the disease progresses with time, it enters into the second stage i.e. the late stage. The early one is dry or atrophic AMD, which is marked by geographic atrophy or sharply demarcated area of depigmentation caused by waste by products of the retinal pigment epithelium (RPE) and photoreceptors. The late stage of disease is called wet AMD as it occurs because of the growth of new blood vessels under the RPE and neurosensory retina, which results in subretinal bleeding and subsequent scar formation [3]. The complete mechanism of age-related macular degeneration (AMD) is not well understood. In recent years, there has been increasing evidence of an inflammatory component in AMD. It has been found to be associated with polymorphism of complement factor H (CFH) [1,2], a polymorphism which leads to an overactivation of the complement system [3], emphasizing the importance of inflammatory mediators in AMD.

During past few years, certain studies have also focused on the role of chemokines in the progression of AMD. Although the mechanisms underlying the regulation of these cytokines in the eye of patients with AMD remain unclear, chemokines like MCP-1, while acting in concert with receptor CCR2, promote recruitment of macrophages [4]. We hypothesized that any dysfunction in the CCL2 and CCR2 results in impaired macrophage recruitment and debris formation under the retinal pigment epithelium (RPE) contributions to AMD. CCL2 gene is located on chromosome 17q11.2 while CCR2 is located on chromosome 3p21.31.We previously described the spontaneous development of CNV in senescent mice deficient in CCL2 or its CCR2 receptor [4]. Besides, many recent reports have suggested that inflammation is the major cellular process that plays main role in the pathogenesis of AMD [5] and its development to CNV [6]. Some RPE cells play essential role in the maintenance of outer retina by secreting cytokines including CCL2 [7], which have been suggested to be

Table 1. Description of SNPs genotyped.

Gene (RefSeq)	SNP	Chromosome position	Position in reference to 5' UTR	Amino acid translation	Minor Allele
CCL2 (NM_0029823)	rs4586	17q11.2	+T974C	Cys35Cys	C
CCR2 (NM_0006482)	rs1799865	3p21.31	+T4439C	Asn260Asn	C

implicated in the pathogenesis of AMD [8]. RPE cells can secrete CCL2 in the direction of choroidal blood vessels during inflammatory reaction suggesting that RPE cells might promote macrophage recruitment to the choroid from circulating monocytes.

There are a few studies which have examined SNPs of the chemokine system with AMD susceptibility but did not find any evidence of association between CCL2, CCR2 and AMD [9,10]. The absence of any such genetic association studies between CCL2 or CCR2 and AMD from Indian patients prompted us to explore the role of these chemokines in these patients. We analyzed whether single nucleotide polymorphism (SNP) variants in the CCL2 or CCR2 loci independently or in combination are associated with AMD as different ethnic groups may exhibit a varying spectrum of SNPs.

Methods

Study Population

The study was approved by the Ethics Committee of Post-Graduate Institute of Medical Education and Research, Chandigarh, India vide letter No Micro/10/1411. The written informed consent was obtained from participants for the study, as well as for the publication of the data obtained after retrieval of medical records, besides use of blood and DNA for AMD related research project. All the patients were scored at the base line. Individuals with AMD in at least one eye were recruited between 2008 to 2011 from Advanced Eye Centre, Post-Graduate Institute of Medical Education and Research, Chandigarh (PGIMER), India.

We included 213 case-control samples consisting of 133 AMD patients from Eye Centre, PGIMER, with 80 genetically unrelated healthy controls as per inclusion and exclusion criteria described below. Out of 133 AMD and 80 control samples, about nine samples were not included in the analysis due to delayed refrigeration. The limited sample size of this study needs to be addressed by larger studies even though many previous investigators have examined comparable sample size [11,12]. The strength of our study, however, lies in the ethnically homogeneous nature of population which was enrolled from a single largest tertiary care centre in the region catering to over 1,50,000 general patients annually.

Inclusion and Exclusion Criteria

The inclusion criteria for patients in both groups included those with age 50 years or older with the diagnosis of AMD. AMD was defined by geographic atrophy and/or choroidal neovascularization with drusen more than five in at least one eye. The controls constituting the study included those that were of age 50 years or older and had no drusen or no more than 5 drusen with absence of other diagnostic criteria for AMD.

The exclusion criteria included the retinal diseases involving the photoreceptors and/or outer retinal layers other than AMD loss such as high myopia, retinal dystrophies, central serous retinopathy, vein occlusion, diabetic retinopathy, uveitis or similar outer retinal diseases that have been present prior to the age of 50 and opacities of the ocular media, limitations of papillary dilation or other problems sufficient to preclude adequate stereo fundus photography. These conditions include occluded pupils due to synechiae, cataracts and opacities due to ocular diseases.

Diagnosis of AMD

A retina specialist diagnosed all patients by ophthalmologic examination for best corrected visual acuity, slit lamp biomicroscopy of anterior segment and dilated fundus examination. All AMD patients were subjected to optical coherence tomography (OCT) and fluorescein fundus angiography (FFA). The diagnosis of AMD was based on FFA and ophthalmoscopic findings.

Demographic Information

The demographic details were obtained by a trained interviewer using a standardized risk factor questionnaire. A written informed consent form signed by each participant, which included the written risk factor questionnaire was taken from each participant. The details such as age, sex, race, smoking etc as self reported by participants were entered in the data base for analysis. Smokers were defined as having smoked at least 1 cigarette per day for at least 6 months and divided into smokers and never smokers. Comorbidity was determined based on the participant's responses

Table 2. Demographic characteristics of Controls and AMD patients.

Variables	AMD	Controls
Total	133	80
Wet AMD	95 (71.4%)	–
Dry AMD	38 (28.6%)	–
Avastin treated	68	
Not treated with Avastin	27	
Duration of disease¥	23 ± 2.6 (M)	
Age†	66.56 ± 7.6	54.24±7.01
Male	88 (66.2%)	57 (71.2%)
Female	45 (33.8%)	23 (28.7%)

Clinical and demographic details of subjects. AMD, age related macular degeneration; M, Months; Age, Age of onset; Values are mean ± SD or (percentage),
†Unpaired, independent 2-tailed student t test analysis showed that mean age differ significantly among the groups (p = 0.02),
¥Duration of disease is the interval between appearance of first symptom of AMD and collection of sample. AMD subjects were asked to provide all clinical and demographic details at the age of disease-onset.

A

B

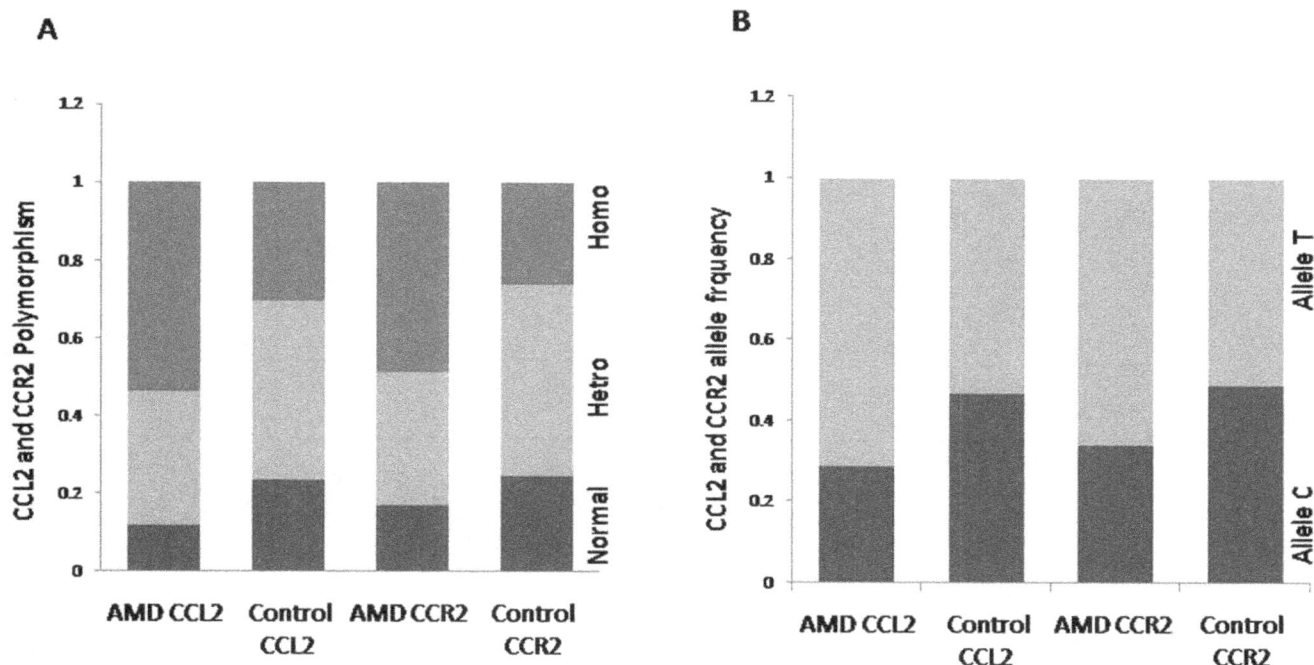

Figure 1. A) Genotype distribution (y-axis) of CCL2 and CCR2 polymorphism in the AMD patients compared to the control group (x-axis) in percentages. B) Allele frequency (y-axis) of CCL2 and CCR2 polymorphism in the AMD patients compared to the control group (x-axis) in percentages.

to whether a physician had ever told them for diagnosis of any major neurological, metabolic or cardiovascular illness.

Selection of Single-nucleotide Polymorphisms

The selected single-nucleotide polymorphisms (SNPs) in our study were either previously studied in other ethnic populations for association with AMD or other inflammatory diseases and chosen due to their reputed functional significance. The details are enumerated in Table 1.

Serum, PBMCs and DNA Isolation

About 8.0 ml of blood sample was collected from all subjects. About 3.0 ml of blood sample was left for 1 hour at 37°C and allowed to clot. Serum was subsequently separated in serum separator tube (BD Biosciences, USA) after centrifugation at 3000 rpm for 30 minutes. From rest of the blood PBMCs were isolated as per Histopaque-1077 (Sigma, USA) instruction sheet provided by the vendor. Briefly, 5.0 ml blood was layered on equal volume of Histopaque-1077 followed by centrifugation at 1800 rpm for 30.0 mins at room temperature. PBMCs were collected from plasma/Histopaque-1077 interface. Aliquots of PBMCs were stored in 90% fetal bovine serum (FBS, HiMedia, India) + 10% dimethyl sulphoxide (DMSO, Sigma, USA) and kept at −80°C until flow cytometry was done. Genomic DNA was extracted from PBMCs using a commercially available genomic DNA extraction and purification kit (INVITROGEN and QIAGEN) according to the manufacturer's protocol. The samples were labeled, coded and stored.

Real Time PCR

SNP (Single neucleotide polymorphism) was analyzed by using real time PCR, and was performed in the 48 wells model Step One™ (Applied Biosystems Inc., Foster city, CA) using published

TaqMan® SNP Genotyping Assays. Real time PCR was carried out for 20.0 µl containing 10 ul master mix, 5 ul Assay (Applied Biosystems), 20 ng DNA and molecular biology grade water was added to make the volume 20.0 µl. All reactions were carried out using TaqMan® SNP Genotyping Assays (Applied Biosystems) according to manufacturer's recommendations. Two reporter dyes VIC and FAM were used to label the Allele 1 and 2 probes and a 5′ Nuclease Assay was carried out. Negative controls included the PCR mix without DNA. Software StepOne™ v 2.0 (Applied Biosystems Inc., Foster city, CA) was used to perform amplification and to estimate SNP. After PCR amplification the Sequence Detection System (SDS) Software was used to import the fluorescence measurements made during the plate read to plot fluorescence (Rn) values.

Total Protein Estimation

Total protein was estimated using Bradford assay. The estimation of total protein was performed according to manufacturer's recommendations. Briefly, serum samples were diluted 1500 times in double distilled water. Bovine Serum Albumin (BSA) served as the standard. Diluted samples and BSA standard protein were mixed with coomassie brilliant blue G–250 dye (Bradford reagent) in 4:1 ratio followed by incubation at room temperature for 10–15 minutes. The absorbance was read at 595 nm in Microplate reader (680XR Biorad, Hercules, CA, USA). The standard curve of BSA was estimated with linear or quadratic fit models.

Enzyme Linked Immunosorbant Assay (ELISA)

The expression of CCL2 was analyzed using commercially available enzyme linked immunosorbant assay (RayBio, Norcross, Cat#: ELH-MCP1-001) as per manufacturer's protocol and absorbance was read at 450 nm in Microplate reader (Biorad

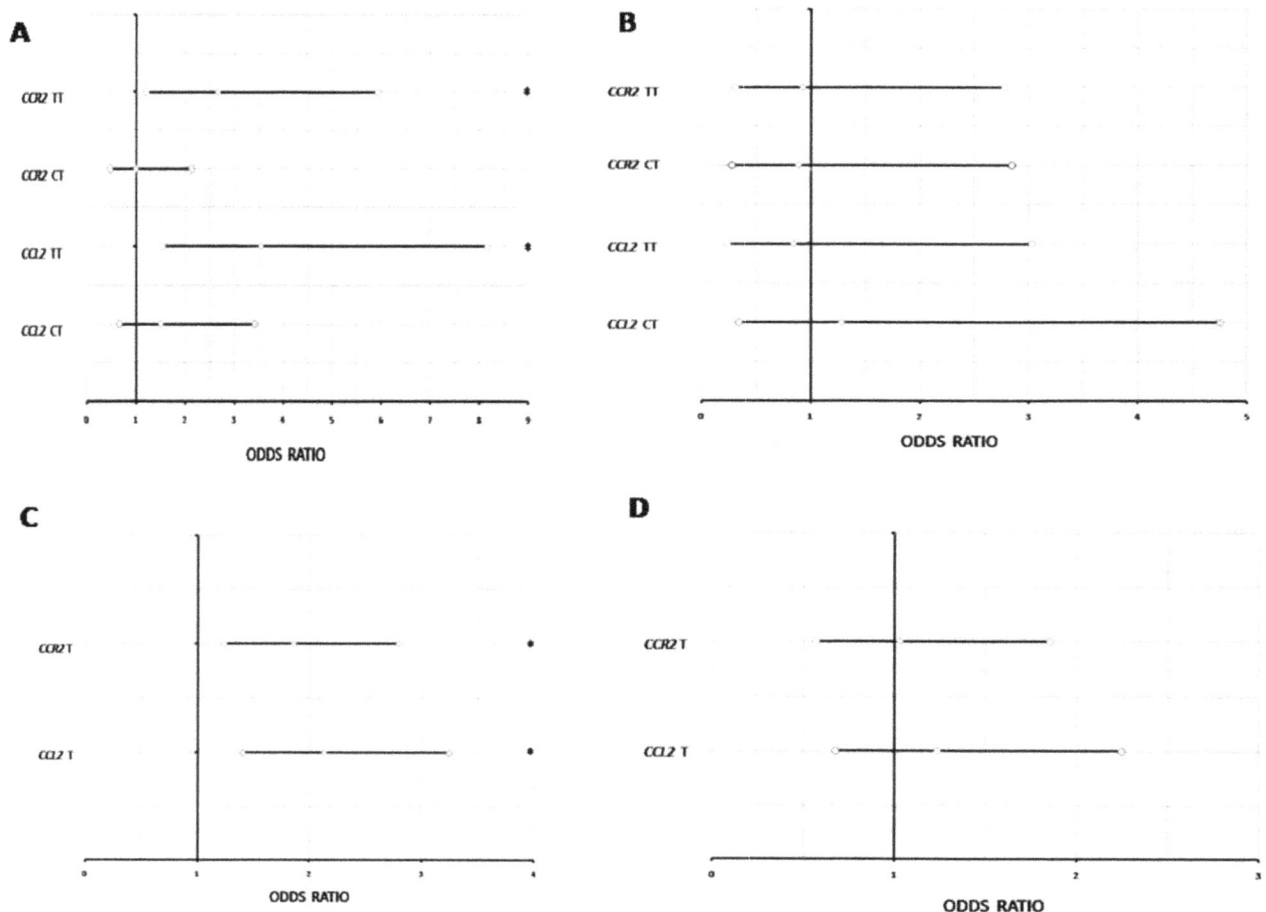

Figure 2. A) Univariate logistic regression analysis in AMD patients with CCL2 and CCR2 polymorphisms as independent and normal controls as a dependent variable. B) Univariate logistic regression analysis in Wet AMD patients with CCL2 and CCR2 polymorphisms as independent and Dry AMD as a dependent variable. C) Univariate logistic regression analysis in AMD patients with CCL2 and CCR2 alleles frequency as independent and normal controls as a dependent variable. D) Univariate logistic regression analysis in Wet AMD patients with CCL2 and CCR2 alleles frequency as independent and Dry AMD as a dependent variable. *p,0.05.

680XR, Hercules, CA, USA). Sample assays were performed in duplicate. This assay recognizes recombinant human CCL2 with minimum detectable dose of CCL2 typically less than 2 pg/ml. The standard curve was plotted using linear model and results were obtained after normalization with total protein.

Flow Cytometry

Flow cytometry was used to study the expression levels of surface receptors namely hCCR2 in PBMCs of normal subjects and AMD patients. $\sim 3 \times 10^5$ PBMCs were initially processed for blocking with Fc blocker (1.0 μg, purified human IgG, R&D Systems Inc., Minneapolis, MN, USA) for 15 mins at room temperature with 0.2 ml of 0.1% sodium azide (Sigma, Germany) in $1 \times$ Ca^{2+} and Mg^{2+} free phosphate buffer saline (PBS) (HiMEDIA, India, pH = 7.2–7.4). Cell suspension was then incubated with primary labeled anti-hCCR2 - Allophycocyanin (0.1 μg, R&D Systems Inc., Minneapolis, MN, USA) antibody for 45 mins on ice in dark in 0.2 ml of fluorescence-activated cell sorter (FACS) buffer. Labeled antibody incubation was followed by two washings with $1 \times$ PBS at 5,000 rpm for 5 mins at 4°C. Finally, the cells were reconstituted in 250.0 μl of 1X PBS and

analyzed in flow cytometer. Approximately 10,000 viable PBMCs were gated based on their forward and side scatter profile, and acquired in each run. PBMCs gate was set to include both lymphocytes and monocytes where maximum CCR2 fluorescence was observed. Same gating was used between the experiments. Background signal was measured for each sample by acquiring unlabeled PBMCs as negative controls and normalized to the signal obtained from anit-hCCR2 labeled PBMCs. Acquired cells were then verified for expression of CCR2. All the analysis was done by acquisition of data within one hour of incubation on FACS CANTO (BD Biosciences, San Jose, CA) flow cytometer using FACS DIVA software (Becton Dickinson).

Statistical Analysis

In order to see whether the data is normally distributed, Normal-quantile (Q-Q) plots were constructed. After establishing the normality for wet AMD cases, a parametric one-way analysis of variance (ANOVA) followed by Fisher's least significant difference (LSD) post-hoc test was applied to compare multiple groups. For comparison of two groups unpaired, student-t test with equal or unequal variance (Welch's correction) was applied. For

Table 3. Effect of CCL2 rs4586 and CCR2 rs1799865 variants on disease phenotype.

Genotype	Number (frequency)		Unadjusted p value			Multivariate analysis, adjusted for age			Multivariate analysis, adjusted for gender		
			OR	95%CI	p-Value	OR	95%CI	p- Value	OR	95%CI	p- Value
CCL2 rs4586											
	AMD	**Controls**									
CC	15 (0.118)	18 (0.236)	Reference			Reference			Reference		
CT	44 (0.346)	35 (0.461)	1.509	0.667–3.413	0.324	0.950	0.227–3.980	0.944	1.523	0.665–3.486	0.320
TT	68 (0.536)	23 (0.303)	3.548	1.543–8.157	0.003	0.517	0.107–2.494	0.411	0.300	0.129–0.695	0.005
	Wet AMD	**Dry AMD**									
CC	11(0.118)	4 (0.118)	Reference			Reference			Reference		
CT	30 (0.323)	14 (0.412)	1.283	0.347–4.749	0.709	2.450	0.388–15.46	0.340	1.254	0.335–4.686	0.737
TT	52 (0.559)	16 (0.471)	0.846	0.237–3.026	0.797	0.334	0.051–2.191	0.253	1.338	0.364–4.915	0.661
CCR2 rs1799865											
	AMD	**Controls**									
CC	22 (0.172)	19 (0.246)	Reference			Reference			Reference		
CT	44 (0.344)	38 (0.494)	1.00	0.472–2.121	1.00	2.147	0.558–8.232	0.267	1.00	0.472–2.212	0.999
TT	62 (0.484)	20 (0.260)	2.677	1.210–5.924	0.015	0.126	0.023–0.679	0.016	0.379	0.171–0.840	0.017
	Wet AMD	**Dry AMD**									
CC	16 (0.168)	6 (0.182)	Reference			Reference			Reference		
CT	33 (0.347)	11 (0.333)	0.889	0.279–2.836	0.842	0.404	0.072–2.249	0.301	0.875	0.275–2.789	0.822
TT	46 (0.484)	16 (0.485)	0.928	0.310–2.779	0.893	1.058	0.210–5.330	0.945	1.108	0.376–3.261	0.853

This table summarizes the genotype frequencies for the single-nucleotide polymorphisms (SNPs) in CCL2 rs4586 and CCR2 rs1799865 among patients with age-related macular degeneration (AMD) and control subjects. Genotype distributions were in Hardy-Weinberg equilibrium. The p-value represents comparison of risk significance between AMD cases and controls. OR indicates odds ratio and CI refers to confidence interval.

Table 4. Allele frequency of CCL2 and CCR2 in AMD and Normal controls.

Allele	Number (frequency)		OR	95%CI	p- Value
CCL2 rs4586					
	AMD	**Controls**			
C	74 (0.29)	71 (0.47)	Reference		
T	180 (0.71)	81 (0.53)	2.132	1.403–3.238	0.0003
	Wet AMD	**Dry AMD**			
C	52 (0.28)	22 (0.32)	Reference		
T	134 (0.72)	46 (0.68)	1.232	0.676–2.246	0.49
CCR2 rs1799865					
	AMD	**Controls**			
C	88 (0.34)	76 (0.49)	Reference		
T	168 (0.66)	78 (0.51)	1.86	1.237–2.796	0.002
	Wet AMD	**Dry AMD**			
C	65 (0.34)	23 (0.35)	Reference		
T	125 (0.66)	43 (0.65)	1.028	0.571–1.852	0.92

This table summarizes the allele frequencies for the single-nucleotide polymorphisms (SNPs) in CCL2 rs4586 and CCR2 rs1799865 among patients with age-related macular degeneration (AMD) and control subjects. The p-value represents comparison of risk significance between AMD cases and controls. OR indicates odds ratio and CI refers to confidence interval.

non-normal data, a non-parametric Kruskal-Wallis H test followed by Mann-Whitney-U test was applied. The real time PCR estimated genotypes for each mutation were stratified for heterozygosity, and homozygosity for the respective allelic variant. Pearson's Chi-square test was applied to study the association between various groups. Genotype distributions were analyzed by logistic regression, integrating adjustments for age and gender. Genotypic associations and odds ratios (ORs) with 95% confidence intervals (CI) were estimated by binary logistic regression. The p ≤0.05 was considered to be significant. Statistical analysis was performed with the help of SPSS 16.0 software.

Results

Summary statistics of all-important variables have been obtained and reported in Table 2.

rs4586 and rs1799865 Polymorphism in AMD Patients

To analyze the spectrum of polymorphism in CCL2 and CCR2 gene, real time PCR was used. The genotypes were in Hardy-Weinberg equilibrium. Genotype and allele frequencies of the polymorphisms of the genes CCL2 and CCR2 have been listed in the Table 3, 4 and Figure 1. The genotype and allele frequency for both CCL2 and CCR2 was found to be significantly different between AMD and normal controls. The TT genotype was more frequent in AMD patients than in controls for both CCL2 and CCR2   (OR = 3.548,   p = 0.003,   CI = 1.543–8.157 and OR = 2.677, p = 0.015, CI = 1.210–5.924, respectively, Table 3; Figure 2A). The study showed that the TT risk variant of CCL2 and CCR2 is associated with AMD (Figure 2A). The individuals having CT genotype in CCL2 and CCR2 revealed no risk of

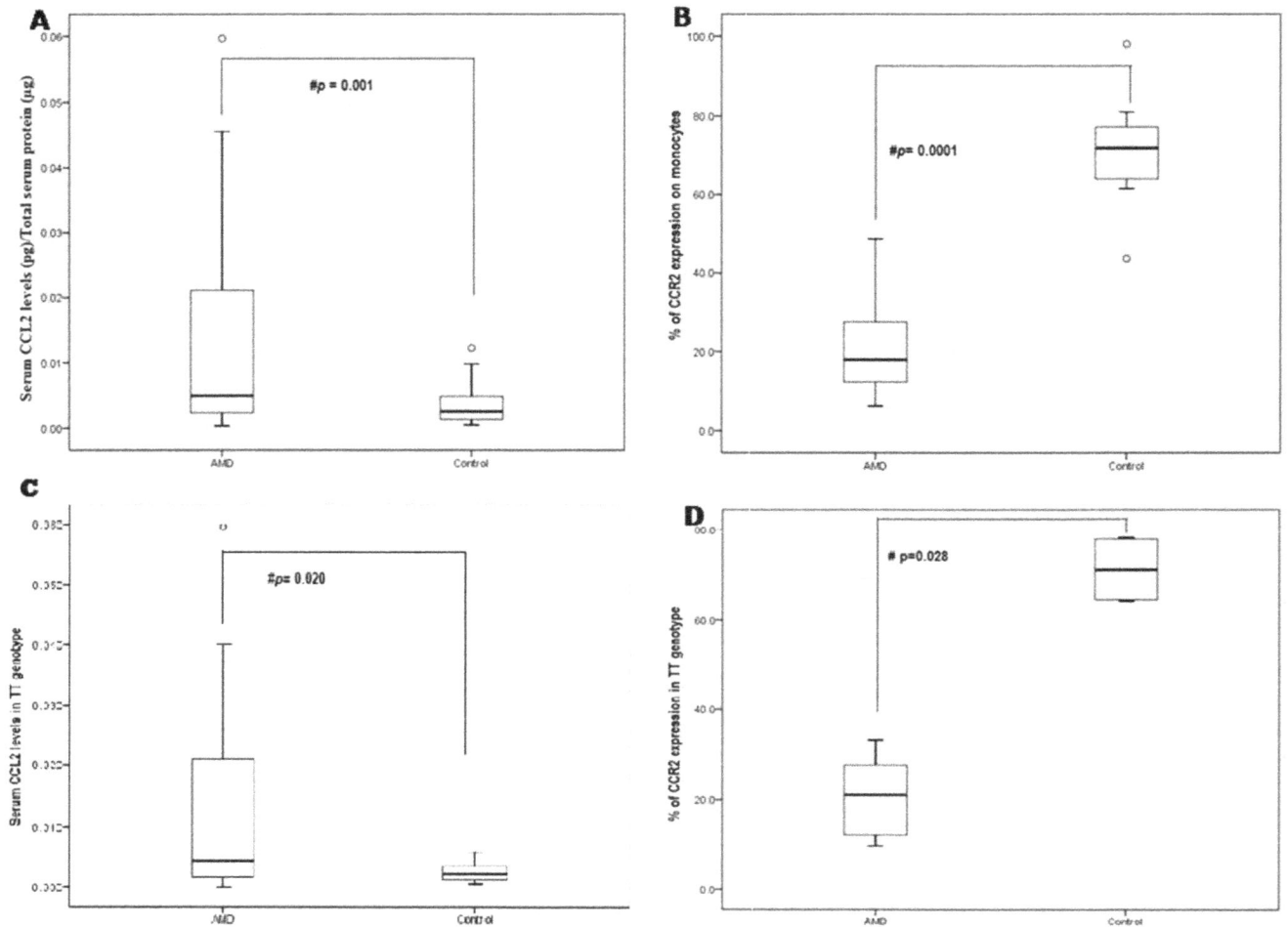

Figure 3. A) Serum levels of CCL2 in AMD and normal controls. B) Percentage (%) of PBMCs expressing CCR2 protein in AMD patients and Normal controls. C) Serum levels of CCL2 in TT genotype of AMD and normal controls. D) Percentage (%) of PBMCs expressing CCR2 protein in TT genotype of AMD patients and Normal controls. Boxes include values from first quartile (25th percentile) to third quartile (75th percentile). Lower and upper error bar refers to 10th and 90th percentile respectively. The thick horizontal line in the box represents median for each dataset. Outliers and extreme values are shown in circles and asterisk respectively. Levels of CCL2 were normalized to total protein. # indicates significant difference (p < 0.05) between the given conditions. Data was analyzed by Mann Whitney U Test. AMD, Age Related Macular Degeneration; CCL2, Chemokine ligand 2; CCR2, Chemokine Receptor 2; pg, picogram; μg, microgram.

developing AMD (Figure 2A). Logistic regression analysis for food habits, existence of comorbidity and smoking habit revealed no significant difference between vegetarian/non-vegetarian, existence of comorbidity/without comorbidity and smokers/non-smokers AMD patients. However, when the comparison was done between AMD and controls, we found that TT genotype was more frequent among vegetarian AMD individuals than in vegetarian controls for CCL2 (OR = 5.574, p = 0.010, CI = 1.510–20.572, Table S1), TT genotype was more frequent in Non-vegetarian AMD than in Non-vegetarian controls for CCR2 (OR = 6.629, p = 0.008, CI = 1.652–26.59 Table S1) emphasizing the association of TT genotype in AMD. The AMD smokers and AMD never smokers showed significant TT frequency as compared to control smokers and control never smokers for CCL2 (OR = 5.80, p = 0.040, CI = 1.081–31.112 and OR = 3.380, p = 0.019, CI = 1.223–9.347, Table S2) and TT frequency was significantly higher in AMD smokers as compared to control smokers for CCR2 (OR = 15.6, p = 0.016, CI = 1.662–146.4, Table S2). However, there was no significant difference on the basis of comorbidity for CCL2 and CCR2 genotypes (Table S3). The

frequency of allele T in CCL2 (rs4586) was found to be significantly higher in AMD patients (0.71%) as compared to the controls (0.53%) (OR = 2.132, p = 0.0003, CI = 1.403–3.238, Table-4, Figure 2C). CCR2 (rs1799865) allele frequency of allele T was also significantly higher in AMD patients (0.66%) as compared to the controls (0.51%) (OR = 1.86, p = 0.002, CI = 1.237–2.792, Table 4, Figure 2C). We did not find any significant difference in genotype and allele frequency between wet and dry AMD patients (Table 3&4; Figure 2B&D). The difference was also not significant when compared between wet AMD patients ie minimally classic, predominantly classic and occult (data not shown). There was no significant difference when compared between those wet variant of AMD patients who received Avastin treatment (dose 1.25 mg in 0.05 ml) and those that did not (data not shown).

Multiple Logistic Regression Analysis

To analyze the association of genetic polymorphism and other risk factors with AMD simultaneously, we performed uncondi-

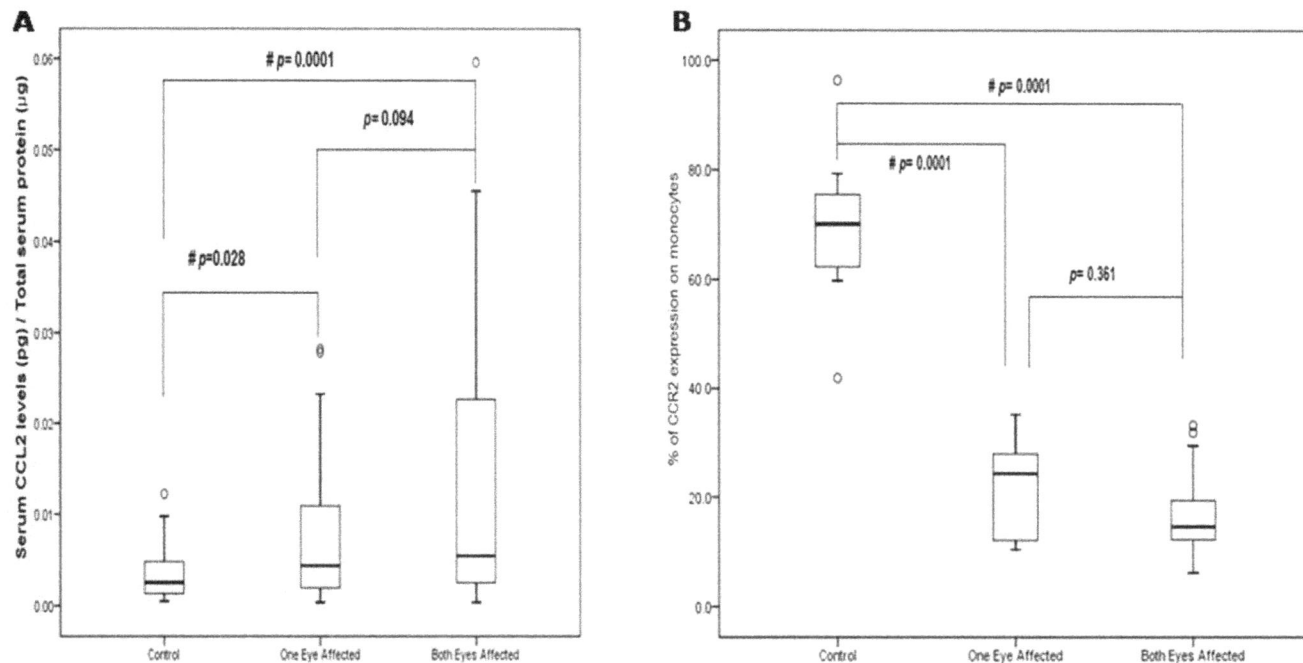

Figure 4. A) Serum levels of CCL2 in normal controls, AMD patients affected in one eye and AMD patients affected in both eyes. B) Percentage (%) of PBMCs expressing CCR2 protein in normal controls, AMD patients affected in one eye and AMD patients affected in both eyes. Boxes include values from first quartile (25th percentile) to third quartile (75th percentile). Lower and upper error bar refers to 10th and 90th percentile respectively. The thick horizontal line in the box represents median for each dataset. Outliers and extreme values are shown in circles and asterisk respectively. Levels of CCR2 were normalized to total protein. # indicates significant difference ($p < 0.05$) between the given conditions. Data was analyzed by Mann Whitney U Test. CCL2, Chemokine ligand 2; CCR2, Chemokine Receptor 2; pg, picogram; μg, microgram.

tional logistic regression analysis and obtained optimized model. We analyzed both age and gender as risk factors which have been shown to be associated with AMD previously. The Hosmer-Lemenshow test shows that the data fits well to the logistic regression ($p = 0.70$). When multiple logistic regression analysis was carried out for age adjustment, we found that TT genotype showed significantly higher frequency for CCR2 rs1799865 in AMD as compared to controls (OR = 0.126, $p = 0.016$, and CI = 0.023–0.679, Table-3) and multiple logistic regression adjustment analysis for gender showed that TT genotype was at significantly higher frequency for CCL2 rs4586 and CCR2 rs1799865 for AMD patients (Table-3). Gender adjustment also showed significant difference in genotype TT for Vegetarian AMD, never smokers AMD (CCL2 rs4586) and comorbidity and smoker AMD (CCR2 rs1799865 Table S1, S2, S3).

Decreased CCR2 and Increased CCL2 Levels

ELISA estimation revealed elevated levels of serum CCL2 in AMD patients as compared to normal controls (Figure 3 A; $p = 0.001$). No difference was observed in CCL2 levels for wet and dry AMD ($p = 0.327$). CCL2 concentration was significantly elevated in the patients affected in one or both eyes with AMD as compare to controls (Figure 4A). However, flow cytometry analysis of PBMCs of AMD patients and normal controls indicates a significant decrease in proportion of CCR2 expressing PBMCs from AMD patients than those from normal controls (Figure 3B & 5; $p = 0.0001$). We found no significant difference in their expression between Dry and Wet AMD samples ($p = 0.934$). CCR2 expression was significantly lower in the patients affected in one eye or both eyes with AMD as compared to controls but the difference was not significant between one eye affected and both

eyes affected (Figure 4B). The CCL2 ELISA and CCR2 FACS levels were not significant when compared between avastin treated & untreated wet AMD patients and between different classes of wet AMD i.e. minimally classic, predominantly classic and occult (data not shown). No association of cigarette smoking, alcohol and meat consumption with CCR2 and CCL2 levels in serum was observed upon univariate and multivariate analysis. The levels of CCL2 determined by ELISA and CCR2 expression estimated by FACS were corresponded to the TT polymorphism in CCL2 and CCR2 in between AMD and controls (Figure 3C&D).

Discussion

The current study suggests that inflammation is essential part of the pathogenesis of AMD in the Indian AMD patients. After examining the involvement of gene polymorphism and levels of inflammatory genes with the risk of AMD, it is suggested that genetic variations in the genes encoding the inflammatory processes might confer susceptibility to AMD by altering the expression of these cytokines. The presence of risk genotype of these genes may increase the risk of AMD.

We examined the levels of CCL2, percentage of cells expressing CCR2 and two variants of these pro-inflammatory cytokine genes which have been studied for other ethnic populations for AMD [9] and shown to be linked with inflammatory diseases [13,14] and were functional variants affecting expression or function of these genes. It must be mentioned that SNPs from CCL2 are previously known to affect CCL2 protein levels [15]. In acute inflammation expression of CCL2 in the retina and RPE increases [16–18], with oxiative stress in the RPE [19]. A recent study had shown that subretinal microglial cells (MCs) induce CCL5 and CCL2 in the

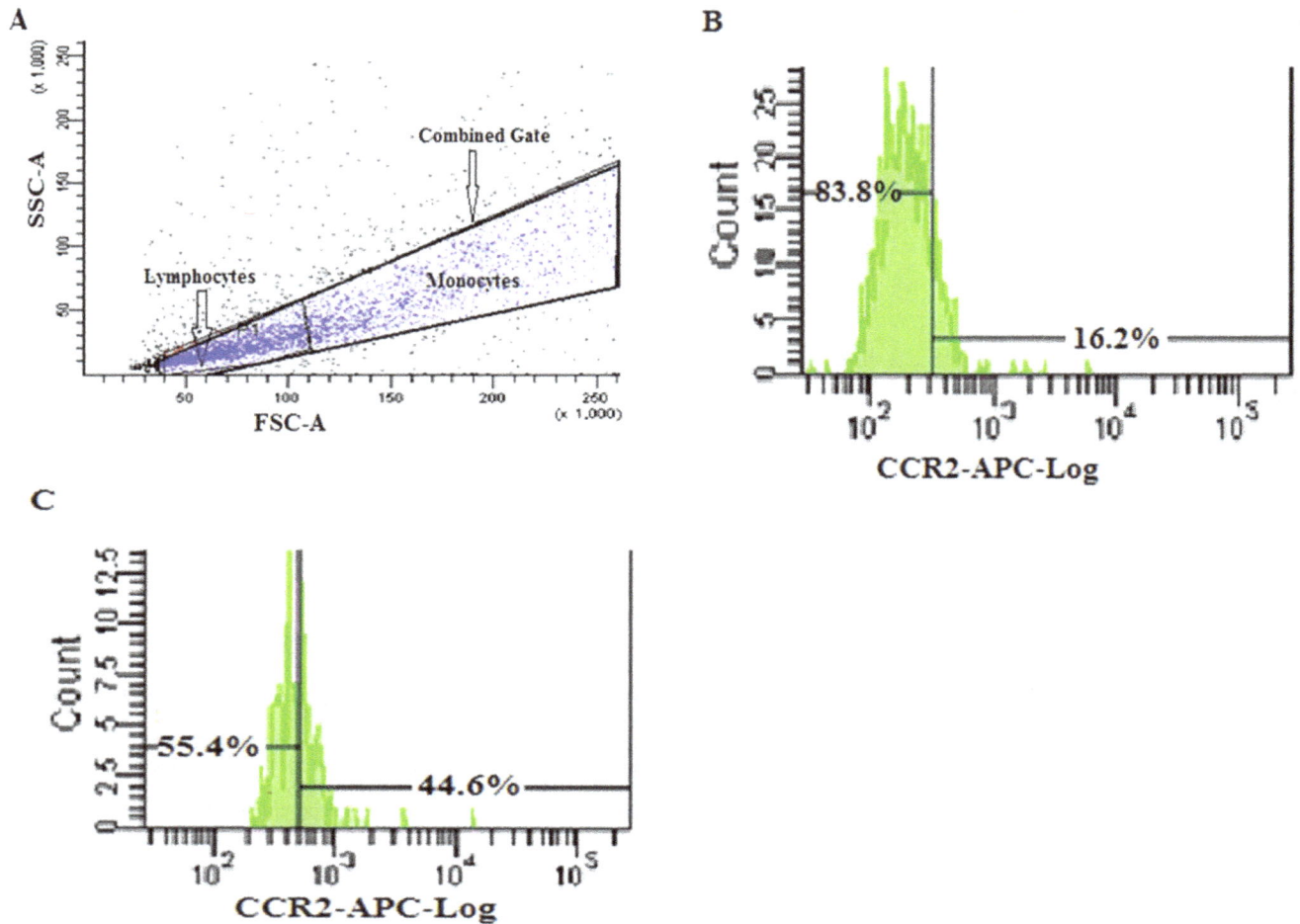

Figure 5. Percentage (%) of CCR2 + PBMCs in AMD patients and normal control subjects as measured by Flow Cytometry. (A) Dot plot showing side and forward scatter analysis of purified unlabeled PBMCs (large combined gate) from a AMD patient. PBMCs consists of two distinct populations namely lymphocytes and monocytes. Approximate lymphocytes and monocytes populations are indicated as smaller gates. Events outside the PBMCs gate represent cell debris and granulocytes. Same gating has been used for PBMCs from each AMD and normal control sample. ~10,000 events have been acquired in each experiment. X-axis represents population cell size in forward scatter (FSC) and y-axis represents population cell granularity in side scatter (SSC). (B,C) Single parameter representative histogram of flow cytometric expression pattern of CCR2 on gated PBMCs is showing decreased number of CCR2 expressing PBMCs in AMD (16.2%; B) as compared to normal control (44.6%; C). Number of cells is represented along y-axis and blue APC fluorescence along x-axis. Appropriate unlabeled PBMCs were used to set marker in histogram and measure background fluorescence. APC, allophycocyanin; CCR2, chemokine receptor 2; PBMCs, peripheral blood mononuclear cells; AMD, Age related macular degeneration.

RPE [20]. CCL2 mainly signals through CCR2 [21]. It has been shown that CCL2/ CCR2 signaling is involved in monocyte or microglial cells enrollment after laser injury [22]. Microglial cells or CCR2-expressing monocytes are present at some point in these models. In a clinical study Jonas et al showed that elevated intraocular levels of CCL2 are associated with exudative AMD [23] and in a mouse model of CNV [16]. CCL2 might therefore play a role in monocyte and MC recruitment to the subretinal space in AMD.

Besides our own work there are numerous reports using CCL2−/− or CCR2−/− mice in an attempt to translate the inflammatory mechanisms of AMD. Recently Chen et al has also shown that aged CCL2 or CCR2 deficient mice develop certain features of atrophic, but not angiogenic AMD-like changes, and represent an animal model for early stage human geographic atrophy [24]. Several studies have examined AMD susceptibility and analyzed SNPs from chemokine family. However, no evidence

has been found for an association between common genetic variations of CCR2 and CCL2 with the etiology of AMD [9,10] but this did not include North Indian patients. However, functional polymorphisms in these genes has been found to play a significant role in the development of other inflammatory diseases [13,25,26]. A family of structurally related chemotactic cytokines comprise chemokines that direct the migration of leukocytes throughout the body, both under pathological and physiological conditions [27]. CCR2 and CCL2 are key mediators in the infiltration of monocytes into foci of inflammation from blood. The CCL2 protein is expressed ubiquitously and exerts its effect after binding to its receptor CCR2 which leads to shape change, actin rearrangement and monocytes movement [28]. As CCL2 and CCR2 genes were considered as potential candidate genes in AMD animal model studies, we analyzed the evidence from genetic variation of CCL2 and CCR2 in human despite conflicting reports. The results of these finding support the postulation that mice deficient in these genes develop hallmarks of AMD [4] (i.e. lipofuscin, accumulation of drusen, photoreceptor atrophy, and CNV). The presence of AMD-like disease in these knockout mice had raised questions of whether CCR2 and CCL2 play a role in human AMD. On examining the two variants of these inflammatory cytokines it was found that these alleles and genotypes are in Hardy-Weinberg Equilibrium in AMD and control subjects. Earlier studies in animal models have shown that CCL2 and CCR2 are involved in the pathogenesis of AMD [4,29,30]. We have examined single polymorphism for CCL2 (rs4586) and CCR2 (rs1799865) with their levels for susceptibility of AMD. The CCL2 transcription may be influenced by the CCL2 (rs4586) SNP, which may act in association with the CCR2 (rs1799865) SNP, impacting the biological activity of the CCR2 receptor, and the CCL2/CCR2 messenger system.

Our study has revealed that the levels of CCL2 were higher and number of cells expressing CCR2 were lower in AMD patients as compared to controls which could be ascribed to the varying physiology of primates and rodents. This might be explained by proposing the activation of a negative feedback seeking to limit the inflammation caused by extravasations of activated monocytes/lymphocytes at the site of macular degeneration. We also found that the levels of CCL2 or percentage of cells expressing CCR2 did not significantly increase or decrease in the patients affected in one eye or those affected in both eyes. We are unable to rule out the local difference in CCL2 and CCR2 because we did not analyze the respective autopsies. The levels of CCL2 in TT genotype of rs4586 was significantly higher in AMD patients as compared to normal controls and the percentage of cells expressing CCR2 were significantly lower in TT genotype of rs1799865 in AMD patients as compared to normal controls which we are unable to explain. The risk of disease increases in individuals 2.6–3.5 times in those who present with genotype TT

as compared to CC within both CCR2 (rs1799865) and CCL2 (rs4586) respectively. Individuals with T allele have higher risk of 1.8–2.1 times for developing AMD as compared to C allele for both CCR2 (rs1799865) and CCL2 (rs4586) respectively. We did not find any significant difference between food habit, comorbidity and smoking for AMD patients which indicates no association with disease.

To the best of our knowledge this is the first study suggesting synergy between the SNPs of CCL2 (rs4586) and its receptor CCR2 (rs1799865) with their protein levels in the development of AMD. Additional studies in larger populations comparing Asian and African and North Americans are needed to validation with larger sample size to allow for the confirmation or negation of an independent role of each of these SNPs on the risk of AMD development or verifying their mutual properties.

Acknowledgments

The study was carried out at Department of Neurology, PGIMER, Chandigarh, India. We are grateful to the volunteers involved in the study, laboratory staff and all those who contributed in terms of time and effort.

Author Contributions

Conceived and designed the experiments: AA. Performed the experiments: NKS. Analyzed the data: AA NKS SKS PKG. Contributed reagents/materials/analysis tools: AA SP. Wrote the paper: AA NKS. Inclusion of patients and clinical scoring: AG RS.

References

1. Haas P, Steindl K, Aggermann T, Schmid-Kubista K, Krugluger W, et al. (2011) Serum VEGF and CFH in Exudative Age-Related Macular Degeneration. Current Eye Research 36(2): 143–148.
2. Simonelli F, Frisso G, Testa F, di Fiore R, Vitale DF, et al. (2006) Polymorphism p.402Y.H in the complement factor H protein is a risk factor for age related macular degeneration in an Italian population. Br J Ophthalmol 90: 1142–1145.
3. Ormsby RJ, Ranganathan S, Tong JC, Griggs KM, Dimasi DP, et al. (2008) Functional and structural implications of the complement factor H Y402H polymorphism associated with age-related macular degeneration. Invest Ophthalmol Vis Sci 49: 1763–1770.
4. Ambati J, Anand A, Fernandez S, Sakurai E, Lynn BC, et al. (2003) An animal model of age related macular degeneration in senescent Ccl-2- or Ccr-2-deficient mice. Nat Med 9(11): 1390–1397.
5. Patel M, Chan CC (2008) Immunopathological aspects of age-related macular degeneration. Semin Immunopathol 30: 97–110.
6. Lommatzsch A, Hermans P, Muller KD, Bornfeld N, Bird AC, et al. (2008) Are low inflammatory reactions involved in exudative age-related macular degeneration? Morphological and immunhistochemical analysis of AMD associated with basal deposits. Graefes Arch Clin Exp Ophthalmol 246: 803–810.
7. Tuo J, Bojanowski CM, Zhou M, Shen D, Ross RJ, et al. (2007) Murine ccl2/cx3cr1 deficiency results in retinal lesions mimicking human age-related macular degeneration. Invest Ophthalmol Vis Sci 48: 3827–3836.
8. Luster AD (1998) Chemokines–chemotactic cytokines that mediate inflammation. N Engl J Med 338: 436–445.
9. Despriet DD, Bergen AA, Merriam JE, Zernant J, Barile GR, et al. (2008) Comprehensive Analysis of the Candidate Genes CCL2, CCR2, and TLR4 in Age-Related Macular Degeneration. Investigative Ophthalmology & Visual Science 49: 364–371.
10. Jonas JB, Tao Y, Neumaier M, Findeisen P (2010) Monocyte Chemoattractant Protein 1, Intercellular Adhesion Molecule 1, and Vascular Cell Adhesion Molecule 1 in Exudative Age-Related Macular Degeneration. Arch Ophthalmol. 128(10): 1281–1286.
11. Scholl HPN, Issa PC, Walier M, Janzer S, Pollok-Kopp B, et al. (2008) Systemic Complement Activation in Age-Related Macular Degeneration. PLoS ONE 3(7): e2593.
12. Kaur I, Hussain A, Hussain A, Das T, Pathangay A, et al. (2006) Analysis of CFH, TLR4, and APOE Polymorphism in India Suggests the Tyr402His Variant of CFH to be a Global Marker for Age-Related Macular Degeneration. Invest. Ophthalmol. Vis. Sci.47: 9 3729–3735.
13. Feng WX, Mokrousov I, Wang BB, Nelson H, Jiao WW, et al. (2011) Tag SNP Polymorphism of CCL2 and its Role in Clinical Tuberculosis in Han Chinese Pediatric Population. PLoS ONE 6(2): e14652.
14. Harmon BT, Orkunoglu-Suer EF, Adham K, Larkin JS, Dressman HG, et al. (2010) CCL2 and CCR2 variants are associated with skeletal muscle strength and change in strength with resistance training. J Appl Physiol 109: 1779–1785.
15. McDermott DH, Yang Q, Kathiresan S, Cupples LA, Massaro JM, et al. (2005) CCL2 polymorphisms are associated with serum monocyte chemoattractant protein-1 levels and myocardial infarction in the Framingham Heart Study. Circulation 112: 1113–1120.
16. Yamada K, Sakurai E, Itaya M, Yamasaki S, Ogura Y (2007) Inhibition of laser induced choroidal neovascularization by atorvastatin by downregulation of monocyte chemotactic protein-1 synthesis in mice. Invest Ophthalmol Vis Sci 48: 1839–1843.
17. Sharma NK, Prabhakar S, Anand A (2009) Age related macular degeneration – advances and trends. Annals of Neurosciences 2: 62–71.
18. Nakazawa T, Hisatomi T, Nakazawa C, Noda K, Maruyama K, et al. (2007) Monocyte chemoattractant protein 1 mediates retinal detachment-induced photoreceptor apoptosis. Proc Natl Acad Sci USA 104: 2425–2430.
19. Higgins GT, Wang JH, Dockery P, Cleary PE, Redmond HP (2003) Induction of angiogenic cytokine expression in cultured RPE by ingestion of oxidized photoreceptor outer segments. Invest Ophthalmol Vis Sci 44: 1775–1782.

20. Ma W, Zhao L, Fontainhas AM, Fariss RN, Wong WT (2009) Microglia in the mouse retina alter the structure and function of retinal pigmented epithelial cells: a potential cellular interaction relevant to AMD. PLoS One 4: e7945.

21. Charo IF, Myers SJ, Herman A, Franci C, Connolly AJ, et al. (1994) Molecular cloning and functional expression of two monocyte chemoattractant protein 1 receptors reveals alternative splicing of the carboxyl-terminal tails. Proc Natl Acad Sci USA 91: 2752–2756.

22. Luhmann UF, Robbie S, Munro PM, Barker SE, Duran Y, et al. (2009) The drusenlike phenotype in aging Ccl2-knockout mice is caused by an accelerated accumulation of swollen autofluorescent subretinal macrophages. Invest Ophthalmol Vis Sci 50: 5934–5943.

23. Jonas JB, Tao Y, Neumaier M, Findeisen P (2010) Monocyte chemoattractant protein 1, intercellular adhesion molecule 1, and vascular cell adhesion molecule 1 in exudative age-related macular degeneration. Arch Ophthalmol 128: 1281–1286.

24. Chen M, Forrester JV, Xu H (2011) Dysregulation in Retinal Para-Inflammation and Age Related Retinal Degeneration in CCL2 or CCR2 Deficient Mice. PLoS ONE 6(8): e22818.

25. Kim MP, Wahl LM, Yanek LR, Becker DM, Becker LC (2007) A monocyte chemoattractant protein-1 gene polymorphism is associated with occult ischemia in a high-risk asymptomatic population. Atherosclerosis 193: 366–372.

26. Jemaa R, Rojbani H, Kallel A, Ben Ali S, Feki M, et al. (2008) Association between the −2518G/A polymorphism in the monocyte chemoattractant protein-1 (MCP-1) gene and myocardial infarction in Tunisian patients. Clin Chim Acta 390: 22–125.

27. Combadiere C, Potteaux S, Rodero M, Simon T, Pezard A, et al. (2008) Combined inhibition of CCL2, CX3CR1, and CCR5 abrogates Ly6C(hi) and Ly6C(lo) monocytosis and almost abolishes atherosclerosis in hypercholesterolemic mice. Circulation 117: 1649–1657.

28. Charo IF, Taubman MB (2004) Chemokines in the pathogenesis of vascular disease. Circ Res 95(9): 858–866.

29. Tuo J, Bojanowski CM, Zhou1 M, Shen D, Ross1 RJ, et al. (2007) Murine Ccl2/Cx3cr1 Deficiency Results in Retinal Lesions Mimicking Human Age-Related Macular Degeneration. Invest Ophthalmol Vis Sci 48(8): 3827–3836.

30. Raoul W, Auvynet C, Camelo S, Guillonneau X, Feumi C, et al. (2010) CCL2/CCR2 and CX3CL1/CX3CR1 chemokine axes and their possible involvement in age-related macular degeneration. Journal Of Neuroinflammation 7: 87.

9

Degeneration Modulates Retinal Response to Transient Exogenous Oxidative Injury

Michal Lederman[1,2], Shira Hagbi-Levi[1], Michelle Grunin[1], Alexey Obolensky[1,2], Eduard Berenshtein[2], Eyal Banin[1], Mordechai Chevion[2], Itay Chowers[1]*

1 Department of Ophthalmology, Hadassah-Hebrew University Medical Center, and the Hebrew University-Hadassah School of Medicine, Jerusalem, Israel, 2 Department of Cellular Biochemistry and Human Genetics, Hadassah-Hebrew University Medical Center, and the Hebrew University-Hadassah School of Medicine, Jerusalem, Israel

Abstract

Purpose: Oxidative injury is involved in retinal and macular degeneration. We aim to assess if retinal degeneration associated with genetic defect modulates the retinal threshold for encountering additional oxidative challenges.

Methods: Retinal oxidative injury was induced in degenerating retinas (rd10) and in control mice (WT) by intravitreal injections of paraquat (PQ). Retinal function and structure was evaluated by electroretinogram (ERG) and histology, respectively. Oxidative injury was assessed by immunohistochemistry for 4-Hydroxy-2-nonenal (HNE), and by Thiobarbituric Acid Reactive Substances (TBARS) and protein carbonyl content (PCC) assays. Anti-oxidant mechanism was assessed by quantitative real time PCR (QPCR) for mRNA of antioxidant genes and genes related to iron metabolism, and by catalase activity assay.

Results: Three days following PQ injections (1 µl of 0.25, 0.75, and 2 mM) the average ERG amplitudes decreased more in the WT mice compared with the rd10 mice. For example, following 2 mM PQ injection, ERG amplitudes reduced 1.84-fold more in WT compared with rd10 mice ($p = 0.02$). Injection of 4 mM PQ resulted in retinal destruction. Altered retina morphology associated with PQ was substantially more severe in WT eyes compared with rd10 eyes. Oxidative injury according to HNE staining and TBARS assay increased 1.3-fold and 2.1-fold more, respectively, in WT compared with rd10 mice. At baseline, prior to PQ injection, mRNA levels of antioxidant genes (*Superoxide Dismutase1, Glutathione Peroxidase1, Catalase*) and of *Transferrin* measured by quantitative PCR were 2.1–7.8-fold higher in rd10 compared with WT mice ($p < 0.01$ each), and catalase activity was 1.7-fold higher in rd10 ($p = 0.0006$).

Conclusions: This data suggests that degenerating rd10 retinas encounter a relatively lower degree of damage in response to oxidative injury compared with normal retinas. Constitutive up-regulation of the oxidative defense mechanism in degenerating retinas may confer such relative protection from oxidative injury.

Editor: Thomas Langmann, University of Cologne, Germany

Funding: This study was supported by a research grant from the Israeli Science Fund (ISF 849/08). The funders had no role in study design, data collection and analysis, decision to publish, or preparation of the manuscript.

Competing Interests: I have read the journal's policy and have the following conflicts: This study was supported by a research grant from the Israeli Science Fund, Grant No. 849/08.

* E-mail: chowers@hadassah.org.il

Introduction

Oxidative damage has been implicated in several neurodegenerative diseases among them Alzheimer's [1], Huntington's [2], Friedreich's ataxia [3] and Parkinson's [4]; as well as in pathologies affecting the retina such as retinitis pigmentosa [5], age related macular degeneration (AMD) [6,7] and glaucoma [8]. The retina is characterized by high oxygen and poly-unsaturated fatty acid content, and by light exposure, which render it vulnerable to oxidative injury [9]. Supplementation of zinc and antioxidants can slow the course of age related macular degeneration in humans [10], and retinal degeneration in mice, further implicating oxidative retinal injury in retinal and macular degeneration [11–14].

Retina and macula undergoing chronic oxidative injury during the course of genetically-driven degenerative processes might encounter additional transient exogenous oxidative stress stemming from exposure to a chemical generating reactive oxygen species (ROS), an inflammatory reaction, or light exposure. Limited data is available with respect to the threshold of the degenerating retina in comparison to the normal retina for such additional oxidative injury. If the degenerating retina is more susceptible to exogenous oxidative challenges then patients with retinal degenerations should be rigorously protected from oxidative challenges which are not harmful to the healthy retina.

We evaluated the extent of retinal damage following exposure to paraquat (PQ), a bipyridium herbicide that selectively generates superoxide radical anions, in mice with genetically–driven retinal degeneration (rd10 mice) and in C57BL/6 wild type (WT) mice [15,16]. We then evaluated the anti oxidative enzymatic defense system and iron homeostasis to explore possible underlying causes for the different susceptibility to oxidative injury between rd10 and

Paraquat= ———— PBS= - - - - -

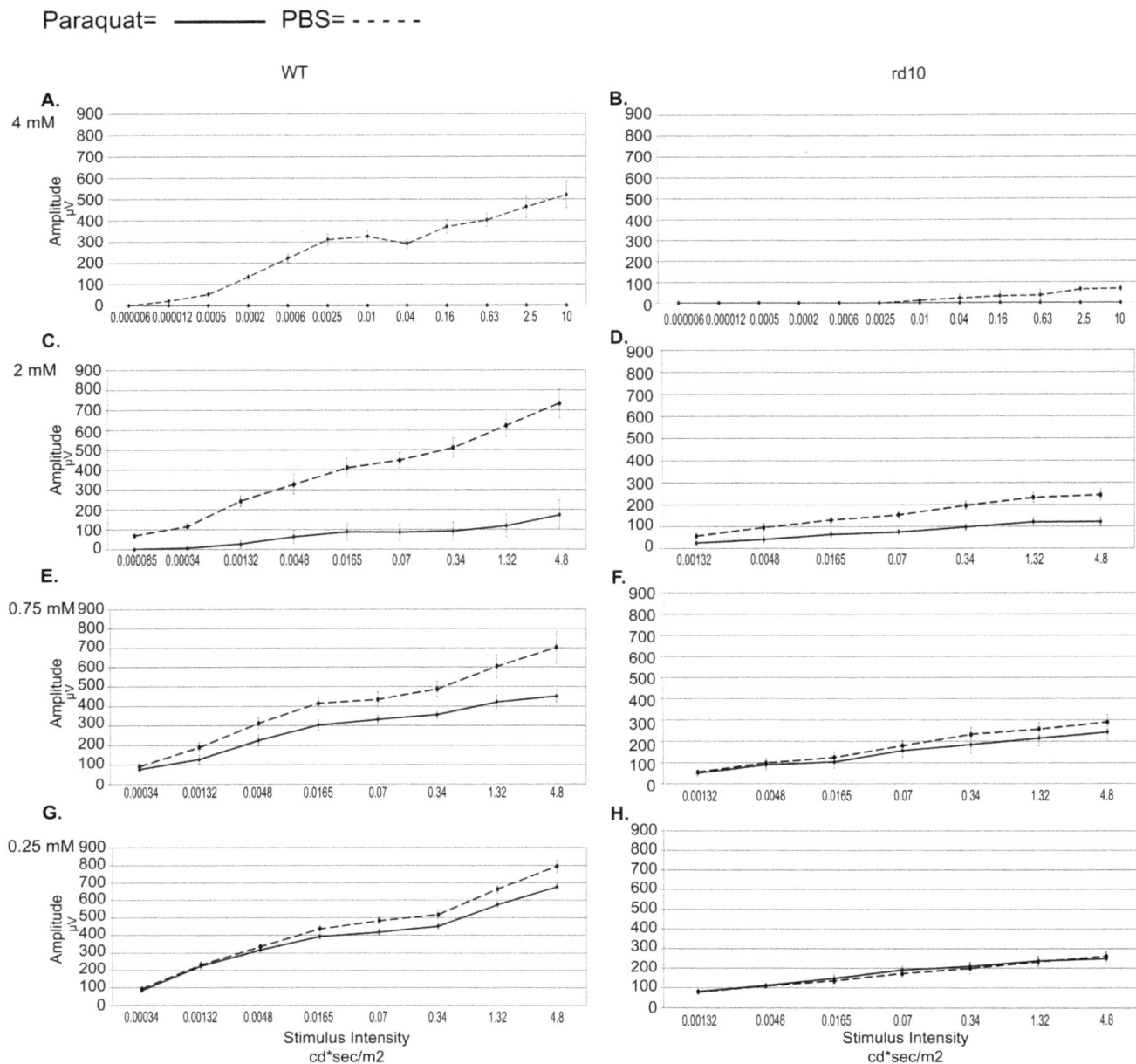

Figure 1. Scotopic b-wave ERG responses following intravitreal injection of PQ. ERGs were recorded three days following injection of 4 mM (A,B), 2 mM (C,D), 0.75 mM (E,F), or 0.25 mM (G,H) of PQ in one eye and PBS in the fellow eye of wild type (WT) and rd10 mice (n = 10–22 in each group). Y-axis shows amplitude in microvolt while the x-axis shows the stimulus intensity.

WT mice. Iron metabolism was characterized as it may contribute to oxidative injury in retinal and macular degeneration through the Fenton reaction [17,18].

Materials and Methods

Mice

rd10 mice (on C57BL/6 background), homozygous for the missense mutation in the β-subunit of the rod phosphodiesterase gene ($Pde6b^{rd10}$), were used as a model for retinal degeneration-accelerates around three weeks of age in this strain and after 60 days of age only few nuclei remain in the outer nuclear layer and the electroretinogram (ERG) is absent or barely recordable

[16,19]. C57BL/6 mice served as controls. Mice were maintained in a specific pathogen free animal facility, with a 12-hour light (white fluorescence, 30 cd/m^2)/dark cycle, and an unlimited food and water supply. Animals were treated in accordance to the guidelines of the Association for Research in Vision and Ophthalmology, and experiments were conducted with the approval of the ethics committee of the Faculty of Medicine of the Hebrew University. Before all procedures mice were anesthetized by intraperitoneal injections of a mixture of ketamine (Bedford Laboratories, Bedford, OH) and xylazine (VMD, Arendonk, Belgium), with doses suitable to their body weight.

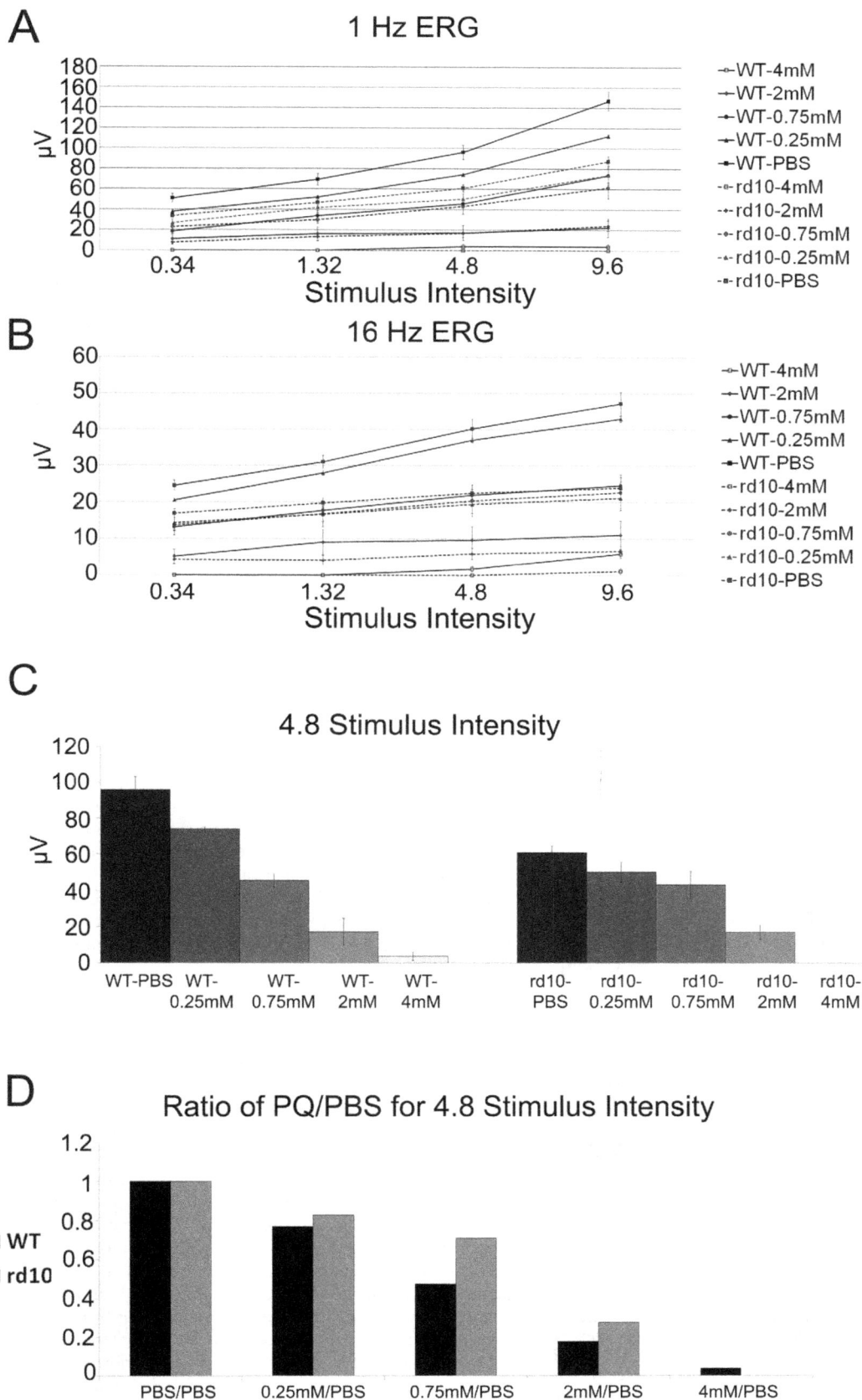

Figure 2. Photopic 1 Hz and 16 Hz ERG amplitudes in wild type (WT) and rd10 mice following PQ or PBS injection. (A) 1 Hz photopic amplitude shows both WT and rd10 mice after PQ or PBS injection. (B) indicates 16 Hz ERG amplitude for same WT and rd10 mice after PQ or PBS

injection. 1 Hz b-wave amplitudes for each experimental group at 4.8 stimulus intensity are displayed in panel C. Average b-wave amplitudes at highest signal intensity divided by b-wave amplitudes from PBS injected eyes for each mouse group at each of the PQ concentrations is summarized in panel D. Larger reduction in ERG amplitudes following PQ injection was observed in WT compared with rd10 mice (please see result section for details). n = 10–22 mice in each group.

Intravitreous Injections

Intravitreous injections were delivered using a PLI-100 Pico-Injector (Medical System Corp., Greenvale, NY), as previously described [20]. Three-week-old mice were anesthetized, and eyelids were drawn back. Under a dissecting microscope, a pulled glass micropipette was passed through the pars plana and mice were injected with 1 µl of 0.25, 0.75, 2 mM or 4 mM PQ (SIGMA-Aldrich, St. Louis, MO) diluted in phosphate buffered saline (PBS) (Biological Industries, Kibbutz Beit Haemek, Israel) in one eye. These concentrations were selected based on a previous report [15]. In that study, the 0.5 mM concentration did not cause retinal damage to wild type mice while 2 mM caused severe retinal injury. Contra-lateral eyes, injected with 1 µl of PBS, served as controls.

Electroretinograms (ERG)

Three days following intraocular injections, full field ERGs were recorded in anesthetized mice following over-night dark adaptation. Pupils were dilated with 1% tropicamide and 2.5% phenylephrine, and benoxinate HCl 0.4% (all from Fisher

Pharmaceuticals, Tel-Aviv, Israel) drops were applied to the corneas as local anesthetics prior to gold-wire active electrode placement on the central cornea. A reference electrode was placed in the tongue and a needle ground electrode was placed intramuscularly in the hip area. ERGs were recorded inside a Faraday cage using the Espion computerized system (Diagnosys Llc, Littleton, MA). Dark adapted ERG responses to a series of white flashes of increasing intensities (from 0.000006 to 9.6 cd*sec/m^2) were recorded with inter-stimulus intervals rising from 10 sec for lowest intensity flashes to 90 sec for highest intensity flashes. Light adaptation was accomplished with a background illumination of 30 cd/m^2. Cone 1 Hz and 16 Hz flicker ERGs to a series of white flashes (from 0.34 to 9.6 cd*sec/m^2) were recorded. All responses were filtered using 0.3 to 500 Hz filters and signal averaging was applied [21]. Amplitudes of a- and b-waves were then measured and analyzed.

Tissue Processing

Mice were euthanized with an overdose of ketamine, followed by cervical dislocation. For frozen sections (used for immuno-staining), five-day post-injection of PQ eyes were enucleated and immediately placed in Davidson solution [25 ml Glacial Acetic acid, 71.25 ml Ethanol (BIO LAB, Jerusalem, Israel), 50 ml 10% neutral buffered formalin (EMS, Hatfield, PA), and 78.75 ml double distilled water] for overnight fixation. The following day, eyes were transferred to 30% sucrose for 24 hours, after which they were frozen in blocks of Tissue-Tek optimum cutting temperature (O.C.T, Sakura, Torrance, CA) embedding compound, and frozen on dry ice. Eyes were sliced into 6 µm thick sections, along the corneal-optic nerve axis, using a Leica CM 1100 cryostat (Heidelberger, Germany). Conventional histology was performed on formalin-fixed, paraffin-embedded sections using hematoxylin and eosin staining.

For all other procedures retinas were gently separated from freshly enucleated eyes under a dissecting microscope, immediately frozen in liquid nitrogen and stored at −80°C until further use.

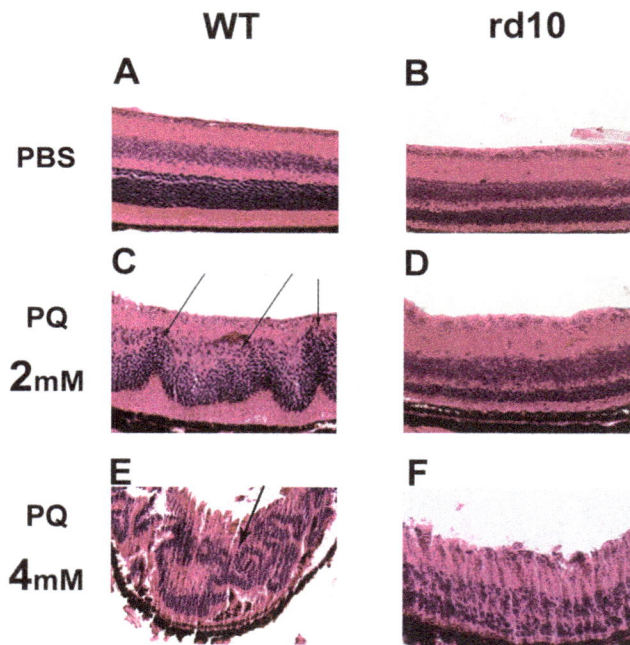

Figure 3. H&E staining of formalin-fixed paraffin-embedded retina sections from rd10 and WT mice injected with 1 µl of 2 mM or 4 mM PQ or PBS. Normal retina morphology was seen in WT mice (A), while the retina appeared disrupted in these mice following PQ injection (C, E). Arrow indicates wavy appearance of nuclear layers and photoreceptor inner and outer segments in WT retina injected with PQ. This wavy appearance appear extreme following injection of 4 mM PQ. Retinas of rd10 mice, already undergoing retinal degeneration, are typically thinner, due to loss of photoreceptors (B). PQ injection in rd10 mice was not associated with structural alterations similar to the one observed in WT mice (D, F). GCL = ganglion cell layer, INL = inner nuclear layer, ONL = outer nuclear layer, RPE = retinal pigmented epithelium.

Immunohistochemistry (IHC)

Immunostaining was performed as we have recently described [17]. Briefly, immunostaining with rabbit anti 4-hydroxy-2-nonenal (HNE; diluted 1:100 in 1% BSA; Alpha Diagnostics, San Antonio, TX) was done to assess the extent of oxidative damage. Cy3-conjugated goat anti rabbit antibody (diluted 1:200; Jackson ImmunoResearch, West Grove, PA), was used as secondary antibody and slides were counterstained with DAPI (Santa Cruz Biotechnology, Santa Cruz, CA) [22]. Sections were viewed through fluorescent microscopy (Olympus BX41, Tokyo, Japan), using appropriate filters. Background was controlled by setting the exposure parameters as such that provide no detectable signal for the control section and these same parameters were maintained while capturing images from the test sections. Images were photographed with an Olympus DP70 digital camera.

Quantification of immunochemistry was performed on digital images using ImageJ Software (http://rsb.info.nih.gov/ij/index. html) [23] by measuring the average staining intensity per pixel in five replicas of sections chosen from each sample at a similar distance from the optic nerve. In each section, staining was

A

B

HNE

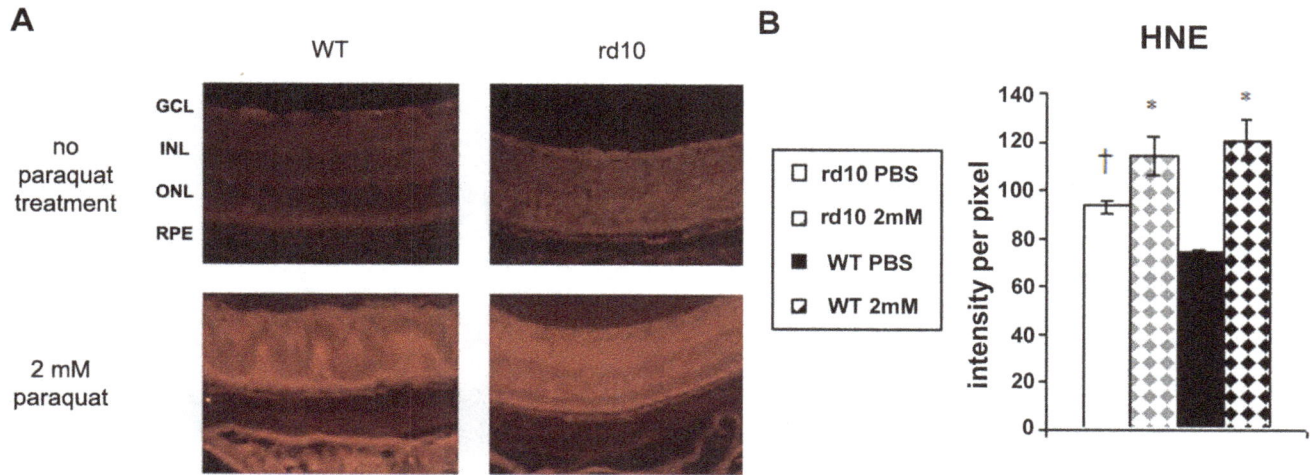

Figure 4. HNE staining of retina sections for assessment of oxidative injury following PQ injection. Retinas of rd10 and WT mice injected with 1 μl of 2 mM PQ or PBS were labeled with anti-HNE antibody (*red*; A). GCL = ganglion cell layer, INL = inner nuclear layer, ONL = outer nuclear layer, RPE = retinal pigmented epithelium. (B) Quantification of HNE staining intensity showed marked oxidative injury following PQ injection in WT and the rd10 mice (*p<0.05 as compared to PBS injected eyes of same strain. † p = 0.0002 comparing control (PBS) eyes between the strains; n = 5 in each group).

measured in an area including the entire thickness of the retina from the inner limiting membrane to the RPE (retinal pigment epithelium).

Quantitative Real-Time RT-PCR (QPCR)

Total RNA was extracted from a pool of two flash-frozen retinas (indicated as paired) using TRI Reagent (SIGMA), according to the manufacturer's instructions, and then treated with DNAase (TURBO DNA-free, Ambion, Austin, TX). Reverse transcriptase polymerase chain reaction was performed using the High Capacity cDNA Reverse Transcription Kits (Applied Biosystems, Foster City, CA) and anchored oligo dT primers on 1 μg of RNA. QPCR

was performed to measure mRNA levels of genes involved in iron metabolism and of anti-oxidant enzymes. Measurement of the anti-oxidant enzymes mRNA levels was performed on retinas prior to injection (4 pairs of WT retinas-8 retinas total, and 7 pairs of rd10 retinas- 14 retinas total), while measurement of the genes involved in iron metabolism was performed on retinas five days after injection with either a PBS control or injection of the contralateral eye with 1 μl of 2 mM PQ. Six pairs (12 retinas total) of rd10 eyes and six pairs of WT eyes were injected with PBS, while six pairs (12 retinas total) of contralateral rd10 or WT eyes were injected with PQ. Measurement of *GAPDH* and *HPRT* mRNA levels served as endogenous controls. All reactions were

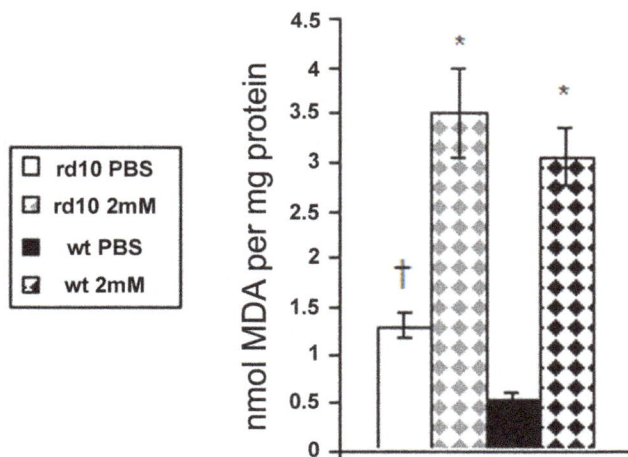

Figure 5. Measurements of TBARS level in mice retinas following PQ injection. TBARS level (nmol MDA per mg protein) indicates the extent of oxidative injury to lipids. TBARS were measured in retinas of rd10 and WT mice following 2 mM paraquat or PBS injections. *p≤0.004 as compared to PBS injected eyes of same strain. † p = 0.001 comparing control (PBS) eyes between the strains (n = 5 in each group).

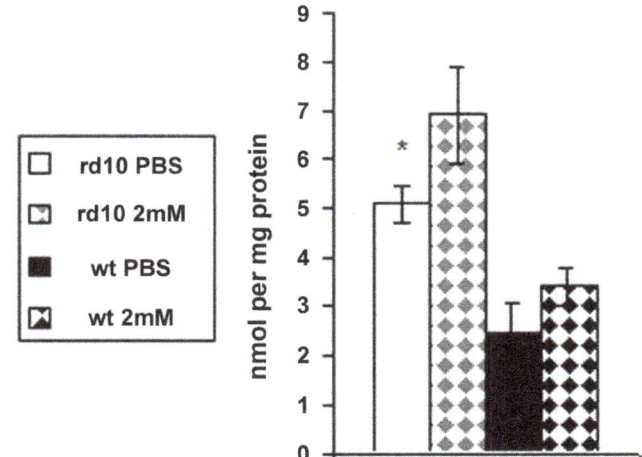

Figure 6. Protein carbonyl content (PCC) in mice retinas following PQ injection. Protein carbonylation was measured to assess oxidative retinal injury to proteins. It was assessed in retinas of rd10 and WT mice injected with 1 μl of 2 mM PQ or PBS. In both strains PQ injections caused an insignificant 1.35 fold increase of PCC. *p = 0.009 comparing control (PBS) rd10 with WT retinas (n = 5 in each group).

A

B

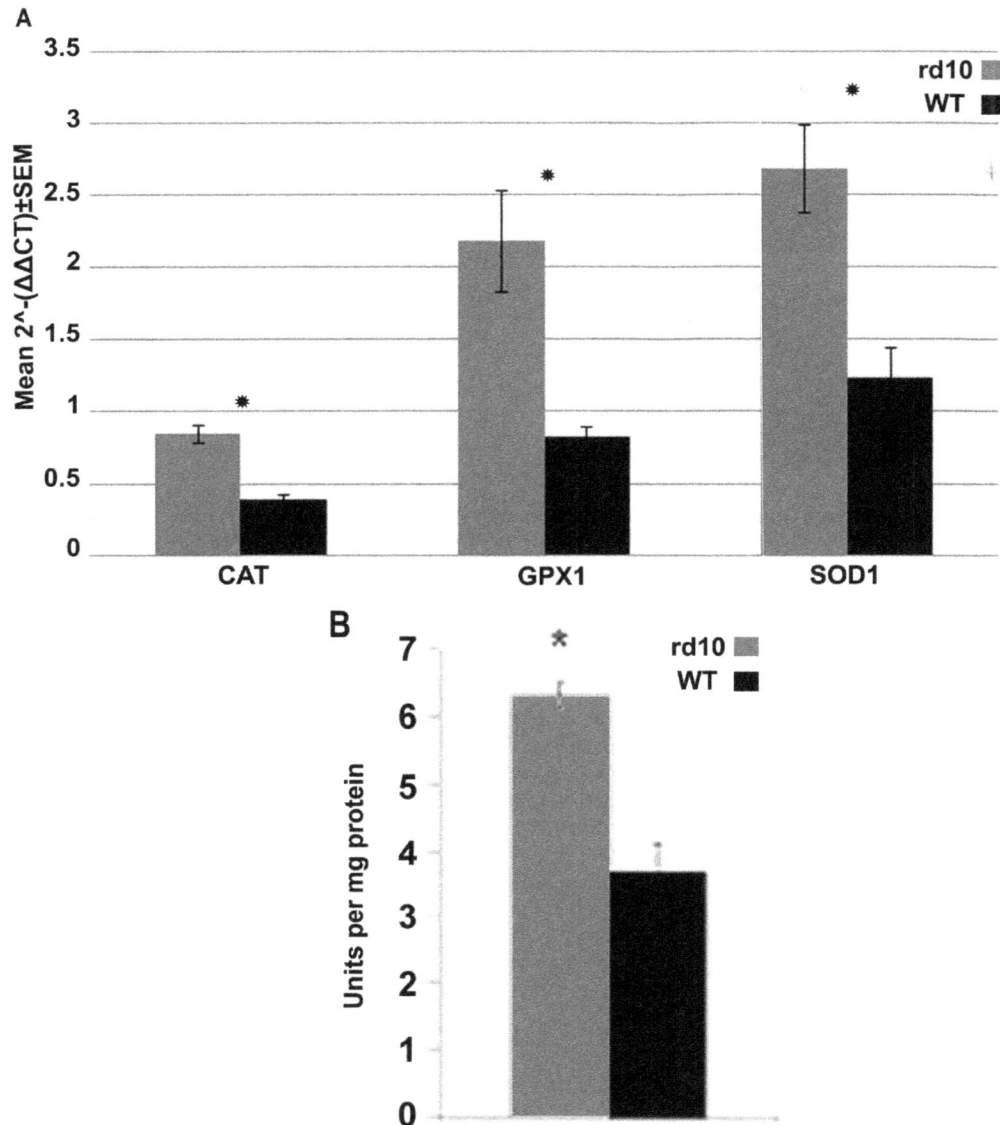

Figure 7. Retinal Expression of antioxidant genes in rd10 and WT mice. (A) mRNA levels of anti-oxidant enzymes in normal and degenerating retinas. *SOD1*, *GPX1*, and *CAT* expression levels were measured using QPCR (rd10 n = 7 pairs, WT n = 4 pairs). (B) Catalase activity evaluated in retinas of three-week-old WT and rd10 mice. *$p < 0.05$ in comparison to WT (n = 5 in each group).

carried out in triplicate at a total volume of 20 µl. Wells contained 40 ng cDNA template, 0.75 µl TaqMan Gene Expression assay [*glyceraldehyde-3-phosphate dehydrogenase (GAPDH)*: Mm99999915_g1; *hypoxanthine guanine phosphoribosyl transferase (HPRT)*: Mm00446968_m1; *catalase (CAT)*: Mm00437992_m1; *superoxide dismutase 1 (SOD1)*: Mm01344233_g1; *glutathione peroxidase 1 (GPX1)*: Mm00656767_g1; *ceruloplasmin (Cp)*: Mm00432654_m1; *transferrin (Tf)*: Mm01230431_m1; *transferrin receptor (Tfrc)*: Mm00441941_m1], 7.5 µl TaqMan Universal PCR Master Mix (Applied Biosystems) and were completed with double distilled water, and standard TaqMan technique was applied. Using 96 well plates, signal amplification was measured throughout 45 cycles of 60°C for 15 seconds, followed by 95°C for 15 seconds. Fluorescent signals were measured by the system StepOnePlus (Applied Biosystems) and analyzed using the Step One Software version 2.2 to obtain threshold cycle (CT) values (Applied

Biosystems), along with spreadsheet software (Excel; Microsoft, Redmond, WA). Expression levels of each gene were compared by using the geometric mean of the endogenous controls [24] according to the standard $2^{(-\Delta\Delta CT)}$ calculation [25], giving results as relative quantification and fold change ± standard error of the mean (SEM).

Protein Isolation

Lysis buffer containing 1% deionized TritonX-100 and 0.1% sodium azide in 50 mM Tris-HCl (SIGMA), pH 7.5, was incubated with Chelex-100 (Bio-Rad, Hercules, CA), for 24 hours. Immediately before use, 0.25 mM Phenyl-Methyl-Sulfonyl-Fluoride was added (1:1000, SIGMA). Pools of retinal tissue were homogenized in the buffer, sonicated at 10 watts for 1 min, and stored on ice for half an hour while vortexing every 5 minutes. Samples were then centrifuged at 2,750 *g*, for 15 min, at 4°C, after

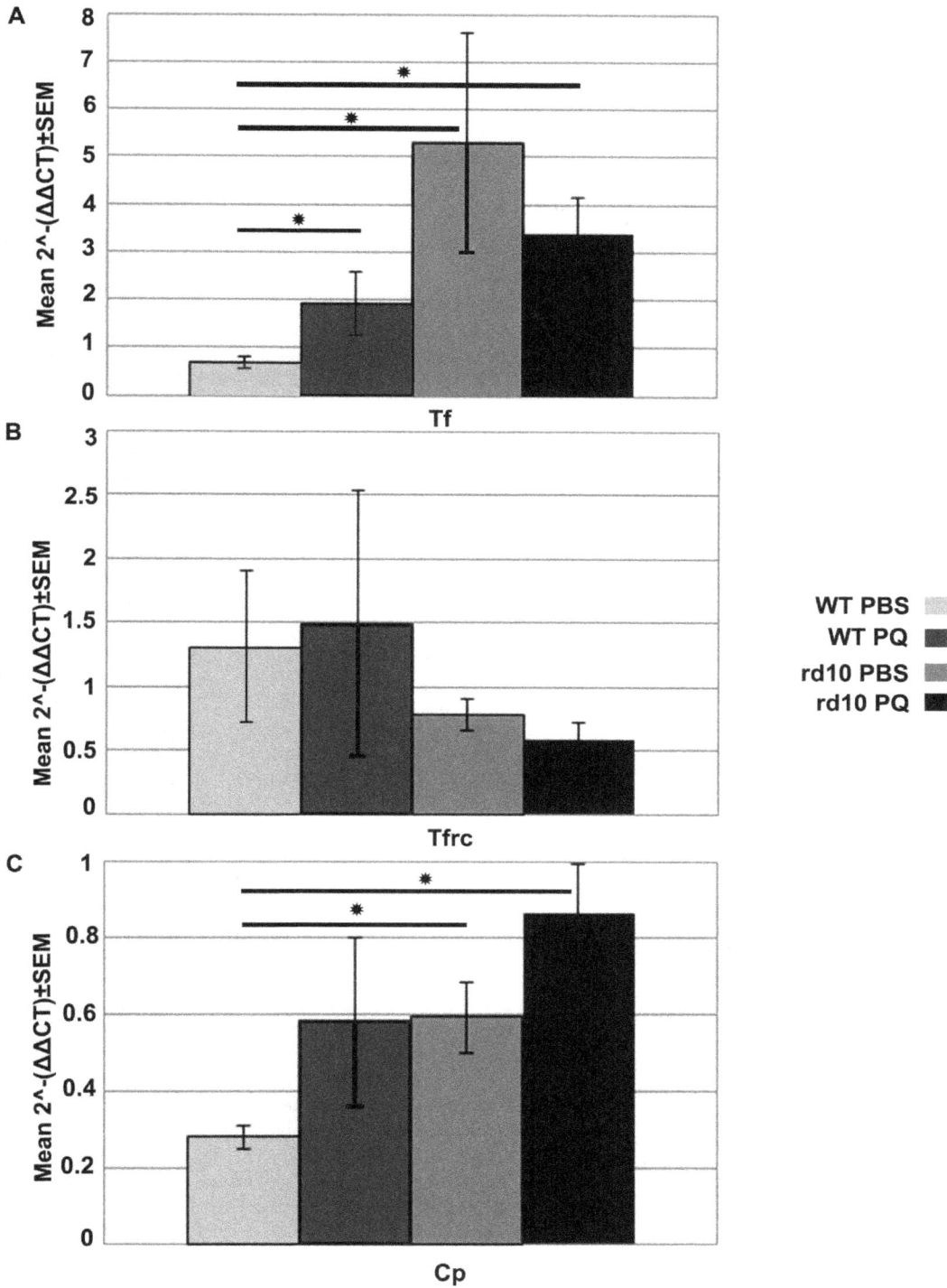

Figure 8. mRNA levels of iron metabolism associated genes. (A) *transferrin (Tf)* expression, (B) *transferrin receptor (Tfrc)* expression, (C) *ceruloplasmin (Cp)* expression, measured in rd10 and WT retinas following intravitreal injection of 1 µl of 2 mM PQ or PBS. Bars = mean relative mRNA levels ± SEM. *p<0.05 as compared to PBS injected eyes (PBS) of same strain. † p<0.05 comparing expression in control eyes between the strains (n = 6 pairs in each group).

which supernatant was separated and refrozen at −80°C. Protein content was estimated using the BCA Protein Assay Kit (Pierce, Rockford, IL). Ferritin levels were measured by ELISA as was previously described [17,26].

Thiobarbituric Acid Reactive Substances (TBARS) Measurement

Lipid peroxidation was evaluated by measuring levels of MDA (Malonaldehyde-bis-DimethylAcetal) [27]. Eight retinas were homogenized in 800 μl lysis buffer (see above) and centrifuged at 10,000 g for 10 min at 4°C. 200 μl of the supernatant were added to 100 μl 8.1% SDS (BDH Chemicals, Poole, UK), 750 μl 20% acetic acid (Frutarom, Haifa, Israel) pH 3.5, and 750 μl 0.8% thiobarbituric acid (SIGMA), and incubated for half an hour at 100°C. After cooling, 1.35 ml n-butanol:pyridine (15:1; BIO LAB:SIGMA) were added, and the mixture was centrifuged at 4,000 g for 15 min at 4°C. Absorbance of the organic phase was measured using a UVKON$_{XL}$ spectrophotometer (Bio-Tek, Winooski, VT) at λ = 532 nm. The amount of TBARS was determined according to a standard calibration curve generated from MDA.

Protein Carbonylation

Protein carbonyl content (PCC) was quantified as an indicator for protein damage in the retina. Samples and controls were each measured in duplicates. Supernatant (100 μl, prepared as described above for TBARS analysis) was reacted with 400 μl 10 mM 2,4-dinitrophenylhydrazine (DNPH, Aldrich) in 2M HCl (Frutarom), or 2M HCl alone (for controls). Reaction tubes were incubated for one hour at room temperature in the dark, while vortexing every 15 min. 500 μl 20% tri chloro-acetic acid (TCA, SIGMA) were added, followed by five min incubation on ice, after which tubes were centrifuged at 10,000 g for 10 min at 4°C. Supernatant was discarded; pellets were re-suspended in 1 ml 10% TCA, and again incubated and centrifuged as described above. Pellets were washed three times with ethanol:ethylacetate (1:1, SIGMA) for 10 min, and centrifuged after each wash. The pellets were re-suspended in 500 μl 6 M guanidine-hydrochloride (BIO LAB) in 0.5 M K$_3$PO$_4$ (SIGMA) pH 2.5, and again centrifuged. Absorbance was measured using a spectrophotometer at λ = 370 nm. Protein carbonyl content was established using the corrected absorbance (CA) that was calculated by subtracting the average absorbance of the controls from that of the samples [28–30].

Catalase Activity

Catalase activity was evaluated by measuring the formaldehyde produced by reacting the samples with methanol in the presence of H$_2$O$_2$, as previously described [31]. Briefly, pairs of retinas were combined and homogenized in 500 μl cold 25 mM KH$_2$PO$_4$ (Riedel-de Haen, Hanover, Germany) pH 7 buffer, centrifuged at 10,000 g for 15 min at 4°C, and stored on ice. 100 μl of the supernatant were transferred into a tube containing 50 μl buffer and 50 μl 100% methanol (BIO LAB). The reaction was initiated by adding 10 μl 0.27% H$_2$O$_2$ (BIO LAB). Samples were incubated for 20 min at room temperature on a shaker. 50 μl 7.8 M KOH (Frutarom) was added to terminate the reaction. 100 μl 34.2 mM purpald (SIGMA) in 480 mM HCl were then added and tubes were again placed on a shaker for 10 min. The perpald was then oxidized by adding 50 μl 65.2 mM potassium periodate (Alfa Aesar, Karlsruhe, Germany) in 470 mM KOH, resulting in the formation of a purple colored product which, after spinning at 9,500 g for 10 min, was quantified by measuring absorption at λ = 550 nm. Amounts of formaldehyde formed were determined by generating a standard calibration curve. One unit of enzymatic activity is defined as the amount of catalase necessary to cause the formation of one nmol formaldehyde per minute at room temperature.

Statistical Analysis

All data are presented as means ± SEM. For ERG analysis statistical significance was calculated using the two tailed paired t-test with Welch correction, when results were of normal distribution, otherwise non-parametric Wilcoxon matched pairs test was performed. Significance of HNE immunostaining and TBARS assay was calculated using two-way ANOVA. The student's t-test or Mann-Whitney test was applied for all other calculations. Statistical calculations were performed using InStat software (GraphPad Software, La Jolla, CA). Differences were considered significant at p-value <0.05.

Results

Retinal Function and Structure Following Intravitreal PQ Injection

Three-week-old C57BL/6 (wild type, WT) and rd10 mice received intravitreal injections of 1 μl of 0.25, 0.75, 2 or 4 mM PQ in one eye, and 1 μl PBS in the fellow eye (n = 10–22 in each group). Three days post injection full field ERGs were recorded to assess retinal function.

As expected, in rd10 mice treated by intravitreal injections of PBS, ERG amplitudes were significantly lower compared to the wild type eyes. A dose-dependent response to PQ injection was observed in both rd10 and WT mice (Fig. 1A–H Fig 2 A–D and Figure S1). Yet, WT mice manifested a more prominent reduction in ERG responses compared with the response of rd10 mice to PQ injection (Fig. 1&2). For example, following 2 mM PQ injection the average scotopic b-wave amplitude at maximal stimulus intensity in WT mice dropped by 79% while in rd10 mice the drop was 47% (p = 0.02). Furthermore, injection of 0.25 mM PQ did not affect the ERG responses of rd10 mice while it significantly reduced responses were recorded in WT mice (Fig. 1). The average scotopic b-wave amplitude at maximal stimulus intensity in WT eyes injected with 0.25 mM PQ was 676±21 μV while in control eyes was 795±34 μV (p = 0.009). Light adapted responses to 1-Hz and 16-Hz stimuli corroborated recordings from dark adapted eyes (Fig. 2). The larger relative decline in ERG recordings from WT mice compared with rd10 mice following PQ injection was highlighted by plotting the ratio of photopic 1 Hz ERG amplitudes at increased concentrations of paraquat injections vs. PBS injection (Fig. 2D). Larger drop in ERG recording is evident in response to injection of 0.25, 0.75, and 2 mM, while injection of 4 mM resulted in flattening of the signal from the rd10 retinas.

Distorted outer nuclear layer (ONL) morphology was evident in sections from 9 of the 11 of the WT mice treated by 2 mM of PQ which were evaluated. By contrast, rd10 mice retinas showed ONL thinning secondary to the degenerative process, but mild distorted morphology was identified only in one eye of the 11 which were evaluated (P = 0.0019; Fig. 3). Similarly, injections of 4 mM PQ resulted in massive alterations in retinal structure in WT retinas while more subtle alterations were detected in rd10 retinas (Fig. 3). Exact quantification of the ONL was hampered by the complete disorganization of the retinal layers due to PQ-associated damage.

Oxidative Retinal Injury

HNE staining and TBARS assay were employed as markers for oxidative injury to fatty acids. Immunostaining for HNE was performed on retinal sections of rd10 and WT mice injected with 2 mM PQ or PBS. Results showed staining in all retinal layers (Fig. 4A). In PBS injected eyes, HNE staining was 1.3-fold higher in rd10 compared with WT retinas (p = 0.0002). Following PQ injection HNE staining intensity increased by 1.2-fold (p = 0.04) in rd10 mice and by 1.6-fold (p = 0.0003) in WT mice. This difference in the fold-increase of HNE staining following PQ injection between WT and rd10 mice was significant (p = 0.04; Fig. 4B).

TBARS levels were 2.4-fold higher in PBS injected rd10 eyes compared to PBS injected C57BL/6 eyes (p = 0.001). Following PQ injection there was a 2.7-fold and 5.7-fold rise in TBARS levels in rd10 (p = 0.004) and WT (p<0.0001) retinas compared to controls, respectively. This difference in the fold-increase of TBARS following PQ injection between WT and rd10 mice was not significant (p = 0.6; Fig. 5).

Oxidative injury to retinal proteins was evaluated by measurement of protein carbonyl content (PCC) in control and 2 mM PQ injected eyes. The PCC measured was 2.1-fold higher in control rd10 retinas compared with WT retinas (p = 0.009; Fig. 6). Both strains showed a 1.3-fold rise in PCC in PQ injected eyes compared with control eyes.

Antioxidant Levels Following Intravitreal PQ Injection

To obtain insight into factors underlying the smaller effect of PQ on retinas from rd10 versus WT mice, we examined the mRNA levels of anti-oxidant enzymes involved in the removal of superoxide radical anion – superoxide dismutase (SOD1), and removal of hydrogen peroxide – catalase (CAT) and glutathione peroxidase (GPX1). mRNA levels of all three genes measured in retinas of three-week-old mice before injection were significantly higher in rd10 mice compared to the WT: SOD1- 2.17-fold (p = 0.04), GPX1–2.65-fold (p = 0.01) and CAT '.1-fold (p = 0.02) (Fig. 7A).

QPCR results were confirmed by assessing catalase enzymatic activity. Results corroborated those of the expression assay, demonstrating a 1.7-fold increase in catalase activity in rd10 mice compared to the WT (p = 0.0006) (Fig. 7B).

Assessment of Iron Metabolism

Alterations in iron homeostasis were evaluated by measurement of mRNA levels of the genes: transferrin (Tf), transferrin receptor (Tfrc), and ceruloplasmin (Cp), along with quantification of ferritin protein level. Tf mRNA levels were higher in PBS-injected rd10 eyes (7.8-fold, p<0.0001), PQ-injected rd10 eyes (5-fold, p = 0.0003), and PQ-injected WT eyes (2.8-fold, p = 0.03) compared with PBS-injected WT eyes, respectively (Figure 8A).

mRNA levels of Tfrc were not affected by PQ or PBS injection in WT or rd10 retinas (Figure 8B). Cp mRNA levels were lower in PBS-injected WT retinas compared with PBS-injected rd10 retinas (2.1-fold, p = 0.082) and PQ-injected rd10 retinas (3.07-fold, p = 0.0017; Figure 8C).

Ferritin protein levels were measured by ELISA in both types of mice after intravitreal injection of 2 mM PQ or PBS. Compared to WT eyes, rd10 mice showed a trend toward higher ferritin levels (1.5-fold, p = 0.07). PQ injection caused a slight rise in mean ferritin content in both strains, however no significant changes were observed (data not shown).

Discussion

PQ injection to the vitreous cavity results in a dose dependent oxidative retinal injury [15,16,32]. In this study we have performed intravitreal injections of four different concentrations of PQ to assess the susceptibility of the degenerating retina for encountering exogenous oxidative stress. The results showed that relative to the pre-injection condition of the retina, rd10 mice suffered less retinal damage following PQ injection compared with WT mice. This relative resilience to PQ-associated damage in rd10 mice manifested in ERG responses, histology, and extent of oxidative injury to lipids as measured by HNE immunostaining

and TBARS assay. The relative resilient of the rd10 retinas to PQ injury was overcome by the 4 mM concentration which resulted in total retinal destruction according to ERG. This last finding suggests that a floor effect did not underline the relative resistance of the rd10 retinas compared with WT retinas which was observed in the 0.25, 0.75, and 2 mM PQ concentrations.

Interestingly, at the time point which we have evaluated retinal lipids seemed to suffer the brunt of the injury, as both assays of lipid peroxidation showed substantial increase in lipid peroxidation following PQ injections, while protein carbonylation did not change significantly. These findings are in agreement with those of Cingolani et al. who demonstrated that protein carbonyl adducts were elevated five days but not three days following intravitreal PQ injections to WT eyes [15]. In that study PQ injections to WT retinas caused superoxide radical levels to rise, resulting in apoptosis and thinning of the inner and outer nuclear layers.

To gain insight into the factors that underlie the relative limited retinal damage in rd10 mice compared with WT mice following PQ injection we evaluated the oxidative defense and iron metabolism systems. Prior to PQ injection there were increased mRNA levels for three anti-oxidative enzymes including superoxide dismutase 1, gluthatione peroxidase 1, and catalase in rd10 mice retinas compared with WT retinas. The functional significance of this increased expression was validated by demonstration of increased catalase activity in rd10 retinas. This data suggests that in retinas undergoing chronic oxidative stress there is up-regulation of the oxidative defense mechanism that may conceivably confer partial protection from transient oxidative challenges. Our results correlate with those of Usui et al. who showed that co-expression of CAT and SOD2, and co-expression of GPX and SOD1 cause a reduction in oxidative damage and delay cone degeneration in rd10 mice [33,34]. Similarly, Dong et al. showed that mice deficient in the SOD1 gene are more sensitive to PQ injury to the retina, hence, identifying this gene as an important component of the defense system of the retina against this type of challenge [35].

Altered iron homeostasis and iron overload were implicated in retinal and macular degeneration, including in rd10 mice, and it was suggested that iron may exacerbate oxidative retinal injury in these diseases by generation of ROS through the Fenton reaction [13,17,21,36–38]. In addition, Chen et al. found alterations in levels of iron metabolism associated proteins in normal aged rodent retinas along with elevated retinal iron. In-vitro studies showed that excess iron increased the susceptibility of retinal neurons to PQ toxicity, leading the authors to conclude that iron may contribute to the progression of age-related neurodegenerative diseases [39].

In the present study we have found increased transferrin mRNA levels and ferritin protein levels in rd10 mice compared with controls. Following PQ injection, levels of Tf increased in WT mice, while ceruloplasmin levels increased in WT and rd10 mice. This data suggests that altered retinal iron metabolism which was reported in the context of genetically driven retinal degeneration [17,20,22,27,37], photic retinal injury in mice [40,41], ageing in rodents [39], and in age related macular degeneration in humans [18,37], also occurs following exposure to oxidative stress.

We previously reported and further validated in the present study that transferrin and ferritin are up-regulated in rd10 mice retinas. Transferrin, an iron transporter, and ferritin, the major intracellular iron storage molecule, may decrease the availability of iron to the Fenton reaction, thereby, ameliorating oxidative injury. This possibility is supported by the fact that ferritin binding sites in the rd10 retina are not saturated [17], as well as by amelioration of retinal injury following intra peritoneal transferrin supplementation in rd10 mice [42].

Additional studies are required to evaluate if our findings may be extended to other sources of oxidative injury such as photic damage and hyperoxia or hypoxia. It would be of particular importance to clarify if transient exposure to environmental sources of oxidative injury, such as light, is harmful to the degenerating human retina in diseases such as macular degeneration and retinitis pigmentosa, and if treatment with anti-oxidants may alter the threshold of the human retina to encounter such stress.

Author Contributions

Conceived and designed the experiments: E. Berenshtein MC IC ML SHL MG AO E. Banin. Performed the experiments: IC ML SHL MG AO E. Berenshtein. Analyzed the data: E. Berenshtein MC IC ML SHL MG AO E. Banin. Contributed reagents/materials/analysis tools: E. Banin MC IC AO E. Berenshtein. Wrote the paper: IC AO E. Banin ML SHL MG MC.

References

1. Zhu X, Su B, Wang X, Smith MA, Perry G (2007) Causes of oxidative stress in Alzheimer disease. Cell Mol Life Sci 64: 2202–2210.
2. Trushina E, McMurray CT (2007) Oxidative stress and mitochondrial dysfunction in neurodegenerative diseases. Neuroscience 145: 1233–1248.
3. Calabrese V, Lodi R, Tonon C, D'Agata V, Sapienza M, et al. (2005) Oxidative stress, mitochondrial dysfunction and cellular stress response in Friedreich's ataxia. J Neurol Sci 233: 145–162.
4. Jenner P (2003) Oxidative stress in Parkinson's disease. Ann Neurol 53 Suppl 3: S26–36; discussion S36–28.
5. Shen J, Yang X, Dong A, Petters RM, Peng YW, et al. (2005) Oxidative damage is a potential cause of cone cell death in retinitis pigmentosa. J Cell Physiol 203: 457–464.
6. Beatty S, Koh H, Phil M, Henson D, Boulton M (2000) The role of oxidative stress in the pathogenesis of age-related macular degeneration. Surv Ophthalmol 45: 115–134.
7. Shen JK, Dong A, Hackett SF, Bell WR, Green WR, et al. (2007) Oxidative damage in age-related macular degeneration. Histol Histopathol 22: 1301–1308.
8. Sacca SC, Izzotti A, Rossi P, Traverso C (2007) Glaucomatous outflow pathway and oxidative stress. Exp Eye Res 84: 389–399.
9. Anderson RE, Kretzer FL, Rapp LM (1994) Free radicals and ocular disease. Adv Exp Med Biol 366: 73–86.
10. Age-Related Eye Disease Study Research Group (2001) A randomized, placebo-controlled, clinical trial of high-dose supplementation with vitamins C and E, beta carotene, and zinc for age-related macular degeneration and vision loss: AREDS report no. 8. Arch Ophthalmol 119: 1417–1436.
11. Dunaief JL (2011) Ironing out neurodegeneration: iron chelation for neuroprotection. Free Radic Biol Med 51: 1480–1481.
12. Komeima K, Rogers BS, Lu L, Campochiaro PA (2006) Antioxidants reduce cone cell death in a model of retinitis pigmentosa. Proc Natl Acad Sci U S A 103: 11300–11305.
13. Obolensky A, Berenshtein E, Lederman M, Bulvik B, Alper-Pinus R, et al. (2011) Zinc-desferrioxamine attenuates retinal degeneration in the rd10 mouse model of retinitis pigmentosa. Free Radic Biol Med 51: 1482–1491.
14. Yoshida N, Ikeda Y, Notomi S, Ishikawa K, Murakami Y, et al. (2013) Laboratory evidence of sustained chronic inflammatory reaction in retinitis pigmentosa. Ophthalmology 120: e5–12.
15. Cingolani C, Rogers B, Lu L, Kachi S, Shen J, et al. (2006) Retinal degeneration from oxidative damage. Free Radic Biol Med 40: 660–669.
16. Chang B, Hawes NL, Pardue MT, German AM, Hurd RE, et al. (2007) Two mouse retinal degenerations caused by missense mutations in the beta-subunit of rod cGMP phosphodiesterase gene. Vision Res 47: 624–633.
17. Deleon E, Lederman M, Berenstein E, Meir T, Chevion M, et al. (2009) Alteration in iron metabolism during retinal degeneration in rd10 mouse. Invest Ophthalmol Vis Sci 50: 1360–1365.
18. Hahn P, Milam AH, Dunaief JL (2003) Maculas affected by age-related macular degeneration contain increased chelatable iron in the retinal pigment epithelium and Bruch's membrane. Arch Ophthalmol 121: 1099–1105.
19. Gargini C, Terzibasi E, Mazzoni F, Strettoi E (2007) Retinal organization in the retinal degeneration 10 (rd10) mutant mouse: a morphological and ERG study. J Comp Neurol 500: 222–238.
20. Mori K, Duh E, Gehlbach P, Ando A, Takahashi K, et al. (2001) Pigment epithelium-derived factor inhibits retinal and choroidal neovascularization. J Cell Physiol 188: 253–263.
21. Obolensky A, Berenshtein E, Konijn AM, Banin E, Chevion M (2008) Ischemic preconditioning of the rat retina: protective role of ferritin. Free Radic Biol Med 44: 1286–1294.
22. Meir T, Dror R, Yu X, Qian J, Simon I, et al. (2007) Molecular characteristics of liver metastases from uveal melanoma. Invest Ophthalmol Vis Sci 48: 4890–4896.

23. Collins TJ (2007) ImageJ for microscopy. Biotechniques 43: 25–30.
24. Vandesompele J, De Preter K, Pattyn F, Poppe B, Van Roy N, et al. (2002) Accurate normalization of real-time quantitative RT-PCR data by geometric averaging of multiple internal control genes. Genome Biol 3: RESEARCH0034.
25. Livak KJ, Schmittgen TD (2001) Analysis of relative gene expression data using real-time quantitative PCR and the 2(-Delta Delta C(T)) Method. Methods 25: 402–408.
26. Konijn AM, Levy R, Link G, Hershko C (1982) A rapid and sensitive ELISA for serum ferritin employing a fluorogenic substrate. J Immunol Methods 54: 297–307.
27. Ohkawa H, Ohishi N, Yagi K (1979) Assay for lipid peroxides in animal tissues by thiobarbituric acid reaction. Anal Biochem 95: 351–358.
28. Reznick AZ, Cross CE, Hu ML, Suzuki YJ, Khwaja S, et al. (1992) Modification of plasma proteins by cigarette smoke as measured by protein carbonyl formation. Biochem J 286 (Pt 2): 607–611.
29. Reznick AZ, Packer L (1994) Oxidative damage to proteins: spectrophotometric method for carbonyl assay. Methods Enzymol 233: 357–363.
30. Chevion M, Berenshtein E, Stadtman ER (2000) Human studies related to protein oxidation: protein carbonyl content as a marker of damage. Free Radic Res 33 Suppl: S99–108.
31. Johansson LH, Borg LA (1988) A spectrophotometric method for determination of catalase activity in small tissue samples. Anal Biochem 174: 331–336.
32. Chen M, Luo C, Penalva R, Xu H (2013) Paraquat-induced retinal degeneration is exaggerated in CX3CR1-deficient mice and is associated with increased retinal inflammation. Invest Ophthalmol Vis Sci 54: 682–690.
33. Usui S, Komeima K, Lee SY, Jo YJ, Ueno S, et al. (2009) Increased expression of catalase and superoxide dismutase 2 reduces cone cell death in retinitis pigmentosa. Mol Ther 17: 778–786.
34. Usui S, Oveson BC, Iwase T, Lu L, Lee SY, et al. (2011) Overexpression of SOD in retina: need for increase in H2O2-detoxifying enzyme in same cellular compartment. Free Radic Biol Med 51: 1347–1354.
35. Dong A, Shen J, Krause M, Akiyama H, Hackett SF, et al. (2006) Superoxide dismutase 1 protects retinal cells from oxidative damage. J Cell Physiol 208: 516–526.
36. He X, Hahn P, Iacovelli J, Wong R, King C, et al. (2007) Iron homeostasis and toxicity in retinal degeneration. Prog Retin Eye Res 26: 649–673.
37. Chowers I, Wong R, Dentchev T, Farkas RH, Iacovelli J, et al. (2006) The iron carrier transferrin is upregulated in retinas from patients with age-related macular degeneration. Invest Ophthalmol Vis Sci 47: 2135–2140.
38. Banin E, Berenshtein E, Kitrossky N, Pe'er J, Chevion M (2000) Gallium-desferrioxamine protects the cat retina against injury after ischemia and reperfusion. Free Radic Biol Med 28: 315–323.
39. Chen H, Liu B, Lukas TJ, Suyeoka G, Wu G, et al. (2009) Changes in iron-regulatory proteins in the aged rodent neural retina. Neurobiol Aging 30: 1865–1876.
40. Hadziahmetovic M, Kumar U, Song Y, Grieco S, Song D, et al. (2012) Microarray analysis of murine retinal light damage reveals changes in iron regulatory, complement, and antioxidant genes in the neurosensory retina and isolated RPE. Invest Ophthalmol Vis Sci 53: 5231–5241.
41. Song D, Song Y, Hadziahmetovic M, Zhong Y, Dunaief JL (2012) Systemic administration of the iron chelator deferiprone protects against light-induced photoreceptor degeneration in the mouse retina. Free Radic Biol Med 53: 64–71.
42. Picard E, Jonet L, Sergeant C, Vesvres MH, Behar-Cohen F, et al. (2010) Overexpressed or intraperitoneally injected human transferrin prevents photoreceptor degeneration in rd10 mice. Mol Vis 16: 2612–2625.

10

Hyperglycaemia Exacerbates Choroidal Neovascularisation in Mice via the Oxidative Stress-Induced Activation of STAT3 Signalling in RPE Cells

Xia Li[1][9], Yan Cai[1][9], Yu-Sheng Wang[1]*, Yuan-Yuan Shi[1], Wei Hou[3], Chun-Sheng Xu[4], Hai-Yan Wang[1], Zi Ye[1], Li-Bo Yao[2], Jian Zhang[2]*

1 Department of Ophthalmology, Xijing Hospital, Fourth Military Medical University, Xi'an, Shaanxi Province, People's Republic of China, 2 State Key Laboratory of Cancer Biology, Department of Biochemistry and Molecular Biology, Fourth Military Medical University, Xi'an, Shaanxi Province, People's Republic of China, 3 Department of Orthopedics, Xijing Hospital, Fourth Military Medical University, Xi'an, Shaanxi Province, People's Republic of China, 4 State Key Laboratory of Cancer Biology, Department of Gastrointestinal Surgery, Xijing Hospital, Fourth Military Medical University, Xi'an, Shaanxi Province, People's Republic of China

Abstract

Choroidal neovascularisation (CNV) that occurs as a result of age-related macular degeneration (AMD) causes severe vision loss among elderly patients. The relationship between diabetes and CNV remains controversial. However, oxidative stress plays a critical role in the pathogenesis of both AMD and diabetes. In the present study, we investigated the influence of diabetes on experimentally induced CNV and on the underlying molecular mechanisms of CNV. CNV was induced via photocoagulation in the ocular fundi of mice with streptozotocin-induced diabetes. The effect of diabetes on the severity of CNV was measured. An immunofluorescence technique was used to determine the levels of oxidative DNA damage by anti-8-hydroxy-2-deoxyguanosine (8-OHdG) antibody, the protein expression of phosphorylated signal transducer and activator of transcription 3 (p-STAT3) and vascular endothelial growth factor (VEGF), in mice with CNV. The production of reactive oxygen species (ROS) in retinal pigment epithelial (RPE) cells that had been cultured under high glucose was quantitated using the 2',7'-dichlorofluorescein diacetate (DCFH-DA) method. p-STAT3 expression was examined using Western blot analysis. RT-PCR and ELISA processes were used to detect VEGF expression. Hyperglycaemia exacerbated the development of CNV in mice. Oxidative stress levels and the expression of p-STAT3 and VEGF were highly elevated both in mice and in cultured RPE cells. Treatment with the antioxidant compound N-acetyl-cysteine (NAC) rescued the severity of CNV in diabetic mice. NAC also inhibited the overexpression of p-STAT3 and VEGF in CNV and in RPE cells. The JAK-2/STAT3 pathway inhibitor AG490 blocked VEGF expression but had no effect on the production of ROS *in vitro*. These results suggest that hyperglycaemia promotes the development of CNV by inducing oxidative stress, which in turn activates STAT3 signalling in RPE cells. Antioxidant supplementation helped attenuate the development of CNV. Thus, our results reveal a potential strategy for the treatment and prevention of diseases involving CNV.

Editor: Lewin Alfred, University of Florida, United States of America

Funding: This work was supported by grants from the National Natural Science Foundation of China (No. 30872818, 81070748) and National Basic Research Program of China (973 Program/No. 2011CB510200). The project was sponsored partly by the equipment donation from the Alexander Von Humboldt Foundation in Germany (to Y.S.W., V8151/02085). The funders had no role in study design, data collection and analysis, decision to publish, or preparation of the manuscript.

Competing Interests: The authors have declared that no competing interests exist.

* E-mail: wangys003@126.com (YSW); biozhangj@yahoo.com.cn (JZ)

❾ These authors contributed equally to this work.

Introduction

Age-related macular degeneration (AMD) is a major cause of visual impairment in elderly people. Choroidal neovascularisation (CNV) beneath the macula, which occurs in the late stage of the disease and is characterised as the "wet form" of AMD, causes rapid central vision loss that has serious effects on the quality of life in older patients [1]. A number of genetic and environmental factors have been identified as being risk factors for neovascular AMD, and knowledge of these factors has helped in both preventing and reducing the occurrence and process of the disease [2].

Because of the effect that diabetes has on vascular systems, epidemiological studies have focused on the relationship between

diabetes and AMD. The similarity of the results that were obtained from an ancillary study to the Women's Health Initiative Sight Exam and a clinical study concerning the association between myocardial infarctions and the development of AMD suggested that diabetes is a risk factor for AMD [3,4]. However, other studies have come to contrary conclusions [5,6,7,8]. In fact, even studies that investigated risk factors that were associated with different types of AMD had inconsistent conclusions regarding whether diabetes was a factor that affected the disease [5,9]. Moreover, two abstracts that were presented at the annual meeting of the Association for Research in Vision and Ophthalmology (ARVO) found that diabetes enhanced the development of laser-induced CNV in mice but suggested that understanding the underlying mechanism for this enhancement required further investigation [10,11]. Therefore, in the present study, we were interested in not only identifying the association between diabetes and CNV but also in attempting to investigate the underlying mechanisms that were responsible for the association.

Increasing evidence has shown that oxidative stress contributes to the development of a wide range of diseases, including age-related diseases, cancer, metabolic diseases and neural diseases. Although the pathogenesis of CNV remains uncertain, it has been suggested that oxidative stress plays a causative role in both the initiation and progression of CNV [12]. It has been reported that mice that are deficient in Cu, Zn-superoxide dismutase (SOD1) have features that are typical of AMD in humans such as the presence of drusen, thickening of Bruch's membrane and CNV [13]. It has been confirmed that the downregulation of NADPH oxidase-mediated ROS production in the retinal pigment epithe-lial (RPE) cells of mice reduces CNV lesions [14]. In addition, studies have demonstrated that the use of antioxidant supplemen-tation to counter cellular oxidative stress results in the suppression of experimental CNV [15]. Meanwhile, diabetes-related investiga-tions have shown that oxidative stress is a key factor in the initiation of structural and functional vascular changes [16,17]. It has been reported that generation of ROS is responsible for early stages of diabetic nephropathy [18]. Other studies have demon-strated that hyperglycaemia results in an increase in the pro-duction of superoxide in retina and ultimately contributes to the pathogenesis of diabetic retinopathy (DR) [19]. Furthermore, treatments that reduce the formation of ROS were successful in preventing DR in a streptozotocin (STZ)-induced diabetic rat model [20].

The signal transducer and activator of transcription-3 (STAT3) protein is important for the regulation of cell differentiation, proliferation, and angiogenesis [21]. Previous studies have verified that STAT3 is a direct transcriptional activator of the vascular endothelial growth factor (VEGF) gene [22]. In a murine model of laser-induced CNV, STAT3 activation was found to be involved in promoting the development of CNV [23]. Recent findings have suggested that diabetes increases the level of STAT3 activation and thereby contributes to the pathophysiology of vascular injury [20].

In the present study, we have investigated the effects of diabetes on the development of laser-induced CNV in mice, and we have also investigated the roles that oxidative stress and STAT3 signalling play in the regulation of VEGF in RPE cells in a high glucose environment.

Results

Blood Glucose and Body Weight after Injection of Streptozotocin

Streptozotocin injection significantly elevated blood glucose levels compared to control mice at 5 time points throughout the experimental period: pretreatment, 1-week, 2-weeks, 3-weeks and 4-weeks post-STZ injection (Fig. 1 A). Body weights of animals were assessed starting on the day of injection and followed thereafter at one-week intervals to observe changes in weights. Control mice showed an increase in body weight over the experimental period, but the diabetic mice had lower weight gain compared with control group (Fig. 1 B).

Hyperglycaemia Promoted the Formation of CNV in Mice

Vascular complexes that formed after the damage to Bruch's membrane extended from the choroid to the subretinal space and caused an appearance of hyperfluorescence in FFA. The leakage reflects the permeability of the neovascularization. Although the

difference between the incidences of CNV at the irradiated spots in the diabetic and control mice was not significant ($P>0.05$), the degree of fluorescence leakage in the eyes of the hyperglycaemic mice was significantly elevated relative to that in the control mice on day 14 after photocoagulation (*$P<0.01$, Fig. 2 A).

Similar results were found in both the flatmount and histopathology assays. Compared with mice in the control group, the average area of CNV was markedly larger in diabetic mice on day 14 (14931 ± 2432 vs. 27162 ± 5197 μm^2 for control and diabetic mice, respectively; *$P<0.01$; Fig. 2 B, C and F). However, analysis of the cross-sectional slices revealed that there was no significant difference between the average thicknesses of CNV in the two groups (27.8 ± 4.2 vs. 29.1 ± 4.6 μm for control and diabetic mice, respectively; $P>0.05$; Fig. 2 D, E and G) and that the CNVs in hyperglycaemic mice were wider than those of the control group (158.6 ± 26.7 vs. 245.9 ± 34.7 μm for control and diabetic mice, respective; *$P<0.01$; Fig. 2 D, E and G).In general, we found that the width and surface area of the CNV lesions had a significant difference but the thicknesses had no difference between the two groups. One possible explanation is that after photocoagulation-induced rupture of Bruch's membrane in mice, vascular complexes began to grow and extend from the choroid to the subretinal space. Because of the relatively tight junctions of the inner retina that possessed, the progression of CNV was mainly located at the external retinal layer. This characteristic causes pathological neovascularization grow parallel to the plane of retinal layer but hard to develop upwards vertically [24]. We thought that this may be the reason that help to explain why there was no significant difference in the thickness of the CNV lesions in the two groups.

Hyperglycaemia Increased Oxidative DNA Damage, Up-regulated VEGF and Phosphorylated STAT3 (p-STAT3) Expression in CNV

Local expression patterns of 8-OHdG, VEGF and p-STAT3 in the initial stage of experimentally induced CNV formation were investigated to determine a potential underlying mechanism for the effects of hyperglycaemia. Compared with the control group, we found evidence of elevated levels of oxidative DNA damage (95.8 ± 9.6 vs. 203.2 ± 30.7 RFI in control and diabetic mice, respectively; *$P<0.01$; Fig. 3 A and C), upregulateion of VEGF (65.7 ± 6.9 vs. 103.9 ± 7.3 RFI in control and diabetic mice, respectively; *$P<0.01$; Fig. 3 A and C) and p-STAT3 (41.5 ± 5.2 vs. 70.8 ± 9.8 RFI in control and diabetic mice, respectively; *$P<0.01$; Fig. 3 B and C) expression in the choroid beneath CNV lesions in the eyes of diabetic mice on day 3 after laser damage. An ELISA further confirmed that the upregulation of VEGF expression was induced by hyperglycaemia (45.5 ± 5.0 vs. 68.5 ± 8.1 pg/eye in control and diabetic mice, respectively; *$P<0.01$; Fig. 3 D).

High Levels of Glucose Promoted Intracellular ROS Formation, STAT3 Activation and VEGF Production in RPE Cells

Because the retinal pigment epithelium has a higher rate of oxygen consumption than any other tissue, RPE cells are vulnerable to oxidative damage [25]. To confirm the role of hyperglycaemia and its subsequent effects on the development of CNV, we investigated the levels of intracellular ROS formation, STAT3 activation and VEGF production in RPE cells. The levels of ROS that were found in the high glucose group are significantly higher than those of the low glucose and mannitol groups (*$P<0.01$, Fig. 4 A).

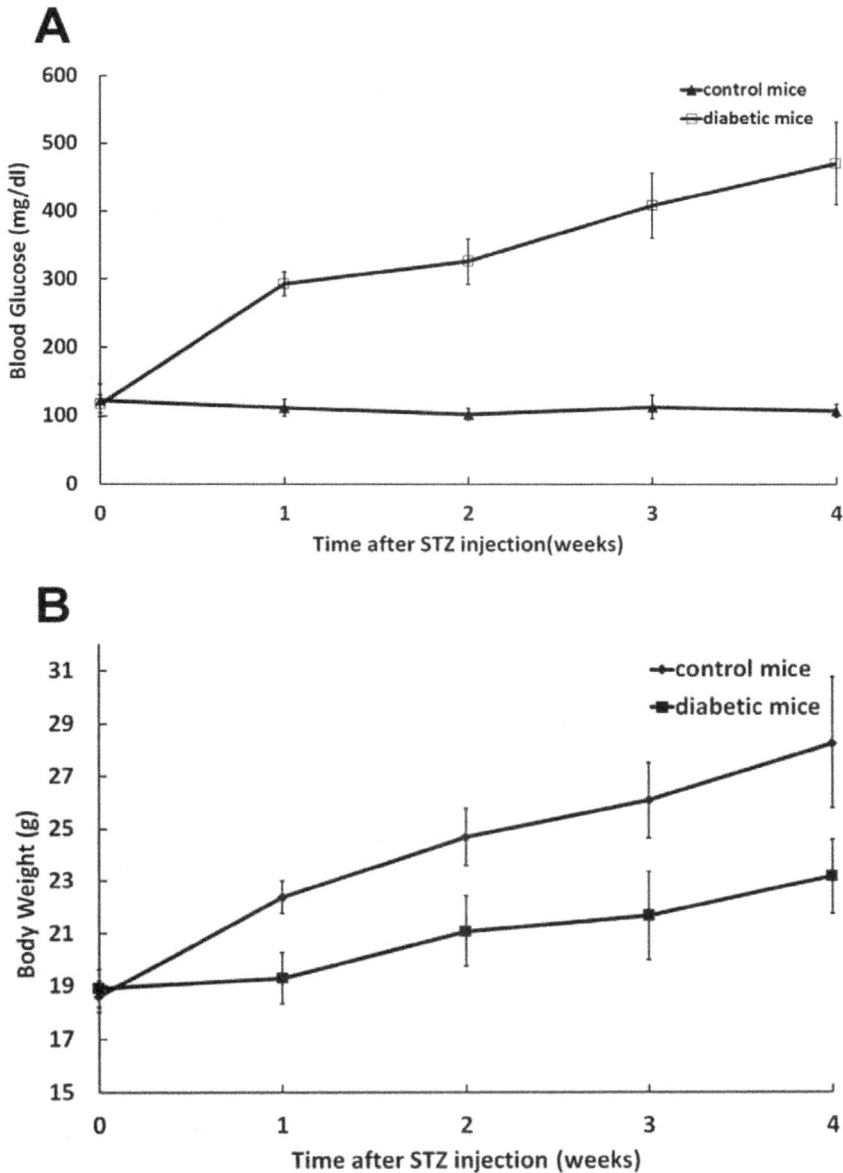

Figure 1. Effects of streptozotocin on blood glucose and body weight of mice. A, STZ injection resulted in elevated blood glucose levels in mice. B, Diabetic mice had lower body weight gain in compared to control group. Error bars represent ± SEM. All diabetic time points are significantly different from control ($P<0.05$).

The level of p-STAT3 protein expression in RPE cells significantly increased in a time-dependent manner; it reached a maximum after 3 hours of exposure to a high-glucose medium and subsequently decreased (*$P<0.01$, #$P<0.05$, Fig.4 B–C), whereas the total level of STAT3 protein expression changed weakly.

In addition, the amount of VEGF mRNA in RPE cells was also up-regulated during exposure to a high glucose medium, and the timecourse of the up-regulation was similar to that of the change in p-STAT3 protein expression (*$P<0.01$, Fig. 4 D–F). After 6 h, the amount of VEGF protein that had been secreted by RPE cells in a culture medium that contained a high concentration of glucose was also higher than the amount of VEGF that had been secreted by RPE cells in a control medium (*$P<0.01$, Fig. 4 F).

NAC-induced Suppression of Oxidative Stress Rescued CNV Severity

NAC is a thiol-containing compound that has been used as a promising antioxidant to counteract oxidative stress in many diseases. In the present study, we assessed the degree to which NAC supplementation was able to reduce or reverse the severity of CNV that formed under hyperglycaemic conditions. As shown in fig. 4, treatment with NAC significantly reduced the amount fluorescence leakage of CNV in diabetic mice (#$P<0.05$, Fig. 5 A). In addition, both the area (25899 ± 5997 vs. 19616 ± 5158 μm^2 in STZ and NAC mice, respectively; #$P<0.05$; Fig. 5 B, C, and F) and width of the CNV lesions in NAC-treated mice (240.3 ± 30.9 vs. 199.1 ± 28.7 μm in STZ and NAC mice, respectively; #$P<0.05$; Fig. 5 D, E, and G) were

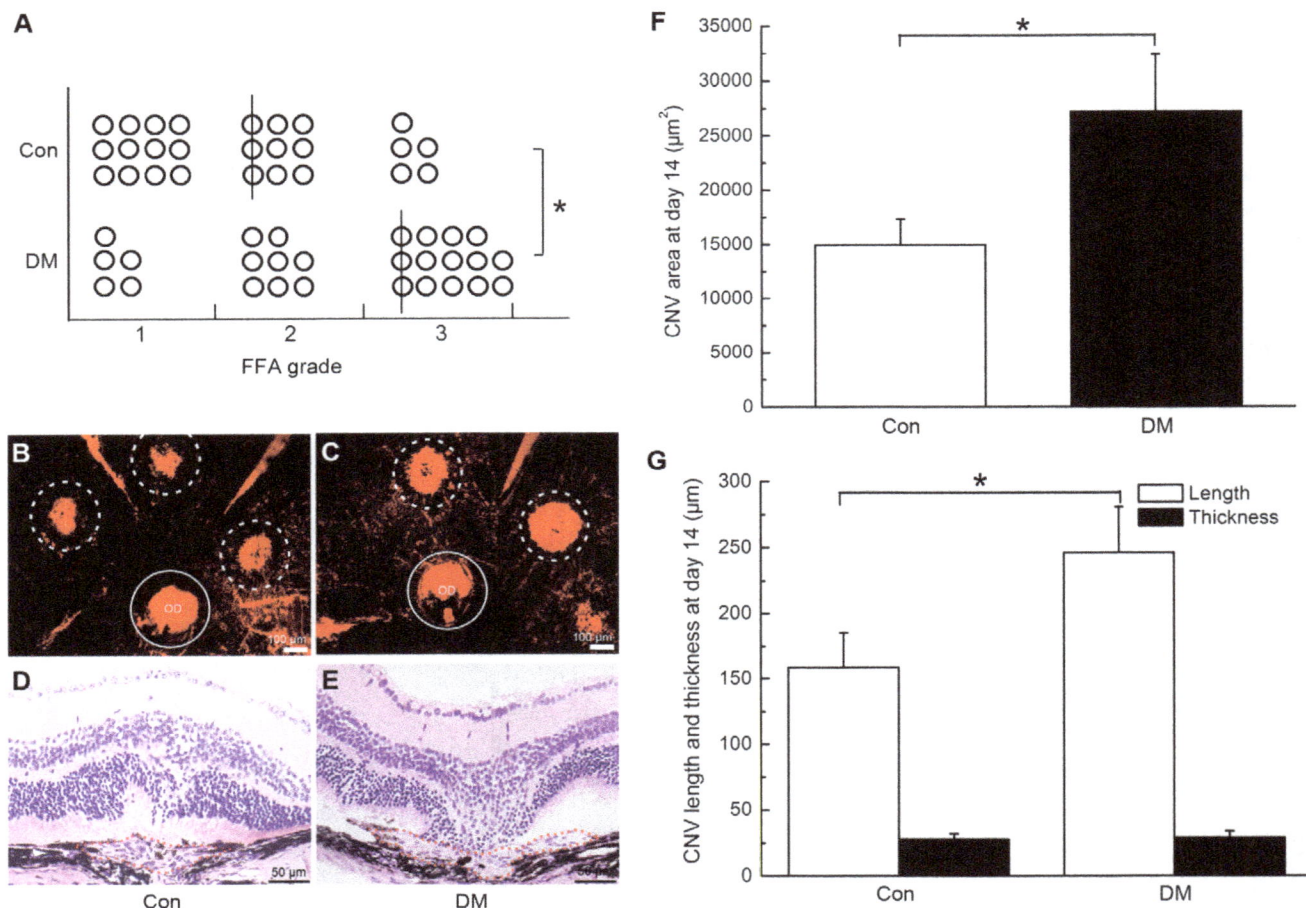

Figure 2. Hyperglycaemia promoted the development of CNV 2 weeks after laser photocoagulation. A, Statistical analysis of the fluorescein leakage in control mice (Con) and diabetic mice (DM) (*P<0.01, lines indicate median leakage levels). B–C, Representative flatmount preparations of the eyecups of control (B) and diabetic (C) mice (Dotted circles: area of CNV; OD: optic disc; Circles: area of OD). D–E, H&E staining images of serial cross-sections of the eye cups of control (D) and diabetic (E) mice. F, Statistical analysis of the data in B and C (*P<0.01); G, Statistical analysis of the data in D and E (*P<0.01).

decreased relative to the CNV characteristics in the control group. However, there was no significant difference in the thicknesses of the CNV lesions in the two groups (28.1±3.7 vs. 26.5±3.7 μmin STZ and NAC mice, respectively; *P*>0.05; Fig. 5 D, E, and G).

NAC Supplementation Inhibited the Hyperglycaemia-induced Oxidative Stress and Expression of p-STAT3 and VEGF

Consistent with our histology findings, NAC supplementation significantly reduced the severity of the hyperglycaemia-induced oxidative DNA damage (199.2±37.2 vs. 129.7±24.3 RFI in diabetic and NAC group, respectively; #*P*<0.05; Fig. 6 A and C), and expression of VEGF (101.8±12.8 vs. 78.1±9.9 RFI in diabetic and NAC group, respectively; #*P*<0.05; Fig. 6 A and C) and p-STAT3 protein (74.3±9.7 vs. 55.8±8.7 RFI in diabetic and NAC group, respectively; #*P*<0.05; Fig. 6 B and C). The NAC-induced decreased in the level of VEGF expression was further confirmed by the ELISA (70.9±8.8 vs. 54.8±6.9 pg/eye in diabetic and NAC group, respectively; #*P*<0.05; Fig. 6 D).

Treatment with NAC and AG490 Inhibited p-STAT3 and VEGF Expression in RPE Cells that were Exposed to High Glucose Conditions

To determine the relationship between oxidative stress and activation of the STAT3 signalling pathway, we tested the effects of NAC and the JAK2/STAT3 pathway inhibitor AG490 on RPE cells that were exposed to high glucose conditions. The administration of NAC reduced the degree of intracellular ROS formation; AG490 administration had no effect (*P<0.01, Fig. 7 A). The induction of p-STAT3 expression in RPE cells that were exposed to high glucose conditions was inhibited by both NAC and AG490 (*P<0.01, Fig. 7 B and C). RT-PCR and ELISA experiments confirmed that VEGF expression was inhibited by both NAC and AG490 (*P<0.01, #*P*<0.05, Fig. 7 D and E). Thus, our data suggest that oxidative stress can be considered an upstream factor that affects STAT3 activity, which in turn leads to the high glucose-mediated transcriptional activation of angiogenic genes such as VEGF (Fig. 8).

Discussion

AMD is the primary cause of blindness among elderly people (those who are 65 years of age and older) in developed countries

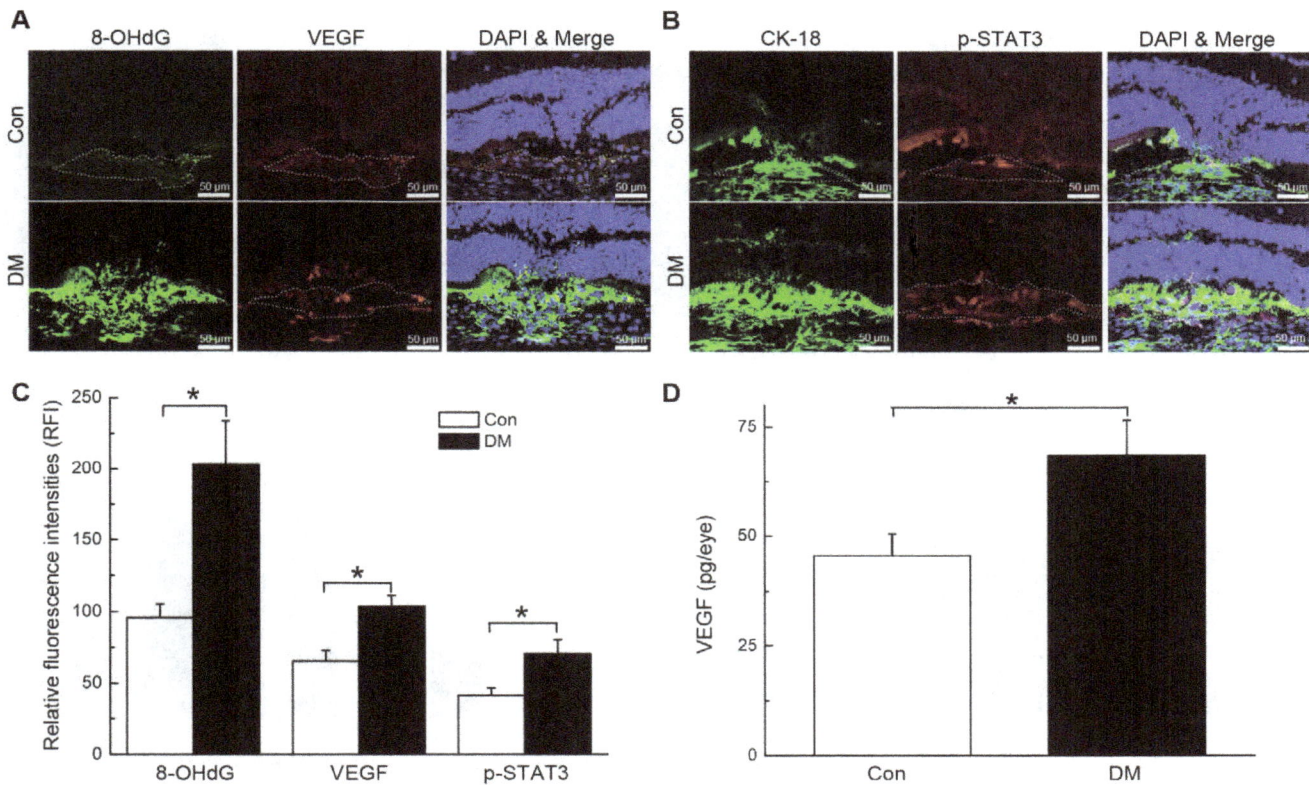

Figure 3. Hyperglycaemia resulted in the up-regulation of 8-OHdG, VEGF and p-STAT3 expression at sites of CNV. A-B, 8-OHdG, VEGF and p-STAT3 expression patterns at CNV sites in control (Con) and diabetic (DM) mice. CNV lesions were encircled with dashed lines. Relative fluorescence intensities (RFI) of targeted proteins were measured by analysing images of the immunofluorescence staining of serial cross sections of the eyecups. C, Statistical analysis of the data in A and B (*P<0.01); D, Statistical analysis of the data from the VEGF ELISA (*P<0.01).

[26,27]. There are two forms of AMD: "dry" AMD, which is characterised by the presence of soft drusen or geographic atrophy, and "wet" AMD, which is characterised by the presence of CNV under the macula. Approximately 10%–15% of dry AMD cases progress to the more advanced and damaging form of AMD, which is characterised by CNV that results in rapid and progressive central vision loss. It has been hypothesised that diabetes-related changes in the structures and functions of the RPE, Bruch's membrane and the choroid layer result in an increased risk of developing AMD [9]. However, disagreement among current results from a number of epidemiological investigations and the limited number of mechanism-specific investigations mean the association between diabetes and AMD remains unclear. Retrospective study of Borrone R et al. found that the prevalence of ARM was lower in diabetic patients and even lower in patients with DR, but the exudative form (CNV) was higher than the atrophic form in diabetic patients compared to the general population [28]. Proctor B et al. have paid attention on the relationship between DR and ARMD [29]. They found that DR patients were much less likely to have CNV, but what's the incidence of CNV in diabetic patients without DR is still unknown. While in the EUREYE study, a positive association of diabetes with CNV was found, but the atrophic form was not relevant with diabetes [7]. Taken together, diabetes with/without DR and different forms of AMD all suggest a different intraocular pathological environment for CNV development. Most of the epidemiological data focused on the relationship between AMD and diabetes remain controversial. Therefore, a lot more

experimental researches focusing on the underlying mechanism needs to be further carried out.

In the current study, we observed that the CNV lesions in STZ-induced diabetic mice were significantly larger than similar lesions in wild-type mice, which indicated that diabetes might have an effect on the development of CNV. Diabetes is characterized by hyperglycaemia due to absolute or relative lack of insulin. Although animal model cannot fully mimic the clinical manifestations and pathological features, animal experiments have contributed much to our understanding of mechanisms of human disease. STZ can selective destruct β-cells of the pancreas, resulting in a lack of insulin secretion and finally increasing the blood glucose level. The model is stable and the effect is significant [30]. It has been reported that the duration of diabetes had no correlation with AMD, but the relationship needs to be further evaluated [1]. We induced CNV in a short period of time after STZ injection in order to observe the effect of hyperglycemia rather than the course of disease or chronic diabetic complications on CNV formation. Diabetes-induced hyperglycaemia has been implicated in the development of diabetes-specific pathology [31]. Histopathological studies of the eyes of diabetic patients have revealed thickening of the basement membranes in the walls of the choriocapillaris, luminal narrowing, dropout of the choriocapillaris, and thickening of Bruch's membrane [32]. Findings from our study suggested that there is a positive relationship between diabetes-induced hyperglycaemia and the development of CNV. Glycaemic control is a very important aspect of diabetes management. Poor control of the blood sugar levels of diabetic patients can accelerate the

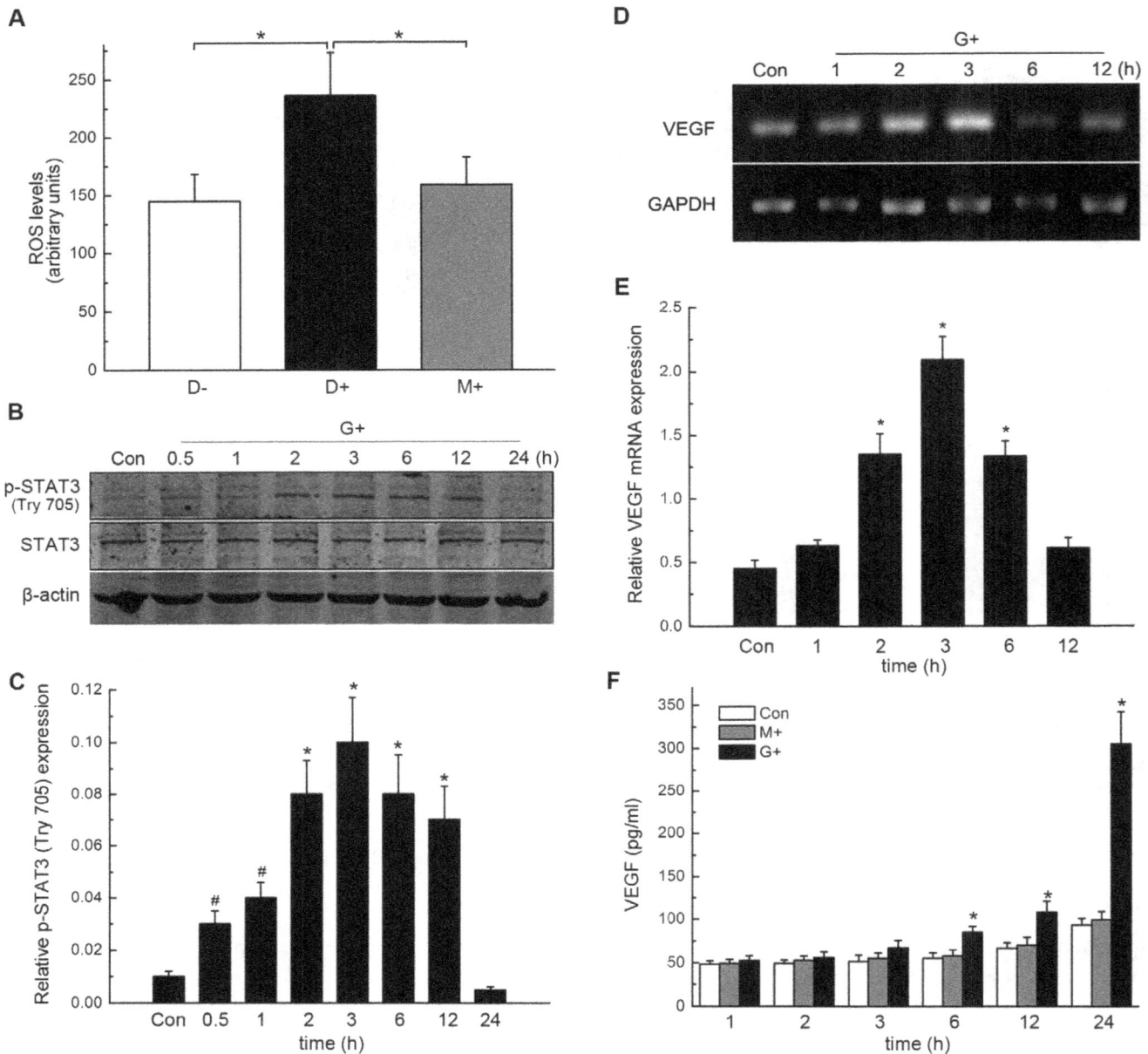

Figure 4. High glucose (HG) promoted intracellular ROS formation, STAT3 activation and VEGF production in RPE cells. A, compared with that were treated with high mannitol (HM) and normal glucose (NG) solutions, treatment with a HG solution increased the ROS level in RPE cells (*P<0.01). B, expression of p-STAT3 and STAT3 in RPE cells after different lengths of exposure to an HG solution as measured by Western Blotting. The results from 3 representative experiments that were performed independently are shown. C, Statistical analysis of the data in B (*P<0.01, #P<0.05). D, Results of representative RT-PCR experiments showing the levels of VEGF mRNA expression at the indicated times. E, Statistical analysis of the data in D (*P<0.01). F, Statistical analysis of the VEGF ELISA data (*P<0.01).

progression of the disease and may increase the risk of diabetes-related complications [31,33,34]. This may help explain the controversial epidemiological results regarding the relation between diabetes and wet AMD. Recruitment biases and differences among study participants, measurement and statistical analyses may account for some of the variation among the results of these studies, but we noticed that most of them did not pay close attention to the control of blood sugar. Therefore, we confirmed for the first time that hyperglycaemia plays an important role in the exacerbation of CNV.

Previous studies have reported that the increased levels of VEGF and inter-cellular adhesion molecule 1 (ICAM-1) expression and the activation of a complementary system were associated with the development CNV in type 1 and type 2 diabetic rodent models [10,11], but the underlying mechanism for these changes was still poorly understood. Hyperglycaemia-induced diabetic vascular damage has been identified as occurring via 4 major pathways: the activation of protein kinase C (PKC) isoforms; the formation of advanced glycation end-products; up-regulation of activity in the polyol pathway; and up-regulation of activity in the hexosamine pathway [35]. In all 4 of these mechanisms, oxidative

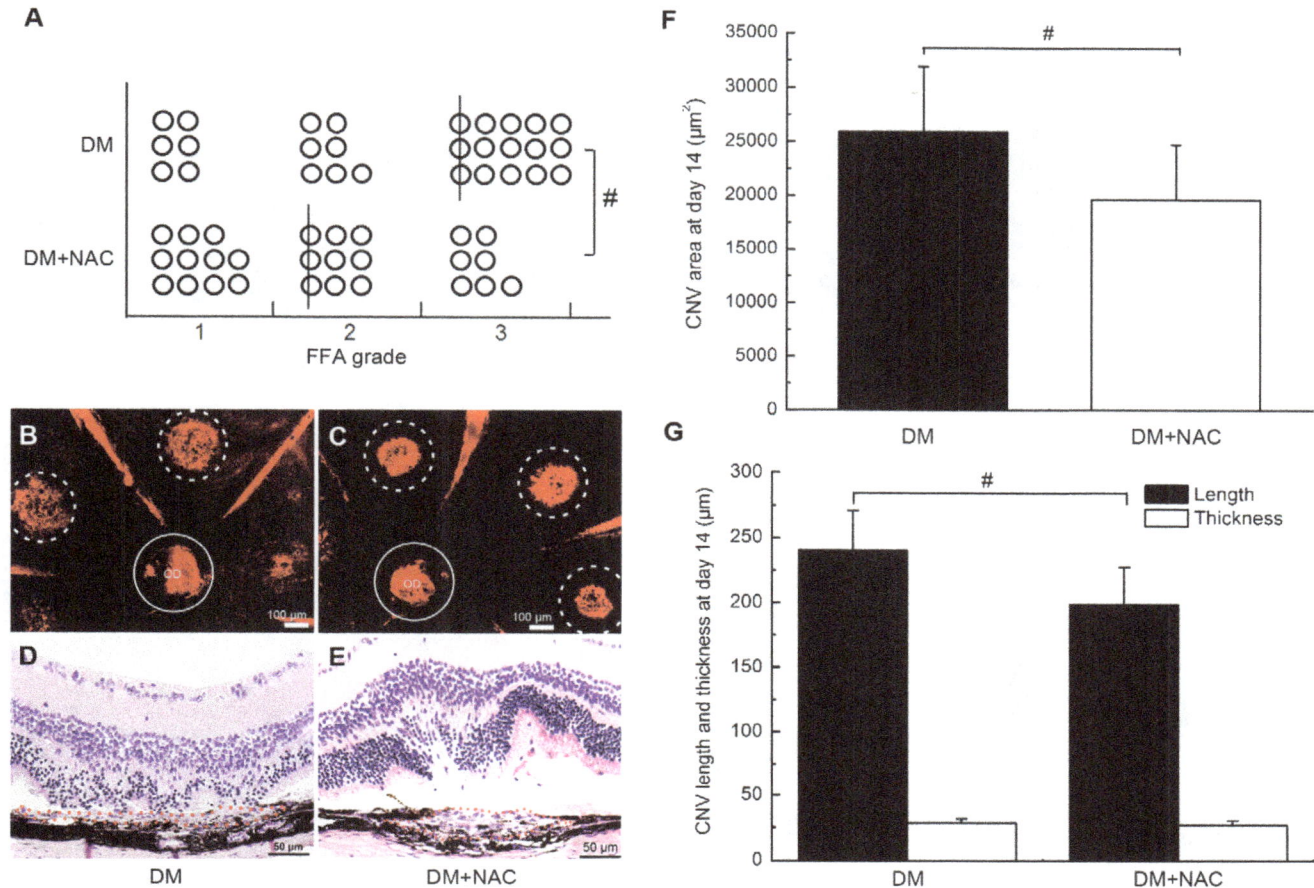

Figure 5. NAC-induced suppression of oxidative stress rescued CNV severity. A, Statistical analysis of the fluorescein leakage in untreated diabetic (DM) and NAC-treated diabetic (NAC) mice (#P<0.05); lines indicate the median CNV grades. B-C, Areas of CNV lesions in the aforementioned groups; D–E, H&E staining of CNV lesions in DM and NAC mice; F, Statistical analysis of the data presented in B and C (#P<0.05). G, Statistical analysis of the data presented in D and E (#P<0.05).

stress has been considered a singular upstream event that is involved in promoting the process of pathology in diabetes and its related vascular complications [31,36]. Moreover, oxidative stress has also been implicated in the up-regulation of VEGF expression and in pathological ocular angiogenesis [37,38]. Thus, we examined the oxidative stress statuses of mice with experimentally induced CNV and the oxidative stress statuses of RPE cells that had been exposed to high-glucose environments. Increased levels of oxidatively modified DNA (8-OHdG), which is one of the most frequently used and reliable indicators of oxidative damage, were most frequently detected in experimentally induced CNV lesions in diabetic mice on the third day after laser injury. Meanwhile, elevated levels of ROS were also confirmed in RPE cells that had been exposed to high-glucose environments in vitro. Taken together, these findings imply that oxidative stress may contribute to the development of CNV in early stages of diabetes.

Because oxidative stress plays pivotal role in high-glucose-induced angiogenesis and CNV development, we sought to investigate whether antioxidant supplementation could hamper the development of CNV in hyperglycaemic conditions. NAC is a potent antioxidant that is known to be a precursor of glutathione (GSH). It has been reported that NAC acted directly as free radical scavengers and is independent of its ability to enhance GSH synthesis [39,40]. A previous study discovered that NAC supplementation in a diabetic mouse model of an incisional

wound resulted in lower levels of oxidative stress among the animals' tissues [41]. It has also been reported that NAC administration prevented oxidative damage to RPE cells that was caused by exposure to a cigarette smoke extract that induced oxidative injury and contributed to the progression of AMD [42]. Our results demonstrated that NAC administration effectively alleviated oxidative stress levels that were exposed to hyperglycaemic conditions in mice and in cultured RPE cells. In addition, we further determined that NAC treatment was able to diminish the severity of CNV in diabetic mice.

RPE cells have the ability to respond quickly and adaptively to environmental stressors by expressing a number of genes that promote the development of CNV. Signalling pathways that regulate the biological functions of RPE cells are useful for understanding the molecular mechanisms that underlie the development of CNV [43]. STAT3 is a cytoplasmic transcription factor that transmits extracellular signals to the nucleus; activated STAT3 in the nucleus then binds to specific DNA promoter sequences and regulates gene expression [44]. In early stages of experimentally induced CNV in diabetic mice and in RPE cells when exposed to hyperglycaemic enviroments, we provided the first evidence that the level of p-STAT3 was dramatically up-regulated and accompanied by increased oxidative stress and upregulation of VEGF. While treatment with NAC was found to suppressed the level of p-STAT3 and

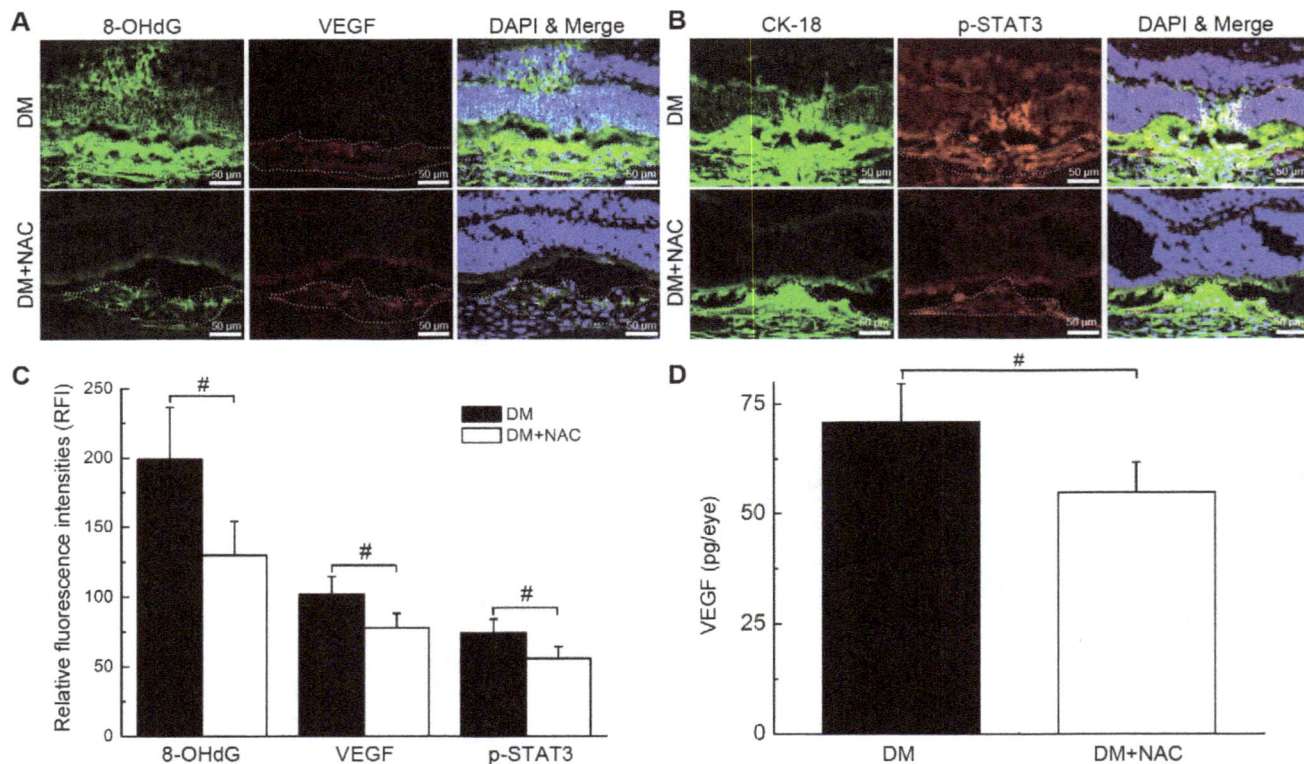

Figure 6. NAC supplementation inhibited hyperglycaemia-induced 8-OHdG, p-STAT3 and VEGF expression. A–B, Expression levels of 8-OHdG, VEGF and p-STAT3 in untreated diabetic (DM) and NAC-treated diabetic (NAC) mice. CNV lesions are indicated by dashed lines. C, Statistical analysis of the data in A and B ($\#P<0.05$); D, Statistical analysis of the data from the VEGF ELISA ($\#P<0.05$).

VEGF overexpression in vivo and in vitro. After exposing to a JAK2/STAT3 pathway inhibitor AG490, STAT3 activation was blocked, which ultimately lead to a decrease in the intracellular level of VEGF mRNA and protein expression in RPE cells, suggesting that the activation of the STAT3 signalling pathway triggers VEGF expression. However, we found that AG490 had no effect on the intracellular level of ROS. Thus, our results indicated that STAT3 signalling may activated by ROS in RPE cells and participate in the development of CNV under hyperglycaemic conditions.

In summary, we confirm for the first time that hyperglycaemia plays a pivotal role in the diabetes-aggravated development of CNV in mice. The underlying mechanism might involve an increase in the level of oxidative stress that results in CNV and the subsequent activation of STAT3-regulated VEGF expression in RPE cells. Furthermore, our data provide evidence that treatment with NAC effectively rescues the severity of experimentally induced CNV in diabetic mice. Our findings suggest that diabetes is a risk factor for disorders that involve the development of CNV, and antioxidant treatment may represent a therapeutic strategy for treating these diseases.

Materials and Methods

Ethics Statement

The experimental protocol that was used in the present study was approved by the Institutional Care and Use Committee at the Fourth Military Medical University (FMMU). All of the mouse studies were approved by the Animal Studies Committee at FMMU.

A total of 108 wild-type C57BL/6J mice, all of which were 8-week-old males and were obtained from the experimental animal centre at FMMU, were used in the present study. The mice were randomly divided into three groups: a control group (n = 27), a diabetic group(n = 54), and a diabetic group that was treated with N-acetyl-cysteine (NAC, n = 27). STZ-induced diabetic mice received daily intraperitoneal injections of the anti-oxidant NAC (Sigma Chemical, St. Louis, MO, 200 mg/kg/day) after laser photocoagulation. After 2 weeks of monitoring diabetes in the diabetic mice, laser induction of CNV was administered to the right eyes of all three groups of mice.

Generation of Diabetic Mice

To induce diabetes in our model animals, mice received daily intraperitoneal injections of STZ (Sigma Chemical, St. Louis, MO, 60 mg/kg of body weight in 0.05 M sodium citrate buffer at a pH of 4.5) for 5 days. Control animals were injected with citrate buffer only. Seven days after the fifth injection, the blood glucose levels of the animals were measured using a glucomonitor. Tail vein blood was used for blood glucose analyses. Mice with glucose levelsabove 300 mg/dl were considered as hyperglyceamic [45].

CNV Induction in Mice

A laser procedure was used to induce CNV in the right eyes of the mice in this study, and the induction of CNV was performed according to a previously reported protocol [46]. Briefly, the mice were anesthetised, and their pupils were dilated. Laser photoco-agulation with a wavelength of 532 nm, a spot size of 75 µm, a duration of 0.1 seconds, and an intensity of 90 mW was delivered using a slit lamp and a corneal contact lens. The burns

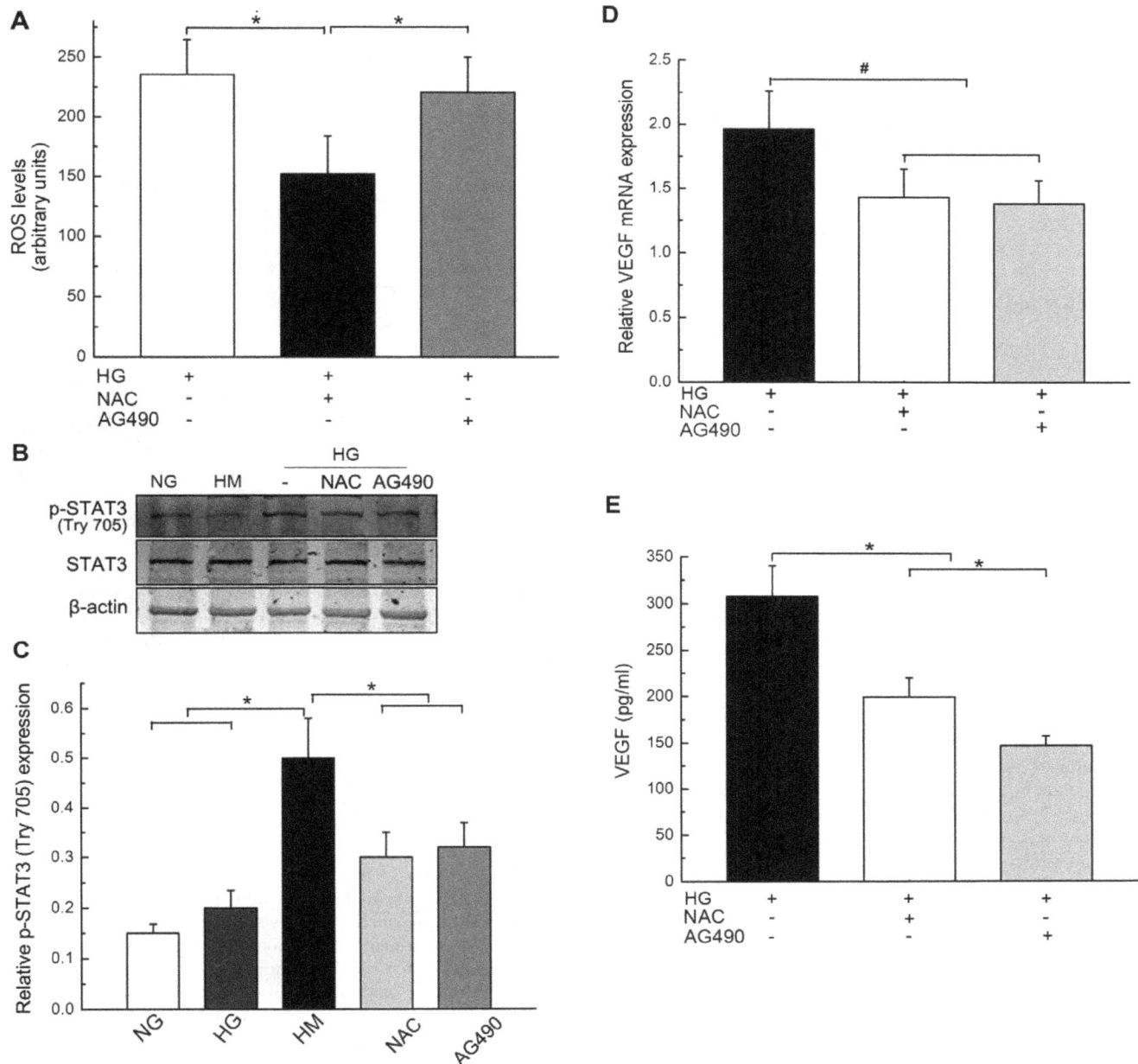

Figure 7. Treatment with NAC and AG490 inhibited p-STAT3 and VEGF expression in RPE cells that were exposed to high glucose (HG) conditions. RPE cells were cultured under normal glucose (NG) or high mannitol (HM) conditions and were subsequently treated with NAC or AG490 in the presence of an HG medium for 3 hours. A, Statistical analysis of the intracellular ROS data (*P<0.01). B, Representative data from Western blot analysis of p-STAT3 and total STAT3 expression in RPE cells. Data presented represent of three iterations of the experiments. C, Statistical analysis of the data in B (*P<0.01). D, Statistical analysis of the VEGF mRNA expression level data that were obtained by RT-PCR (*P<0.01). E, Statistical analysis of the VEGF ELISA data (*P<0.01, #P<0.05).

were performed at positions that were 1.5–2 disc diameters away from the optic nerve. Only those laser spots at which the rupture of Bruch's membrane was confirmed via the presence of a vaporisation bubble and the absence of haemorrhaging were considered successful and were included in the study.

CNV Severity Evaluation

CNV (6 spots per eye) was evaluated using fundus fluorescence angiography (FFA) 2 weeks after the photocoagulation procedure. The mice were anesthetised and were given intraperitoneal injections that contained 0.1 ml of 2.5% sodium fluorescein (Wuzhou Pharmaceutical, Guangxi, China). FFA recording began 3 min after the injection, and recordings were performed with a digital imaging system (Heidelberg Engineering, Heidelberg, Germany). The presence of a hyperfluorescent lesion at a site of laser irradiation that increased in size was defined as leakage and was indicative of both the incidence of CNV and the leaking grade of it. Two examiners graded fluorescence leakage independently using reference angiograms. Fluorescein leakage intensity scores

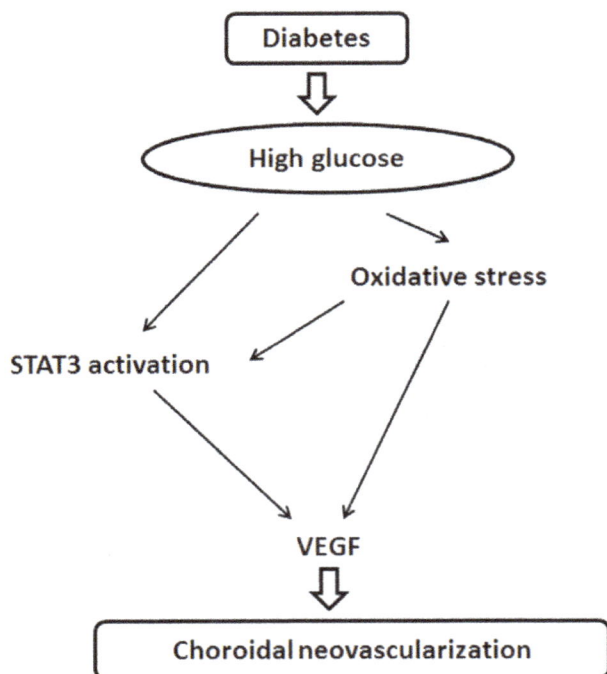

Figure 8. Mechanism for the diabetes-induced exacerbation of choroidal neovascularisation. Hyperglycaemia-increased oxidative stress is an upstream factor that promotes STAT3 activity, which in turn leads to the activation of VEGF transcription and eventually exacerbates the development of CNV.

Table 1. Numbers of animals per group and laser spots per eye that were included in each CNV assay.

Assay	Eyes	Laser spots per eye	Statistical analysis method
FFA	7	6	Mann-Whitney U test
HE staining	3	6	Student's t test
Choroidal flatmount	4	6	Student's t test
Immunofluorescence	3	6	Student's t test
ELISA	10	10	Student's t test

and eosin. Serial slices were examined, and the specimens that contained the thickest and/or widest lesions among the set of specimens that was obtained for each instance of CNV were evaluated. Sections that had been stained with hematoxylin and eosin were digitised using a light microscope (Olympus Corporation, Tokyo, Japan) that was connected to a colour video camera equipped with a frame grabber. IPP 6.0 was used to calculate the maximum thicknesses and lengths of each CNV from the selected hematoxylin and eosin-stained specimens.

8-OHdG, p-STAT3 and VEGF Immunofluorescence

On day 3 after photocoagulation (6 spots per eye), anesthetised mice were transcardially perfused with a 0.9% saline solution followed by a 4% paraformaldehyde solution. Eyes were then enucleated and post-fixed. Alternate sets of serial vertical sections of the eye were cut and mounted. To detect the level of oxidative DNA damage and the expression of p-STAT3 and VEGF protein in or near sites at which CNV occurred, serial cross sections of the eyes were incubated with primary antibodies against 8-OHdG (1:200, Biosynthesis Biotechnology Company, Beijing, China), p-STAT3 (1:200, Santa Cruz Biotechnology, CA, USA), VEGF (1:200, Santa Cruz Biotechnology, CA, USA) and CK18, which is an RPE marker (1:100, Biosynthesis Biotechnology Company, Beijing, China). Prepared sections were then incubated with FITC and TRITC-conjugated secondary antibodies, counterstained with DAPI, and examined with confocal laser scanning microscope using identical intensity of laser stimulation. IPP 6.0 was used to assess the relative fluorescence intensities (RFI) by dividing the average luminosity within the lesion by the average luminosity of the nomal choroid away from the CNV.

Cell Culture

Human RPE cells were obtained from a mature cell line that had been preserved in our laboratory as has been previously described [43]. Experimentation was carried out on subconfluent RPE cells in passage numbers three through eight. Cells in the control group were cultured and maintained in Dulbecco's Modified Eagle Medium (DMEM) with a normal glucose concentration (NG, 5.5 mM D-glucose) that was supplemented with 10% newborn serum in a humidified 5% CO_2 incubator at 37°C. Cultured RPE cells in other experimental groups were treated with a high mannitol control medium (HM, 5.5 mM D-glucose+24.5 mM D-mannitol), a high glucose medium (HG, 30 mM D-glucose), an antioxidant (1 mM NAC with HG), or a Janus kinase (JAK)-specific inhibitor (30 µM AG490 with HG).

ELISA for VEGF

The ocular levels of VEGF protein expression on day 3 after photocoagulation (10 spots per eye) were determined using a mouse

were graded as follows: 0 = no leakage; 1 = slight leakage; 2 = moderate leakage; 3 = prominent leakage.

Choroidal flat mounts were prepared on day 14 after CNV induction (6 spots per eye) in accordance with a previously described protocol [47]. Anesthetised mice were transcardially perfused with a 0.9% saline solution followed by a 4% paraformaldehyde solution. The entire ocular globes were enucleated, and the anterior segment and neural retina were removed from each globe. The remaining RPE-choroid-sclera complex was flatmounted using six or more radial cuts, after which the flatmount preparations were permeabilised in a 0.2% Triton X-100 solution for a period of 24 h prior to transferring them to a 1:1000 solution of rhodamine-conjugated Ricinus communis agglutinin (Vector Laboratories, Burlingame, CA, USA). Choroidal preparations were incubated with the agglutinin for 24 h and were subsequently washed in a 0.01 M Tris-Buffered Saline Tween-20 (TBST) solution for another 24 h. Flatmounts were subsequently examined and photographed using confocal laser scanning microscopy (Olympus Corporation, Tokyo, Japan), and the CNV area of each preparation was assessed using the image pro plus software program (IPP 6.0). Individual lesions with surface areas of more than 0.50 disc areas (DAs) were defined as having CNV.

Histopathological analysis was performed according to a previously described procedure [48]. Mice that were examined using light microscopy were killed on the 14th day after photocoagulation (6 spots per eye), and their eyes were enucleated. Eyecup preparations were fixed via incubation in Bouin's fixative (Zhongshan Biotechnology Company, Beijing, China) at 4°C for a period of 24 h. The fixed tissues were embedded in paraffin, serially sectioned into 3-µm slices, and stained with hematoxylin

VEGF ELISA kit (USCN Life Science and Technology, Wuhan, China). On the third day after photocoagulation, the eyes were removed and prepared for ELISA according to a previously reported protocol [46]. The eyes were quick-frozen in 200 µl of phosphate-buffered saline solution (pH 7.4) that contained 0.05% phenylmethylsulfonyl fluoride, and they were then manually homogenised on ice and exposed to three freeze-thaw cycles in liquid nitrogen and wet ice. The homogenates were centrifuged in a refrigerated desktop centrifuge to pellet any insoluble material, and the supernatants were collected. ELISA was performed according to the instructions from the manufacturer.

A human ELISA kit was used to measure the expression levels of VEGF protein that were secreted by human RPE cells in various culture media at the appropriate times (USCN Life Science and Technology, Wuhan, China) in accordance with the manufacturer's instructions.

Representative results were taken from three independent experiments and were expressed in picograms/millilitre.

Measurement of Intracellular Oxidative Stress by Flow Cytometry

Analysis of high glucose-induced generation of intracellular oxidative stress was determined by flow cytometry using the 2′,7′-dichlorofluorescein diacetate (DCFH-DA) probe (Beyotime Institute of Biotechnology, Shanghai, China). DCFH-DA is a oxidation-sensitive nonfluorescent precursor dye that can be oxidized by H_2O_2, other ROS and low molecule weight peroxides to fluorescent DCFH. DCFH is generally considered a probe not only for H_2O_2 in presence of cellular peroxidases but also for the determination of ONOO•, and HO•. When used in cellular systems, DCFH is a general marker of oxidative stress rather than a specific indicator H_2O_2 formation or other ROS and reactive nitrogen species [49].

RPE cells were seeded on 6-well plates at 1×10^5 cells per well and cultured for 24 h. After maintained in DMEM with different glucose concentration and various agents, cells were detached by means of trypsinisation, and a FAC Scan flow cytometer (BD, San Jose, CA) was used to measure the intensity of the cellular fluorescence intensity after a 30-min incubation in a 10 µmol/l DCFH-DA solution. The excitation and emission wavelengths were set at 488 nm and 525 nm respectively. Three independent experiments were performed and the results were expressed as the means ± SDs in arbitrary units of DCFH fluorescence intensity.

RNA Preparation and Semi-quantitative RT-PCR Analysis

Trizol (Takara, Kyoto, Japan) was used to extract the total cellular RNA from RPE cells, and the extracted RNA was subsequently quantified. Two micrograms of total RNA was reverse-transcribed to cDNA using the Exscript RT Reagent kit (Takara, Kyoto, Japan). All of the PCR experiments were performed using Taq polymerase (Promega, Madison, WI, USA); the primers 5′-AGGAGGGCAGAATCATCACG-3′ and 5′-CAAGGCCCACAGGGATTTTCT-3′ were used in PCR for VEGF, and 5′-GCCTCAAGATCATCAGCAAT-3′ and 5′-AGGTCCACCACTGACACGTT-3′ were used for the GAPDH control. Agarose gels that had been stained with ethidium bromide (1%) were scanned using a Fluor-Multimager (BioRad). IPP 6.0 was used to quantitate the band intensities of the PCR products. All experiments were repeated at least three times.

Western Blot Analysis

RPE cells were collected and lysed, and the expression levels of various proteins in the RPE cells were measured. Standard techniques were used to assess the expression levels of p-STAT3, STAT3 and β-actin. The following primary antibodies were used: monoclonal mouse anti-STAT3 (1:200, Santa Cruz Biotechnology, USA), monoclonal mouse anti-p-STAT3 (1:200, Santa Cruz Biotechnology, USA) and polyclonal rabbit anti-β-actin (1:100, Santa Cruz Biotechnology, USA). All experiments were repeated at least three times.

Statistical Analysis

Statistical analyses were performed using the SPSS 13.0 software program. Data from several experiments were pooled and subsequently presented as the means and standard deviations. One-way analyses of variance (ANOVAs) followed by LSD-t tests were used to make comparisons between pairs of groups. Student's t tests were used for the remaining statistical analyses. All of the experimental datasets were scrutinised to ensure that the sample variance was normally distributed, and appropriate non-parametric tests were applied when necessary. A two-tailed p-value of $P<0.05$ was considered significant.

The numbers of animals in each group and laser spots per eye have been summarised in Table 1; the statistical analyses that were used in each assay are also summarised in Table 1.

Acknowledgments

We appreciate Dr Bin Li(Shaanxi DONGAO Biosciences, LTD, Shaanxi,-China) for thoughtful comments and suggestions during the course of this project.

Author Contributions

Conceived and designed the experiments: XL YSW. Performed the experiments: XL YC WH. Analyzed the data: YC CSX. Contributed reagents/materials/analysis tools: YYS ZY HYW LBY JZ. Wrote the paper: XL YC.

References

1. Calabrese A, Bernard JB, Hoffart L, Faure G, Barouch F, et al. (2011) Wet versus dry age-related macular degeneration in patients with central field loss: different effects on maximum reading speed. Invest Ophthalmol Vis Sci 52: 2417–2424.

2. Guymer RH, Chong EW (2006) Modifiable risk factors for age-related macular degeneration. Med J Aust 184: 455–458.

3. Klein R, Deng Y, Klein BE, Hyman L, Seddon J, et al. (2007) Cardiovascular disease, its risk factors and treatment, and age-related macular degeneration: Women's Health Initiative Sight Exam ancillary study. Am J Ophthalmol 143: 473–483.

4. Duan Y, Mo J, Klein R, Scott IU, Lin HM, et al. (2007) Age-related macular degeneration is associated with incident myocardial infarction among elderly Americans. Ophthalmology 114: 732–737.

5. Topouzis F, Anastasopoulos E, Augood C, Bentham GC, Chakravarthy U, et al. (2009) Association of diabetes with age-related macular degeneration in the EUREYE study. Br J Ophthalmol 93: 1037–1041.

6. Fraser-Bell S, Wu J, Klein R, Azen SP, Hooper C, et al. (2008) Cardiovascular risk factors and age-related macular degeneration: the Los Angeles Latino Eye Study. Am J Ophthalmol 145: 308–316.

7. Tomany SC, Wang JJ, Van Leeuwen R, Klein R, Mitchell P, et al. (2004) Risk factors for incident age-related macular degeneration: pooled findings from 3 continents. Ophthalmology 111: 1280–1287.

8. Klein R, Klein BE, Moss SE (1992) Diabetes, hyperglycemia, and age-related maculopathy. The Beaver Dam Eye Study. Ophthalmology 99: 1527–1534.

9. Choi JK, Lym YL, Moon JW, Shin HJ, Cho B (2011) Diabetes mellitus and early age-related macular degeneration. Arch Ophthalmol 129: 196–199.

10. Ito M, Sakurai E, Hirano Y, Itaya M, Ogura Y (2008) Effect of Diabetes on the Development of Laser-Induced Choroidal Neovascularization in Mice. Invest Ophthalmol Vis Sci 49: 540.

11. Lyzogubov VV, Tytarenko RG, Bora PS, Bora NS (2010) Relationship Between Complement Activation and Choroidal Neovascularization in Type II Diabetes. Invest Ophthalmol Vis Sci 51: 6182.

12. Beatty S, Koh H, Phil M, Henson D, Boulton M (2000) The role of oxidative stress in the pathogenesis of age-related macular degeneration. Surv Ophthalmol 45: 115–134.
13. Imamura Y, Noda S, Hashizume K, Shinoda K, Yamaguchi M, et al. (2006) Drusen, choroidal neovascularization, and retinal pigment epithelium dysfunction in SOD1-deficient mice: a model of age-related macular degeneration. Proc Natl Acad Sci U S A 103: 11282–11287.
14. Li Q, Dinculescu A, Shan Z, Miller R, Pang J, et al. (2008) Downregulation of p22phox in retinal pigment epithelial cells inhibits choroidal neovascularization in mice. Mol Ther 16: 1688–1694.
15. Hara R, Inomata Y, Kawaji T, Sagara N, Inatani M, et al. (2010) Suppression of choroidal neovascularization by N-acetyl-cysteine in mice. Curr Eye Res 35: 1012–1020.
16. Yan M, Mehta JL, Zhang W, Hu C (2011) LOX-1, oxidative stress and inflammation: a novel mechanism for diabetic cardiovascular complications. Cardiovasc Drugs Ther 25: 451–459.
17. Pop-Busui R, Sima A, Stevens M (2006) Diabetic neuropathy and oxidative stress. Diabetes Metab Res Rev 22: 257–273.
18. Brezniceanu ML, Lau CJ, Godin N, Chenier I, Duclos A, et al. (2010) Reactive oxygen species promote caspase-12 expression and tubular apoptosis in diabetic nephropathy. J Am Soc Nephrol 21: 943–954.
19. Du Y, Miller CM, Kern TS (2003) Hyperglycemia increases mitochondrial superoxide in retina and retinal cells. Free Radic Biol Med 35: 1491–1499.
20. Al-Shabrawey M, Bartoli M, El-Remessy AB, Ma G, Matragoon S, et al. (2008) Role of NADPH oxidase and Stat3 in statin-mediated protection against diabetic retinopathy. Invest Ophthalmol Vis Sci 49: 3231–3238.
21. Chen Z, Han ZC (2008) STAT3: a critical transcription activator in angiogenesis. Med Res Rev 28: 185–200.
22. Xu Q, Briggs J, Park S, Niu G, Kortylewski M, et al. (2005) Targeting Stat3 blocks both HIF-1 and VEGF expression induced by multiple oncogenic growth signaling pathways. Oncogene 24: 5552–5560.
23. Izumi-Nagai K, Nagai N, Ozawa Y, Mihara M, Ohsugi Y, et al. (2007) Interleukin-6 receptor-mediated activation of signal transducer and activator of transcription-3 (STAT3) promotes choroidal neovascularization. Am J Pathol 170: 2149–2158.
24. Miller H, Miller B, Ishibashi T, Ryan SJ (1990) Pathogenesis of laser-induced choroidal subretinal neovascularization. Invest Ophthalmol Vis Sci 31: 899–908.
25. Strunnikova N, Zhang C, Teichberg D, Cousins SW, Baffi J, et al. (2004) Survival of retinal pigment epithelium after exposure to prolonged oxidative injury: a detailed gene expression and cellular analysis. Invest Ophthalmol Vis Sci 45: 3767–3777.
26. Zarbin MA (2004) Current concepts in the pathogenesis of age-related macular degeneration. Arch Ophthalmol 122: 598–614.
27. Campa C, Harding SP (2011) Anti-VEGF compounds in the treatment of neovascular age related macular degeneration. Curr Drug Targets 12: 173–181.
28. Borrone R, Saravia M, Bar D (2008) Age related maculopathy and diabetes. Eur J Ophthalmol 18: 949–954.
29. Proctor B, Ambati J (2007) Age-Related Macular Degeneration and Diabetic Retinopathy: Is Diabetic Retinopathy Protective Against ARMD? ARVO 2149(supple).
30. Wei M, Ong L, Smith MT, Ross FB, Schmid K, et al. (2003) The streptozotocin-diabetic rat as a model of the chronic complications of human diabetes. Heart Lung Circ 12: 44–50.
31. Lachin JM, Genuth S, Nathan DM, Zinman B, Rutledge BN (2008) Effect of glycemic exposure on the risk of microvascular complications in the diabetes control and complications trial–revisited. Diabetes 57: 995–1001.
32. Hidayat AA, Fine BS (1985) Diabetic choroidopathy. Light and electron microscopic observations of seven cases. Ophthalmology 92: 512–522.
33. Zhang L, Krzentowski G, Albert A, Lefebvre PJ (2001) Risk of developing retinopathy in Diabetes Control and Complications Trial type 1 diabetic patients with good or poor metabolic control. Diabetes Care 24: 1275–1279.
34. Ryan CM, Freed MI, Rood JA, Cobitz AR, Waterhouse BR, et al. (2006) Improving metabolic control leads to better working memory in adults with type 2 diabetes. Diabetes Care 29: 345–351.
35. Brownlee M (2005) The pathobiology of diabetic complications: a unifying mechanism. Diabetes 54: 1615–1625.
36. Giacco F, Brownlee M (2010) Oxidative stress and diabetic complications. Circ Res 107: 1058–1070.
37. Yildirim Z, Ucgun NI, Yildirim F (2011) The role of oxidative stress and antioxidants in the pathogenesis of age-related macular degeneration. Clinics (Sao Paulo) 66: 743–746.
38. Dong A, Xie B, Shen J, Yoshida T, Yokoi K, et al. (2009) Oxidative stress promotes ocular neovascularization. J Cell Physiol 219: 544–552.
39. Awad N, Khatib N, Ginsberg Y, Weiner Z, Maravi N, et al. (2011) N-acetyl-cysteine (NAC) attenuates LPS-induced maternal and amniotic fluid oxidative stress and inflammatory responses in the preterm gestation. Am J Obstet Gynecol 204: 450 e415–420.
40. Zhang F, Lau SS, Monks TJ (2011) The cytoprotective effect of N-acetyl-L-cysteine against ROS-induced cytotoxicity is independent of its ability to enhance glutathione synthesis. Toxicol Sci 120: 87–97.
41. Aktunc E, Ozacmak VH, Ozacmak HS, Barut F, Buyukates M, et al. (2010) N-acetyl cysteine promotes angiogenesis and clearance of free oxygen radicals, thus improving wound healing in an alloxan-induced diabetic mouse model of incisional wound. Clin Exp Dermatol 35: 902–909.
42. Bertram KM, Baglole CJ, Phipps RP, Libby RT (2009) Molecular regulation of cigarette smoke induced-oxidative stress in human retinal pigment epithelial cells: implications for age-related macular degeneration. Am J Physiol Cell Physiol 297: C1200–1210.
43. Zhu J, Wang YS, Zhang J, Zhao W, Yang XM, et al. (2009) Focal adhesion kinase signaling pathway participates in the formation of choroidal neovascularization and regulates the proliferation and migration of choroidal microvascular endothelial cells by acting through HIF-1 and VEGF expression in RPE cells. Exp Eye Res 88: 910–918.
44. Jung JE, Lee HG, Cho IH, Chung DH, Yoon SH, et al. (2005) STAT3 is a potential modulator of HIF-1-mediated VEGF expression in human renal carcinoma cells. FASEB J 19: 1296–1298.
45. Motyl K, McCabe LR (2009) Streptozotocin, type I diabetes severity and bone. Biol Proced Online 11: 296–315.
46. Hou HY, Liang HL, Wang YS, Zhang ZX, Wang BR, et al. (2010) A therapeutic strategy for choroidal neovascularization based on recruitment of mesenchymal stem cells to the sites of lesions. Mol Ther 18: 1837–1845.
47. Hou HY, Wang YS, Xu JF, Wang BR (2008) Nicotine promotes contribution of bone marrow-derived cells to experimental choroidal neovascularization in mice. Exp Eye Res 86: 983–990.
48. Shi YY, Wang YS, Zhang ZX, Cai Y, Zhou J, et al. (2011) Monocyte/macrophages promote vasculogenesis in choroidal neovascularization in mice by stimulating SDF-1 expression in RPE cells. Graefes Arch Clin Exp Ophthalmol 249: 1667–1679.
49. Gomes A, Fernandes E, Lima JL (2005) Fluorescence probes used for detection of reactive oxygen species. J Biochem Biophys Methods 65: 45–80.

11

Association between Reproductive Factors and Age-Related Macular Degeneration in Postmenopausal Women: The Korea National Health and Nutrition Examination Survey 2010-2012

Bum-Joo Cho[1,2], Jang Won Heo[1,2]*, Jae Pil Shin[3], Jeeyun Ahn[1,4], Tae Wan Kim[1,4], Hum Chung[1,2]

1 Department of Ophthalmology, Seoul National University College of Medicine, Seoul, Korea, 2 Department of Ophthalmology, Seoul National University Hospital, Seoul, Korea, 3 Department of Ophthalmology, Kyungpook National University School of Medicine, Daegu, Korea, 4 Department of Ophthalmology, Seoul Metropolitan Government Seoul National University Boramae Medical Center, Seoul, Korea

Abstract

Purpose: To examine the association between female reproductive factors and age-related macular degeneration (AMD) in postmenopausal women.

Design: Nationwide population-based cross-sectional study.

Methods: A nationally representative dataset acquired from the 2010–2012 Korea National Health and Nutrition Examination Survey was analyzed. The dataset involved information for 4,377 postmenopausal women aged ≥50 years with a fundus photograph evaluable for AMD in either eye. All participants were interviewed using standardized questionnaires to determine reproductive factors including menstruation, pregnancy, parity, lactation, and hormonal use. The association between reproductive factors and each type of AMD was investigated.

Results: The mean age of the study participants was 63.1±0.2 years. Mean ages at menarche and menopause were 16.1±0.0 and 49.2±0.1 years, respectively. The overall prevalence rates of early and late AMD were 11.2% (95% confidence interval [CI], 10.1–12.5) and 0.8% (95% CI, 0.5–1.2), respectively. When adjusted for age, neither smoking nor alcohol use was associated with the presence of any AMD or late AMD. Multivariate logistic regression analysis revealed age (OR, 1.12 per 1 year), duration of lactation (OR, 0.91 per 6 months), and duration of use of oral contraceptive pills (OCP) (OR, 1.10 per 6 months) as associated factors for late AMD. The other variables did not yield a significant correlation with the risk of any AMD or late AMD.

Conclusion: After controlling for confounders, a longer duration of lactation appeared to protect against the development of late AMD. A longer duration of OCP use was associated with a higher risk of late AMD.

Editor: Demetrios Vavvas, Massachusetts Eye & Ear Infirmary, Harvard Medical School, United States of America

Funding: The authors have no support or funding to report.

Competing Interests: The authors have declared that no competing interests exist.

* Email: jangwonheo@gmail.com

Introduction

The leading cause of blindness and visual impairment in elderly individuals of developed countries is age-related macular degeneration (AMD) [1,2]. With the expanding human lifespan, AMD has garnered increasing interest among researchers. Several risk factors have been identified for this condition, including cigarette smoking, hyperopia, and genetic variation in complement factor H [3–5].

Among those risk factors, female sex has been associated with a higher prevalence of AMD in many population-based studies [6]. Recent researches have suggested gender differences in the pathophysiology of AMD arising from dissimilar hormonal status [5,6]. However, there have not been sufficient data on the association between female own risk factors and AMD. Only a few epidemiological studies were performed, and the results have been inconclusive to date [7–10]. Identification of female risk factors for AMD would help to understand the pathogenesis of the disease and screen the patients at risk. Because most female patients at risk for AMD are post-menopausal, the associated hormonal changes must be examined closely as well.

Therefore, in this study, we investigated the association between female reproductive factors and each type of AMD in postmenopausal women. Various factors related to menstruation, pregnancy, delivery, lactation, and the use of hormonal drugs were explored. To acquire representative data for the general population, we analyzed the nationwide data obtained as part of the Korea National Health and Nutrition Examination Survey (KNHANES) on behalf of the Korean Ophthalmological Society (KOS) [11]. The ethnic homogeneity of Korea might facilitate to reveal the risk factors of AMD by minimizing the bias resulting from interracial differences [12]. To the authors' knowledge, this is the first study to analyze this association in an Asian population.

Materials and Methods

Study population

The data analyzed in this study were obtained from the fifth cycle of the KNHANES which was performed from 2010 through 2012. The KNHANES is an ongoing nationally representative cross-sectional survey to examine the health, physical, and nutritional status of the general Korean population [11,12]. The survey was first administered in 1998 and has been conducted annually since 2007 by the Korea Center for Disease Control and Prevention (KCDC). Ophthalmologic examinations were included since the second half of 2008. Details relating to the KNHANES design and methods have been presented elsewhere [11,12]. To summarize briefly, the study methodology involves stratified multistage cluster-sampling to prevent subject omission or overlap. The rolling-sampling method makes each annual survey results representative for the entire Korean population and mergeable with the past results. During the period from 2010–2012, the KNHANES annually included 3,800 households from 192 enumeration districts. From each household, all family members aged ≥1 year were included as eligible subjects [11]. The eligible subjects were asked to take part in health interviews and physical examinations including comprehensive ophthalmologic assessments in mobile centers by trained teams. Non-mydriatic 45° color fundus photographs were obtained for each subject aged ≥19 years in a dark room using a digital fundus camera (TRC-NW6S; Topcon, Tokyo, Japan). When the non-mydriatic photograph was of insufficient quality for grading due to media opacity or a small pupil, mydriatic fundus photographs were obtained at the point of maximal pupillary dilation, with the patients' consent.

Among the participants, only postmenopausal women were included in this study. As suggested previously, premenopausal women, women aged <50 years, women who experienced menopause before the age of 30, or those who did not report the age of menopause were excluded [10,13]. Subjects without any fundus photograph evaluable for the presence of AMD were also excluded from this study. Ultimately, only postmenopausal women who were aged ≥50 years and who had ≥1 assessable fundus photograph were included. The study described here adhered to the tenets of the Declaration of Helsinki, and written informed consent was obtained from all participants. The survey protocol was approved by the Institutional Review Board of the KCDC (IRB No: 2010-02CON-21-C, 2011-02CON-06-C, 2012-01EXP-01-2C).

Assessment of Reproductive factors

Female reproductive factors, demographic variables, and health behavioral factors were assessed on the basis of self-reported answers to a standardized questionnaire. The reproductive factors evaluated included the following: age at menarche, age at menopause, type of menopause, number of pregnancies, number of spontaneous and/or artificial abortions, parity (the number of children given birth to), lactation, use of oral contraceptive pills

(OCP), and use of postmenopausal female hormone replacement therapy (HRT).

The type of menopause was dichotomized as natural vs. artificial (e.g., hysterectomy or oophorectomy). The duration of lactation, OCP use, or HRT use was recorded as the total number of experienced months. The drug components of HRT and/or OCP were not specified. Length of the reproductive period was calculated as follows: age at menopause − age at menarche. Duration of the postmenopausal period was designated as follows: age − age at menopause. Duration of lactation per child was calculated from the division of duration of lactation by the number of parity.

Assessment of AMD

The presence of each AMD type was determined on the fundus photographs [11]. Each fundus photograph was preliminarily evaluated for the presence of AMD on site by dispatched ophthalmologists who were trained for grading by the National Epidemiologic Survey Committee of the KOS and used the International Age-related Maculopathy Epidemiological Study Group grading system [14]. Detailed grading was later performed by nine retina specialists with experience in grading AMD, who were masked to the patients' characteristics. Any discrepancy between the preliminary and detailed grading was resolved by an independent ophthalmologist (J.P.S.). Drusen were classified on the basis of size, appearance, and edge sharpness [14]. Retinal pigmentary abnormalities were graded as hypo- or hyperpigmentation [14]. Patients were defined as having early AMD if they met any one of the following criteria: (1) the presence of soft indistinct drusen or reticular drusen; (2) the presence of hard or soft distinct drusen with pigmentary abnormalities in the absence of late AMD [14]. Late AMD was defined as either the presence of neovascularization or geographic atrophy [14]. AMD was classified as neovascular if associated with detachment of the retinal pigment epithelium (RPE), serous detachment of the neurosensory retina, subretinal or sub-RPE hemorrhages, or subretinal fibrous scars [14]. Geographic atrophy was defined as a circular area with a sharp edge ≥175 μm in diameter showing hypopigmented RPE and apparent choroidal vessels, in the absence of signs for neovascular AMD [14]. When the severity of AMD differed between eyes, the subject was assigned the more advanced grade, and when only one eye could be assessed, the subject was assigned the grade of that eye. The presence of any AMD was defined as having either early AMD or late AMD. The quality of the grading was verified by the KOS. Grading agreement between the preliminary graders and the standard reading specialists ranged from 94.1–96.2%.

Statistical Analysis

Statistical estimations were performed using the sampling weights adjusted for response rate, extraction rate, and the distribution of the general Korean population. Continuous variables were expressed as mean ± standard error or mean with 95% confidence intervals (CIs). Categorization was performed for some of the continuous variables. In order to assess the association with AMD, the odds ratios (ORs) of continuous and categorical variables were calculated.

Prior to main analyses, the confounders for the risk of AMD were investigated among demographic and health behavioral variables by age-adjusted univariate logistic regression analyses. Next, univariate logistic regression analyses were performed to screen the potential reproductive risk factors for any AMD or late AMD after controlling for confounders. Risk factors with P<0.1 were selected, and multicollinearity among them was examined by calculating the variance inflation factors (VIFs). Those with a VIF ≥5 were excluded from subsequent analyses. Finally, multivariate logistic regression analyses were performed using a stepwise selection method. Final models for the presence of AMD were constructed using the set of risk factors with P<0.05 in the multivariate analysis. All statistical analyses were performed using SPSS 20.0 for Windows (SPSS Inc., Chicago, IL).

Results

During the period from 2010–2012, among 16,593 eligible women, 13,298 women were interviewed and underwent physical examinations (response rate, 80.1%) (Fig. 1). Participation rates during the period from 2010–2012 ranged from 79.5–80.5%. Of these, 4,922 subjects were postmenopausal and aged ≥50 years old. Among these, 4,377 (88.9%) subjects with a fundus photograph for either eye that could be used to assess the presence of AMD were ultimately included in this study.

Demographics of Study Participants

The mean age of the all study participants was 63.1±0.2 years (range, 50–97 years). Mean ages at menarche and menopause were 16.1±0.0 years (range, 8–28 years) and 49.2±0.1 years (range, 30–72 years), respectively. The age-stratified reproductive characteristics of the study group are presented in Table 1. In younger generations, reproductive years were longer and the numbers of pregnancy and parity were smaller compared to those in older generations (P<0.001 for all). Duration of lactation was shorter in the younger generations than in the older generations (P<0.001), while both the periods of OCP use and HRT use tended to be longer in the younger generations than in the older generations (P<0.001).

The overall prevalence rates of early, late, and any AMD among the study participants were 11.2% (95% CI, 10.1–12.5), 0.8% (95% CI, 0.5–1.2), and 12.0% (95% CI, 10.8–13.2), respectively. The overall prevalence of neovascular AMD and geographic atrophy was 0.6% (95% CI, 0.4–1.0) and 0.1% (95% CI, 0.0–0.5).

Data pertaining to demographic and reproductive characteristics are presented according to the type of AMD in Table 2. Both early AMD subjects and late AMD subjects were significantly older than those without any AMD (P<0.001 and P=0.006, respectively). Postmenopausal period was also significantly longer in early AMD subjects and in late AMD subjects than in those without any AMD (P<0.001 and P=0.010, respectively).

Univariate binary logistic regression analysis showed that age was highly associated with the presence of any AMD and that of late AMD (OR 1.08; 95% CI, 1.07–1.09 and OR 1.07; 95% CI, 1.02–1.14, respectively). When adjusted for age, the presence of any AMD was not associated with a history of ever smoking, current smoking, or current alcohol use (P=0.826, P=0.139, and P=0.701, respectively). The same trend was observed for late AMD (P=0.439, P=0.795, and P=0.798, respectively).

Association between Reproductive Factors and AMD

The association of reproductive factors with any AMD and late AMD is summarized in Table 3. Age-adjusted univariate logistic regression analysis did not reveal any associated factor (P<0.1) for the presence of any AMD. On the other hand, age-adjusted univariate logistic regression analysis showed that the following factors were correlated with the presence of late AMD (P<0.1): number of pregnancy, number of parity, duration of lactation per child, duration of lactation, and duration of OCP use. Among these variables, the VIFs of number of parity, duration of lactation

per child, and duration of lactation were ≥5 (5.618, 5.025, and 10.000, respectively). Duration of lactation per child was excluded from next analyses, because it was obtained from the calculation with number of parity and duration of lactation, and the authors reached a consensus that it would be a less meaningful variable than total duration of lactation in the development of AMD. After the exclusion, the corresponding VIFs of number of pregnancy, number of parity, duration of lactation, and duration of OCP use were all <5 (1.852, 3.300, 2.538, and 1.009, respectively).

In a multivariate logistic regression analysis using these variables, number of pregnancy and number of parity yielded insignificant correlations. Ultimately, the final regression model for late AMD included age (OR, 1.12 per year; 95% CI, 1.06–1.18), duration of lactation (OR per 6 months, 0.91; 95% CI 0.86–0.95), and duration of OCP use (OR, 1.10 per 6 months; 95% CI, 1.02–1.18) as associated factors. Among these, duration of lactation was shown to protect against late AMD, with a 9% risk reduction per 6-month breast-feeding. The other factors were positively correlated with the risk of late AMD (Table 4).

Discussion

The present study examined the association of various reproductive factors with the risk of AMD, in a representative population of postmenopausal Korean women. The investigated factors included menstruation, pregnancy, abortion, parity, lactation, as well as the use of OCP and HRT. After controlling for confounders, the duration of lactation was inversely associated with the risk of late AMD. In contrast, the use of OCP increased the risk of late AMD.

An interesting finding in this study is that breast-feeding has a protective effect against late AMD. More specifically, a 6-month increment in the total duration of lactation was associated with a 9% decrease in the risk of late AMD. This finding was first suggested by Erke et al in a recent research [7]. The authors stated that an increase in the total duration of lactation was significantly associated with a reduced risk of late AMD (OR per 3 months, 0.84) and a 1-month increase in the duration of lactation per child decreased the risk of late AMD by 20% [7]. The current study consisted with this result and identified the protective effect in a period-dependent manner. The amount of protective effect was less than that in the previous study [7]. Thus far, no other prior study has explored the association between lactation and AMD in the literature. Notably, the duration of lactation appeared to be significantly higher in the early AMD group in this study compared to that in the control group. However, this difference was eliminated in the regression analysis after age-adjustment, indicating that the increase in the duration of lactation in the early AMD group may have arisen from the increased age of the group.

The mechanism underlying the association between lactation and AMD is not well understood, but it might be approached in consideration of the protective effect of breast-feeding against several cardiovascular diseases [7,15]. In Women's Health Initiative study that included 139,681 postmenopausal women, those who had breastfed for >12 months were less likely to have hypertension (OR, 0.88), diabetes mellitus (OR, 0.80), hyperlipidemia (OR, 0.81), and cardiovascular disease (OR, 0.91) than those who had never breastfed [15]. In a Norwegian prospective population-based cohort study, lactation for ≥24 months decreased the cardiovascular mortality significantly among parous women aged <65 years (hazard ratio, 0.36) [16]. Additionally, lactation is known to improve the subclinical vascular indices of cardiovascular disease [17], to promote lipid metabolism [18], and to reduce serum concentrations of C-reactive protein [19].

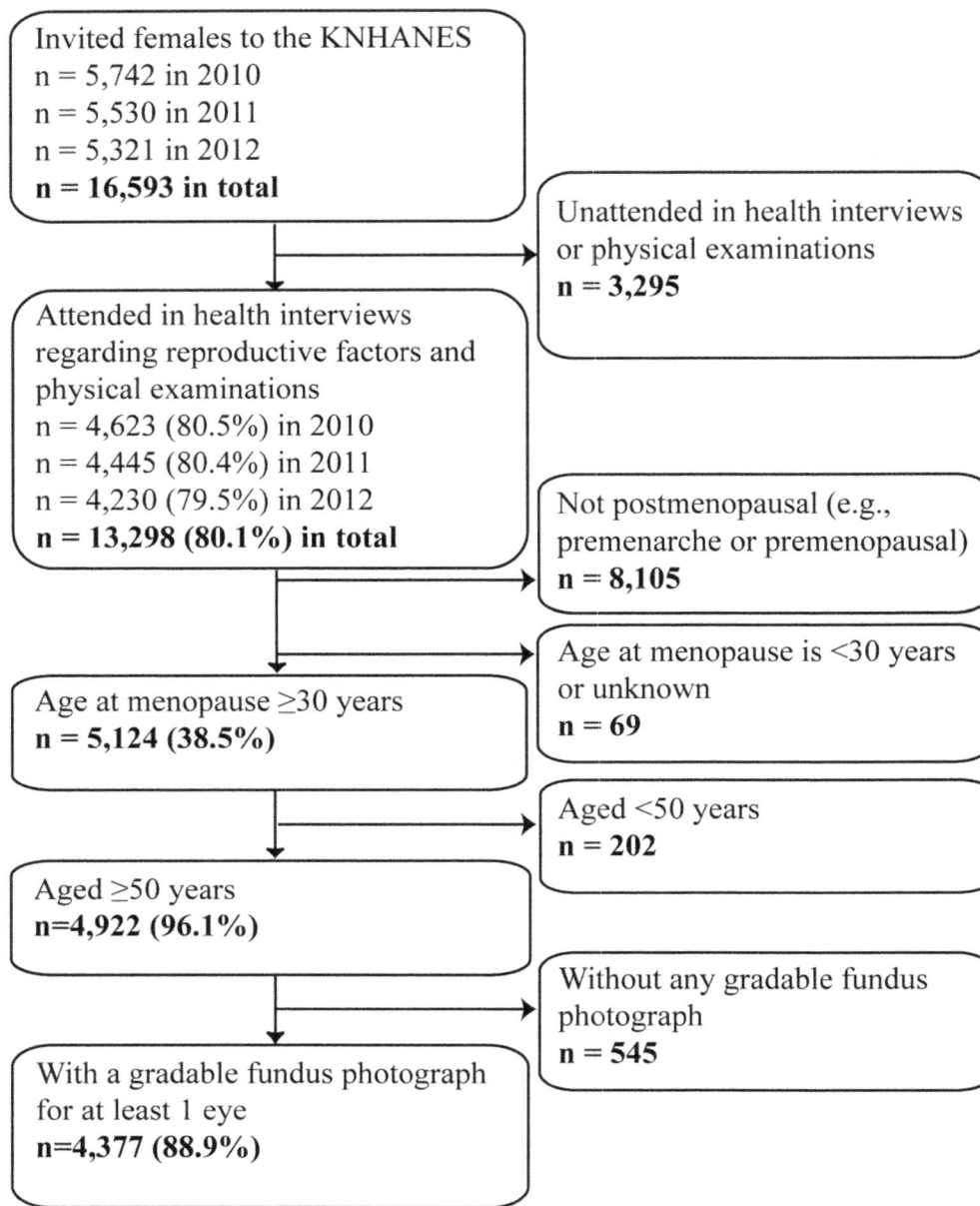

Figure 1. Participation flow-chart for the Korea National Health and Nutrition Examination Survey (KNHANES) during the period from 2010–2012.

Moreover, these effects were found to be long-lasting in a large cohort study [20]. Late AMD has been associated with cardio-vascular diseases in several studies [21,22], thus the protective effect of lactation against cardiovascular diseases might also help to reduce the risk of late AMD. This might be mediated by the effects on the microvasculature of choroid or retina. On the other hand, lactation has an inhibitory effect on the female hormonal axis, including estrogen exposure [15]. Considering that estrogen exposure has shown a protective effect against development of AMD in some previous studies [23], the protective effect of lactation against late AMD described above may override the anti-protective effect mediated by the inhibition of the hormonal axis.

Another novel finding presented here is the positive correlation between the use of OCP and the risk of late AMD. The present

study showed a 10% increase in the risk of late AMD per 6-month increase of OCP use. Thus far, there have been only a few studies on the association between AMD and OCP use [5,7,10,24]. One study reported a reduced risk of neovascular AMD (OR, 0.55) in women who had used OCP at least once [5], and another found a decreased risk of early AMD (OR, 0.5) in those who had used OCP ever [24]. Other researchers have reported that the use of OCP was not associated with the risk of early or late AMD in postmenopausal women [7,10]. On the other hand, since the introduction of OCP, a variety of vascular complications have been reported to be associated with it [25]. The risky diseases associated with OCP include deep-vein thrombosis, pulmonary embolism, stroke, and myocardial infarction (MI) [25]. A recent meta-analysis revealed a three-fold increase in the risk of venous

Table 1. Age-based stratification of postmenopausal women aged ≥50 years in the KNHANES 2010–2012.

	50–59[a] (n = 1586)	60–69[a] (n = 1516)	70–79[a] (n = 1080)	≥80[a] (n = 195)	P Value
Age, y	54.6±0.1	64.3±0.1	74.1±0.1	82.6±0.2	<0.001[b]
Prevalence of early AMD, %	4.8±0.7	11.8±1.0	20.7±1.7	22.2±4.0	<0.001[c]
Prevalence of late AMD, %	0.3±0.2	0.7±0.3	1.1±0.3	3.4±1.6	0.002[c]
Age at menarche, y	15.7±0.1	16.3±0.1	16.7±0.1	16.6±0.2	<0.001[b]
Age at menopause, y	49.4±0.1	49.9±0.2	48.0±0.2	47.7±0.5	<0.001[b]
Reproductive years, y	33.7±0.1	33.6±0.2	31.3±0.2	31.2±0.5	<0.001[b]
Postmenopausal period, y	5.2±0.1	14.4±0.2	26.1±0.2	34.9±0.5	<0.001[b]
Number of pregnancy	3.9±0.1	5.0±0.1	6.2±0.1	6.2±0.2	<0.001[b]
Number of spontaneous abortion	0.3±0.0	0.3±0.0	0.3±0.0	0.3±0.1	0.988[b]
Number of artificial abortion	1.3±0.0	1.5±0.1	1.4±0.1	0.6±0.1	<0.001[b]
Number of parity	2.3±0.0	3.2±0.0	4.5±0.1	5.2±0.2	<0.001[b]
Duration of lactation, m	25.2±0.8	50.0±1.2	90.8±2.1	107.9±5.4	<0.001[b]
Duration of OCP use, m	4.1±0.6	7.6±0.7	6.0±0.7	1.0±0.5	<0.001[b]
Duration of HRT use, m	5.3±0.5	7.4±0.8	1.8±0.5	0.9±0.6	<0.001[b]

AMD = age-related macular degeneration; OCP = oral contraceptive pills; HRT = hormone replacement therapy.
[a]Age in years.
[b]General linear model for complex samples.
[c]Pearson's chi-square test for complex samples.

thromboembolism, a two-fold increase in the risk of ischemic stroke, and an indeterminate effect on the risk of MI [25]. The positive association between OCP use and late AMD in this study is in line with the increased rate of cardiovascular disease observed for OCP users.

The pathophysiology of the association of OCP with cardiovascular diseases or late AMD is not clearly elucidated yet. OCP are typically either a combination of progestin and lower doses of estrogen or progestin only [26]. OCP increase the levels of prothrombin fragments, fibrinogen, plasmin–antiplasmin complex, and protein C activity, and decrease antithrombin activity and the level of tissue-plasminogen activator [27,28]. These hemostatic effects are known to be modulated by the progestin's potency as an androgen [27]. Progestin is also suggested to increase the level of aminopeptidase P and the breakdown of bradykinin, and thereby to increase blood pressure [29]. The hemodynamic and hemostatic effects of OCP might contribute to the risk of cardiovascular disease, and thus affect the development

Table 2. Demographics of postmenopausal women aged ≥50 years by the type of age-related macular degeneration (AMD) in the KNHANES 2010–2012.

	No AMD (n = 3845)	Early AMD (n = 500)	P value[a]	Late AMD (n = 32)	P value[a]
Age, y	62.4±0.2	68.9±0.5	<0.001	69.6±2.7	0.006
Age at menarche, y	16.1±0.0	16.4±0.1	0.005	16.9±0.4	0.084
Age at menopause, y	49.2±0.1	48.9±0.3	0.242	48.8±0.9	0.661
Reproductive years, y	33.1±0.1	32.5±0.3	0.044	32.0±0.8	0.141
Postmenopausal period, y	13.2±0.2	20.0±0.6	<0.001	20.8±3.0	0.010
Number of pregnancy	4.7±0.0	5.5±0.1	<0.001	4.4±0.4	0.369
Number of spontaneous abortion	0.3±0.0	0.3±0.0	0.657	0.2±0.1	0.220
Number of artificial abortion	1.3±0.0	1.3±0.1	0.708	1.0±0.4	0.485
Number of parity	3.1±0.0	3.8±0.1	<0.001	3.1±0.2	0.948
Duration of lactation, m	48.4±1.1	69.7±3.1	<0.001	44.5±6.7	0.565
Duration of OCP use, m	5.2±0.4	5.9±0.9	0.495	27.7±21.5	0.296
Duration of HRT use, m	5.0±0.4	4.5±0.9	0.570	4.1±2.6	0.724

OCP = oral contraceptive pills; HRT = hormone replacement therapy.
[a]Comparison with no AMD group, not adjusted for any covariate.

Table 3. Age-adjusted odds ratios (ORs) of age-related macular degeneration (AMD) for reproductive risk factors in postmenopausal women in the KNHANES 2010–2012.

Reproductive risk factors	Increment	Any AMD			Late AMD		
		OR	95% CI	P Value	OR	95% CI	P Value
Age at menarche	1 year	1.01	0.96-1.06	0.705	1.13	0.90-1.41	0.289
Age at menopause	1 year	1.00	0.98-1.03	0.746	1.00	0.94-1.07	0.911
Reproductive years	1 year	1.00	0.98-1.02	0.878	0.99	0.94-1.04	0.634
Postmenopausal period	1 year	1.00	0.97-1.02	0.744	1.00	0.94-1.06	0.908
Number of pregnancy	1	1.00	0.95-1.04	0.911	0.81	0.67-0.97	0.025
Number of spontaneous abortion	1	0.97	0.82-1.14	0.677	0.79	0.47-1.32	0.364
Number of artificial abortion	1	1.00	0.94-1.06	0.963	0.92	0.64-1.32	0.644
Number of parity	1	1.00	0.92-1.08	0.999	0.74	0.62-0.88	0.001
Duration of lactation per child	1 month	1.00	0.98-1.01	0.415	0.96	0.91-1.00	0.053
Duration of lactation[a]	6 months	1.00	0.98-1.01	0.616	0.91	0.87-0.95	<0.001
Duration of OCP use[a]	6 months	1.03	0.99-1.07	0.149	1.09	1.01-1.18	0.025
Duration of HRT use[a]	6 months	1.01	0.99-1.04	0.436	1.00	0.93-1.09	0.881
Artificial menopause	Yes	0.92	0.62-1.37	0.667	0.87	0.26-2.91	0.818
Bilateral oophorectomy	Yes	1.08	0.61-1.90	0.798	1.66	0.45-6.16	0.449

CI = confidence interval; OCP = oral contraceptive pills; HRT = hormone replacement therapy.
[a]Total years of experience.

Table 4. Multivariate-adjusted odds ratios (ORs) of late age-related macular degeneration (AMD) for reproductive risk factors in postmenopausal women in the KNHANES 2010–2012.

	Risk factors	Increment	OR	95% CI	P Value
Model 1	Age	1 year	1.12	1.06–1.17	<0.001
	Number of pregnancy	1	0.82	0.53–1.28	0.386
	Number of parity	1	1.11	0.61–2.02	0.725
	Duration of lactation[a]	6 months	0.92	0.85–1.00	0.043
	Duration of OCP use[a]	6 months	1.10	1.02–1.19	0.013
Model 2[b]	Age	1 year	1.12	1.06–1.18	<0.001
	Duration of lactation[a]	6 months	0.91	0.86–0.95	<0.001
	Duration of OCP use[a]	6 months	1.10	1.02–1.18	0.019

CI = confidence interval; OCP = oral contraceptive pills.
[a]Total years of experience.
[b]Final multivariate model consisted of risk factors of p value<0.05.

of AMD. However, further studies with larger sample sizes will be necessary in the future to validate the findings of this study.

Estrogen is considered one of the most important reproductive hormones in women. Endogenous exposure to estrogen starts with the release of estrogen from the ovary, and is related to the age at menarche, age at menopause, and the number of pregnancies [23]. The Aravind Comprehensive Eye Survey showed age at menarche ≥14 years, which means the late start of estrogen release, is a risk factor for overall AMD (OR, 2.3) [30], and the Rotterdam Study showed an increased risk of AMD in those who experienced early menopause following oophorectomy (OR, 3.8) [3]. The Blue Mountain Eye Study reported that a long reproductive period was associated with a decreased prevalence of early AMD [31]. These findings provide further support for the notion that a shorter duration of estrogen exposure may increase the risk of AMD. However, no such association was found in this study.

The association between AMD and exogenous exposure to estrogen in the form of HRT has been inconsistent in previous studies [5,9,13,23,32]. A 34% increase in the risk of early AMD was observed among current HRT users in one report as compared to that in individuals who had never used HRT [10]. To the contrary, HRT was associated with a lower risk of neovascular AMD (RR, 0.52) among female nurses aged 30–55 years [10], and reduced the risk of exudative AMD (OR, 0.6) in the Eye Disease Case–Control Study [33]. A postulated explanation for this association is that estrogen deficiency results in a down-regulation of matrix metalloproteinase–2 activity and an up-regulation of YKL-40 protein which may accelerate choroidal neovascularization [24,34]. However, most studies to date have reported no association between estrogen treatment and early or late AMD [3,7,8,24,30,32]. In the current study, we were also unable to find an association between HRT and any AMD or late AMD. This result might stem from our limited sample size.

The present study has several limitations. As it was a cross-sectional survey, the association between risk factors and late AMD does not guarantee causality. The result means only a cross-sectional distribution of AMD in a certain population, and a survivorship bias may intervene. Therefore, a longitudinal cohort study is required to validate the findings presented here and disclose the causality. It will also help to examine the incidence of AMD in the population at risk. In addition, as the information for

several reproductive factors in this survey was based on self-reported answers from the participants, and not on their medical records, there could be an intervening recall bias. To minimize biases, the health interviews in this survey were performed using a standardized questionnaire by trained teams. However, because most participants were old, there may be some recall bias remaining in this study. Moreover, although we tried to control for several potential confounders, the possibility of a confounding effect between the risk factors studied and AMD still remains. The small number of late AMD patients represents another limitation that may have reduced the statistical power of our conclusions. Regarding OCP use, more specific data such as the drug components were not investigated in the current survey. Future studies involving the drug components of OCP are necessary in order to reveal the association of OCP use with AMD more clearly. Lastly, subjects who could not have an evaluable fundus photograph taken due to mature cataract or other media opacity were excluded. Because these patients tended to be older [12] and thus were more likely to have had AMD, the prevalence of AMD may have been underestimated. The strength of this study derives largely from our use of data from a large, nationally representative sample population.

In conclusion, the current study suggests a longer period of lactation might protect against late AMD. We also presented our novel finding that a longer use of OCP increases the risk of late AMD. These findings could elucidate the development of AMD and help the screening of patients at risk as well as the prevention of AMD among postmenopausal women in public health.

Acknowledgments

The authors appreciate the Epidemiologic Survey Committee of the Korean Ophthalmological Society for the dedication to designing and accomplishment of the Korea National Health and Nutrition Examination Survey, acquisition and verification of the data, and opening of the data to the public.

Author Contributions

Conceived and designed the experiments: BJC JWH HC. Performed the experiments: BJC JWH JPS TWK. Analyzed the data: BJC JA TWK. Contributed reagents/materials/analysis tools: BJC JWH JPS. Contributed to the writing of the manuscript: BJC JA.

References

1. Pascolini D, Mariotti SP, Pokharel GP, Pararajasegaram R, Etya'ale D, et al. (2004) 2002 global update of available data on visual impairment: a compilation of population-based prevalence studies. Ophthalmic Epidemiol 11: 67–115.

2. Congdon N, O'Colmain B, Klaver CC, Klein R, Munoz B, et al. (2004) Causes and prevalence of visual impairment among adults in the United States. Arch Ophthalmol 122: 477–485.

3. Tomany SC, Wang JJ, Van Leeuwen R, Klein R, Mitchell P, et al. (2004) Risk factors for incident age-related macular degeneration: pooled findings from 3 continents. Ophthalmology 111: 1280–1287.

4. Gemmy Cheung CM, Li X, Cheng CY, Zheng Y, Mitchell P, et al. (2013) Prevalence and risk factors for age-related macular degeneration in Indians: a comparative study in Singapore and India. Am J Ophthalmol 155: 764–773, 773 e761–763.

5. Edwards DR, Gallins P, Polk M, Ayala-Haedo J, Schwartz SG, et al. (2010) Inverse association of female hormone replacement therapy with age-related macular degeneration and interactions with ARMS2 polymorphisms. Invest Ophthalmol Vis Sci 51: 1873–1879.

6. Rudnicka AR, Jarrar Z, Wormald R, Cook DG, Fletcher A, et al. (2012) Age and gender variations in age-related macular degeneration prevalence in populations of European ancestry: a meta-analysis. Ophthalmology 119: 571–580.

7. Erke MG, Bertelsen G, Peto T, Sjolie AK, Lindekleiv H, et al. (2013) Lactation, female hormones and age-related macular degeneration: the Tromso Study. Br J Ophthalmol 97: 1036–1039.

8. Klein BE, Klein R and Lee KE (2000) Reproductive exposures, incident age-related cataracts, and age-related maculopathy in women: the beaver dam eye study. Am J Ophthalmol 130: 322–326.

9. Haan MN, Klein R, Klein BE, Deng Y, Blythe LK, et al. (2006) Hormone therapy and age-related macular degeneration: the Women's Health Initiative Sight Exam Study. Arch Ophthalmol 124: 988–992.

10. Feskanich D, Cho E, Schaumberg DA, Colditz GA, Hankinson SE (2008) Menopausal and reproductive factors and risk of age-related macular degeneration. Arch Ophthalmol 126: 519–524.

11. Yoon KC, Mun GH, Kim SD, Kim SH, Kim CY, et al. (2011) Prevalence of eye diseases in South Korea: data from the Korea National Health and Nutrition Examination Survey 2008–2009. Korean J Ophthalmol 25: 421–433.

12. Cho BJ, Heo JW, Kim TW, Ahn J, Chung H (2014) Prevalence and risk factors of age-related macular degeneration in Korea: the Korea National Health and Nutrition Examination Survey 2010–2011. Invest Ophthalmol Vis Sci 55: 1101–1108.

13. Snow KK, Cote J, Yang W, Davis NJ, Seddon JM (2002) Association between reproductive and hormonal factors and age-related maculopathy in postmenopausal women. Am J Ophthalmol 134: 842–848.

14. Bird AC, Bressler NM, Bressler SB, Chisholm IH, Coscas G, et al. (1995) An international classification and grading system for age-related maculopathy and age-related macular degeneration. The International ARM Epidemiological Study Group. Surv Ophthalmol 39: 367–374.

15. Schwarz EB, Ray RM, Stuebe AM, Allison MA, Ness RB, et al. (2009) Duration of lactation and risk factors for maternal cardiovascular disease. Obstet Gynecol 113: 974–982.

16. Natland Fagerhaug T, Forsmo S, Jacobsen GW, Midthjell K, Andersen LF, et al. (2013) A prospective population-based cohort study of lactation and cardiovascular disease mortality: the HUNT study. BMC Public Health 13: 1070.

17. McClure CK, Catov JM, Ness RB, Schwarz EB (2012) Lactation and maternal subclinical cardiovascular disease among premenopausal women. Am J Obstet Gynecol 207: 46. e41–48.

18. Kjos SL, Henry O, Lee RM, Buchanan TA, Mishell DR Jr (1993) The effect of lactation on glucose and lipid metabolism in women with recent gestational diabetes. Obstet Gynecol 82: 451–455.

19. Williams MJ, Williams SM, Poulton R (2006) Breast feeding is related to C reactive protein concentration in adult women. J Epidemiol Community Health 60: 146–148.

20. Stuebe AM, Rich-Edwards JW, Willett WC, Manson JE, Michels KB (2005) Duration of lactation and incidence of type 2 diabetes. Jama 294: 2601–2610.

21. Klein R, Klein BE, Tomany SC, Cruickshanks KJ (2003) The association of cardiovascular disease with the long-term incidence of age-related maculopathy: the Beaver Dam eye study. Ophthalmology 110: 636–643.

22. van Leeuwen R, Ikram MK, Vingerling JR, Witteman JC, Hofman A, et al. (2003) Blood pressure, atherosclerosis, and the incidence of age-related maculopathy: the Rotterdam Study. Invest Ophthalmol Vis Sci 44: 3771–3777.

23. Connell PP, Keane PA, O'Neill EC, Altaie RW, Loane E, et al. (2009) Risk factors for age-related maculopathy. J Ophthalmol 2009: 360764.

24. Fraser-Bell S, Wu J, Klein R, Azen SP, Varma R (2006) Smoking, alcohol intake, estrogen use, and age-related macular degeneration in Latinos: the Los Angeles Latino Eye Study. Am J Ophthalmol 141: 79–87.

25. Peragallo Urrutia R, Coeytaux RR, McBroom AJ, Gierisch JM, Havrilesky LJ, et al. (2013) Risk of acute thromboembolic events with oral contraceptive use: a systematic review and meta-analysis. Obstet Gynecol 122: 380–389.

26. Christin-Maitre S (2013) History of oral contraceptive drugs and their use worldwide. Best Pract Res Clin Endocrinol Metab 27: 3–12.

27. Sitruk-Ware R, Nath A (2013) Characteristics and metabolic effects of estrogen and progestins contained in oral contraceptive pills. Best Pract Res Clin Endocrinol Metab 27: 13–24.

28. Wiegratz I, Lee JH, Kutschera E, Winkler UH, Kuhl H (2004) Effect of four oral contraceptives on hemostatic parameters. Contraception 70: 97–106.

29. Cilia La Corte AL, Carter AM, Turner AJ, Grant PJ, Hooper NM (2008) The bradykinin-degrading aminopeptidase P is increased in women taking the oral contraceptive pill. J Renin Angiotensin Aldosterone Syst 9: 221–225.

30. Nirmalan PK, Katz J, Robin AL, Ramakrishnan R, Krishnadas R, et al. (2004) Female reproductive factors and eye disease in a rural South Indian population: the Aravind Comprehensive Eye Survey. Invest Ophthalmol Vis Sci 45: 4273–4276.

31. Smith W, Mitchell P, Wang JJ (1997) Gender, oestrogen, hormone replacement and age-related macular degeneration: results from the Blue Mountains Eye Study. Aust N Z J Ophthalmol 25 Suppl 1: S13–15.

32. Abramov Y, Borik S, Yahalom C, Fatum M, Avgil G, et al. (2004) The effect of hormone therapy on the risk for age-related maculopathy in postmenopausal women. Menopause 11: 62–68.

33. The Eye Disease Case-Control Study Group (1992) Risk factors for neovascular age-related macular degeneration. Arch Ophthalmol 110: 1701–1708.

34. Rakic JM, Lambert V, Deprez M, Foidart JM, Noel A, et al. (2003) Estrogens reduce the expression of YKL-40 in the retina: implications for eye and joint diseases. Invest Ophthalmol Vis Sci 44: 1740–1746.

12

T Cells and Macrophages Responding to Oxidative Damage Cooperate in Pathogenesis of a Mouse Model of Age-Related Macular Degeneration

Fernando Cruz-Guilloty[1,2*¤], Ali M. Saeed[1], Stephanie Duffort[1], Marisol Cano[3], Katayoon B. Ebrahimi[3], Asha Ballmick[1], Yaohong Tan[1], Hua Wang[4], James M. Laird[4], Robert G. Salomon[4], James T. Handa[3], Victor L. Perez[1,2*]

1 Bascom Palmer Eye Institute, Department of Ophthalmology, University of Miami Miller School of Medicine, Miami, Florida, United States of America, 2 Department of Microbiology and Immunology, University of Miami Miller School of Medicine, Miami, Florida, United States of America, 3 Wilmer Eye Institute, Department of Ophthalmology, Johns Hopkins University School of Medicine, Baltimore, Maryland, United States of America, 4 Department of Chemistry, Case Western Reserve University, Cleveland, Ohio, United States of America

Abstract

Age-related macular degeneration (AMD) is a major disease affecting central vision, but the pathogenic mechanisms are not fully understood. Using a mouse model, we examined the relationship of two factors implicated in AMD development: oxidative stress and the immune system. Carboxyethylpyrrole (CEP) is a lipid peroxidation product associated with AMD in humans and AMD-like pathology in mice. Previously, we demonstrated that CEP immunization leads to retinal infiltration of pro-inflammatory M1 macrophages before overt retinal degeneration. Here, we provide direct and indirect mechanisms for the effect of CEP on macrophages, and show for the first time that antigen-specific T cells play a leading role in AMD pathogenesis. In vitro, CEP directly induced M1 macrophage polarization and production of M1-related factors by retinal pigment epithelial (RPE) cells. In vivo, CEP eye injections in mice induced acute pro-inflammatory gene expression in the retina and human AMD eyes showed distinctively diffuse CEP immunolabeling within RPE cells. Importantly, interferon-gamma (IFN-γ) and interleukin-17 (IL-17)-producing CEP-specific T cells were identified ex vivo after CEP immunization and promoted M1 polarization in co-culture experiments. Finally, T cell immunosuppressive therapy inhibited CEP-mediated pathology. These data indicate that T cells and M1 macrophages activated by oxidative damage cooperate in AMD pathogenesis.

Editor: Alfred S. Lewin, University of Florida, United States of America

Funding: This work was supported by The Edward N. & Della L. Thome Memorial Foundation Bank of America N.A. Trustee Award Program in Macular Degeneration Research (VLP, JTH); NIH P30EY14801 (Center Grant); Research to Prevent Blindness (Unrestricted Grant to the Bascom Palmer Eye Institute); NIH R01-GM21249 (RGS), NIH EY14005 (JTH), EY019904 (JTH), and RPB Senior Scientist Award (JTH). JTH is the Robert Bond Welch Professor. A.M.S. acknowledges partial support and assistance from the Sheila and David Fuente Graduate Program in Cancer Biology, Sylvester Comprehensive Cancer Center. FCG was supported by a Howard Hughes Medical Institute Fellowship of the Life Sciences Research Foundation. The funders had no role in study design, data collection and analysis, decision to publish, or preparation of the manuscript.

Competing Interests: The authors have read the journal's policy and have the following conflicts: This study was partly supported by a Bank of America N.A. Trustee Award Program. The mouse model for dry AMD described in this study is protected for commercialization by SKS Ocular. R.G.S. and V.L.P. are co-inventors. The CEP model patent name and number is the following: "Non-human model of autoimmune disease," number 20090155243. There are no further patents, products in development or marketed products to declare.

* E-mail: fcruzguilloty@gmail.com (FCG); Vperez4@med.miami.edu (VLP)

¤ Current address: Immucor, Inc., Norcross, Georgia, United States of America

Introduction

Age-related macular degeneration (AMD) is a complex and heterogeneous collection of retinal diseases representing the leading cause of blindness in industrialized countries [1,2]. There are two major classifications of AMD: dry and wet AMD. Dry AMD is a result of dysfunctional retinal pigment epithelial (RPE) cells, which are in charge of nourishing and protecting the retina, especially the photoreceptor (PR) cells [3]. Clinical features of dry AMD include the presence of drusen (accumulated debris in the form of visible yellow spots), geographic atrophy (focal loss of the RPE layer), PR cell death and ultimately loss of central vision. In contrast, wet AMD is a more severe, end-stage form of the disease

that occurs in ~10% of total cases when blood vessels from the underlying choroid abnormally grow into the outer retina, a process called choroidal neovascularization (CNV) [4,5]. Laser-induced CNV (although technically involving a wound healing response) serves as a valuable model of wet AMD in many species, and intraocular anti-VEGF therapy, which inhibits the angiogenesis associated with CNV, is useful for the treatment of wet AMD [6]. Unfortunately, there is no treatment for dry AMD and the pathogenic mechanisms remain to be fully elucidated. Recent evidence now implicates the immune system in the development of AMD [7,8], as immune-related proteins are found in drusen from AMD eyes [9] and genome-wide association studies have linked specific polymorphisms in complement factor genes with the development of AMD [10–15]. In this light, it has been suggested that AMD can be viewed as a chronic inflammatory disease [16–19]. Thus, the detailed analysis of immune responses at the onset of disease opens the door for a greater understanding of AMD etiology mechanisms.

The immune system can be broadly divided into innate (general, non-specific immune system) and adaptive (specific) immunity. While many aspects of the interplay between innate and adaptive immune systems have been studied in the setting of acute bacterial or viral infections [20,21], much less is known about their mechanistic crosstalk in the context of chronic inflammatory diseases, such as cancer, atherosclerosis and heart disease [22]. Information related to the AMD disease process could apply to chronic inflammation in general. Two relevant cell types that merit attention are macrophages and T cells. Macrophages are essential components of the innate immune system and have been the subject of close inspection in the context of AMD [23–29], although their specific roles at different stages of disease progression remain controversial. Macrophage differentiation is mostly dictated by the microenvironment and has profound implications for proper activation and function [30,31]. Pro-inflammatory M1 macrophages produce tumor necrosis factor-alpha (TNF-α) and interleukin-12 (IL-12), and are associated with tissue destruction, whereas M2 macrophages, characterized by production of the immunosuppressive cytokine IL-10, play a role in tissue homeostasis and repair. On the other hand, T cells are major effector cells of the adaptive immune response, providing the antigen specificity required for proper immune responses. Two major classes of T cells include CD4+ helper T (Th) cells and CD8+ cytotoxic T lymphocytes (CTLs) [32,33]. Th cells mainly shape the type of response based on the cytokines they release and help the recruitment and function of other immune cells, while CTLs are capable of directed killing of target cells. Our present knowledge regarding the role of T cells in AMD is surprisingly limited. Robert Nussenblatt and colleagues have shown that complement component 5a (C5a) induces the expression of IL-17 and IL-22 by human CD4+ T cells and that blood from AMD patients contains higher levels of these cytokines compared to controls [34]. Recently, AMD was also associated with age-related changes in peripheral T cells in humans, lending support to the idea that AMD can be a systemic disease [35]. However, the identity of antigen-specific T cells that potentially mediate AMD pathology and how they may interact with other immune cells (e.g. macrophages and B cells) in chronic retinal inflammation remains to be determined.

A potential link between innate and adaptive immune responses in disease is oxidative stress, a known contributing factor in the development of pathological inflammatory conditions, including atherosclerosis and AMD [36]. Lipid peroxidation has been shown to produce oxidation specific epitopes (OSEs) that can function as new antigens for immune recognition [37]. One of the best-characterized OSEs in the context of AMD is carboxyethylpyrrole (CEP) a protein adduct resulting from an oxidation fragment of docosahexaenoic acid (DHA) [38]. AMD donor eyes contain more CEP-modified proteins in the outer retina and drusen than age-matched controls [9], although the precise histological localization patterns of CEP within the healthy or diseased human retina have not been described. CEP-modified proteins and CEP autoantibodies are also more abundant in AMD plasma than in control samples [38,39]. Our laboratory immunized mice with CEP-adducted mouse serum albumin (CEP-MSA) and produced a novel mouse model with dry AMD-like pathology [40,41], effectively making the connection between an adaptive immune

response (due to the presence of CEP-specific antibodies) and the onset of AMD. Furthermore, we recently showed that pro-inflammatory M1 macrophages are recruited to the retina of CEP-immunized mice prior to overt degeneration [26]. While the laser-induced CNV model of wet AMD has provided great insight into the disease process and potential therapies (especially in the context of angiogenesis), the CEP model is to date the only one available for the immunological study of the dry form of the disease in genetically unmanipulated animals.

Here we provide evidence that CEP serves as an initiating signal for the cooperation of innate and adaptive immunity in the pathogenesis of AMD. CEP acts directly and indirectly to influence M1 macrophage polarization. It can directly activate macrophages, leading to M1 gene expression. We also find CEP-specific T cells from CEP-immunized mice that produce the inflammatory cytokines interferon-gamma (IFN-γ) and IL-17 that are able to induce M1 macrophage polarization *in vitro*. Surprisingly, we observed CEP-mediated retinal pathology in mice lacking mature B cells, indicating that AMD-like pathology in our model is antibody-independent and T cell-mediated. Analysis of mice with defects in several T cell differentiation pathways suggests that Th1 (IFN-γ producing) cells are important for development of disease. Finally, pharmacological inhibition of T cell activation prevents retinal pathology in our model, providing proof of concept for the use of immunotherapy in AMD treatment. This study provides cellular and molecular mechanisms that explain the role of inflammation in AMD: M1 macrophages and antigen-specific T cells activated by oxidative damage-induced products work together at the early onset stage of dry AMD. Disruption of this cooperation could lead to innovative therapies for this highly prevalent disease.

Materials and Methods

Ethics Statement

Protocols for use of experimental animals in this study adhered to the ARVO Statement for the Use of Animals in Ophthalmic and Vision Research and were approved by the Institutional Animal Care and Use Committee of the University of Miami Miller School of Medicine (Protocol 11–321). All surgical procedures were performed under anesthesia and all efforts were made to minimize suffering.

Mice

The following mice were obtained from The Jackson Laboratory: BALB/cJ (stock #000651) wild type mice, C57BL/6J (stock #000664) wild type mice, μMT−/− (B6.129S2-Ighm<tm1Cgn>/J, stock #002288), Stat6−/− (BALB/c background, C.129S2-Stat6< tm1Gru>/J, stock #002828), and Tbx21−/− (B6.129S6-Tbx21< tm1Glm>/J, stock #004648). Tlr2−/− (B6) mice were kindly provided by Dr. Dmitry Ivanov, along with corresponding littermate controls (Bascom Palmer Eye Institute). Il17a−/− (BALB/c) mice were kindly provided by Dr. Abul Abbas (UCSF). All mice were housed in a room exposed to 300 lux (outside the cage) in a 12 hr dark/light cycle.

Antigen

CEP-MSA was prepared from commercially available mouse serum albumin (Sigma-Aldrich), which was converted to CEP-modified MSA following previously published procedures [42].

Immunizations

The CEP-MSA immunization protocol has been described previously [40]. In summary, mice were primed by hind leg injections of 200 µg CEP-MSA in complete Freund's adjuvant (CFA; from DIFCO) at 8–12 weeks of age. At day 10 post-immunization (p.i.), the mice were challenged in the neck with 100 µg CEP-MSA in incomplete Freund's adjuvant (IFA; from DIFCO), followed by a final boost with 100 µg CEP-MSA in CFA in the neck seven days before harvest. As described in Cruz-Guilloty et al., 2013 [26], mice harvested at 40–90 days p.i. were defined as early recovery times, those harvested at 100–200 days p.i. were defined as intermediate recovery times, while those harvested after day 200 p.i. were considered late recovery times. Anti-CEP antibody titers at days 40–60 p.i. were quantified by ELISA as previously described [40] and used to determine efficiency of immunization. All immunized mice were compared with age-matched naïve, sham-MSA or CFA only controls. As previously reported [26,40], there are no significant differences among the control mice (with low to undetectable anti-CEP titers) in terms of retinal pathology and are therefore used interchangeably, depending on experimental setup, and collectively labeled as "control". For each mouse strain that was analyzed in this study, 2 or 3 independent experiments were performed with n = 3–5 mice per group per time point.

Histology

Eyes were harvested at early (40–90 days), intermediate (100–200 days) and late (over 200 days) recovery times post-immunization (p.i.). Right eyes were used for histology and were fixed in 2% paraformaldehyde and 2.5% glutaraldehyde in 0.1M PO_4 buffer (pH = 7.4) overnight and dehydrated in graded ethanol and propylene oxide. After polymerization in a resin mixture containing Polybed 812 (Polysciences) and Araldite 502 (Polysciences), semi-thin (0.7 µm) sagittal sections of each eye were stained with toluidine blue and analyzed for histopathology with light microscopy using a Zeiss microscope (equipped with an AxioCam digital camera) using a 63x oil-immersion lens.

Pathology Scoring: Quantification of Lesions and Inflammatory Cells in the IPM

Each individual mouse in this study was scored for retinal pathology on a masked fashion, using 10 sections of the right eye with at least 25–30 µm intervals between each section. Scoring was divided in 2 subclasses: 1) the retinal lesion count represents the sum of RPE areas showing abnormal vesiculation, swelling, thinning, pyknosis, and cell lysis; 2) inflammatory cells were defined as dark nuclear stains of macrophage-like cells observed and counted only within the interphotoreceptor matrix (IPM) compartment at the level of the photoreceptor outer segments and the apical border of the RPE. The overall pathology score for each eye is the sum of the two subclasses. The data is always presented as pathology (cells and lesions combined) per section unless specified otherwise. A total of 3–5 mice were used in the analysis at each time point. At least two independent experiments were performed for each strain reported in this study. Repeat experiments with similar results were analyzed separately because of the use of independent batches of CEP-MSA.

Immunohistochemistry

Identification of inflammatory cells in the mouse retinas was performed as previously described (Cruz-Guilloty et al, 2013).

The following was the protocol for analysis of human eyes. Autopsy eyes (n = 10) were obtained from the Wilmer Eye Institute Pathology Division after approval from the Human Subjects Committee at Johns Hopkins University. "Unaffected" eyes (n = 5) had no AMD history or microscopic evidence of drusen, basal deposits, or loss of RPE cuboidal epithelial morphology. Early AMD donors (n = 5) had an AMD history and macular drusen, but no late stage disease. Eyes were fixed in 4% formaldehyde, paraffin embedded, sectioned to 4 µm thickness, and deparaffinized with xylene and an ethanol gradient. Antigens were retrieved with the Target Retrieval System (Dako, Inc., Carpinteria, CA). Sections were incubated with blocking serum for 1 h; with mouse monoclonal anti-CEP antibody (30 µg/ml) or equivalent concentrations of mouse IgG1 isotype control overnight at 4°C; with biotinylated anti-mouse IgG for 60 min, and then with ABC-AP (Vector labs, Burlingame, CA) for 30 min. The chromagen was developed with blue substrate working solution (Vector labs) supplemented with levamasole. The IgG1 monoclonal anti-CEP antibody described here was produced by our lab in conjunction with Genscript, Inc. (Piscataway, NJ) following our standard immunization protocol and was tested (by ELISA and Western blots) for specificity against a variety of CEP-modified proteins and lacked recognition of other lipid-derived modifications (data not shown).

Enzyme-linked Immunosorbent Assay (ELISA) for the Quantification of Cytokines in Culture and Serum

ELISAs for cytokine detection were performed, as per manufacturer's instructions, using paired antibodies against IFN-γ, IL-17A, IL-2, IL-4, IL-1β, IL-12, TNF-α and IL-10 (all purchased from eBioscience, San Diego, CA). Purified recombinant cytokines from the same vendor were used to develop standard curves. In summary, flat bottom, high binding 96-well plates were coated with 100 µl of primary (capture) antibody in PBS, and washed with 150 µl of washing solution (PBS, 0.1% Tween-20). Blocking was done with 100 µl of the dilution buffer (PBS, 0.1% Tween-20, 1% BSA) followed by additional washes before adding 100 µl per well of protein (purified cytokine) standards or samples (undiluted CEP culture supernatants or 1:25 serum dilution). After incubation and washing, 100 µl per well of secondary (biotin-labeled) antibody were added, followed by addition of 50 µl per well of Avidin-Alkaline Phosphatase (Sigma-Aldrich). After incubation, 50 µl of developing solution (Phosphatase Substrate from Sigma-Aldrich in DEA buffer at 1 mg/ml) were loaded per well and the absorbance was measured in a microplate reader at 405 nm.

Gene Expression Analysis of Acute Retinal Inflammation by Quantitative Real Time PCR (RT-PCR)

Intravitreal injections were performed as follows. C57BL/6j mice (male and female, 2 months old) were anesthetized and the pupils dilated. Using a dissecting microscope, intravitreous injections into one eye of each mouse (n = 5 per group) were performed with a pump microinjection apparatus (Harvard Apparatus, Holliston, MA) and a glass micropipette that was calibrated to deliver 1 µl of vehicle containing either BSA (2 µg), CEP-BSA (2 µg), MSA (2.44 µg), or CEP-MSA (2.44 µg) on depression of the foot switch. Mice were sacrificed 6 and 24 hours later, eyes were enucleated, and the RPE/choroid and retinas were dissected. Total RNA was extracted using the RNeasy mini kit (Qiagen, Valencia, CA) according to the manufacturers protocol, and reverse transcription was perform using the High Capicity RNA-to-cDNA kit (Life Technologies, Grand Island, NY) following the manufacturer's protocol. Analyses of selected genes were performed with TaqMan Gene Expression Assays (Life Technologies, Grand Island, NY), using the StepOnePlus TaqMan System Fast Mode (Life Technologies, Grand Island, NY). Data were analyzed using the comparative CT method. Primer and probe sets were as follows: *IL-1β*, Mm01336189_m1; *TNF-α*, Mm00443258_m1; *IL-6*, Mm00446190_m1; *IL-12*, Mm00434165_m1; *Ccl2*, Mm00441242_m1; *IL-10*, Mm00439614_m1; *KC*, Mm 04207460_m1.

In vitro Culture and Stimulation of Primary Macrophages, RPE Cells and Splenocytes (CEP-specific T cells)

For *in vitro* macrophage cultures, bone marrow-derived macrophages (BMDM) were used. Bone marrow cells were differentiated in DMEM (Invitrogen) supplemented with 10% heat-inactivated FBS (Atlanta Biologicals) and 15% L929 cell-conditioned media (as a source of M-CSF) for seven days. Macrophage culture purity was determined by flow cytometry and cultures were >97% double positive for F4/80 and CD11b. Macrophages were stimulated in fresh DMEM with CEP-MSA (100 µg/ml), sham-MSA (100 µg/ml), or left untreated for 4–24 hours. The CEP-MSA and sham-MSA preparations were tested for endotoxin contamination using the ToxinSensor Chromogenic LAL Endotoxin Assay Kit (GenScript) and endotoxin levels were determined to be below 1 endotoxin unit (EU)/mL, with similar levels in both solutions. Lipopolysaccharide (LPS; from Sigma) at 100 ng/ml and Pam3CSK4 (InvivoGen) at 500 ng/ml were used as controls. After stimulation, the cells were used for RNA extraction (4–6 hr time point), while the supernatant was used for detection of secreted factors (24 hr time point). For detection of secreted proteins (TNF-α, IL-12 and IL-1β), ELISAs were performed as described above using antibody pairs and recombinant protein standard curves as per manufacturer's instructions (eBioscience).

For *in vitro* RPE cultures, eyes were enucleated from mice and bisected along the ora serrata. The anterior portions (cornea, lens, etc.) were discarded and the neuronal retina was carefully removed and separated from the posterior eyecups. Next, the posterior eyecups were incubated in 0.25% trypsin-EDTA (Invitrogen) at 37°C for 1 h. Then, the RPE cells were removed from the posterior eye cups, pelleted and washed with DMEM/F12 (Invitrogen) containing 20% heat-inactivated FBS (Atlanta Biologicals). RPE cells were seeded into 12-well culture plates in DMEM/F12 containing 20% heat-inactivated FBS and cultured for 4–8 weeks. RPE cells were stimulated in fresh DMEM with CEP-MSA (100 µg/ml), sham-MSA (100 µg/ml), or left untreated for 4 hours.

To isolate CEP-specific T cells, splenocytes from mice immunized with CEP-MSA (or control mice) were stimulated *in vitro* with 100 µg/ml of antigen (CEP-MSA or Sham-MSA) in complete DMEM media. After 4 days, cultures were divided in two, with recombinant human IL-2 (20 units/ml; eBioscience) added to one of the two samples, followed by two more days of incubation. Flow cytometry acquisition (FACS Diva software on LSR-II cytometer) and analysis (FlowJo software) were performed at different time points using antibodies specific for CD3, CD4, CD8, B220, CD19, CD11b, NK1.1, CD69, F4/80 (all from eBioscience). For T cell-macrophage co-culture experiments, CEP-specific T cells and naïve BMDM were co-cultured at different ratios and different time points (6, 12, 24 and 48 hr). Data shown here were obtained from the optimal conditions of 1:1 T cell-BMDM ratio and 24 hr co-culture period. The supernatants were collected to measure cytokine production by ELISA. For RT-PCR analysis of macrophage gene expression (as described below), T cells were removed from the cultures by vigorous pipetting and extensive washes in PBS (5 times), considering that BMDM are extremely adherent cells. Purity of the BMDM (~95% F4/80+ cells) after co-culture was confirmed by flow cytometry.

Gene Expression Analysis of BMDM by Quantitative Real Time PCR (RT-PCR)

Total RNA was isolated from cells using the RNeasy kit (Qiagen), then cDNA was generated with the Maxima First Strand cDNA Synthesis Kit (Fermentas). Gene expression was measured by real-time quantitative PCR (qPCR) using various primers (see below). qPCR was performed using iQ SYBR Green Supermix (Bio-Rad) on a Roche Light Cycler real-time PCR instrument. Relative gene expression was calculated using the $\Delta\Delta C_t$ method, with gene expression normalized to Gapdh expression. Each treatment is represented as relative-expression (i.e., fold-expression over reference group), where the control sample served as the reference with a set value of 1.

The following primer sets were used:

iNOS (**For:** GTTCTCAGCCCAACAATACAAGA, **Rev:** GTGGACGGGTCGATGTCAC).

TNF-α (**For:** CTGAACTTCGGGGTGATCGG, **Rev:** GGCTTGTCACTCGAATTTTGAGA).

IL-12A (**For:** CAATCACGCTACCTCCTCTTTT, **Rev:** CAGCAGTGCAGGAATAATGTTTC).

IL-1b (**For:** GCAACTGTTCCTGAACTCAACT, **Rev:** ATCTTTTGGGGTCCGTCAACT).

IL-10 (**For:** GCTCTTACTGACTGGCATGAG, **Rev:** CGCAGCTCTAGGAGCATGTG).

Arginase-1 (**For:** CTCCAAGCCAAAGTCCTTAGAG, **Rev:** AGGAGCTGTCATTAGGGACATC).

HO-1 (**For:** AAGCCGAGAATGCTGAGTTCA, **Rev:** GCCGTGTAGATATGGTACAAGGA).

Srxn1 (**For:** CCCAGGGTGGCGACTACTA, **Rev:** GTGGACCTCACGAGCTTGG).

Ccl2 (**For:** TTAAAAACCTGGATCGGAACCAA, **Rev:** GCATTAGCTTCAGATTTACGGGT).

IL-6 (**For:** CTGCAAGAGACTTCCATCCAG, **Rev:** AGTGGTATAGACAGGTCTGTTGG).

KC (**For:** ACTGCACCCAAACCGAAGTC, **Rev:** TGGGGACACCTTTTAGCATCTT).

Vegf-A (**For:** GCACATAGAGAGAATGAGCTTCC, **Rev:** CTCCGCTCTGAACAAGGCT).

Vegf-B (**For:** GCCAGACAGGGTTGCCATAC, **Rev:** GGAGTGGGATGGATGATGTCAG).

Gapdh (**For:** AGGTCGGTGTGAACGGATTTG, **Rev:** TGTAGACCATGTAGTTGAGGTCA).

Animal Treatment with the Immunosuppressive Drugs Cyclosporine A and Rapamycin

Wild-type (8-week old) BALB/cJ mice were immunized with CEP-MSA in CFA and treated with a combination therapy of cyclosporine A (CsA; "Sandimmune" from Novartis, East Hanover, NJ) and rapamycin (Rapa; "Rapamune" from Wyeth Pharmaceuticals, Philadelphia, PA) with daily intraperitoneal (i.p.) injections for 21 or 40 days (starting on the first day of immunization). Blood was collected at day 50 p.i. for anti-CEP titer evaluation and eyes were harvested at day 60–100 p.i. (early recovery time) for histological analysis. The stock solutions where diluted in sterile PBS for 100 µl i.p. injections at the following doses: CsA = 5 mg/kg/day; Rapa = 0.5 mg/kg/day.

Statistics

Results shown in graphs are presented as means +/− S.D. Data for direct comparison of two samples were analyzed using two-tailed Student's t test with Prism software (GraphPad). Analyses for 3 groups or more were performed using one-way analysis of variance (ANOVA) followed by Newman-Keuls multiple comparison tests, also with Prism software. P-values <0.05 were considered significant.

Results

CEP Directly Activates Macrophages, Leading to M1 Polarization *In vitro*

We recently reported that CEP immunization in mice leads to Ccl2/Ccr2-mediated M1 macrophage recruitment to the outer retina before AMD-like pathology ensues [26]. However, the mechanisms by which CEP promotes M1 polarization remained to be elucidated. Because oxidized phospholipids and their resulting protein modifications have been shown to activate macrophages [29,43], we tested whether CEP has a direct effect on macrophage activation using an *in vitro* system. Bone-marrow derived macrophages (BMDM) were differentiated *in vitro* and stimulated with CEP-MSA, Sham-MSA (non-adducted MSA) or left untreated, followed by quantitative PCR (qPCR) analysis of gene expression. We used two different wild type strains (BALB/c and C57BL/6J), since we have shown that both develop CEP-mediated pathology [26,40]. As shown in **Fig. 1**, CEP-MSA specifically induced the expression of M1 marker genes (iNOS, IL-1β, TNF-α, IL-12) in both BALB/c (**Fig. 1A**) and C57BL/6J (**Fig. 1B**) macrophages, but did not have a significant effect on the expression of M2 markers (Arg-1, IL-10) or genes (HO-1, Srxn1) expressed in a recently described class of macrophages activated by oxidized phospholipids termed Mox cells [43] (Figure S1). In addition to the M1 marker genes mentioned above, CEP induced macrophage expression of other pro-inflammatory cytokines such as IL-6 and KC, but did not have an effect on the pro-angiogenic genes Vegf-A and Vegf-B (Figure S2). Furthermore, the CEP-induced M1 polarization was confirmed at the protein level, as stimulated cells secreted IL-1β, TNF-α, and IL-12 (**Fig. 2**).

CEP Promotes Acute Inflammatory Responses in RPE Cells *In vivo* and *In vitro*

As previously described [40], systemic CEP immunization leads to a chronic, low-grade inflammatory response in the mouse retina, but experimental evidence for its *in situ* effects has not been reported to date. This is particularly relevant for the effects of CEP on the RPE, the cell type mostly affected in AMD. To further probe the ability of CEP to induce pro-inflammatory conditions in the retina, we performed intravitreal injections of CEP-MSA or Sham-MSA, followed by gene expression analysis of M1-associated transcripts in RPE/choroid samples isolated 6 hrs post-injection. As shown in **Fig. 3A**, injection of CEP-MSA (but not Sham-MSA) specifically induced the expression of a subset of M1-related genes (such as IL-1β, IL-12 and Ccl2), but not others (such as TNF-α, Figure S3). In addition, *in vitro* CEP stimulation of primary RPE cells (in the absence of choroid) also led to pro-inflammatory gene expression, including the production of the monocyte chemoattractant Ccl2 (**Fig. 3B**). Taken together, these data show that CEP can indeed promote a retinal microenvironment conducive to the recruitment of circulating monocytes (through the Ccl2/Ccr2 axis) and M1 polarization.

CEP is Distinctively Localized within the RPE of Human AMD Eyes, but not in Healthy Eyes

Our CEP mouse model of dry AMD is based on observations from human AMD patients that show elevated levels of CEP in drusen and CEP autoantibodies [9,38]. However, a detailed description of the CEP localization patterns in normal versus dry (non-neovascular) AMD retinas is still lacking. We took advantage of a new mouse IgG1 monoclonal antibody against CEP developed in our laboratory to perform CEP immunolabeling in human retinas (**Fig. 4**). Distinct differences in CEP immunolabeling were observed between maculas of unaffected control (n = 5; average age 85.4 yrs) and dry (non-neovascular) AMD donors (n = 5; average age 73.8 yrs). To our surprise, CEP was identified in unaffected control donor maculas, including the ganglion cell layer, inner plexiform layer, inner nuclear layer, and photoreceptor outer segments (**Fig. 4A–B**). Within the PR cells, CEP was more prominent in cones relative to rods. The RPE had minimal, if any, CEP labeling. When present, CEP was seen in inner Bruch's membrane. Minimal labeling for CEP was present in the choroid. Like unaffected controls, CEP was identified in the inner retinal layers of AMD maculas, including the ganglion cell layer, inner plexiform layer, and inner nuclear layer (**Fig. 4C**). However, CEP immunolabeling was more prominent in the inner aspect of photoreceptors compared to outer segments. In addition, immunolabeling for CEP was diffusely seen within RPE cells of dry AMD eyes (**Fig. 4C–G**). CEP immunolabeling within drusen ranged from absent to prominent labeling. The presence of CEP within RPE of dry AMD patients complements our data on CEP-induced retinal inflammation in mice by suggesting that CEP signaling in the RPE associates with AMD pathology.

CEP-induced Retinal Pathology is Antibody-independent and T Cell-mediated

Besides the apparent deleterious role of innate cells (M1 macrophages) in our CEP model of dry AMD [26], we have already published evidence for the role of the adaptive immune system. Not only does CEP immunization result in elevated titers of anti-CEP autoantibodies in wild type mice, but the same immunization protocol in RAG−/− mice (which lack mature T and B cells) fails to produce retinal pathology [40]. We now provide evidence for a leading role of antigen-specific T cells in the immune response against CEP. We observed specific antibody isotype switching (indicative of a T cell-dependent humoral response) from IgM (which was detected early at day 20 post-immunization, data not shown) to IgG1 (**Fig. 5A**), but not IgG2a or IgG2b (data not shown), in CEP immunized mice on both C57BL/6 and BALB/c backgrounds. Anti-CEP antibody production requires complete Freund's adjuvant (CFA), as other adjuvants, such as Alum, fail to induce high titers (Figure S4). Because T cells are known for their ability to secrete cytokines, we quantified several types of cytokines in serum by ELISA and found elevated levels of the pro-inflammatory cytokines IFN-γ (44.5 ng/ml vs undetectable) and IL-17A (2.8 ng/ml vs 0.97 ng/ml) in serum of CEP-immunized compared to control mice (**Fig. 5B**). In addition, we observed a similar pattern of cytokine production *ex vivo* when splenocytes from CEP-immunized or control mice were stimulated with the cognate antigen (**Fig. 5C**). Production of the Th2-type cytokine IL-4 was not detected in these cultures (data not shown). To confirm the presence of CEP-specific T cells, we performed flow cytometric analysis of the *in vitro* stimulated splenocytes and found a clear population of activated T cells (gate in forward and side scatter plots) when cells from CEP-immunized mice (but not control mice such as mice immunized with CFA only) were cultured in the presence of CEP-MSA (**Fig. 5D**). T cell activation was absent in control conditions with Sham-MSA, irrelevant antigen (ovalbumin) and media only (data not shown). Both CD4+ and CD8+ T cells were present in the CEP-specific cultures, with increased expansion of the CD8+ population when IL-2 (a T cell growth and differentiation factor) was added to the cultures, most likely due to the known increased sensitivity for IL-2 and proliferation ability of CD8+ CTLs [44].

A   BALB/c Macrophages

B   C57BL/6J Macrophages

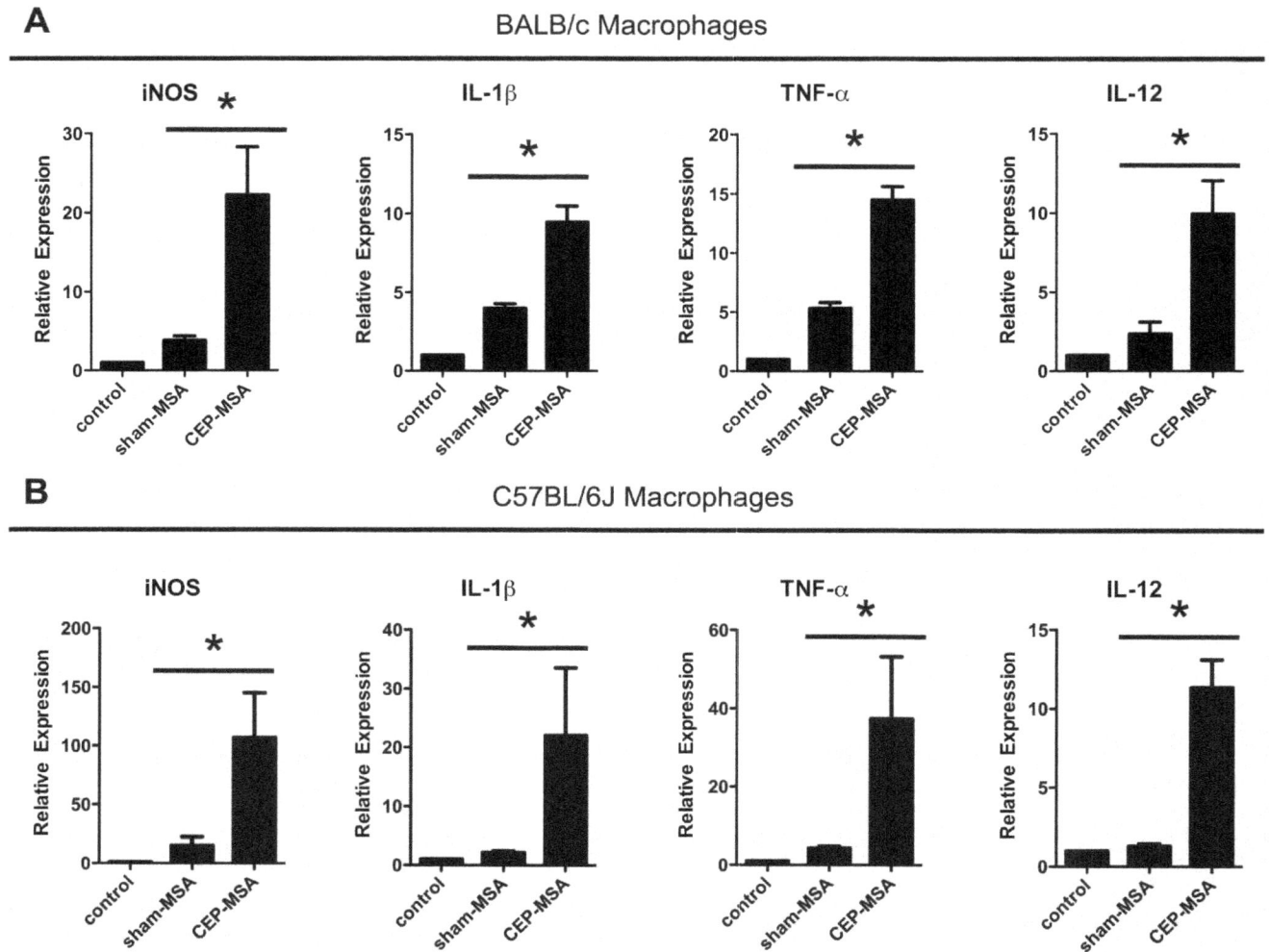

Figure 1. CEP directly activates macrophages *in vitro*, leading to M1 polarization. (A) Bone marrow-derived macrophages (BMDM) from BALB/c mice were stimulated for 4 hrs with CEP-MSA (100 μg/ml), Sham-MSA (100 μg/ml) or left untreated. RNA was isolated and qPCR was used for gene expression analysis. Each treatment is represented as relative-expression (i.e., fold-expression over reference group), where the control (untreated) sample served as the reference with a set value of 1. CEP specifically induced the expression of M1 markers (iNOS, IL-1β, TNF-α and IL-12A) but had no effect on M2 or Mox marker genes (Figure S1). **(B)** BMDM from C57BL/6 mice were stimulated and analyzed as described above. Data from 4 independent experiments were pooled and two-tailed Student's t tests were used for statistical analysis (* denotes p<0.05); error bars represent S.D.

To formally test the role of antibody-producing B cells in our model, we immunized mice lacking only mature B cells (μMT−/− mice) with CEP-MSA (**Fig. 6**). While, as expected, anti-CEP antibody titers were not detectable in CEP-immunized μMT−/− mice (data not shown), CEP-specific T cell activation was observed, with most cells being CD8+ T cells (**Fig. 6A,** left panel). This result proves that T cells can be activated in the absence of B cells, which also function as antigen presenting cells (APCs). Importantly, CEP-mediated retinal pathology was observed in μMT−/− mice (**Fig. 6B,** quantification in **Fig. 6C,** left panel), indicating that AMD-like pathology in our model does not require antibodies and can be mediated by T cells only. To dissect which pathways of T cell differentiation may be more relevant to CEP-induced pathology, we immunized several knockout (ko) mice with specific defects in Th1, Th2 and Th17 responses. Anti-CEP antibody titers were not significantly affected in any of the tested ko mice (data not shown). Mice with impaired Th2 differentiation (Stat6 ko mice) or lacking IL-17A production (IL-

17A ko mice) developed CEP-mediated pathology similar to WT mice (all on the BALB/c background; data now shown). However, T-bet ko mice (on the B6 background), with known defects in Th1 differentiation and IFN-γ production, did not develop retinal pathology after CEP immunization (**Fig. 6C**, right panel), even though CEP-specific T cells with increased IL-17A production were detected *ex vivo* (**Fig. 6A**, right panel and data now shown). Taken together, these results indicate that T cells, not B cells or antibodies, lead the adaptive immune response to CEP and are required for development of disease. Furthermore, Th1 differentiation (or IFN-γ production in general) seems to play an essential role in this process.

CEP-specific T Cells Induce M1 Macrophage Polarization in Co-culture Experiments

Our combined data suggests that both macrophages and T cells are needed to generate CEP-mediated retinal degeneration. Activation or function of just one of the two cell types is not

BALB/c Macrophages ELISA

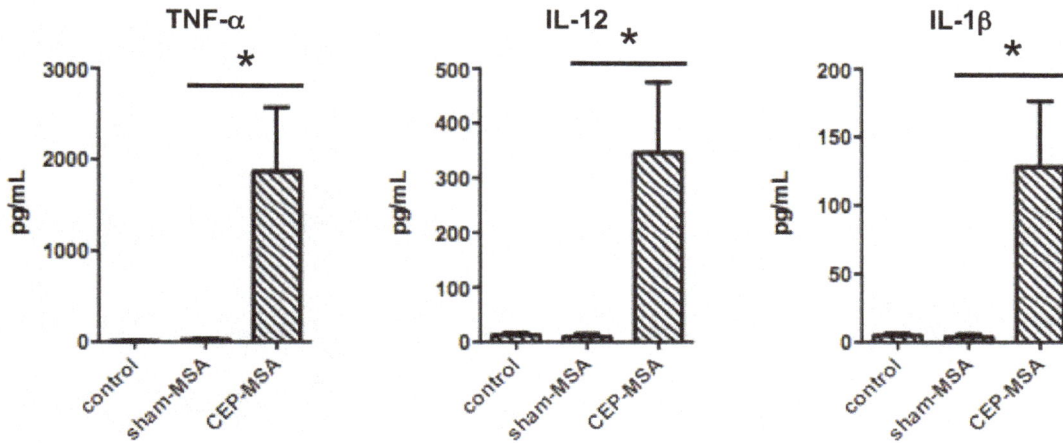

Figure 2. CEP induces secretion of M1-type cytokines by activated macrophages. Bone marrow-derived macrophages from BALB/c mice were stimulated for 24 hrs with CEP-MSA (100 µg/ml), Sham-MSA (100 µg/ml) or left untreated. Supernatants were collected and used for detection of secreted proteins by ELISA. CEP specifically induced the secretion of M1 cytokines (TNF-α, IL-12 and L-1β). Data from at least 2 independent experiments were pooled and ANOVA was used for statistical analysis (* denotes p<0.05); error bars represent S.D.

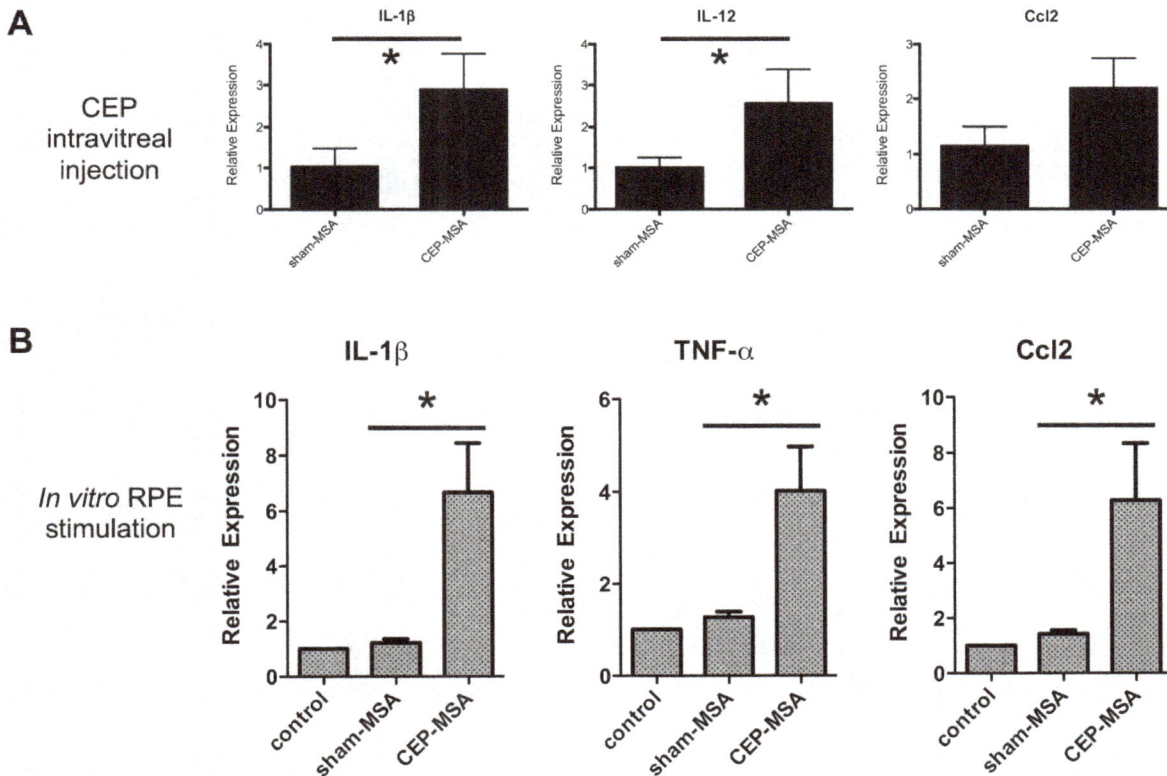

Figure 3. CEP induces pro-inflammatory gene expression in RPE cells *in vivo* and *in vitro*. (**A**) Intravitreal injections of CEP-MSA or Sham-MSA (2 µg total) were performed, RNA was isolated after 6 hrs from the RPE/choroid, followed by Taqman gene expression analysis (n = 5). Mean values from one of two independent experiments are shown; error bars represent S.D. (*) denotes statistically significant differences (p<0.05) based on two-tailed Student's t tests. (**B**) Primary mouse RPE cultures were stimulated for 4 hrs with CEP-MSA (100 µg/ml), Sham-MSA (100 µg/ml) or left untreated. RNA was isolated and qPCR was used for gene expression analysis. Each treatment is represented as relative-expression (i.e., fold-expression over reference group), where the control (untreated) sample served as the reference with a set value of 1. Data are pooled from at least 2 independent experiments and include RPE cells from both BALB/c and B6 mice. Mean values from a total of four experiments are shown; error bars represent S.D. (*) denotes statistically significant differences (p<0.05) based on two-tailed Student's t tests.

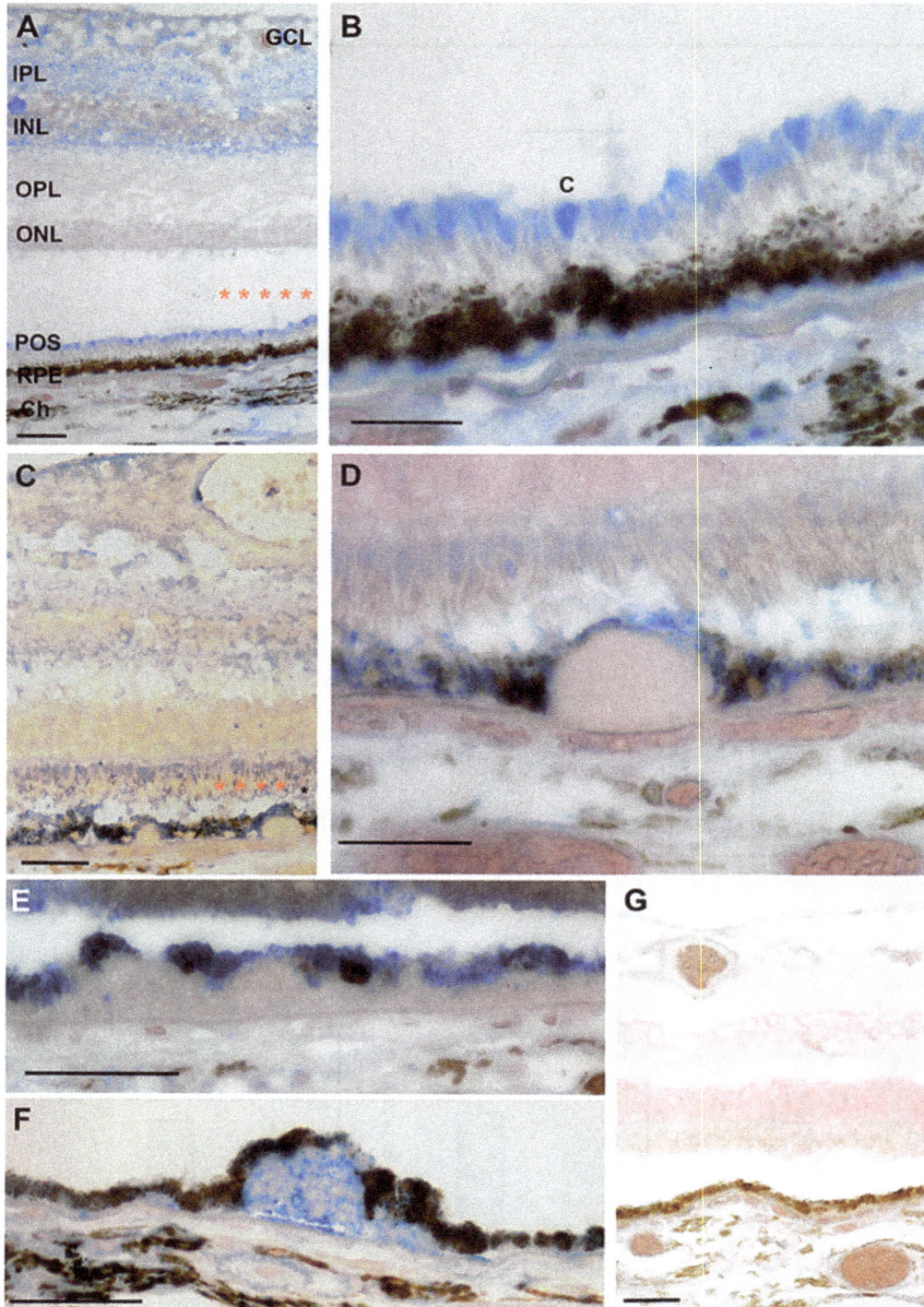

Figure 4. CEP immunolabeling in normal healthy eyes and dry AMD eyes. (**A**) Macula from a 77 yo unaffected female with CEP immunolabeling (blue) in the ganglion cell layer (GCL), inner plexiform layer (IPL), inner nuclear layer (INL), and photoreceptor outer segments (POS). Minimal labeling is seen in the RPE. Thin immunolabeling is seen at the RPE basement membrane. (**B**) Magnified view of the region labeled with red asterisks in A. POS are prominently labeled, especially cones (c). CEP immunolabeling at the basal RPE in inner Bruch's membrane is more obvious. (**C**) Macula from a 51 yo male with dry (non-neovascular) AMD with CEP immunolabeling in the nerve fiber layer and GCL, IPL, INL, and photoreceptors. Labeling in photoreceptors is more prominent in the inner regions than in the POS. The RPE is diffusely labeled. (**D**) Magnified view of the region labeled with red asterisks in C shows diffusely labeled RPE. A prominent drusen is minimally labeled for CEP. (**E**) 69 yo female with non-neovascular AMD. The RPE cells overlying a large drusen are diffusely labeled for CEP. The drusen has a speckled labeling pattern for CEP. (**F**) 83 yo female with dry AMD. The drusen has prominent CEP immunolabeling with diffuse labeling within the overlying RPE. (**G**) IgG control from a 61 yo male with non-neovascular AMD. Ch, choroid; Bar = 25 μm.

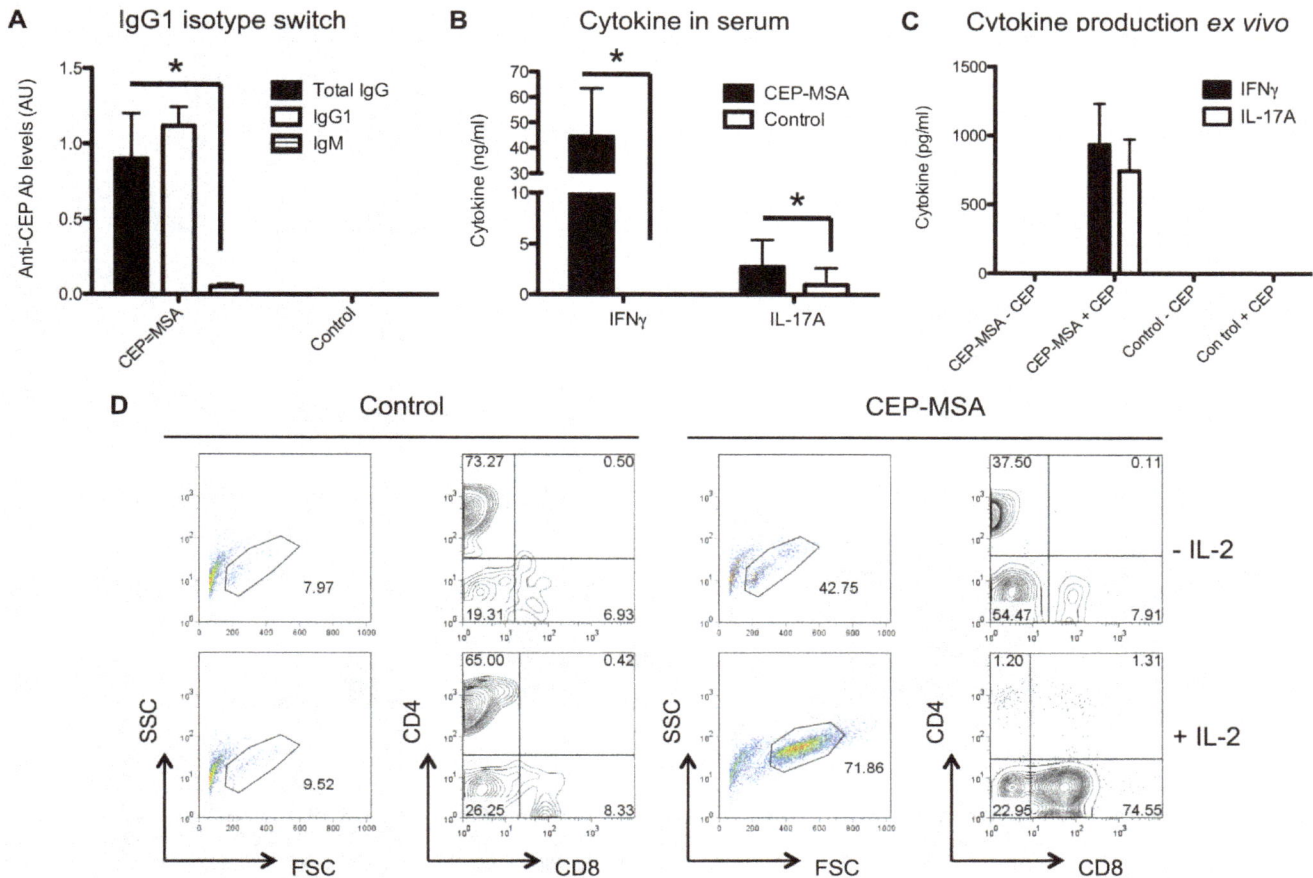

Figure 5. IgG1 isotype switch, pro-inflammatory cytokine production and CEP-specific T cell priming in CEP-MSA immunized mice.
(**A**) Significant amounts of anti-CEP antibody titers are detected in serum from immunized mice. Isotype switch to IgG1 from IgM (undetectable levels) was observed. Naïve controls show undetectable levels of anti-CEP titers. ANOVA was used for statistical analysis (* denotes p<0.05). (**B**) Serum levels of IFN-γ and IL-17A were measured by ELISA. While both cytokines were present at higher levels in serum from CEP-immunized mice compared to control (naïve) mice, IFN-γ levels were predominantly elevated. Two-tailed Student's t test was used for statistical analysis (* denotes p< 0.05). (**C**) T cells from CEP-MSA immunized, but not naïve, mice produce IFN-γ and IL-17A when stimulated *in vitro* with the CEP-MSA antigen. (**D**) Splenocytes from WT B6 mice immunized with either CEP-MSA or CFA only were stimulated in vitro with CEP-MSA for 6 days *ex vivo*. At day 4 the cultures were divided in two, and IL-2 was added to the indicated samples. Cells were stained with anti-CD4 and anti-CD8 and analyzed by flow cytometry. Forward and side scatters are shown on the left with a "live lymphocyte" gate, CD8-CD4 plots show cells within this gate. Results shown here are mean values representative of more than 5 independent experiments for C57BL/6 mice (with n>3 for each experiment); error bars represent S.D. Similar results are observed with BALB/c mice (not shown).

sufficient for disease development. M1 macrophages are the main effector cells at the site of injury [26]; we have not detected T cells of any kind within the outer retina, although some T cells are present in the choroid of CEP-immunized mice (data not shown). Macrophages need to be recruited to the retina for the pathology to ensue, even if CEP-specific T cell activation and antibody production are normal, as is the case in Ccr2-deficient mice ([26] and data not shown). On the other hand, T cell activation is required for pathology even if a normal monocyte/macrophage compartment is present, as is the case in RAG−/− mice [40] and T-bet ko mice (this study). Therefore, we addressed the issue of T cell-macrophage interactions by setting up a simplified co-culture system using CEP-specific T cells and "naïve" bone marrow-derived macrophages (BMDM). As shown in **Fig. 7A**, CEP-specific T cells promote (in an antigen-specific manner) a distinct pattern of M1 polarization *in vitro* by inducing the expression of at least a subset of M1-related genes (iNOS and IL-12A but not TNF-α). The effect of CEP-specific T cells on M1 macrophage polarization does not require cell-cell contacts, as T cell-secreted

factors (in purified CEP stimulation supernatants) induce a similar pattern of gene expression in BMDM (**Fig. 7B**). Notably, the supernatant effect is not simply due to the presence of IFN-γ or IL-17A in the supernatants (Fig. 5C), since similar concentrations of the purified cytokines fails to reproduce this effect. Importantly, expression of M2-related genes (such as Arg-1) is not significantly enhanced in the presence of T cells or their secreted factors (**Figure 7**).

Proof-of-principle: Pharmacological Inhibition of T Cell Activation Prevents CEP-induced Retinal Pathology

One of the ultimate goals of our research program is to learn the basic mechanisms involved in the AMD disease process so that we can attempt to translate such information into meaningful therapeutic strategies in the future. While immunotherapy has been proposed as an alternative for the treatment of AMD [16], there is no current published data formally proving the efficacy of this approach. As a proof-of-concept, we treated CEP-immunized mice with a combination drug therapy aimed at suppressing T cell

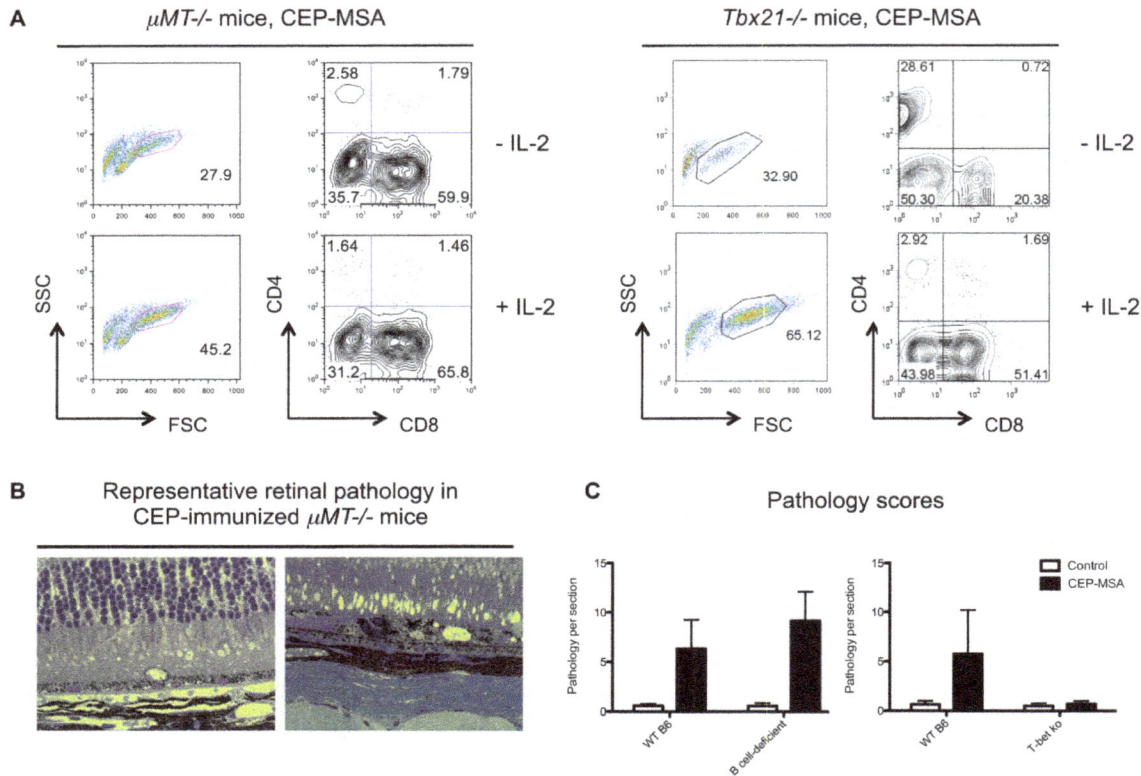

Figure 6. CEP-induced retinal pathology is antibody-independent and Th1 cell-mediated. (**A**) B cell deficient ($\mu MT-/-$) or T-bet deficient (*Tbx21-/-*) mice were immunized with CEP-MSA and splenocytes were activated *ex vivo* with CEP-MSA as described above. Forward and side scatters are shown on the left with a "live lymphocyte" gate, CD8-CD4 plots show cells within this gate. CEP-specific T cells were observed in the cultures for both strains. (**B**) CEP-MSA immunized $\mu MT-/-$ mice develop AMD-like pathology. Pictures are representative of histological analysis using plastic sections as described in Ref. 24. (**C**) Retinal pathology scores for the indicated groups at the late time point (day 200+ p.i.; n = 3). Mean values are shown; error bars represent S.D. Data from one representative experiment for each strain were used for this analysis; similar results were obtained in at least one separate independent experiment per strain.

responses [45]. In general, T cells require two signals for complete activation: T cell receptor (TCR) signaling and co-stimulation. Cyclosporine A (CsA) is an inhibitor of calcineurin, a phosphatase downstream of TCR signaling required for activation of NFAT and IL-2 production. Rapamycin (Rapa, also known as Sirolimus) inhibits the mTOR pathway, which is downstream of co-stimulatory molecules (such as CD28) and cytokine receptors. Treatment of CEP-immunized BALB/c mice with both CsA and Rapa lead to two important results: downregulation of anti-CEP titers (**Fig. 8A**) and prevention of CEP-induced retinal pathology (**Fig. 8B**).

Discussion

This report provides several novel findings of great potential significance for the study of AMD pathogenesis, specifically, and chronic inflammatory diseases in general. We show that the innate and adaptive immune systems work in concert for disease development over extended periods of time, and we provide precise cellular and molecular mechanisms for this cooperation (**Fig. 9**). The lipid peroxidation product CEP serves as the functional link, capable of directly activating both M1 macrophages and antigen-specific T cells. CEP eye injections can also induce acute inflammation in the retina and human eyes have a distinctive CEP localization pattern in the retina, with diffuse presence within RPE of dry AMD patients. Our data help to

clarify the role of antibodies in the CEP model of dry AMD by showing that CEP immunization leads to retinal lesions even in the absence of B cells. Moreover, CEP-specific T cells can induce M1 macrophage polarization *in vitro* and pharmacological suppression of T cell function prevents AMD-like pathology.

Previous evidence, including data from our lab, suggests that macrophages play a crucial role in the AMD disease process, but there is still controversy in this regard. It is possible that this discrepancy is partly due to the different stages of AMD progression: macrophages could have varied roles at the onset of dry AMD in response to oxidative damage, during the accumulation of drusen and during the transition from dry to wet AMD. It has been shown that iNOS-expressing macrophages infiltrate the Bruch's membrane of AMD patients [46]. In addition, an intriguing pilot study by Chi-Chao Chan and colleagues showed that human AMD eyes had more M1 macrophages compared to normal eyes, which contained more M2 macrophages [47]. However, we cannot rule out the possibility that, in some instances, M2 or other types of macrophages (e.g. Mox?) can drive the dry AMD pathology. For instance, the important distinction between retinal resident microglia and macrophages recruited from the circulation awaits the development of microglia-specific markers. Regardless, the likely determining factor in macrophage polarization and AMD outcomes will be the patient-specific onset factors, which in our case is CEP. Our data on CEP tilting the balance toward M1 polarization *in vivo* and

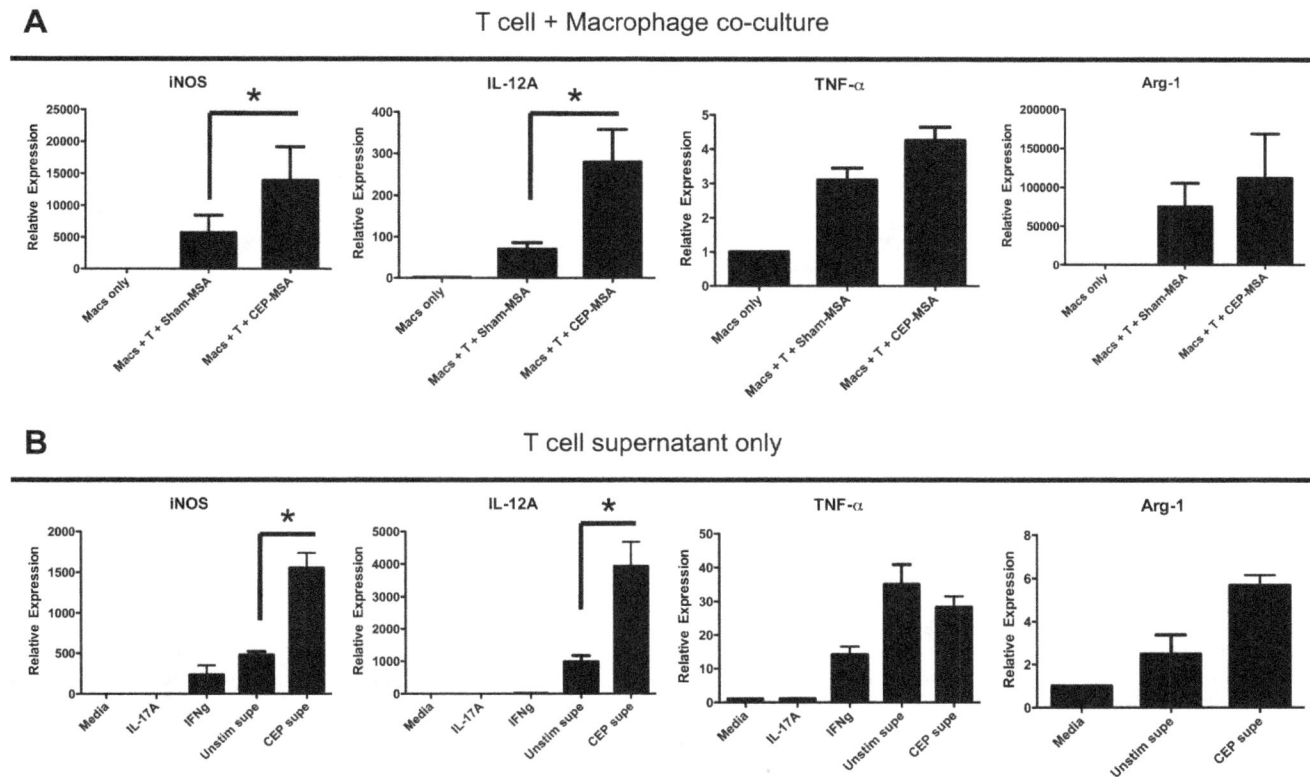

Figure 7. CEP-specific T cells induce M1 macrophage polarization *in vitro*. (A) Splenocytes from CEP-immunized mice were stimulated *in vitro* with CEP-MSA (or left unstimulated). At day 4 of stimulation, live cells were isolated and used for co-culture with primary macrophages for 24 hrs. After co-culture period, macrophages were isolated, RNA was extracted and qPCR used for gene expression analysis. Each treatment is represented as relative expression (fold-expression over Macrophage only). IL-10 showed no CEP effect (data not shown). Data from at least 3 independent experiments were pooled for each analysis. Two-tailed Student's t test was used for statistical analysis (* denotes $p<0.05$). (B) Supernatants (secreted factors) from CEP-stimulated or unstimulated splenocytes were used for primary macrophage stimulation for 4 hrs. Purified IL-17A (1 ng/ml) and purified IFN-γ (1 ng/ml) were used for control stimulations. Each treatment is represented as relative expression (fold-expression over macrophages stimulated in Media only). Data from at least 3 independent experiments were pooled for each analysis. ANOVA was used for statistical analysis (* denotes $p<0.05$).

in vitro, in conjunction with the specific localization of CEP in the RPE of dry AMD eyes reported here, may explain the increased M1/M2 ratios observed in AMD patients [47]. Differences in drusen CEP patterns may also explain the focal nature of RPE lesions and geographic atrophy. Drusen with high CEP content could be hubs of inflammatory microenvironment. It was also interesting to find increased levels of CEP in cone photoreceptor (PR) cells of healthy donors, since the macula contains the highest concentration of cone cells in the eye. Is this a potential signal of propensity to develop AMD? The precursor for CEP, DHA, has been shown to be increased in cone versus rod PR cells in the gecko [48], but the specific content of CEP itself within PR subtypes of humans (and mice) requires further investigation. Unfortunately, we could not perform a similar CEP immunolabeling analysis in eyes from CEP-immunized and control mice due to high non-specific background using our mouse monoclonal antibody.

The first type of cells shown to directly respond to CEP were endothelial cells, which promote angiogenesis through TLR2 signaling [49]. Here, we show that two cell types relevant to dry AMD, macrophages and RPE cells, can directly respond to CEP. Doyle et al. [50] recently reported that macrophages could respond to CEP *in vitro*, priming the NLRP3 inflammasome through TLR2 ligation. While they report that NLRP3 is active in

CEP-MSA-immunized mice, its role in macrophage differentiation is not known. Here we clearly show that CEP activation leads to an (M1) inflammatory response associated with tissue damage, which correlates with our published *in vivo* findings [26]. Whether there is a connection between macrophage polarization and inflammasome priming/activation in the context of AMD remains to be determined. Further characterization of the CEP receptor-mediated signaling events and transcriptional regulation in macrophages and RPE cells is under current experimentation in our lab.

What about the role of the adaptive immune system in AMD? Most of the evidence for adaptive immunity in AMD comes from the presence of anti-retinal autoantibodies in AMD patients [51–53], which is recapitulated in our CEP mouse model [40]. However, it is not clear if these antibodies (in humans) have deleterious or protective effects, or if they arise as secondary events and have no direct role in disease pathogenesis or progression. We have addressed this major question in our model by immunizing mice deficient in mature B cells *(μMT/*mice), which resulted in strong retinal lesions, indicating that the CEP-induced pathology is independent of antibodies. Because RAG-deficient mice do not develop AMD-like lesions [40], this result indicates that T cells are the major players within the adaptive immune system associated with disease in our model. This result, however, does not eliminate

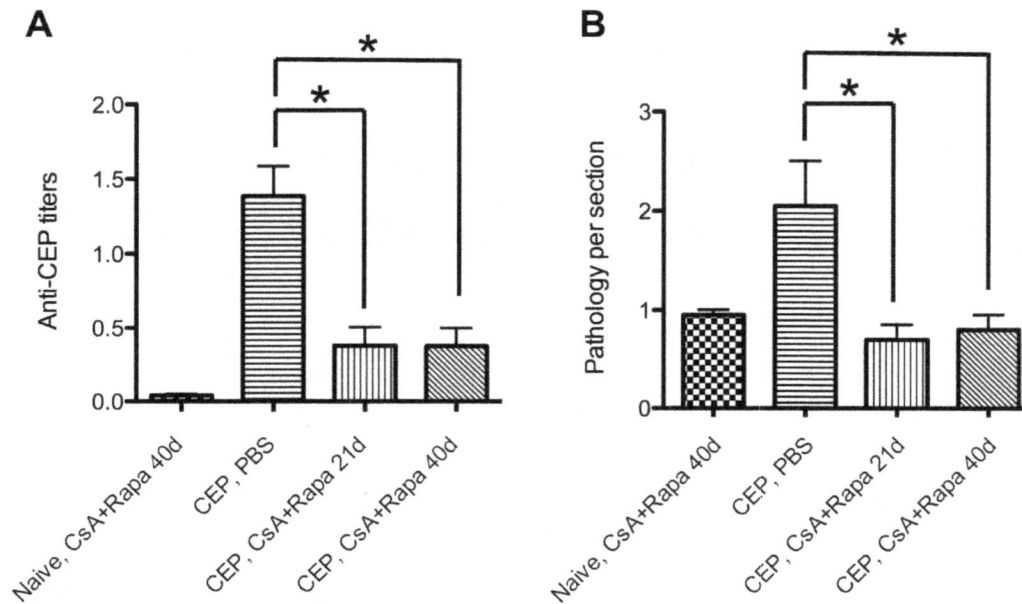

Figure 8. Proof of concept experiment showing that T cell inhibitory drugs Cyclosporin A and Rapamycin prevent CEP-induced retinal pathology. (A) WT BALB/c mice were immunized with CEP-MSA and treated every day (starting at day of immunization) with combined CsA+Rapa for either 21 or 40 days p.i. Control PBS injections were also performed. Serum was isolated at day 47 p.i. and anti-CEP titers were evaluated by ELISA. **(B)** Eyes were harvested at day 60 p.i. Retinal pathology scores for the indicated groups are shown (n = 3). ANOVA was used for statistical analysis (* denotes p<0.05). Results are representative of two independent experiments.

the possibility that antibodies may be involved in the AMD disease process. It may be possible for some anti-retinal antibodies to fix complement in the outer retina or to induce macrophages to damage the RPE. Conversely, some autoantibodies could actually serve a protective role. Regardless of their specific functions, autoantibodies represent useful targets for the development of AMD biomarkers. In this context, we suggest profiling autoantibody signatures, instead of single antibodies, to gain a better diagnostic and therapeutic picture.

To our knowledge, CEP-specific T cells are the second example of OSE-specific T cells in the literature. Malondialdehyde (MDA) is another lipid peroxidation product that serves as a marker of oxidative stress. MDA is formed upon peroxidation of polyunsaturated fatty acids present in phospholipids of low density lipoprotein (LDL), and has been associated with a number of oxidative stress-related diseases, such as atherosclerosis and AMD [29,54]. Binder et al. [54] showed that immunization of mice with MDA-modified LDL (MDA-LDL) leads to an adaptive T cell-dependent immune response, with expansion of antigen-specific Th2 cells that mainly secrete IL-5. Therefore, these lipid modifications of self-proteins function as haptens and can actually dictate the T cell differentiation pathways (cytokine production profiles) of the responding cells. Recognition of oxidation by-products by T cells is an emerging paradigm in disease development, as it has also been shown that immune responses against oxidized lipoprotein is associated with atherosclerosis [55]. In the case of AMD, pro-inflammatory cytokine production by CEP-specific T cells contributes to the polarization of macrophages toward the M1 phenotype, providing a functional link between adaptive and innate immunity in the onset of disease.

T cell-produced cytokines can also integrate the antibody production to complete the response against CEP, as we have detected specific class isotype switching to IgG1. This switch is usually associated with Th2 (IL-4-mediated) responses, but we

have not detected IL-4 production by CEP-specific T cells. In this regard, IFN-γ may not influence class switching but could certainly impact macrophage M1 polarization. This is supported by the lack of retinal macrophages in CEP-immunized T-bet ko mice. We attribute this result to the absence of Th1 cell differentiation and not to an intrinsic effect on T-bet ko macrophages, which have been reported to behave normally [56]. On the other hand, IL-17A may be more relevant to the antibody response, as there is some evidence that Th17 cells can promote IgG1 switching [57]. Even if IL-17A ko mice develop CEP-induced pathology, we do believe that IL-17 does play a significant role in AMD because IL-17 levels are elevated in AMD patients [34] and the *IL-17RC* promoter region is preferentially hypomethylated in AMD patients [58]. In fact, it has been shown in a retinal disease model that either Th1 or Th17 cells are capable of mediating disease [59]. Examining the role of IL-17-family cytokines (such as IL-17A and IL-17F) and their relationship with IFN-γ in AMD pathogenesis should clarify this issue in the future.

The use of pharmacological inhibition of T cell-mediated pathology in our model is a significant novel aspect of this work. We selected a strategy aimed at maximizing the possibility of T cell immunosuppression using both CsA and rapamycin. While we recognize that these two drugs may have other targets besides T cells, our interpretation of their effects in our model are based on complementary data, such as the results on B cell-deficient and T-bet ko mice. We have been careful in analyzing control mice and have seen no effect of this treatment on the retina. Specifically, control (CsA+rapa treated, without CEP immunization) mice remained healthy throughout the dosing period and their retinas looked normal. Similar results have been published in the context of the retina [60], at least in the case of i.p. rapamycin treatment (at higher doses of 3 mg/kg). To substantiate our approach, it is important to note that there are several ongoing clinical trials testing immunotherapy for AMD, including treatments that target

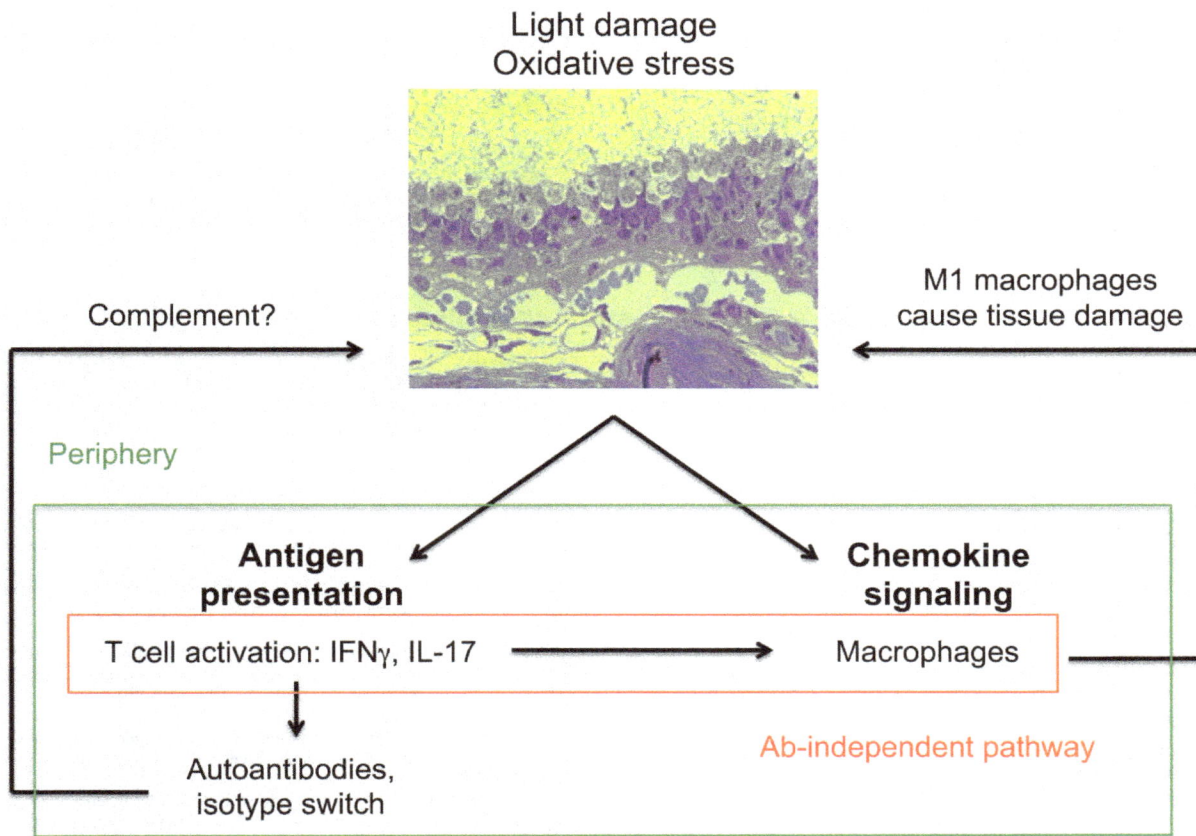

Figure 9. Working model for the cooperation of antigen-specific T cells and M1 macrophages in the development of AMD. Oxidative damage in the outer retina initiates a cascade of events that activate both innate and adaptive immune responses that ultimately lead to retinal damage.

TNF-α (one of the key effector molecules upregulated by CEP) and mTOR (the molecular target of rapamycin) [8]. Of course, there are important questions that need answers to complete our understanding of the macrophage and T cell pathways involved in the AMD disease process. What is the identity of the CEP receptor(s) in macrophages? Do macrophages reciprocally influence T cells? The precise mechanisms of antigen presentation of OSEs and TCR signaling dynamics are not known. Cloning OSE-specific TCR and generating transgenic mice (efforts currently underway in our lab) will certainly help address these issues. The subsequent analysis of such transgenic mice should provide valuable insight into the molecular mechanisms underlying initiation of immune-mediated AMD and could be used to test immunotherapies. Our proof-of-concept experiment with T cell suppression is a first step. Since we used a systemic, non-specific immunosuppressive approach, it would be interesting to develop antigen-specific therapies, such as depletion/suppression of CEP-specific T cells. Targeting the macrophage arm of the immune response could also have a beneficial outcome. For example, strategies that specifically prevent recruitment of blood-borne monocytes to the retina or that inhibit M1 polarization *in situ* may prove useful as AMD treatments. Our CEP model provides a great setting to test these and other protocols in future pre-clinical studies.

Supporting Information

Figure S1 CEP does not induce M2 or Mox gene expression in BALB/c macrophages *in vitro*. Bone marrow-derived macrophages from BALB/c mice were stimulated for 4 hrs with CEP-MSA (100 μg/ml), Sham-MSA (100 μg/ml) or left untreated. RNA was isolated and qPCR was used for gene expression analysis. Each treatment is represented as relative-expression (i.e., fold-expression over reference group), where the control (untreated) sample served as the reference with a set value of 1. CEP did not influence expression of M2-related genes (Arg-1 and IL-10) or Mox-related genes (HO-1 and SXRN-1).

Figure S2 CEP induces pro-inflammatory, but not angiogenic, gene expression in BALB/c macrophages *in vitro*. Bone marrow-derived macrophages from BALB/c mice were stimulated for 4 hrs with CEP-MSA (100 μg/ml), Sham-MSA (100 μg/ml) or left untreated. RNA was isolated and qPCR was used for gene expression analysis. Each treatment is represented as relative-expression (i.e., fold-expression over reference group), where the control (untreated) sample served as the reference with a set value of 1. CEP specifically induced the expression of inflammation genes (IL-6 and KC) but had no effect on angiogenesis-related genes (Vegf-A and Vegf-B). As opposed to RPE cells, CEP did not induce Ccl2 expression in BMDM *in vitro*. Two-tailed Student's t test was used for statistical analysis.

Figure S3 CEP induces selective pro-inflammatory gene expression in RPE cells *in vivo*. Intravitreal injections of CEP-MSA or Sham-MSA (2 μg total) were performed, RNA was isolated after 6 hrs from the RPE/choroid, followed by Taqman gene expression analysis (n = 5). While TNF-α expression was not upregulated upon CEP injections, KC levels were elevated in response to CEP. Mean values from one of two independent experiments are shown; error bars represent S.D. (*) denotes statistically significant differences (p<0.05) based on two-tailed Student's t tests.

Figure S4 Anti-CEP antibody production is maximized with CFA adjuvant. WT BALB/c mice were immunized with CEP-MSA in the presence of either complete Freund's adjuvant (CFA) or Alum. Anti-CEP titers were measured 40 days post-immunization (p.i.) (n = 5 per group). (*) denotes statistically

significant differences (p<0.05) based on two-tailed Student's t tests.

Acknowledgments

We thank B. Ksander, T. Malek, Z. Chen, C. Binder, R. Apte and members of the Perez Lab for valuable discussions, L. Buffa and M. Abdulreda for critical comments on the manuscript, E. Hernandez for expert animal care, G. Gaidosh for help with confocal microscopy, and D. Ivanov for reagents and technical help/discussions.

Author Contributions

Conceived and designed the experiments: FCG VLP. Performed the experiments: FCG AMS SD MC KBE AB YT JTH. Analyzed the data: FCG JTH VLP. Contributed reagents/materials/analysis tools: HW JML RGS. Wrote the paper: FCG VLP.

References

1. Bird AC (2010) Therapeutic targets in age-related macular disease. J Clin Invest 120: 3033–3041.
2. Coleman HR, Chan CC, Ferris FL 3rd, Chew EY (2008) Age-related macular degeneration. Lancet 372: 1835–1845.
3. Buschini E, Piras A, Nuzzi R, Vercelli A (2011) Age related macular degeneration and drusen: neuroinflammation in the retina. Prog Neurobiol 95: 14–25.
4. Bressler SB, Maguire MG, Bressler NM, Fine SL (1990) Relationship of drusen and abnormalities of the retinal pigment epithelium to the prognosis of neovascular macular degeneration. The Macular Photocoagulation Study Group. Arch Ophthalmol 108: 1442–1447.
5. Sarks SH, Van Driel D, Maxwell L, Killingsworth M (1980) Softening of drusen and subretinal neovascularization. Trans Ophthalmol Soc U K 100: 414–422.
6. Ambati J, Fowler BJ (2012) Mechanisms of age-related macular degeneration. Neuron 75: 26–39.
7. Ambati J, Atkinson JP, Gelfand BD (2013) Immunology of age-related macular degeneration. Nat Rev Immunol 13: 438–451.
8. Whitcup SM, Sodhi A, Atkinson JP, Holers VM, Sinha D, et al. (2013) The role of the immune response in age-related macular degeneration. Int J Inflam 2013: 348092.
9. Crabb JW, Miyagi M, Gu X, Shadrach K, West KA, et al. (2002) Drusen proteome analysis: an approach to the etiology of age-related macular degeneration. Proc Natl Acad Sci U S A 99: 14682–14687.
10. Edwards AO, Ritter R 3rd, Abel KJ, Manning A, Panhuysen C, et al. (2005) Complement factor H polymorphism and age-related macular degeneration. Science 308: 421–424.
11. Gold B, Merriam JE, Zernant J, Hancox LS, Taiber AJ, et al. (2006) Variation in factor B (BF) and complement component 2 (C2) genes is associated with age-related macular degeneration. Nat Genet 38: 458–462.
12. Hageman GS, Anderson DH, Johnson LV, Hancox LS, Taiber AJ, et al. (2005) A common haplotype in the complement regulatory gene factor H (HF1/CFH) predisposes individuals to age-related macular degeneration. Proc Natl Acad Sci U S A 102: 7227–7232.
13. Haines JL, Hauser MA, Schmidt S, Scott WK, Olson LM, et al. (2005) Complement factor H variant increases the risk of age-related macular degeneration. Science 308: 419–421.
14. Klein RJ, Zeiss C, Chew EY, Tsai JY, Sackler RS, et al. (2005) Complement factor H polymorphism in age-related macular degeneration. Science 308: 385–389.
15. Yates JR, Sepp T, Matharu BK, Khan JC, Thurlby DA, et al. (2007) Complement C3 variant and the risk of age-related macular degeneration. N Engl J Med 357: 553–561.
16. Nussenblatt RB, Ferris F 3rd (2007) Age-related macular degeneration and the immune response: implications for therapy. Am J Ophthalmol 144: 618–626.
17. Nussenblatt RB, Liu B, Li Z (2009) Age-related macular degeneration: an immunologically driven disease. Curr Opin Investig Drugs 10: 434–442.
18. Parmeggiani F, Romano MR, Costagliola C, Semeraro F, Incorvaia C, et al. (2012) Mechanism of inflammation in age-related macular degeneration. Mediators Inflamm 2012: 546786.
19. Tuo J, Grob S, Zhang K, Chan CC (2012) Genetics of immunological and inflammatory components in age-related macular degeneration. Ocul Immunol Inflamm 20: 27–36.
20. Iwasaki A, Medzhitov R (2010) Regulation of adaptive immunity by the innate immune system. Science 327: 291–295.
21. Palm NW, Medzhitov R (2009) Pattern recognition receptors and control of adaptive immunity. Immunol Rev 227: 221–233.
22. Lichtman AH, Binder CJ, Tsimikas S, Witztum JL (2013) Adaptive immunity in atherogenesis: new insights and therapeutic approaches. J Clin Invest 123: 27–36.
23. Ambati J, Anand A, Fernandez S, Sakurai E, Lynn BC, et al. (2003) An animal model of age-related macular degeneration in senescent Ccl-2- or Ccr-2-deficient mice. Nat Med 9: 1390–1397.
24. Apte RS, Richter J, Herndon J, Ferguson TA (2006) Macrophages inhibit neovascularization in a murine model of age-related macular degeneration. PLoS Med 3: e310.
25. Cousins SW, Espinosa-Heidmann DG, Csaky KG (2004) Monocyte activation in patients with age-related macular degeneration: a biomarker of risk for choroidal neovascularization? Arch Ophthalmol 122: 1013–1018.
26. Cruz-Guilloty F, Saeed AM, Echegaray JJ, Duffort S, Ballmick A, et al. (2013) Infiltration of proinflammatory m1 macrophages into the outer retina precedes damage in a mouse model of age-related macular degeneration. Int J Inflam 2013: 503725.
27. Kelly J, Ali Khan A, Yin J, Ferguson TA, Apte RS (2007) Senescence regulates macrophage activation and angiogenic fate at sites of tissue injury in mice. J Clin Invest 117: 3421–3426.
28. Sene A, Khan AA, Cox D, Nakamura RE, Santeford A, et al. (2013) Impaired cholesterol efflux in senescent macrophages promotes age-related macular degeneration. Cell Metab 17: 549–561.
29. Weismann D, Hartvigsen K, Lauer N, Bennett KL, Scholl HP, et al. (2011) Complement factor H binds malondialdehyde epitopes and protects from oxidative stress. Nature 478: 76–81.
30. Biswas SK, Mantovani A (2010) Macrophage plasticity and interaction with lymphocyte subsets: cancer as a paradigm. Nat Immunol 11: 889–896.
31. Sica A, Mantovani A (2012) Macrophage plasticity and polarization: in vivo veritas. J Clin Invest 122: 787–795.
32. Kaech SM, Cui W (2012) Transcriptional control of effector and memory CD8+ T cell differentiation. Nat Rev Immunol 12: 749–761.
33. Yamane H, Paul WE (2012) Cytokines of the gamma(c) family control CD4+ T cell differentiation and function. Nat Immunol 13: 1037–1044.
34. Liu B, Wei L, Meyerle C, Tuo J, Sen HN, et al. (2011) Complement component C5a promotes expression of IL-22 and IL-17 from human T cells and its implication in age-related macular degeneration. J Transl Med 9: 1–12.
35. Faber C, Singh A, Kruger Falk M, Juel HB, Sorensen TL, et al. (2013) Age-Related Macular Degeneration Is Associated with Increased Proportion of CD56 T Cells in Peripheral Blood. Ophthalmology.
36. Cruz-Guilloty F, Perez VL (2011) Molecular medicine: Defence against oxidative damage. Nature 478: 42–43.
37. Handa JT (2012) How does the macula protect itself from oxidative stress? Mol Aspects Med 33: 418–435.
38. Gu X, Meer SG, Miyagi M, Rayborn ME, Hollyfield JG, et al. (2003) Carboxyethylpyrrole protein adducts and autoantibodies, biomarkers for age-related macular degeneration. J Biol Chem 278: 42027–42035.
39. Gu J, Pauer GJ, Yue X, Narendra U, Sturgill GM, et al. (2010) Proteomic and Genomic Biomarkers for Age-Related Macular Degeneration. Adv Exp Med Biol 664: 411–417.
40. Hollyfield JG, Bonilha VL, Rayborn ME, Yang X, Shadrach KG, et al. (2008) Oxidative damage-induced inflammation initiates age-related macular degeneration. Nat Med 14: 194–198.
41. Hollyfield JG, Perez VL, Salomon RG (2010) A hapten generated from an oxidation fragment of docosahexaenoic acid is sufficient to initiate age-related macular degeneration. Mol Neurobiol 41: 290–298.
42. Lu L, Gu X, Hong L, Laird J, Jaffe K, et al. (2009) Synthesis and structural characterization of carboxyethylpyrrole-modified proteins: mediators of age-related macular degeneration. Bioorg Med Chem 17: 7548–7561.
43. Kadl A, Meher AK, Sharma PR, Lee MY, Doran AC, et al. (2010) Identification of a novel macrophage phenotype that develops in response to atherogenic phospholipids via Nrf2. Circ Res 107: 737–746.

44. Pipkin ME, Sacks JA, Cruz-Guilloty F, Lichtenheld MG, Bevan MJ, et al. (2010) Interleukin-2 and inflammation induce distinct transcriptional programs that promote the differentiation of effector cytolytic T cells. Immunity 32: 79–90.

45. Barshes NR, Goodpastor SE, Goss JA (2004) Pharmacologic immunosuppression. Front Biosci 9: 411–420.

46. Cherepanoff S, McMenamin P, Gillies MC, Kettle E, Sarks SH (2010) Bruch's membrane and choroidal macrophages in early and advanced age-related macular degeneration. Br J Ophthalmol 94: 918–925.

47. Cao X, Shen D, Patel MM, Tuo J, Johnson TM, et al. (2011) Macrophage polarization in the maculae of age-related macular degeneration: a pilot study. Pathol Int 61: 528–535.

48. Yuan C, Chen H, Anderson RE, Kuwata O, Ebrey TG (1998) The unique lipid composition of gecko (Gekko Gekko) photoreceptor outer segment membranes. Comp Biochem Physiol B Biochem Mol Biol 120: 785–789.

49. West XZ, Malinin NL, Merkulova AA, Tischenko M, Kerr BA, et al. (2010) Oxidative stress induces angiogenesis by activating TLR2 with novel endogenous ligands. Nature 467: 972–976.

50. Doyle SL, Campbell M, Ozaki E, Salomon RG, Mori A, et al. (2012) NLRP3 has a protective role in age-related macular degeneration through the induction of IL-18 by drusen components. Nat Med 18: 791–798.

51. Morohoshi K, Goodwin AM, Ohbayashi M, Ono SJ (2009) Autoimmunity in retinal degeneration: autoimmune retinopathy and age-related macular degeneration. J Autoimmun 33: 247–254.

52. Morohoshi K, Ohbayashi M, Patel N, Chong V, Bird AC, et al. (2012) Identification of anti-retinal antibodies in patients with age-related macular degeneration. Exp Mol Pathol 93: 193–199.

53. Morohoshi K, Patel N, Ohbayashi M, Chong V, Grossniklaus HE, et al. (2012) Serum autoantibody biomarkers for age-related macular degeneration and possible regulators of neovascularization. Exp Mol Pathol 92: 64–73.

54. Binder CJ, Hartvigsen K, Chang MK, Miller M, Broide D, et al. (2004) IL-5 links adaptive and natural immunity specific for epitopes of oxidized LDL and protects from atherosclerosis. J Clin Invest 114: 427–437.

55. Hermansson A, Ketelhuth DF, Strodthoff D, Wurm M, Hansson EM, et al. (2010) Inhibition of T cell response to native low-density lipoprotein reduces atherosclerosis. J Exp Med 207: 1081–1093.

56. Lugo-Villarino G, Maldonado-Lopez R, Possemato R, Penaranda C, Glimcher LH (2003) T-bet is required for optimal production of IFN-gamma and antigen-specific T cell activation by dendritic cells. Proc Natl Acad Sci U S A 100: 7749–7754.

57. Mitsdoerffer M, Lee Y, Jager A, Kim HJ, Korn T, et al. (2010) Proinflammatory T helper type 17 cells are effective B-cell helpers. Proc Natl Acad Sci U S A 107: 14292–14297.

58. Wei L, Liu B, Tuo J, Shen D, Chen P, et al. (2012) Hypomethylation of the IL17RC promoter associates with age-related macular degeneration. Cell Rep 2: 1151–1158.

59. Luger D, Silver PB, Tang J, Cua D, Chen Z, et al. (2008) Either a Th17 or a Th1 effector response can drive autoimmunity: conditions of disease induction affect dominant effector category. J Exp Med 205: 799–810.

60. Zhao C, Yasumura D, Li X, Matthes M, Lloyd M, et al. (2013) mTOR-mediated dedifferentiation of the retinal pigment epithelium initiates photoreceptor degeneration in mice. J Clin Invest 121(1): 369–383.

13

Biological Effects of Cigarette Smoke in Cultured Human Retinal Pigment Epithelial Cells

Alice L. Yu[1]*, Kerstin Birke[2], Johannes Burger[1], Ulrich Welge-Lussen[2]

1 Department of Ophthalmology, Ludwig-Maximilians-University, Muenchen, Germany, **2** Department of Ophthalmology, Friedrich-Alexander-University, Erlangen, Germany

Abstract

The goal of the present study was to determine whether treatment with cigarette smoke extract (CSE) induces cell loss, cellular senescence, and extracellular matrix (ECM) synthesis in primary human retinal pigment epithelial (RPE) cells. Primary cultured human RPE cells were exposed to 2, 4, 8, and 12% of CSE concentration for 24 hours. Cell loss was detected by cell viability assay. Lipid peroxidation was assessed by loss of *cis*-parinaric acid (PNA) fluorescence. Senescence-associated ß-galactosidase (SA-ß-Gal) activity was detected by histochemical staining. Expression of apolipoprotein J (Apo J), connective tissue growth factor (CTGF), fibronectin, and laminin were examined by real-time PCR, western blot, or ELISA experiments. The results showed that exposure of cells to 12% of CSE concentration induced cell death, while treatment of cells with 2, 4, and 8% CSE increased lipid peroxidation. Exposure to 8% of CSE markedly increased the number of SA-ß-Gal positive cells to up to 82%, and the mRNA expression of Apo J, CTGF, and fibronectin by approximately 3–4 fold. Treatment with 8% of CSE also increased the protein expression of Apo J and CTGF and the secretion of fibronectin and laminin. Thus, treatment with CSE can induce cell loss, senescent changes, and ECM synthesis in primary human RPE cells. It may be speculated that cigarette smoke could be involved in cellular events in RPE cells as seen in age-related macular degeneration.

Editor: Michael E. Boulton, University of Florida, United States of America

Funding: These authors have no support or funding to report.

Competing Interests: The authors have declared that no competing interests exist.

* E-mail: alice.yu@med.uni-muenchen.de

Introduction

Age-related macular degeneration (AMD) is the major cause of legal blindness in industrialized nations [1,2,3,4]. It is a multifactorial disease leading to the loss of central vision at the final stage. Both genetic and environmental factors may play a fundamental role in the disease development and progression [5,6]. Cigarette smoke is the single most important environmental risk factor for AMD [7,8,9]. Recent studies have detected a two- to threefold increased risk for AMD in smokers compared to non-smokers [8,10]. One reason for these adverse effects could be attributed to the various potent oxidants, which are contained in cigarette smoke [11,12]. Therefore, it is assumed that cigarette smoke mediates its toxic effects via increased production of reactive oxygen species (ROS) and thus oxidative stress [10].

Oxidative stress plays the key role in the process of ageing and age-related diseases. In age-related diseases, it induces a number of biological events such as cell death, advanced senescence, and extracellular matrix (ECM) production [13]. These characteristic findings can also be found in ocular age-related diseases such as AMD. In the setting of massive deposition of extracellular debris, the loss of retinal pigment epithelial (RPE) cells is the key event of the atrophic form of AMD leading to the loss of central vision [14]. In early AMD, advanced cellular senescence of the RPE may represent an initial step in the pathogenesis of AMD [15]. Cellular senescence can be identified by increased senescence-associated ß-galactosidase (SA-ß-Gal) activity and elevated expression of senescence-associated biomarkers such as apolipoprotein J (Apo

J), connective tissue growth factor (CTGF), and fibronectin [16,17,18]. ApoJ, also called clusterin, is abundant in drusen [19]. CTGF and fibronectin accumulate in the Bruch's membrane, in drusen and in basal linear deposits of AMD eyes [20,21,22]. Fibronectin and also the basement membrane component laminin have been shown to be secreted by senescent human RPE cells [23]. In AMD donor eyes, increased ECM accumulation can lead to a diffuse thickening of the Bruch's membrane beneath the RPE, and thus an impaired diffusion of oxygen towards the retina [23,24].

In this study, we hypothesized that cigarette smoke is responsible for these cellular changes in the RPE of AMD patients. In our experiments, we used cigarette smoke extract (CSE) as a well-established *in vitro* model of cigarette smoke exposure [25,26,27]. We first examined at which concentration CSE could induce cell death in primary cultured human RPE cells. Furthermore, we wanted to known whether or not CSE could increase lipid peroxidation in human RPE cells. In addition, we investigated the effects of CSE on senescence-associated changes and the synthesis of ECM components. These data should reveal further information about the potential role of cigarette smoke in cellular events of AMD.

Materials and Methods

Isolation of human RPE cells

For the total study, five human donor eyes were obtained from the eye bank of the Ludwig-Maximilians-University, Munich,

Germany, and were processed within 4 to 16 hours after death. The donors ranged in age between 30 and 43 years. None of the donors had a history of eye disease. Methods of securing human tissue were humane, included proper consent and approval, complied with the declaration of Helsinki, and was approved by the Department of Medicine of the Ludwig-Maximilians-University, Munich. The consent statement was written. Human retinal pigment epithelial (RPE) cells were harvested following the procedure as described previously [28,29,30]. In brief, whole eyes were thoroughly cleansed in 0.9% NaCl solution, immersed in 5% polyvinylpyrrolidone iodine (Jodobac; Bode-Chemie, Hamburg, Germany), and rinsed again in NaCl solution. The anterior segment from each donor eye was removed, and the posterior poles were examined with the aid of a binocular stereomicroscope to confirm the absence of gross retinal disease. Next, the neural retinas were carefully peeled away from the RPE-choroid-sclera using fine forceps. The eyecup was rinsed with Ca^{2+} and Mg^{2+} - free Hank's balanced salt solution, and treated with 0.25% trypsin (GIBCO, Karlsruhe, Germany) for 1 hour at 37°C. The trypsin was aspirated and replaced with Dulbecco's modified Eagles medium (DMEM, Biochrom, Berlin, Germany) supplemented with 20% fetal calf serum (FCS) (Biochrom). Using a pipette, the media was gently agitated, releasing the RPE into the media by avoiding damage to Bruch's membrane.

Human RPE cell culture

The human RPE cell suspension was added to a 50 ml flask (Falcon, Wiesbaden, Germany) containing 20 ml of DMEM supplemented with 20% FCS and maintained at 37°C and 5% CO_2. Epithelial origin was confirmed by immunohistochemical staining for cytokeratin using a pan-cytokeratin antibody (Sigma-Aldrich, Deisenhofen, Germany) [31]. RPE cells were characterized by positive immunostaining with RPE65-antibody, a RPE-specific marker (anti-RPE65, Abcam, Cambridge, UK), and quantified by flow cytometry showing that nearly 100% of cells were RPE65 positive in each cell culture. The cells were tested and found free of contaminating macrophages (anti-CD11, Sigma-Aldrich) and endothelial cells (anti-von Willbrand factor, Sigma-Aldrich). The expression of zonula occludens-1 (ZO-1; Molecular Probes, Darmstadt, Germany) was used as a marker of RPE tight junctions. After reaching confluence, primary RPE cells were subcultured and maintained in DMEM supplemented with 10% FCS at 37°C and in 5% CO_2. Confluent primary RPE cells of passage 3 to 5 were exposed to cigarette smoke extract (CSE) in a concentration from 2, 4, 8 and 12% for 24 hours.

To generate aqueous CSE, the smoke of commercially available filter cigarettes (Marlboro, Philip Morris GmbH, Berlin, Germany; nicotine: 0.8 mg; tar: 10 mg) was bubbled through 25 ml pre-warmed (37°C) serum-free DMEM as described in Bernhard et al. [26]. The cigarettes were syringe-smoked in a similar apparatus as described by Carp and Janoff [32] at a rate of 35 ml/2 sec followed by a pause of 28 sec. This rate of smoking should simulate the smoking habits of an average smoker [33]. The resulting suspension was adjusted to pH 7.4 with concentrated NaOH and then filtered through a 0.22-μM-pore filter (BD biosciences filter Heidelberg, Germany) to remove bacteria and large particles. This solution, considered to be 100% CSE, was applied to RPE cultures within 30 min of preparation. CSE concentrations in the current study ranged from 2 to 12%. CSE preparation was standardized by measuring the absorbance (OD, 0.86±0.05) at a wavelength of 320 nm. The pattern of absorbance (spectrogram) observed at λ_{320} showed insignificant variation between different preparations of CSE. The nicotine in the CSE was determined by high-performance liquid chromatography with

ultraviolet detection and resulted in 47.1 ng nicotine/ ml cigarette smoke on average. This concentration was similar to the plasma nicotine concentration of an average smoker [43.7 ng/ml+/−38] [34]. After exposure to CSE, cells were kept for 72 hours under serum free conditions. For control experiments, air was bubbled through the serum-free DMEM, pH was adjusted to 7.4, and sterile filtered as described earlier. The medium was changed at the same time points.

Cell viability assay

Cell viability was quantified based on a two-colour fluorescence assay, in which the nuclei of non-viable cells appear red because of staining by the membrane-impermeable dye propidium iodide (Sigma-Aldrich), whereas the nuclei of all cells were stained with the membrane-permeable dye Hoechst 33342 (Intergen, Purchase, NY). Confluent cultures of RPE cells growing on coverslips in four well tissue culture plates were either non-stressed or exposed to CSE. For evaluation of cell viability, cells were washed in PBS and incubated with 2.0 μg/ml propidium iodide and 1.0 μg/ml Hoechst 33342 for 20 minutes at 37°C. Subsequently, cells were analyzed with a fluorescence microscope (Leica DMR, Leica Microsystems, Wetzlar, Germany). Representative areas were documented with Leica IM 1000 software (Leica Microsystems, Heerbrugg, Switzerland), with three to five documented representative fields per well. The labelled nuclei were then counted in fluorescence photomicrographs, and dead cells were expressed as a percentage of total nuclei in the field. All experiments were run in triplicate in RPE cultures from three donors and repeated three times.

Assessment of lipid peroxidation

Oxidative stress can be assessed by markers of lipid peroxidation. A sensitive and specific assay for lipid peroxidation is based on metabolic incorporation of the fluorescent oxidation-sensitive fatty acid, cis-parinaric acid (PNA), a natural 18-carbon fatty acid with four conjugated double bonds, into membrane phospholipids of cells [35,36]. Oxidation of PNA results in disruption of the conjugated double bond system that cannot be re-synthesized in mammalian cells. Therefore, lipid peroxidation was estimated by measuring loss of PNA fluorescence. Briefly, treated cells were incubated with 10 μM PNA (Molecular Probes, Invitrogen, UK) at 37°C for 30 minutes in the dark. The media was then removed and cells washed three times with phosphate-buffered saline (PBS). Afterwards, cells were scraped into 2 ml PBS using a rubber policeman. The suspension was then added to a fluorescence cuvette and measured at 312-nm excitation and 455-nm emission. A blank (unlabelled cells) was measured and subtracted from all readings. This method has been validated by treating the RPE cultures with different concentrations of hydrogen peroxide. A dose-dependent loss of fluorescence could be observed (data not shown). All experiments were run in triplicate in RPE cultures from three donors and repeated three times.

Senescence-associated ß-galactosidase activity

The proportion of RPE cells positive for the senescence-associated ß-galactosidase (SA-ß-Gal) activity was determined as described by Dimri et al. [37]. Briefly, treated RPE cells were washed twice with PBS and fixed with 2% formaldehyde and 0.2% glutaraldehyde in PBS at pH 6.0 at room temperature (RT) for 4 minutes. Cells were then washed twice with PBS and incubated under light protection for 8 hours at 37°C with fresh SA-ß-Gal staining solution (1 mg/ml 5-bromo-4-chloro-3-indoyl-ß-D-galactopyranoside (X-gal), 40 mM citric acid/sodium phosphate, pH 6.0, 5 mM potassium ferrocyanide, 5 mM potassium ferricyanide, 150 mM NaCl, 2 mM MgCl$_2$ diluted in PBS). Cells were then examined for the development of blue color and photographed at low magnification (200×) using a light microscope. All experiments were run in triplicate in RPE cultures from three donors and repeated three times.

RNA isolation and real-time PCR

Total RNA was isolated from 10 mm petri dishes by the guanidium thiocyanate-phenol-chloroform extraction method (Stratagene, Heidelberg, Germany). Structural integrity of the RNA samples was confirmed by electrophoresis in 1% Tris-acetate-EDTA (TAE)-agarose gels. Yield and purity were determined photometrically. After RNA isolation, mRNA was transcribed to cDNA via reverse transcriptase. This cDNA was then used for specific real-time PCR. Quantification of human mRNA was performed with specific primers during 40 cycles with a LightCycler Instrument (LightCycler System, Roche Diagnostics, Mannheim, Germany). The primers selected were apolipoprotein J (Apo J) forward primer 5'- ggacatccacttccacagc -3' and reverse primer 5'- ggtcatcgtcgccttctc -3'; connective tissue growth factor (CTGF) forward primer 5'- ctgcaggctagagaagcagag -3' and reverse primer 5'- gatgcacttttttgcccttct -3'; fibronectin forward primer 5'-ctggccgaaaatacattgtaaa-3' and reverse primer 5'-ccacagtcgggtcaggag-3'; and GAPDH forward primer 5'-agccacatcgctcagacac-3' and reverse primer 5'-gcccaatacgaccaaatcc-3'. Primers and probes were found with the programme ProbeFinder Version: 2.04. The standard curve was obtained from probes of three different untreated human RPE cell cultures. To normalize differences of the amount of total RNA added to each reaction, GAPDH was simultaneously processed in the same sample as an internal control. The level of Apo J, CTGF and fibronectin mRNA was determined as the relative ratio (RR), which was calculated by dividing the level of Apo J, CTGF and fibronectin mRNA by the level of the GAPDH housekeeping gene in the same samples. All experiments were run in triplicate in RPE cultures from three donors and repeated three times.

Protein extraction and western blot analysis

For nuclear extracts, cells were washed twice with ice-cold PBS, collected, and lysed in three times packed cell volumes of low-salt hypotonic cell lysis buffer [20 mM HEPES pH 7.5, 10 mM KCl, 5 mM MgCl2, 0.5 mM EDTA, 0.1% TritonX-100, 10% glycerol, protease inhibitor cocktail (Roche)] for 10 min on ice. After centrifugation (19,000 g for 30 minutes at 4°C) in a microfuge, the supernatants were transferred to fresh tubes and stored at −70°C for future use. The protein content was measured by the bicinchoninic acid (BCA) protein assay (Pierce, Rockford, IL). Denatured proteins (2 μg) were separated under reducing conditions by electrophoresis using 10% SDS-polyacrylamide gels. Thereafter, the proteins were transferred with tank blotting onto a nitrocellulose membrane (Protran Ba-183; Whatman, Dassel, Germany) and probed with a mouse monoclonal anti-human ApoJ antibody (Abcam) and rabbit polyclonal anti-human CTGF antibody (Abcam) as described previously [38]. These antibodies were used at a dilution of 1:1000, respectively. Secondary alkaline phosphatase (AP)-conjugated goat anti-mouse IgG (Sigma-Aldrich) or AP-conjugated goat anti-rabbit IgG antibodies (Sigma-Aldrich) were incubated for 30 minutes at a dilution of 1:2500 at room temperature. After substrate incubation (CDP-star; Roche) the signals were visualized by exposure to light sensitive films (Hyperfilm ECL; GE Healthcare, Munich, Germany), which were digitized and densitometrically quantified with the Multi Gauge V3.1 software (Fujifilm, Duesseldorf, Germany). All experiments

were run in triplicate with three different RPE cultures from three donors.

Analysis of fibronectin and laminin secretion into culture media

Release of fibronectin and laminin into culture media of RPE cells was measured using corresponding QuantiMatrixTM Human Fibronektin ELISA kits (Millipore, Billerica, MA, USA) and QuantiMatrixTM Human Laminin ELISA kits (Millipore) according to the manufacturer's instructions. All experiments were run in triplicate with three different RPE cultures from three donors.

Statistical analysis

Results for the analyses of RPE cell death, lipid peroxidation, SA-ß-Gal activity, real-time PCR, western blot and ELISA experiments are expressed as the mean ± s.d. For comparison of means between two groups, an unpaired t-test was employed. Statistical significance was defined as $P < 0.05$.

Results

ZO-1 expression in cultured human RPE cells

The expression and localization of ZO-1 was used to define the tight junction structure of the cultured human RPE cells. Each RPE cell was outlined by the expression of ZO-1 (Figure 1).

Cigarette smoke extract induced cell death

To determine the cytotoxic effects of cigarette smoke extract (CSE), primary cultured human retinal pigment epithelial (RPE) cells were treated with 2, 4, 8 and 12% of CSE (Fig. 2). In this cell viability assay, untreated control cells demonstrated almost no dead cells staining red by propidium iodide (Fig. 2B). Incubation of cultured human RPE cells with 2, 4, and 8% of CSE led to elevated proportions of non-viable cells with 5.1+/−2.4%, 12.0+/−1.7%, and 14.0+/−2.4% of total cells (Fig. 2E). The most pronounced effect was seen after treatment with 12% of CSE, which significantly increased the proportion of non-viable RPE cells to 86.2+/−11.4% of total cells (Figs. 2D, 2E). Based on these results, only concentrations of 2, 4, and 8% of CSE were used in the subsequent experiments.

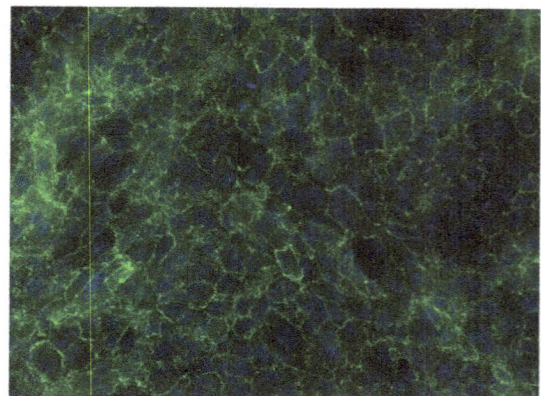

Figure 1. ZO-1 immunofluorescence staining in primary human RPE cultures. DAPI nuclear counterstaining.

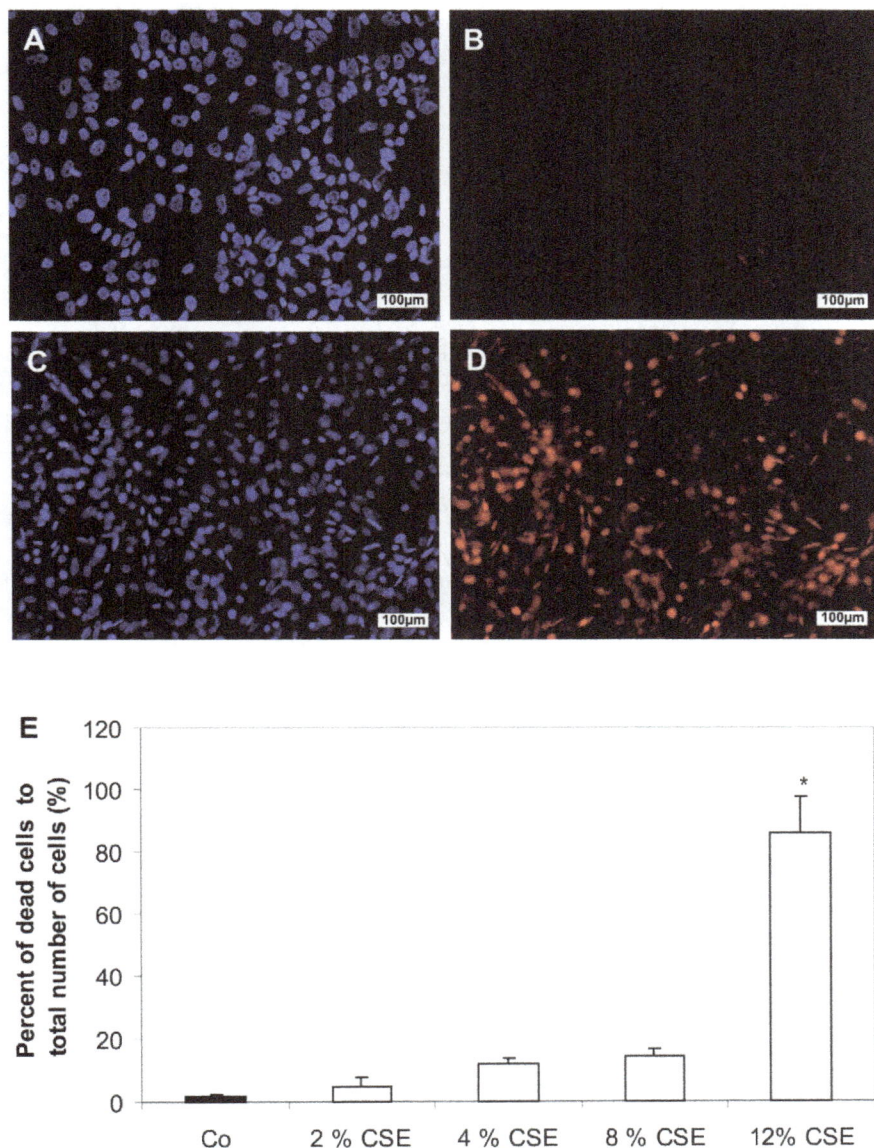

Figure 2. CSE induced cell death detected by live dead assay. Representative fluorescence photomicrographs of Hoechst 33342-stained RPE cells in (**A**) untreated controls or (**C**) cells treated with 12% of CSE for 24 hours. Scale bar: 100 μm. (**B, D**) Non-viable cells in the corresponding field. Scale bar: 100 μm. (**E**) Quantification of the number of non-viable cells. The percentage of dead cells was scored by counting at least 700 cells in fluorescence photomicrographs of representative fields. Data presented as a mean ± s.d. of nine experiments with three different cell cultures from different donors (*P<0.05). Co, control.

Cigarette smoke extract increased lipid peroxidation

Lipid peroxidation of the cytoplasm membrane of primary cultured human RPE cells was assessed by increased loss of *cis*-parinaric acid (PNA) fluorescence (Fig. 3). The PNA fluorescence of untreated cells was set to 100%. We could observe a decrease of PNA fluorescence after treatment of RPE cells with 2 and 4% concentration of CSE for 24 hours to 91.3+/−4.7% and 84.7+/−5.3% as compared to untreated control cells. The most significant decrease of PNA fluorescence to 81.7+/−7.3% was observed after exposure of RPE cells to 8% of CSE (Fig. 3).

Cigarette smoke extract induced SA-ß-Gal activity

Human RPE cells were treated for 2, 4, and 8% concentration of CSE for 24 hours (Fig. 4). Untreated control cells showed 3.5+/

−0.6% of senescence-associated ß-Galactosidase (SA-ß-Gal) positive RPE cells (Figs. 4A, 4C). Exposure to 2% and 4% of CSE increased the number of SA-ß-Gal positive RPE cells to 12.0+/−1.4% and 16.0+/−1.7% of all treated cells (Fig. 4C). The most pronounced effect was observed after exposure of cells to 8% of CSE with a proportion of 82.0+/−12.0% SA-ß-Gal positive cells (Figs. 4B, 4C). We have not observed any differences in SA-ß-Gal staining in RPE cell cultures from different donors (data not shown).

Cigarette smoke extract induced mRNA expression of Apo J, CTGF, and fibronectin

The mRNA expressions of apolipoprotein J (Apo J), connective tissue growth factor (CTGF), and fibronectin were detected by

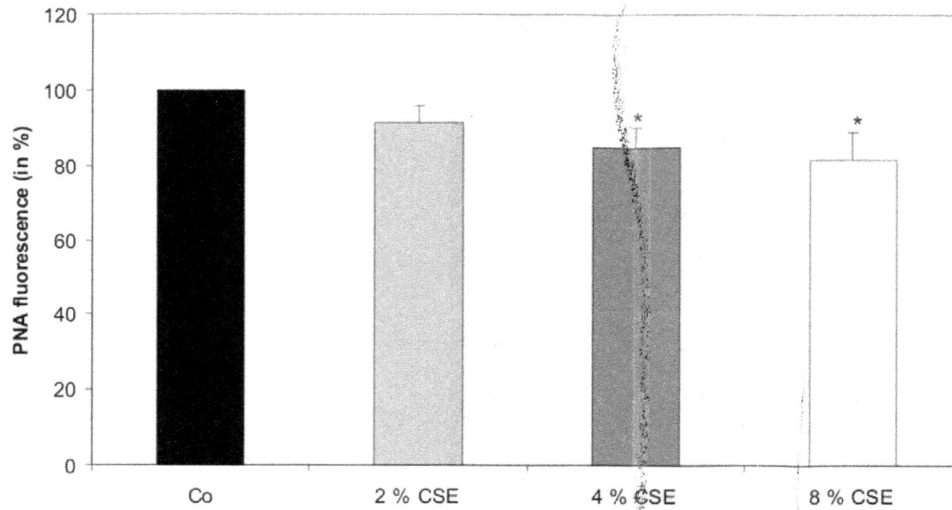

Figure 3. CSE increased lipid peroxidation. *cis*-parinaric acid (PNA) fluorescence was analysed after 2, 4, and 8% concentration of CSE for 24 hours. Data are expressed as the percentage of PNA fluorescence of untreated control cells kept for 24 hours and represent the mean $\pm$ s.d of results of nine experiments with three different cell cultures from different donors (*$P<0.05$). Co, control.

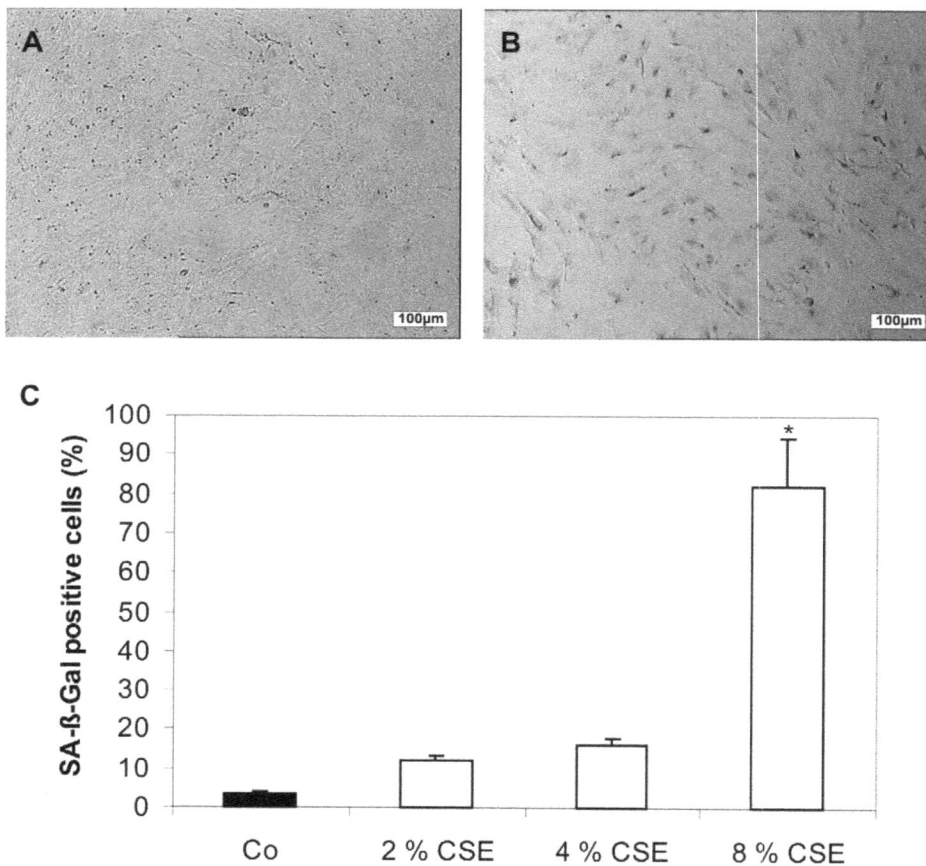

Figure 4. CSE induced SA-ß-Gal activity in cultured human RPE cells. (**A**) Morphology and SA-ß-Gal activity of untreated human RPE cells. Only single cells were stained blue indicating SA-ß-Gal activity. Scale bar: 100 µm. (**B**) In contrast, RPE cells of the same passage exposed to 8% of CSE showed a marked increase of SA-ß-Gal activity. Scale bar: 100 µm. (**C**) Quantification of the number of SA-ß-Gal positive cells. The percentage of SA-ß-Gal activity was analyzed after exposure to 2, 4, and 8% of CSE and scored by counting at least 300 cells in phase contrast photomicrographs of representative fields. Data (mean $\pm$ s.d.) are based on the sampling of 6 to 10 photomicrographs per condition from nine experiments with three different cell cultures from different donors (*$P<0.05$). Co, control.

real-time PCR analysis. The signals generated in untreated control cells were set to 100% (Figs. 5A, 5B, 5C). Expressions of Apo J (Fig. 5A), CTGF (Fig. 5B), and fibronectin (Fig. 5C) were measured after treatment with 2, 4, and 8% of CSE. Exposure to 2% and 4% of CSE increased the expression of Apo J to 1.2+/−0.2 fold and 1.9+/−0.3 fold, the expression of CTGF to 2.8+/−0.4 fold and 3.3+/−0.4 fold, and the expression of fibronectin to 1.5+/−0.2 fold and 3.0+/−0.4 fold, as compared to untreated control cells. The most significant effects were seen after exposure to 8% of CSE. In these cells, the Apo J mRNA expression increased by 2.9+/−0.3 fold (Fig. 5A), the CTGF expression by 4.8+/−0.6 fold (Fig. 5B), and the fibronectin expression by 3.5+/−0.6 fold (Fig. 5C), as compared to untreated control cells.

Cigarette smoke extract induced protein expression of Apo J and CTGF

The protein expression of Apo J and CTGF was analysed by western blot analysis. Data are expressed as x-fold changes compared to the signals of untreated control cells (Figure 6). Protein expressions of Apo J and CTGF were measured after treatment with 2, 4, and 8% of CSE. There was a marked increase of Apo J protein expression after treatment of cultured human RPE cells with 4 and 8% of CSE as compared to untreated control cells (2% CSE: 1.0 ± 0.1 fold; 4% CSE: 1.8 ± 0.1 fold; 8% CSE: 2.2 ± 0.8 fold) (Figure 6A). Similarly, CTGF protein expression was significantly elevated after exposure to 4 and 8% of CSE compared to untreated control cells (2% CSE: 1.1 ± 0.5 fold; 4% CSE: 1.6 ± 0.3 fold; 8% CSE: 2.0 ± 0.6 fold) (Figure 6B).

Cigarette smoke extract induced fibronectin and laminin secretion

To determine the fibronectin and laminin secretion of cultured human RPE cells by CSE exposure, we have used commercially available ELISA assays. Data are expressed as x-fold changes compared to the basal secretion levels of untreated control cells (Figure 7). Treatment of human RPE cells with 2, 4 and 8% of CSE increased the fibronectin secretion by 1.1 ± 0.1 fold, 1.1 ± 0.1 fold and 1.6 ± 0.2 fold, as compared to untreated control cells. Furthermore, exposure of RPE cells to 2, 4 and 8% of CSE also led to increased levels of laminin secretion by 1.4 ± 0.3 fold, 1.6 ± 0.4 fold and 1.6 ± 0.2 fold, compared to untreated control cells (Figure 7).

Discussion

Previous epidemiological studies have demonstrated that cigarette smoking significantly increases the risk of age-related macular degeneration (AMD) [7,8,9]. However, the impact of cigarette smoke on pathogenic processes of AMD is still unknown. One reason for the harmful effects of cigarette smoke on human cells is the generation of reactive oxygen species (ROS) and therefore oxidative stress [10]. Oxidative stress is also an important risk factor for ocular age-related diseases such as AMD. The loss of retinal pigment epithelial (RPE) cells is the major characteristic event of the atrophic form of AMD [39]. Previous *in vitro* studies have already demonstrated cytotoxic effects of cigarette smoke [40,41]. Cigarette smoke is known to contain an abundant number of toxic compounds. In ARPE-19 cells, specific toxic elements of cigarette smoke such as acrolein and benzopyrene may lead to reduced cell viability [40,41]. Cadmium, which is found in higher amounts in retinal tissues of AMD eyes, is also released from cigarette smoke and can induce RPE cell death [42]. In our experiments, treatment of primary human RPE cells with 2, 4, and 8% of cigarette smoke extract (CSE) had no significant effects on

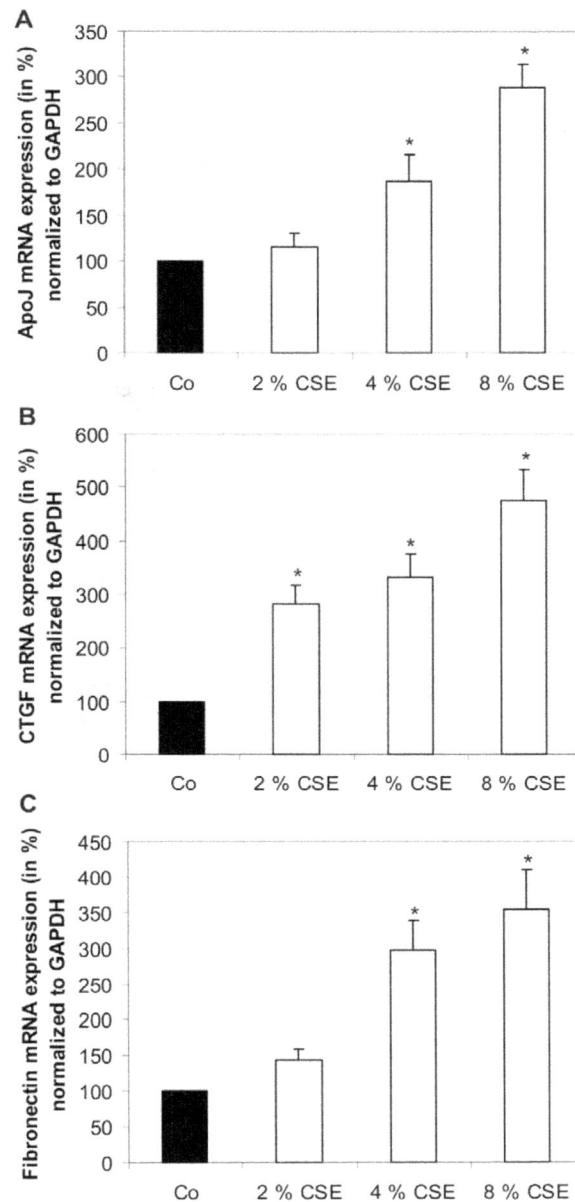

Figure 5. CSE increased Apo J, CTGF, fibronectin mRNA expression. mRNA expression of (**A**) Apo J, (**B**) CTGF, (**C**) fibronectin. Real-time PCR analysis was conducted after treatment with 2, 4, and 8% of CSE. Results were normalized to GAPDH as reference. The steady-state mRNA levels of these senescence-associated genes in untreated control cells were set to 100%. Results are given as mean ± s.d. of nine experiments with three different cell cultures from different donors (*P<0.05). Co, control.

RPE cell loss. However, exposure of cells to 12% of CSE markedly induced RPE cell death. At the first glance, these results are in contrast to previous investigations with ARPE-19 cells, which showed a decreased viability after 0.5% of CSE [43]. However, it must be taken into account that in Bertram et al. [43], CSE was generated by the smoke of research-grade cigarettes (Kentucky Tobacco Research Council, Lexington, KY, U.S.A.), which contain a much higher nicotine concentration than commercially available filter cigarettes. Therefore, CSE may be toxic for RPE

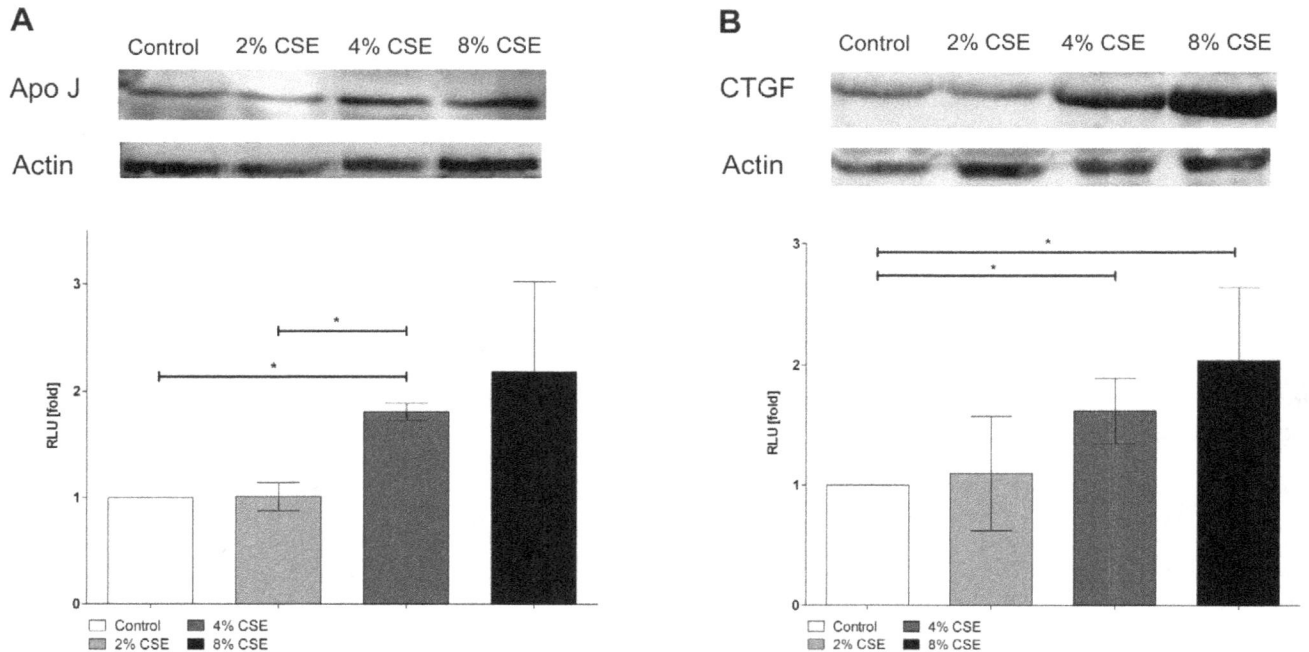

Figure 6. CSE increased Apo J, CTGF protein expression. Protein expression of (**A**) Apo J, (**B**) CTGF. Data are expressed as x-fold changes compared to the signals of untreated control cells and represent the mean ± s.d. of results of three experiments with three different cell cultures from different donors (*P<0.05).

cells at higher concentrations. Interestingly, Patil et al. [44] did not find decreased cell viability of human ARPE-19 cells after treatment with nicotine itself. This observation may be explained by the fact that not only nicotine itself but also other toxic elements of cigarette smoke influence the RPE viability. Furthermore, in our subsequent experiments, treatment of primary human RPE cells with 2, 4, and 8% of CSE increased lipid peroxidation

estimated by the loss of *cis*-parinaric acid (PNA) fluorescence. These results suggest that lower concentrations of CSE can induce the release of ROS and thus cause oxidative stress in primary human RPE cells.

At the cellular level, oxidative stress can trigger the so-called 'stress-induced premature senescence' (SIPS) [15,45]. There is a growing body of evidence suggesting that RPE cells also undergo

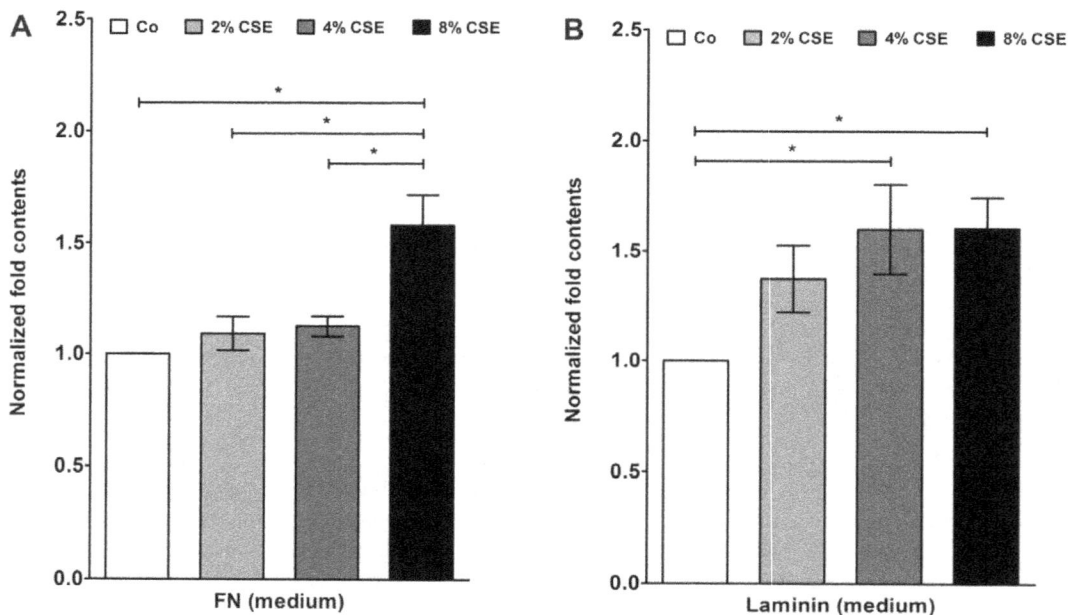

Figure 7. CSE increased fibronectin, laminin protein secretion. Protein secretion of (**A**) fibronectin (FN) and (**B**) laminin into culture media. Error bars: ± s.d. of results from three experiments with three different cell cultures (*P<0.05). Co, control.

an accelerated ageing process in AMD [24,46,47,48]. We have previously shown that sublethal concentrations of hydrogen peroxide induced senescence-associated ß-Galactosidase (SA-ß-Gal) activity in primary cultured RPE cells [29]. In the experiments of the current study, treatment of primary human RPE cultures with CSE could significantly increase the proportion of SA-ß-Gal positive cells. Positive staining of SA-ß-Gal has also been detected *in vitro* in late passage RPE cultures [49,50] and *in vivo* in the RPE cells of old primate eyes [51]. In human RPE cells, an increased expression of SA-ß-Gal staining could be triggered by mild hyperoxia-mediated ROS release [52]. Furthermore, cellular senescence can also be identified by increased expression of senescence-associated biomarkers such as Apo J, CTGF, and fibronectin. All three biomarkers are inducible by oxidative stress [16,18]. In our experiments, exposure of primary human RPE cells to CSE could lead to a significant elevation of Apo J, CTGF, and fibronectin expression. The cellular chaperone Apo J has been previously detected in the RPE of AMD donor eyes, although its role and function in the RPE is still unclear [19,53]. In contrast, CTGF and fibronectin have been found in the Bruch's membrane, in drusen and in basal linear deposits of AMD eyes [20,21,22]. Furthermore, we could show that treatment of human RPE cells with CSE also increased the secretion of fibronectin and laminin into the culture media. Laminin is a basement membrane protein, which is involved in the formation of basal laminar deposits of the ageing macula [24]. Both laminin and fibronectin have been shown to be secreted by senescent human RPE cells [23]. In the pathogenesis of AMD, it is assumed that cellular senescence and dysfunction of the RPE lead to an increased aggregation of ECM [15,54]. Therefore, CSE-induced levels of CTGF and fibronectin

represent senescence-associated changes and demonstrate increased ECM synthesis in cultured human RPE cells. A similar effect could also be observed after treatment of RPE cells with hypoxia/reoxygenation [55]. Furthermore, exposure to cigarette smoke could increase the formation of sub-RPE ECM deposits in an experimental mouse model [56,57]. An induction of CTGF levels was previously observed during cutaneous wound healing in smoke-exposed mice [58]. Whether or not CSE is responsible for the ECM accumulation in the RPE of AMD patients awaits further investigations.

Based on these results, we conclude that cigarette smoke may be responsible for the cell loss, senescent changes, and synthesis of ECM components in primary cultured human RPE cells. Therefore, cigarette smoke may induce cellular events, which may resemble pathogenic changes in AMD. Hence, these results may provide one explanation for the adverse effects of cigarette smoke on the pathogenesis and progression of AMD.

Acknowledgments

The authors thank Katja Obholzer and Jerome Moriniere for excellent technical assistance.

Author Contributions

Conceived and designed the experiments: ALY KB JB UWL. Performed the experiments: ALY KB JB UWL. Analyzed the data: ALY KB UWL. Contributed reagents/materials/analysis tools: ALY UWL. Wrote the paper: ALY UWL. Obtained permission for the use of cell line: ALY UWL.

References

1. Congdon N, O'Colmain B, Klaver CC, Klein R, Muñoz B, et al. (2004) Causes and prevalence of visual impairment among adults in the United States. Arch Ophthalmol 122: 477–485.

2. Ferris FL 3rd (1983) Senile macular degeneration: review of epidemiologic features. Am J Epidemiol 118: 132–151.

3. Klein R, Wang Q, Klein BE, Moss SE, Meuer SM (1995) The relationship of age-related maculopathy, cataract, and glaucoma to visual acuity. Invest Ophthalmol Vis Sci 36: 182–191.

4. Leibowitz HM, Krueger DE, Maunder LR, Milton RC, Kini MM, et al. (1980) The Framingham Eye Study monograph: An ophthalmological and epidemiological study of cataract, glaucoma, diabetic retinopathy, macular degeneration, and visual acuity in a general population of 2631 adults, 1973–1975. Surv Ophthalmol 24: 335–610.

5. Chen Y, Bedall M, Zhang K (2010) Age-related macular degeneration: genetic and environmental factors of disease. Mol Interv 10: 271–281.

6. Francis PJ, Klein ML (2011) Update on the role of genetics in the onset of age-related macular degeneration. Clin Ophthalmol 5: 1127–1133.

7. Chakravarthy U, Wong TY, Fletcher A, Piault E, Evans C, et al. (2010) Clinical risk factors for age-related macular degeneration: a systemic review and meta-analysis. BMC Ophthalmol 10: 31.

8. Khan JC, Thurlby DA, Shahid H, Clayton DG, Yates JR, et al. (2006) Smoking and age related macular degeneration: the number of pack years of cigarette smoking is a major determinant of risk for both geographic atrophy and choroidal neovascularisation. Br J Ophthalmol 90: 75–80.

9. Klein R, Knudtson MD, Cruickshanks KJ, Klein BE (2008) Further observations on the association between smoking and the long-term incidence and progression of age-related macular degeneration: the Beaver Dam Eye Study. Arch Ophthalmol 126: 115–121.

10. Thornton J, Edwards R, Mitchell P, Harrison RA, Buchan I, et al. (2005) Smoking and age-related macular degeneration: a review of association. Eye 19: 935–944.

11. Smith CJ, Hansch C (2000) The relative toxicity of compounds in mainstream cigarette smoke condensate. Food Chem Toxicol 38: 637–646.

12. Solberg Y, Rosner M, Belkin M (1998) The association between cigarette smoking and ocular diseases. Surv Ophthalmol 42: 535–547.

13. Terman A (2001) Garbage catastrophe theory of aging: imperfect removal of oxidative damage? Redox Rep 6: 15–26.

14. Sarks JP, Sarks SH, Killingsworth MC (1988) Evolution of geographic atrophy of the retinal pigment epithelium. Eye 2: 552–577.

15. Roth F, Bindewald A, Holz FG (2004) Keypathophysiologic pathways in age-related macular disease. Graefes Arch Clin Exp Ophthalmol 242: 710–716.

16. Dumont P, Burton M, Chen QM, Gonos ES, Frippiat C, et al. (2000) Induction of replicative senescence biomarkers by sublethal oxidative stresses in normal human fibroblast. Free Radic Biol Med 28: 361–373.

17. Kim KH, Park GT, Lim YB, Rue SW, Jung JC, et al. (2004) Expression of connective tissue growth factor, a biomarker in senescence of human diploid fibroblasts, is up-regulated by a transforming growth factor-beta-mediated signaling pathway. Biochem Biophys Res Commun 318: 819–825.

18. Toussaint O, Medrano EE, von Zglinicki T (2000) Cellular and molecular mechanisms of stress-induced premature senescence (SIPS) of human diploid fibroblasts and melanocytes. Exp Gerontol 35: 927–945.

19. Wang L, Clark ME, Crossman DK, Kojima K, Messinger JD, et al. (2010) Abundant lipid and protein components of drusen. PLoS One 5: e10329.

20. Löffler KU, Lee WR (1986) Basal linear deposit in the human macula. Graefes Arch Clin Exp Ophthalmol 224: 493–501.

21. Nagai N, Klimava A, Lee WH, Izumi-Nagai K, Handa JT (2009) CTGF is increased in basal deposits and regulates matrix production through the ERK (p42/p44mapk) MAPK and the p38 MAPK signaling pathways. Invest Ophthalmol Vis Sci 50: 1903–1910.

22. Newsome DA, Hewitt AT, Huh W, Robey PG, Hassell JR (1987) Detection of specific extracellular matrix molecules in drusen, Bruch's membrane, and ciliary body. Am J Ophthalmol 104: 373–381.

23. An E, Lu X, Flippin J, Devaney JM, Halligan B, et al. (2006) Secreted Proteome Profiling in human RPE cell cultures derived from donors with age related macular degeneration and age matched healthy donors. J Proteome Res 5: 2599–2610.

24. van der Schaft TL, Mooy CM, de Bruijn WC, Bosman FT, de Jong PT (1994) Immunohistochemical light and electron microscopy of basal laminar deposit. Graefe's Arch Clin Exp Ophthalmol 232: 40–46.

25. Baglole CJ, Sime PJ, Phipps RP (2008) Cigarette smoke-induced expression of heme oxygenase-1 in human lung fibroblasts is regulated by intracellular glutathione. Am J Physiol Lung Cell Mol Physiol 295: L624–L636.

26. Bernhard D, Pfister G, Huck CW, Kind M, Salvenmoser W, et al. (2003) Disruption of vascular endothelial homeostasis by tobacco smoke: impact on atherosclerosis. FASEB J 17: 2302–2304.

27. Shapiro SD (2004) Smoke gets in your cells. Am J Respir Cell Mol Biol 31: 481–482.

28. Campochiaro PA, Jerdon JA, Glaser BM (1986) The extracellular matrix of human retinal pigment epithelial cells in vivo and its synthesis in vitro. Invest Ophthalmol Vis Sci 27: 1615–1621.

29. Yu AL, Fuchshofer R, Kook D, Kampik A, Bloemendal H, et al. (2009) Subtoxic oxidative stress induces senescence in retinal pigment epithelial cells via TGF-beta release. Invest Ophthalmol Vis Sci 50: 926–935.

30. Yu AL, Lorenz RL, Haritoglou C, Kampik A, Welge-Lussen U (2009) Biological effects of native and oxidized low-density lipoproteins in cultured human retinal pigment epithelial cells. Exp Eye Res 88: 495–503.

31. Leschey KH, Hackett SF, Singer JH, Campochiaro PA (1990) Growth factor responsiveness of human retinal pigment epithelial cells. Invest Ophthalmol Vis Sci 31: 839–846.

32. Carp H, Janoff A (1978) Possible mechanisms of emphysema in smokers. In vitro suppression of serum elastase-inhibitory capacity by fresh cigarette smoke and its prevention by antioxidants. Am Rev Respir Dis 118: 617–621.

33. Djordjevic M, Fan J, Ferguson S, Hoffmann D (1995) Self-regulation of smoking intensity. Smoke yields of the low-nicotine, low-"tar" cigarettes. Carcinogenesis 16: 2015–2021.

34. Zuccaro P, Altieri I, Rosa M, Passa AR, Pichini S, et al. (1993) Determination of nicotine and four metabolites in the serum of smokers by high performance liquid chromatography with ultraviolet detection. J Chromatogr 621: 257–261.

35. Carini M, Aldini G, Piccone M, Facino RM (2000) Fluorescent probes as markers of oxidative stress in keratinocyte cell lines following UVB exposure. Farmaco 55: 526–534.

36. Hodges NJ, Green RM, Chipman JK, Graham M (2007) Induction of DNA strand breaks and oxidative stress in HeLa cells by ethanol is dependent on CYP2E1 expression. Mutagenesis 22: 189–194.

37. Dimri GP, Lee X, Basile G, Acosta M, Scott G, et al. (1995) A biomarker that identifies senescent human cells in culture and in aging skin in vivo. Proc Natl Acad Sci USA 92: 9363–9367.

38. Welge-Lüssen U, May CA, Eichhorn M, Bloemendal H, Lütjen-Drecoll E (1999) AlphaB-crystallin in the trabecular meshwork is inducible by transforming growth factor-beta. Invest Ophthalmol Vis Sci 40: 2235–2241.

39. Petrukhin K (2007) New therapeutic targets in atrophic age-related macular degeneration. Expert Opin Ther Targets 11: 625–639.

40. Jia L, Liu Z, Sun L, Miller SS, Ames BN, et al. (2007) Acrolein, a toxicant in cigarette smoke, causes oxidative damage and mitochondrial dysfunction in RPE cells: Protection by (R)-alpha-lipoic acid. Invest Ophthalmol Vis Sci 48: 339–348.

41. Sharma A, Neekhra A, Gramajo AL, Patil J, Chwa M, et al. (2008) Effects of benzo(e)pyrene, a toxic component of cigarette smoke, on human retinal pigment epithelial cells in vitro. Invest Ophthalmol Vis Sci 49: 5111–5117.

42. Kalariya NM, Wills NK, Ramana KV, Srivastava SK, van Kuijk FJ (2009) Cadmium-induced apoptotic death of human retinal pigment epithelial cells is mediated by MAPK pathway. Exp Eye Res 89: 494–502.

43. Bertram KM, Baglole CJ, Phipps RP, Libby RT (2009) Molecular regulation of cigarette smoke induced-oxidative stress in human retinal pigment epithelial cells: implications for age-related macular degeneration. Am J Physiol Cell Physiol 297: C1200–C1210.

44. Patil AJ, Gramajo AL, Sharma A, Seigel GM, Kuppermann BD, et al. (2009) Differential effects of nicotine on retinal and vascular cells in vitro. Toxicology 259: 69–76.

45. Chen J, Goligorsky MS (2006) Premature senescence of endothelial cells: Methusaleh's dilemma. Am J Physiol Heart Circ Physiol 290: 1729–1739.

46. Ehrlich R, Kheradiya NS, Winston DM, Moore DB, Wirostko B, et al. (2009) Age-related ocular vascular changes. Graefes Arch Clin Exp Ophthalmol 247: 583–591.

47. Kaarniranta K, Salminen A, Eskelinen EL, Kopitz J (2009) Heat shock proteins as gatekeepers of proteolytic pathways-Implications for age-related macular degeneration (AMD). Ageing Res Rev 8: 128–139.

48. Zarbin MA (2004) Current concepts in the pathogenesis of age-related macular degeneration. Arch Ophthalmol 122: 598–614.

49. Matsunaga H, Handa JT, Aotaki-Keen A, Sherwood SW, West MD, et al. (1999) Beta-galactosidase histochemistry and telomere loss in senescent retinal pigment epithelial cells. Invest Ophthalmol Vis Sci 40: 197–202.

50. Wang XF, Cui JZ, Nie W, Prasad SS, Matsubara JA (2004) Differential gene expression of early and late passage retinal pigment epithelial cells. Exp Eye Res 79: 209–221.

51. Mishima K, Handa JT, Aotaki-Keen A, Lutty GA, Morse LS, et al. (1999) Senescence-associated beta-galactosidase histochemistry for the primate eye. Invest Ophthalmol Vis Sci 40: 1590–1593.

52. Honda S, Hjelmeland LM, Handa JT (2002) Senescence associated beta galactosidase activity in human retinal pigment epithelial cells exposed to mild hyperoxia in vitro. Br J Ophthalmol 86: 159–162.

53. Sakaguchi H, Miyagi M, Shadrach KG, Rayborn ME, Crabb JW (2002) Clusterin is present in drusen in age-related macular degeneration. Exp Eye Res 74: 547–549.

54. Young RW (1987) Pathophysiology of age-related macular degeneration. Surv Ophthalmol 31: 291–306.

55. Fuchshofer R, Yu AL, Teng HH, Strauss R, Kampik A, et al. (2009) Hypoxia/reoxygenation induces CTGF and PAI-1 in cultured human retinal pigment epithelium cells. Exp Eye Res 88: 889–899.

56. Espinosa-Heidmann DG, Suner IJ, Catanuto P, Hernandez EP, Marin-Castano ME, et al. (2006) Cigarette smoke–related oxidants and the development of sub-RPE deposits in an experimental animal model of dry AMD. Invest Ophthalmol Vis Sci 47: 729–737.

57. Fujihara M, Nagai N, Sussan TE, Biswal S, Handa JT (2008) Chronic cigarette smoke causes oxidative damage and apoptosis to retinal pigmented epithelial cells in mice. PLoS ONE 3: e3119.

58. Cardoso JF, Mendes FA, Amadeu TP, Romana-Souza B, Valença SS, et al. (2009) Ccn2/Ctgf overexpression induced by cigarette smoke during cutaneous wound healing is strain dependent. Toxicol Pathol 37: 175–182.

14

Modelling the Genetic Risk in Age-Related Macular Degeneration

Felix Grassmann[1], Lars G. Fritsche[1], Claudia N. Keilhauer[2], Iris M. Heid[3,4], Bernhard H. F. Weber[1]*

1 Institute of Human Genetics, University of Regensburg, Regensburg, Germany, **2** University Eye Hospital Würzburg, Würzburg, Germany, **3** Institute of Epidemiology and Preventive Medicine, University Hospital Regensburg, Regensburg, Germany, **4** Institute of Genetic Epidemiology, Helmholtz Zentrum München, German Research Center for Environmental Health, Neuherberg, Germany

Abstract

Late-stage age-related macular degeneration (AMD) is a common sight-threatening disease of the central retina affecting approximately 1 in 30 Caucasians. Besides age and smoking, genetic variants from several gene loci have reproducibly been associated with this condition and likely explain a large proportion of disease. Here, we developed a genetic risk score (GRS) for AMD based on 13 risk variants from eight gene loci. The model exhibited good discriminative accuracy, area-under-curve (AUC) of the receiver-operating characteristic of 0.820, which was confirmed in a cross-validation approach. Noteworthy, younger AMD patients aged below 75 had a significantly higher mean GRS (1.87, 95% CI: 1.69–2.05) than patients aged 75 and above (1.45, 95% CI: 1.36–1.54). Based on five equally sized GRS intervals, we present a risk classification with a relative AMD risk of 64.0 (95% CI: 14.11–1131.96) for individuals in the highest category (GRS 3.44–5.18, 0.5% of the general population) compared to subjects with the most common genetic background (GRS −0.05–1.70, 40.2% of general population). The highest GRS category identifies AMD patients with a sensitivity of 7.9% and a specificity of 99.9% when compared to the four lower categories. Modeling a general population around 85 years of age, 87.4% of individuals in the highest GRS category would be expected to develop AMD by that age. In contrast, only 2.2% of individuals in the two lowest GRS categories which represent almost 50% of the general population are expected to manifest AMD. Our findings underscore the large proportion of AMD cases explained by genetics particularly for younger AMD patients. The five-category risk classification could be useful for therapeutic stratification or for diagnostic testing purposes once preventive treatment is available.

Editor: Florian Kronenberg, Innsbruck Medical University, Austria

Funding: This work was supported in part by a grant from the Deutsche Forschungsgemeinschaft WE 1259/19-2. No additional external funding was received for this study. The funders had no role in study design, data collection and analysis, decision to publish, or preparation of the manuscript.

Competing Interests: The authors have declared that no competing interests exist.

* E-mail: bweb@klinik.uni-regensburg.de

Introduction

Age-related macular degeneration (AMD) is a common degenerative disease of the central retina and a leading cause of severe vision impairment in Western societies [1]. Advanced forms of AMD (late-stage AMD) are known as geographic atrophy (GA) of the retinal pigment epithelium (RPE) or neovascular (NV) complications with RPE detachment, scar formation, and subretinal hemorrhage [2,3]. To date, effective therapeutic intervention is available for active NV, while GA still remains untreatable [4,5].

AMD is a complex disease influenced by genetic and environmental factors with estimates of heritability varying from 45% to 71% [6]. So far, several AMD susceptibility loci have been identified. Two loci are accounting for an estimated 50% of AMD cases: complement factor H (*CFH*) on 1q32 and age-related maculopathy susceptibility 2 (*ARMS2*)/HtrA serine peptidase 1 (*HTRA1*) on 10q26 [7,8]. Fine-mapping studies and functional analyses at the *CFH* locus indicate at least three independent risk variants [8–13]. At the *ARMS2/HTRA1* region, a single risk haplotype was found to fully explain the observed association [14].

A crucial role of the complement system in AMD pathogenesis was further supported by subsequent candidate gene studies.

These studies identified risk-associated variants in or near three additional complement genes including the complement component 2 (*C2*)/complement factor B (*CFB*) [15], complement component 3 (*C3*) [16,17] and complement factor I (*CFI*) [18]. In addition, variants in genes involved in the cholesterol and lipid metabolism were also implicated in AMD susceptibility [19,20]. Strongest signals peaked near the hepatic lipase gene (*LIPC*) on chromosome 15q22 [19,20], the cholesterylester transfer protein (*CETP*) and the lipoprotein lipase precursor (*LPL*) genes [19]. Also, among the most replicated AMD risk variants are two coding SNPs in the apolipoprotein E (*APOE*) gene [21,22]. A recent genome wide association study established a significant association of AMD with rs9621532, a variant intronic to synapsin III (*SYN3*) and approximately 100 kb upstream of the tissue inhibitor of metalloproteinases-3 gene (*TIMP3*) [19]. Finally, common variations near VEGFA and FRK/COL10A1 were associated with AMD, further implicating angiogenesis as well as extracellular matrix metabolism in AMD pathogenesis [23].

To predict the genetic risk in complex diseases, testing of single susceptibility variants is generally of limited value [24]. In contrast, genotyping and evaluating a series of independent disease associated variants, a process also known as genetic profiling, may be more appropriate [24]. This can be facilitated by a genetic risk score (GRS) which could simply represent the sum of risk associated variants found in each individual. However, such an approach may not be particularly effective in the presence of greatly differing effect sizes of the respective variants [25]. Therefore, an extension to this model weighs each additional risk allele by its effect size. For example, Seddon et al. (2009) calculated a risk score for AMD based on 6 known genetic risk variants and additional environmental factors. Their model revealed good discriminatory power with a reported area-under-curve (AUC) of the receiver-operating characteristic of 0.82 [26]. Other studies reporting a GRS [19,20,23] primarily aimed at identifying novel variants without using independent data or a cross-validation approach and are thus likely biased to overestimate the effect of these variants. The quantification of the genetic risk based on frequently replicated AMD loci in a single study which is independent from locus identification is still lacking.

Here, we present a genetic risk model for AMD, specifically the late-stage forms of AMD, based on a large and well characterized AMD case-control study group including 986 cases and 796 controls. We selected 13 genetic variants from eight gene loci that have repeatedly been shown to be associated with AMD and computed a genetic risk score. This was used to establish a classification system that allows for discriminating subjects at high and low genetic risk. Environmental variables such as smoking or diet were not included in the model building.

Results

SNP selection based on published data and linkage disequilibrium structure

Eight loci (CFH, ARMS2/HTRA1, CFI, CFB, C3, APOE, LIPC and TIMP3) with 13 SNPs and established association with AMD were included into our genetic risk score modeling (**Table S1**). There were three further SNPs with reportedly established association, which we did not select for the model: (i) at the CFH locus, an association of four variants with AMD is known (rs1410996, rs800292, rs1061170, rs6677604); however, rs1410996 is present on two distinct haplotypes, each of which is tagged by rs800292 (correlation $r^2 = 0.473$ to rs1410996 [27]) or rs6677604 ($r^2 = 0.283$ to rs1410996 [27]), respectively [13], while rs800292 and rs667604 are uncorrelated ($r^2 = 0.008$ [27]), (ii) among the three highly correlated ARMS/HTRA variants (rs10490924, rs11200638, and c.del443ins54; pairwise $r^2 = 1$), rs10490924 was reported to fully capture the disease risk at this locus [28]. We therefore selected rs1061170, rs800292 and rs667604 at CFH and rs10490924 at the ARMS2/HTRA1 locus yielding the 13 SNPs for model building.

Genotyping of SNPs in the Lower Frankonian AMD case-control study

We genotyped the selected 13 SNPs as well as the three highly correlated SNPs (to validate the correlations) in 986 cases and 796 controls from the Lower Frankonian AMD case-control study (**Table 1**). All variants showed high genotyping quality with an average call rate >99.5%. With the exception of rs1061170 at CFH, all genotypes were in Hardy-Weinberg equilibrium in controls (HWE, p>0.04). The variant rs1061170 was genotyped twice with two independent assays yielding identical genotypes and therefore persistent HWE violation in controls (p = 0.002) [29]. There were no missing genotypes at the 13 variants for any individual in the study.

Table 1. Summary characteristics of the case-control study.

	Cases	Controls	Total
Subjects	986	796	1782
GA[1]	229	-	
NV[2]	581	-	
Mixed GA+NV[3]	176	-	
Mean Age (S.D.) [in years]	78.7 (6.5)	78.3 (5.1)	78.5 (5.9)
Men [%]	34.1	39.3	36.4
Fraction smoker [%][4,5]	15.9	14.3	

[1]Geographic atrophy.
[2]Neovascular AMD.
[3]Mixed GA+NV: GA and NV in the same eye or GA in one and NV in the second eye.
[4]Smoking was defined as ever smoked more than 20 pack years.
[5]This variable was surveyed incompletely in cases and controls and thus was not further considered in the analysis.

Association of the selected 13 SNPs with AMD

For each SNP, association with AMD was computed using a logistic regression model, unadjusted for age or gender (**Table 2**). Sensitivity analysis additionally adjusting for age and gender yielded similar results. Odds ratio (OR) estimates per AMD risk increasing variant ranged from 1.14 [95% CI: 1.00–1.30] for rs2285714 to 3.13 [95% CI: 2.68–3.68] for rs10490924 and were significantly different from unity for all 13 variants demonstrating sufficient statistical power in our study (**Table 2**). In a subgroup analysis, AMD cases with GA (n = 229) or NV (n = 581) or mixed GA+NV in one or both eyes (n = 176) were compared to controls using logistic regression for each variant separately (**Figure S1**).

Computing the genetic risk score

Based on the data from the 13 SNPs, we fit a multiple logistic regression model (**Figure 1**). The odds ratios in this model ranged from 1.070 to 4.063. This is, to our knowledge, the first study to report these 13 variants together in one multiple logistic regression accounting for other AMD risk variants. We computed a GRS for each individual as the sum of AMD risk increasing alleles weighted by the relative effect size of each SNP from the logistic model. We added the alpha estimate of −10.13 to center the GRS on zero for our study (see Methods). Cases had a significantly higher mean GRS (1.61, 95% CI: 1.53–1.69) compared to controls (−0.03, 95% CI: −0.12–0.06, p<0.01). The relative risk of AMD per GRS unit approximated by the OR was 2.72 (95% CI: 2.46–3.01). The mean GRS of our controls was slightly lower than the one for the HapMap data representing a general population (0.00, 95% CI: −0.14–0.14), which is in-line with our controls being selected for having no AMD.

Good discriminative ability of the GRS

Computing the area-under-the-curve (AUC) of the receiver-operating characteristic for the 13-SNP GRS, we observed good ability to correctly classify those with and without the disease (AUC = 0.820, **Figure 2**). We also computed the AUC per locus demonstrating that the impact by gene varied substantially, as expected. The three SNPs at the CFH locus alone (rs800292, rs1061170, rs6677604) showed the highest classification efficiency (AUC = 0.710), followed by rs10490924 at ARMS2/HTRA1 (AUC = 0.684), and the remaining variants (AUC from 0.512 to 0.571) (**Figure 2**).

Table 2. Association results for the 13 known AMD associated variants in the lower Frankonian case-control study (986 cases, 796 controls) using single logistic regression.

| Nearby gene(s) | Marker | ID | Impact/effect of variant | Odds ratio | 95% CI[1] | P-value[2] | Non risk allele | Risk allele[3] | Frequency of risk allele in | | AUC[4] of variant | correlation[5] |
									Controls (N=796)	Cases (N=986)		
CFH	rs1061170	1	p.Y402H	2.74	2.36-3.18	1.66E-45	T	C	0.365	0.600	0.676	
	rs800292	2	p.I62V	2.43	2.02-2.92	6.95E-23	A	G	0.761	0.888	0.606	0.150
	rs6677604	3	proxy for ΔCFHR3/CFHR1	2.19	1.82-2.64	1.42E-17	A	G	0.777	0.884	0.590	0.203
ARMS2	rs10490924	4	p.A69S	3.13	2.68-3.68	7.97E-54	G	T	0.189	0.441	0.684	
CFB	rs4151667	5	p.L9H	2.82	1.90-4.28	1.41E-07	A	T	0.951	0.982	0.530	
	rs438999	6	proxy for rs641153 (p.R32Q)	2.31	1.73-3.11	5.75E-09	C	T	0.915	0.962	0.542	0.01
C3	rs2230199	7	p.R102G	1.52	1.29-1.80	4.71E-07	G	C	0.175	0.245	0.556	
APOE	rs7412	8	p.R158C	1.41	1.12-1.80	0.003613	C	T	0.079	0.107	0.526	
	rs429358	9	p.C112R	1.35	1.09-1.69	0.006812	C	T	0.881	0.908	0.528	0.783
PLA2G12A	rs2285714	10	synonymous exonic, unknown	1.14	1.00-1.30	0.04839	C	T	0.409	0.443	0.523	
LIPC	rs493258	11	intergenic (36 kb upstream)	1.18	1.04-1.35	0.01277	T	C	0.538	0.580	0.531	
	rs10468017	12	intergenic (46 kb upstream)	1.26	1.08-1.46	0.002992	T	C	0.707	0.751	0.536	0.367
SYN3/TIMP3	rs9621532	13	intronic, unknown	1.58	1.09-2.30	0.01246	C	A	0.96	0.974	0.512	

[1]CI = confidence interval.
[2]P-values were derived from a logistic regression model with one SNP as covariate.
[3]Risk allele is the allele that is associated with increased risk of AMD.
[4]AUC = area-under-curve of the receiver-operating characteristic.
[5]r² values representing the correlation with the first SNP in each gene/locus based on 1000 genomes data (build 1) or HapMap release 22 [27].

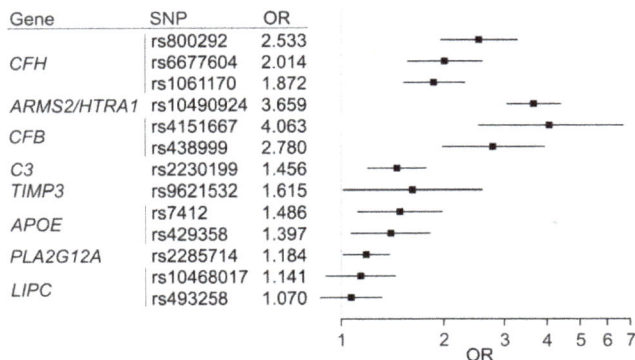

Figure 1. Risk estimates for each of thirteen AMD risk variants from eight gene loci. Odds ratios (OR) per risk allele were derived from multiple logistic regression models. Horizontal lines indicate 95% confidence intervals.

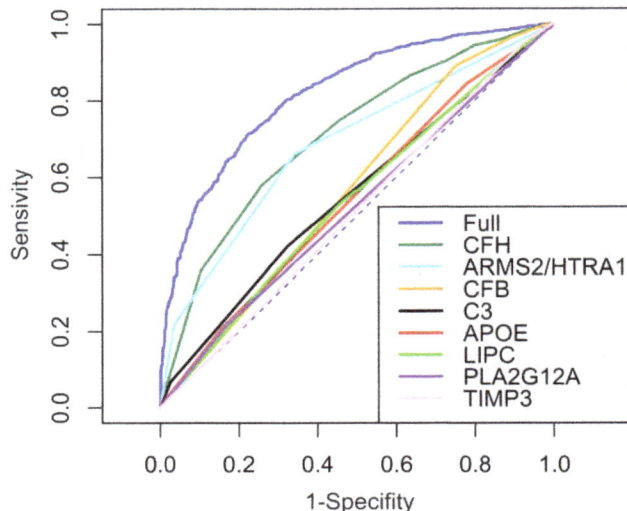

Figure 2. Area-under-the-curve of the receiver operating characteristic for the 13-SNP genetic risk score and by gene locus. Observed AUC was 0.820 and the locus-specific AUCs were 0.513, 0.524, 0.536, 0.547, 0.555, 0.571, 0.686 and 0.710 from bottom to top.

Although we specifically avoided selecting the SNPs based on association in our own data set but rather from the literature, there could be a potential overestimation of the AUC: We estimated the effect sizes per variant from our data and used these as weights for the GRS. To evaluate this potential over-estimation, we performed a sensitivity analysis via a cross-validation approach by repeated (i = 2000) random sub-sampling with 2/3rd of the data for model building and 1/3rd for testing. The cross validated AUC of 0.813 (95% CI: 0.813–0.814) is close to the one described in our initial study (AUC = 0.820).

Developing a parsimonious genetic risk score model

We evaluated whether a parsimonious model based on our data could be developed. We thus explored several models by subsequently excluding the loci with the weakest AUC and found a model restricted to 10 variants with equally discriminatory ability (AUC 0.820) and equal model fit ($R^2 = 0.247$) (**Table 3**). This model could be of value for translational studies minimizing the genotyping burden. Whether this is specific to our data set or holds true for other study populations needs to be evaluated further. It should be noted that all further analyses are based on the 13-SNPs-GRS.

Distribution of the genetic risk score

The distribution of GRS for cases and controls as observed in our study is given in **Figure 3A**. To provide a more realistic view of the GRS distribution, the proportion of cases were weighted to reflect a general distribution. For this modeling, an AMD prevalence of 15% was assumed as reported for the general population aged >85 years [30–32] (**Figure 3B**). The derived GRS is comparable to the distribution estimated from individual HapMap data (**Figure 3B**).

Genetic risk score by age groups, gender and AMD subtype

We further investigated differences of the GRS between age-groups (below or older than 75 years), men and women, or types of AMD (GA, NV, or mixed GA+NV) using a significance level of 0.05/3 to account for the three subgroup tests performed.

Significant differences in mean GRS were found between younger (1.87, 95% CI: 1.69–2.05) and older (1.45, 95% CI: 1.36–1.54) AMD cases (p = 8.7×10^{-5}), but there was no difference between the age-groups among controls (p = 0.18). The OR per

GRS unit was 3.06 (95%CI: 2.64–3.59) for younger and 2.71 (95% CI: 2.44–3.05) for older individuals. We also found that the AUC restricted to the younger subjects (cases and controls) was higher (0.852) than when only older subjects (cases and controls) were included in the calculations (0.809).

Cases with mixed GA+NV had a significantly higher mean GRS (1.87, 95% CI: 1.69–2.04) compared to NV cases (1.44, 95% CI: 1.34–1.55, p = 6.6×10^{-5}). It was also higher when compared to GA cases (1.65, 95% CI: 1.48–1.83, p = 0.03), although the latter was statistically not significant when applying a conservative Bonferroni-adjusted significance level of 0.05/3. The OR per GRS unit was also higher for mixed GA+NV cases (OR = 3.79, 95% CI: 3.13–4.67) than for NV cases (OR = 3.79, 95% CI: 3.13–4.67) or for GA cases (OR = 2.84, 95% CI: 2.44–3.33). This effect appeared to be independent of age, since mean age in GA (78.8 years, 95% CI: 77.9–79.6), NV (78.5 years, 95% CI: 77.9–79.0) and mixed GA+NV (79.4 years, 95% CI: 78.4–80.3) was similar. There was no significant difference in the GRS means between men and women neither among cases nor among controls.

Table 3. Model fit and discriminative accuracy of parsimonious models.

Model[1]	Variants[2]	R^2	AUC
13-SNP model	1,2,3,4,5,6,7,8,9,10,11,12,13	0.2475	0.820
- TIMP3	1,2,3,4,5,6,7,8,9,10,11,12	0.2475	0.820
- PLA2G12A	1,2,3,4,5,6,7,8,9,11,12	0.2454	0.819
- APOE	1,2,3,4,5,6,7,10,11,12	0.2411	0.816
- LIPC[3]	1,2,3,4,5,6,7,8,9,10	0.2457	0.820

[1]SNPs from one additional locus at a time were omitted from the 13-SNP model by starting with the locus with the smallest risk.
[2]Numbering corresponds to IDs in Table 2.
[3]This model contained the least number of SNPs without compromising R^2 or AUC values.

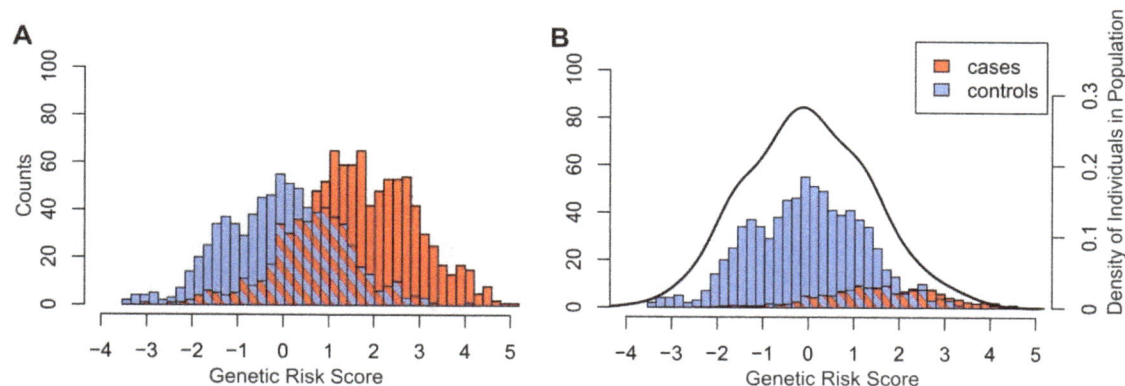

Figure 3. Genetic risk score distribution in the study population and in a modeled population. AMD cases are shown in red, controls in blue, while overlapping bars are shaded blue/red. (**A**) Genetic risk score distribution for cases (N = 986) and controls (N = 796) in the present study. (**B**) Counts of cases in (A) were scaled to represent 15% of the total population (assumed as AMD prevalence of the 85–90 year old general population). The density curve represents the risk score distribution in 381 European ancestry samples available through the 1000 Genomes Project (Release 20110521).

These subgroup analyses demonstrate a higher genetic risk of the younger AMD patients compared to the older patients as well as a higher genetic risk for those with mixed late-stage manifestations (GA+NV) when compared to NV or GA alone.

Genetic risk groups and relative risk estimates

To establish a classification scheme, we formed five equally sized intervals for the GRS spectrum (≤−1.79, (−1.79)–(−0.05), (−0.05)–1.70, 1.60–3.44, and >3.44; **Table 4**). The highest GRS category (no. 5) contained 7.92% of AMD cases, but only 0.13% of controls. In contrast, the two lowest GRS categories (nos. 1+2) jointly contained only 9.8% of cases, but 48.7% of controls. According to the HapMap data reflecting a general population, the proportion of subjects in the two lowest risk groups combined was 48.9% and 0.5% in the highest risk group. This is consistent with the general population being a mixture of mostly controls and only few cases.

The relative risks were approximated as ORs for each GRS category using the middle category (no. 3) as reference (**Table 4**). It can be seen that the OR is dramatically increased for category four (OR = 5.44, 95% CI = 4.03–7.46) and even more for category five (OR = 64.00, 95% CI = 14.11–1132.96). The odds ratios are substantially decreased for categories two and one (OR = 0.22, CI = 0.17–0.29 and OR = 0.12, 95% CI = 0.05–0.24) compared to the reference. Thus, these GRS categories can effectively describe genetic risk groups for AMD.

Due to the substantial differences found in mean GRS for younger compared to older cases (see above), we derived these ORs also separately by age-group. To avoid scarce data, risk group one and two as well as four and five were combined to a low and a high risk group, respectively (**Table 4**). This highlights the higher genetic relative risk for AMD when restricting the analysis to the younger (OR = 12.66, 95% CI: 6.76–25.65) compared to the older (OR = 5.18, 95% CI: 3.70–7.38) subjects. Although the 95% confidence intervals overlap slightly, we observed a significant difference (p = 0.0194).

Modeled absolute risk for late-stage AMD

To reflect the anticipated situation in the general population and to compute the absolute risk of AMD per GRS group, we computed the fraction of late-stage AMD cases per GRS category by (i) utilizing the fraction of cases and controls as observed in each GRS category (**Table 4**) and (ii) weighting the fraction of cases assuming various AMD prevalences (1%–15%). The fraction of cases and the fraction of subjects of the modeled general population (also for comparison in the HapMap sample) by GRS category are shown in **Table 5**. The fraction of late-stage AMD in the highest GRS group (absolute AMD risk) ranged from 38.6–91.7% depending on the assumed AMD prevalence which were chosen to correspond to the various age-groups as reported [30–32]. For example, in a general population with an AMD prevalence of 10% approximately 90% of the persons in the highest GRS group are expected to be affected by late-stage AMD. Consequently, the genetic relative risk for subjects in the highest GRS group (compared to the middle GRS group) is higher for younger compared to the older AMD cases. However, the absolute risk of AMD among subjects in the highest GRS group is higher for the older population due to the higher AMD prevalence among the older persons.

We again adopted the same cross-validation approach to compute absolute risks since the effect sizes of the variants in the GRS model, on which the absolute risk estimates are based, were estimated from our study data. This approach yielded overall similar estimates (**Table S2**).

Discussion

Based on a genetic risk score including 13 reported SNPs from eight established AMD gene loci, we propose a five-category classification system that effectively differentiates subjects with high or low genetic risk. With this, we extend on earlier efforts to predict the genetic risk for late-stage AMD [26,33–35]. Seddon et al. described a risk score model for six genetic variants in four loci also including environmental factors like BMI, smoking, age and diet (sample size was 1.446 individuals of which 279 progressed to AMD) [26]. Similarly, a study from Gibson et al. included 470 cases and 470 controls and reported an AUC of 0.83 (95% CI 0.81 to 0.86) using six SNPs in four loci and two environmental factors [33]. A study by Spencer et al. investigated one variant in each of four loci as well as age and smoking as environmental factors and found an AUC of 0.84 (95% CI: 0.81–0.88) [35]. Jakobsdottir et al. reported an AUC of 0.79 based on one SNP in each of three loci [34]. This study consisted of around 1.000 family-based cases and 429 controls as well as a case-control study with 187 cases and

Table 4. Five genetic risk groups and relative risk of AMD (ORs and 95% confidence intervals).

GRS category	Genetic risk groups				
	1	**2**	**3**	**4**	**5**
Sample size	N = 63	N = 417	N = 761	N = 450	N = 79
GRS interval	≤−1.79	]−1.79,−0.05]	]−0.05,1.70]	]1.70,3.44]	>3.44
Cases [%]	0.81	9.00	42.5	39.7	7.92
Cases <75 years [%]	1.70	6.20	34.0	42.3	15.8
Cases >75 years [%]	0.54	9.96	45.2	38.9	5.38
Controls [%]	6.99	41.7	43.6	7.50	0.13
Frequency in HapMap[1]	8.92	40.2	41.2	9.18	0.53
OR (95% CI)	0.12 (0.05–0.24)	0.22 (0.17–0.29)	reference	5.44 (4.02–7.46)	64.00 (14.11–1131.96)
GRS categories	**low (1+2)**		**3**		**high (4+5)**
Sample size	N = 480		N = 761		N = 529
GRS interval	≤−0.05		]−0.05,1.70]		>1.70
OR (95% CI)	0.21 (0.16–0.27)		reference		6.41 (4.76–8.76)
<75 years: OR (95% CI)	0.19 (0.10–0.33)		reference		12.66 (6.76–25.65)
>= 75 years: OR (95% CI)	0.22 (0.16–0.29)		reference		5.18 (3.70–7.38)

[1]Fraction of individuals in 1000 Genome Project European Ancestry Samples residing in risk groups.

168 controls. We evaluated 13 SNPs from 8 AMD loci in a well characterized and well powered case-control study and observed an AUC of 0.820, which is sufficient to classify AMD patients and controls into high risk and low risk groups [24]. Our study has not contributed to the identification of any of the 13 SNPs as AMD risk-increasing variants and would thus not be subject to winner's curse regarding the effect size. To our knowledge, this is a first study to include most of the currently known genetic loci for their value to predict late-stage AMD risk in a study that is independent of the identification of any of these loci.

Interestingly, we find a higher relative risk of the CFB SNP rs4151667 compared to CFH and ARMS2/HTRA1 risk-increasing SNPs particularly in the multivariable logistic regression model. This can also be seen in a previously published study (Seddon et al., Table 4) [36], although it needs to be noted that the models used in our and the published study differ in the sense that

Table 5. Absolute risks for AMD by modeling a general population for various prevalences of AMD (reflecting various age-groups).

	Modeled prevalence (age-group [yrs])[1]	Absolute risk of AMD by genetic risk group [%]				
		1 (low)	**2**	**3**	**4**	**5 (high)**
GRS interval		≤−1.79	]−1.79,−0.05]	]−0.05,1.70]	]1.70,3.44]	>3.44
% cases, modeled general population						
	1% (65–69)	0.12	0.22	0.97	5.08	38.6
	2.5% (70–74)	0.30	0.55	2.44	12.0	61.5
	5% (75–79)	0.61	1.13	4.87	21.8	76.6
	10% (80–84)	1.30	2.40	9.80	37.0	87.4
	15% (>85)	2.00	3.70	14.7	48.3	91.7
% subjects, modeled general population						
	1%	6.84	40.9	43.6	8.31	0.32
	2.5%	6.68	40.1	43.8	8.50	0.34
	5%	6.69	40.1	43.6	9.12	0.52
	10%	6.38	38.5	43.5	10.7	0.91
	15%	6.10	36.8	43.5	12.3	1.30
% subjects, HapMap population[2]		8.92	40.2	41.2	9.18	0.53

[1]Approximate age-groups corresponding to the modeled prevalences for 65 and 79 years [30,31] and for those above 80 years [32].
[2]see Table 4.

ours considers exclusively genetic factors while the other work largely focused on non-genetic factors. The smaller allele frequency of the CFB SNP (1.8% in our cases, 6.7% in the European ancestry 1000G individuals) compared to SNP frequencies in CFH and ARMS2/HTRA1 results in a reduced power to detect association and may explain why CFB SNP rs4151667 was not among those detected first by AMD GWAS.

As expected, the mean GRS was significantly higher in cases when compared to controls. Importantly, patients with late-stage AMD diagnosed at an earlier age had a significantly higher mean GRS than individuals that developed AMD later in life. This strongly suggests that genetic predisposition influences disease onset, which is also reflected in the higher relative AMD risk for younger subjects with an OR of 12.66 (95% CI: 6.76–25.65) when compared to older individuals with an OR of 5.18 (95% CI: 3.70–7.38). The mean genetic risk score in our control group was slightly lower but similar to the mean score in the HapMap sample (including a total of 381 European subjects from CEU, GBR, IBS, TSI and FIN, 1000 Genomes Project (Release 20110521, http://www.1000genomes.org, accessed 2 May 2012).). The slight discrepancy would be in-line with the fact that our controls were specifically selected to reveal no signs of early or late-stage AMD.

Limitations of our study for risk prediction should be acknowledged. First, the analysis was based on a case-control study, which has no element of a prospective study or a nested case-control study. The controls were often spouses of AMD patients and thus non-genetic risk factors could not be studied due to the known similarities among spouses regarding life style factors. However, our AMD patients were virtually incident AMD cases and thus the age at study entry is likely the age-at-diagnosis and the best possible proxy for age-of-onset (allowing for a delay of about 1–2 years between onset and diagnosis). In a case-control setting, absolute risk or positive/negative predictive values cannot be derived without making assumptions on the overall AMD prevalence, which a prospective cohort study could estimate directly. Thus, the predictive ability of the risk score groups greatly depends on those assumptions. Second, it might be considered a limitation but also a strength that our study included exclusively late-stage AMD with NV or GA in one or both eyes as well as highly-matched controls with no signs of early or late-stage AMD in any eye. A strength as our data might exhibit less disease misclassification than other studies, but a limitation as the genetic relative risk could be overestimated if the genetic risk is larger for subjects with both eyes affected than for those with only one affected eye. Third, we had no independent and equally well characterized data set available to separate model building from testing although this is also the case for all other studies published on AMD risk score model building [26,33,34]. Only one study [35] reported a small replication study. We avoided selecting SNPs for our model based on association signals in our own data but rather selected SNPs from the literature. However, the SNP-specific effect sizes utilized as weights in the genetic risk score computation were still estimated in our data set. Thus, estimations of AUC or absolute risk in the same data could lead to a slight over-estimation of risk. We therefore adopted a cross-validation approach as sensitivity analysis, which did not provide evidence of remarkable over-estimation.

The highest genetic risk group of our proposed five-category classification scheme can effectively identify subjects at high risk for AMD. The specificity in this risk group was 99.9% (95% CI: 99.3%–100%). For example, our data and model suggest that 87.4% of subjects testing positive at some time in life for a high genetic risk are likely to develop AMD in their mid-eighties (positive predictive value). Thus, this group of individuals could

greatly profit from a sight-saving prevention or early intervention program while only 13% of (false-positive) subjects would be alarmed and treated unnecessarily. However, still a large number of cases would be missed if this was established as a screening method (sensitivity 8.0% (95% CI: 6.5%–9.9%), i.e. 92% of all AMD cases would not be found in the highest risk group). Also individuals in the second highest risk group could possibly profit from early intervention, which would increase sensitivity to 47.6% and decrease specificity to 91.2%. However, this would only be acceptable, if the prevention/intervention is not harmful to the 59.9% of subjects treated and alarmed unnecessarily (40.1% positive predictive value). These numbers are well in the range of established screening tests, e.g. for prostate cancer by prostate specific antigen (PSA) (positive predictive value = 25.1%, sensitivity = 72.1%, specificity = 93.2%, [37]), albeit with a higher predictive value at the cost of reduced sensitivity. Abnormal levels of PSA are detected in about 10% of the male population, which is comparable to the coverage of high risk group four and five [37]. Offering an effective prevention program to individuals in the highest AMD risk group (approximately 400,000 individuals in Germany alone), almost 10% of incident late-stage AMD could be avoided. If individuals in risk groups four and five are included (about 10% of the general population), up to 50% of future AMD patients could be addressed.

So far, only the progression of the neovascular complications in AMD can be slowed by treatment [38]. If disease progression to an advanced neovascular form is detected early in high risk patients, immediate intervention might prove essential to sustain full vision for a more extended time. Accordingly, high risk individuals could be advised to seek clinical follow-ups more frequently and could also benefit from dietary recommendations, including the intake of antioxidants [39] or omega-3 fatty acids [40,41]. Identification of individuals at high risk for developing AMD may also help to include defined candidates in clinical AMD trials and thus may allow a better assessment of therapeutic effects.

In conclusion, our study provides a genetic risk score for late-stage AMD from a well characterized case-control study emphasizing the large proportion of disease explained by genetic markers particularly for younger subjects. We propose a classification scheme to identify subjects at high or low genetic risk that might be suitable for risk stratification in therapy studies or genetic screening once preventive treatment is available.

Methods

Ethics statement

This study followed the tenets of the declaration of Helsinki and was approved by the Ethics Review Board at the University of Würzburg, Germany. Informed written consent was obtained from each patient after explanation of the nature and possible consequences of the study.

The study subjects

The case-control sample includes 986 AMD patients and 796 controls recruited from the Lower Frankonian area at the University Eye Clinic of Würzburg, Germany [14]. Controls were often unaffected spouses or nonrelated acquaintances of cases of similar age as the patient. All patients and controls were examined by a trained ophthalmologist (CNK). Stereo fundus photographs were graded according to standardized classification systems as described previously [9,42,43]. Only patients with severe forms of AMD (GA or NV) in at least one eye and signs of early AMD (e.g. large soft drusen) in the other eye were included. The patients were divided into three subgroups according to their type of late-stage AMD: patients with GA in the severe eye, patients with NV in the severe eye and patients that had either GA in one eye and NV in the other eye or that showed both late-stage forms in the same eye (mixed GA+NV). Mean age in cases was 78.7 (±6.5) years and 78.3 (±5.1) in controls. A total of 34.1% of cases and 39.1% of controls were male. Study characteristics are summarized in **Table 1**.

Genotyping

Genomic DNA was extracted from peripheral blood leukocytes according to established protocols. Genotyping of SNPs was achieved by direct sequencing, restriction enzyme digestion of PCR products, TaqMan SNP Genotyping (Applied Biosystems, Foster City, USA) or primer extension of multiplex PCR products with detection of the allele-specific extension products by the matrix-assisted laser desorption/ionization time of flight (MALDI-TOF) mass spectrometry method (Sequenom, San Diego, USA) (**Table S3**). Direct sequencing was performed with the Big Dye Terminator Cycle Sequencing Kit Version 1.1 (Applied Biosystems, Foster City, USA) according to the manufacturer's instructions. Reactions were analyzed with an ABI Prism Model 3130xl Sequencer (Applied Biosystems). TaqMan Pre-Designed SNP Genotyping Assays (Applied Biosystems) were performed according to the manufacturer's instructions. Additionally, some variants were genotyped by PCR followed by restriction enzyme digestion (New England Biolabs, Ipswich, USA) and subsequent restriction fragment length analysis. The c.del443ins54 variant in the 3′-region of the *ARMS2* locus was genotyped by a single PCR with oligonucleotide primers 5′-ACTCATCACGTCATCAC-CAAT-3′ and 5′-CTCTCTGCAGCCCTCATTTG-3′ resulting in distinct fragment sizes due to the presence or absence of the deletion/insertion polymorphism.

Estimating genetic risk and model fit

Genotypes were coded as the number of AMD risk increasing alleles (0, 1, and 2). Logistic regression analyses were carried out using the R software [44]. Odds ratios (OR) per risk allele and 95% confidence intervals (95% CI) were calculated from the estimated beta-coefficients to derive an approximate relative risk. The goodness-of-fit of each model was assessed by calculating McFaddens pseudo R^2 [45], which however, does not reflect the variance explained by the model [46].

Computing the genetic risk score

Based on the intercept "a" and the single-SNP beta-coefficients estimated using the logistic regression model including all SNPs at once, the genetic risk score (GRS) was calculated as

$$GRS = a + \sum_{i=1}^{k} b_i * x_i \qquad (1)$$

with k being the number of SNPs in the model and x_i the genotype of the ith SNP. Here, "a" denotes a constant that centers the risk score distribution around zero and b_i relates to the ith variant. The odds ratio of the effect of the ith variant is thus given by $\exp(b_i)$ [19,23,26]. The mean GRS by age-group, sex, or AMD subtype were compared based on the independent samples t test using the R software [44] and differences were considered as significant, if P<0.05/3 accounting for the three comparisons performed.

Assessing the discriminative ability

To estimate the ability of a potential genetic screening test to discriminate between AMD cases and healthy subjects, we computed the receiver-operating-characteristic (ROC) curve. This involves ranking all subjects according to their GRS starting with the smallest, computing sensitivity and specificity at each possible GRS cut-off, and plotting sensitivity versus 1-specificity. The area-under-the-curve (AUC) is a measure of how well the GRS cut-offs can separate AMD cases from controls. We used the package EPICALC [47] for AUC computations and forest plots were generated with RMETA [48].

Internal validation by cross-validation

Although we have not selected the SNPs into the model based on their association in our data set but rather with information from the literature, there is a potential overestimation of the AUC due to the fact that we used the SNP effect sizes to weigh the risk alleles when computing the GRS. Thus, we conducted a sensitivity analysis using a cross-validation approach to derive AUC estimates that are not subject to this bias to compare with the original data AUC. We randomly assigned 2/3rd of the data to the model building (to compute the effect sizes and thus establish the GRS model) and 1/3rd of the data to testing (to compute the AUC and positive predictive values) ([49,50]). We repeated this 2000 times and computed the average AUC as an unbiased estimate.

Modeling of the absolute risk by GRS group

In order to derive the fraction of cases in the five GRS categories as expected in the general population (corresponding to the absolute AMD risk) from the number of cases (N_cases = 986) and controls (N_controls = 796) in our case-control study, we weighted the number of AMD cases in our study by

$$weight = \frac{prevalence * N\_controls}{(1\text{-}prevalence) * N\_cases} \qquad (2)$$

where prevalence denotes the fraction of AMD cases in the general population, that we chose to reflect previously reported prevalences of AMD in the various age groups (65–69 years: 1%, 70–74 years: 2.5%, 75–79 years: 5%, 80–84 years: 10% and >85 years: 15%) [30–32]. These were also used to compute positive and negative predictive value for the highest GRS category as a screening test for AMD. The cross-validation approach described above was also adopted for a sensitivity analysis to compute unbiased absolute risk.

Supporting Information

Figure S1 Risk estimates for 16 AMD associated variants by disease subtypes. Logistic regression models were fitted with all patients (N = 986), GA cases only (N = 229), NV cases only (N = 581) or mixed GA+NV cases (N = 176) versus controls (N = 796). Odds ratio estimates (OR) are given per risk allele; horizontal bars indicate 95% confidence intervals and the arrow indicates that the boundary extends below 1 or above 6.

Table S1 Published genetic variations associated with AMD.

Table S2 Cross validated absolute risks for late stage AMD in different risk groups in the modeled population.

Table S3 Primers and methods used for genotyping.

Acknowledgments

We thank Teresa Leist and Kerstin Meier for excellent technical support in genotyping the samples.

References

1. Congdon N, O'Colmain B, Klaver CCW, Klein R, Muñoz B, et al. (2004) Causes and prevalence of visual impairment among adults in the United States. Archives of ophthalmology 122: 477–485. Available:http://www.ncbi.nlm.nih.gov/pubmed/15078664.

2. de Jong PTVM (2006) Age-related macular degeneration. The New England journal of medicine 355: 1474–1485. Available:http://www.ncbi.nlm.nih.gov/pubmed/17021323.

3. Jager RD, Mieler WF, Miller JW (2008) Age-related macular degeneration. The New England journal of medicine 358: 2606–2617. Available:http://www.ncbi.nlm.nih.gov/pubmed/18550876.

4. Rosenfeld PJ, Brown DM, Heier JS, Boyer DS, Kaiser PK, et al. (2006) Ranibizumab for neovascular age-related macular degeneration. The New England journal of medicine 355: 1419–1431. Available:http://www.ncbi.nlm.nih.gov/pubmed/17021318.

5. Brown DM, Kaiser PK, Michels M, Soubrane G, Heier JS, et al. (2006) Ranibizumab versus verteporfin for neovascular age-related macular degeneration. The New England journal of medicine 355: 1432–1444. Available:http://www.ncbi.nlm.nih.gov/pubmed/17021319. Accessed 2011 Sept 28.

6. Seddon JM, Cote J, Page WF, Aggen SH, Neale MC (2005) The US twin study of age-related macular degeneration: relative roles of genetic and environmental influences. Archives of ophthalmology 123: 321–327. Available:http://www.ncbi.nlm.nih.gov/pubmed/15767473. Accessed 2012 Mar 21.

7. Fisher SA, Abecasis GR, Yashar BM, Zareparsi S, Swaroop A, et al. (2005) Meta-analysis of genome scans of age-related macular degeneration. Human molecular genetics 14: 2257–2264. Available:http://www.ncbi.nlm.nih.gov/pubmed/15987700. Accessed 2010 Jul.

8. Klein RJ, Zeiss C, Chew EY, Tsai J-yue, Sackler RS, et al. (2005) Complement factor H polymorphism in age-related macular degeneration. Science (New York, NY) 308: 385–389. Available:http://www.pubmedcentral.nih.gov/articlerender.fcgi?artid=1512523&tool=pmcentrez&rendertype=abstract. Accessed 2001 Jun 16.

9. Hageman GS, Anderson DH, Johnson LV, Hancox LS, Taiber AJ, et al. (2005) A common haplotype in the complement regulatory gene factor H (HF1/CFH) predisposes individuals to age-related macular degeneration. Proceedings of the National Academy of Sciences of the United States of America 102: 7227–7232. Available:http://www.pubmedcentral.nih.gov/articlerender.fcgi?artid=1088171&tool=pmcentrez&rendertype=abstract.

10. Li M, Atmaca-sonmez P, Othman M, Branham KEH, Khanna R, et al. (2006) CFH haplotypes without the Y402H coding variant show strong association with susceptibility to age-related macular degeneration. Nature Genetics 38: 1049–1054. doi:10.1038/ng1871.

11. Hughes AE, Orr N, Esfandiary H, Diaz-torres M, Goodship T, et al. (2007) A common CFH haplotype, with deletion of CFHR1 and CFHR3, is associated with lower risk of age-related macular degeneration. Nature Genetics 38: 1173–1178. doi:10.1038/ng1890.

12. Schmid-kubista KE, Tosakulwong N, Wu Y, Ryu E, Hecker LA, et al. (2009) Contribution of Copy Number Variation in the Regulation of Complement Activation Locus to Development of Age-Related Macular Degeneration. Investigative Ophthalmology. pp 5070–5079. doi:10.1167/iovs.09-3975.

13. Fritsche LG, Lauer N, Hartmann A, Stippa S, Keilhauer CN, et al. (2010) An imbalance of human complement regulatory proteins CFHR1, CFHR3 and factor H influences risk for age-related macular degeneration (AMD). Human molecular genetics 19: 4694–4704. Available:http://www.ncbi.nlm.nih.gov/pubmed/20843825. Accessed 11 April 2011.

14. Rivera A, Fisher SA, Fritsche LG, Keilhauer CN, Lichtner P, et al. (2005) Hypothetical LOC387715 is a second major susceptibility gene for age-related macular degeneration, contributing independently of complement factor H to disease risk. Human molecular genetics 14: 3227–3236. Available:http://www.ncbi.nlm.nih.gov/pubmed/16174643. Accessed 2011 Aug 1.

15. Gold B, Merriam JE, Zernant J, Hancox LS, Taiber AJ, et al. (2006) Variation in factor B (BF) and complement component 2 (C2) genes is associated with age-related macular degeneration. Nature genetics 38: 458–462. Available:http://www.ncbi.nlm.nih.gov/pubmed/16518403.

16. Yates JRW, Sepp T, Matharu BK, Khan JC, Thurlby DA, et al. (2007) Complement C3 variant and the risk of age-related macular degeneration. The New England journal of medicine 357: 553–561. Available:http://www.ncbi.nlm.nih.gov/pubmed/17634448.

17. Maller JB, Fagerness JA, Reynolds RC, Neale BM, Daly MJ, et al. (2007) Variation in complement factor 3 is associated with risk of age-related macular degeneration. Nature genetics 39: 1200–1201. Available:http://www.ncbi.nlm.nih.gov/pubmed/17767156.

18. Fagerness Ja, Maller JB, Neale BM, Reynolds RC, Daly MJ, et al. (2009) Variation near complement factor I is associated with risk of advanced AMD. European journal of human genetics: EJHG 17: 100–104. Available:http://www.pubmedcentral.nih.gov/articlerender.fcgi?artid=2985963&tool=pmcentrez&rendertype=abstract.

19. Chen W, Stambolian D, Edwards AO, Branham KE, Othman M, et al. (2010) Genetic variants near TIMP3 and high-density lipoprotein-associated loci influence susceptibility to age-related macular degeneration. Proceedings of the National Academy of Sciences of the United States of America 107: 7401–7406. Available:http://www.ncbi.nlm.nih.gov/pubmed/20385819.

20. Neale BM, Fagerness J, Reynolds R, Sobrin L, Parker M, et al. (2010) Genome-wide association study of advanced age-related macular degeneration identifies a role of the hepatic lipase gene (LIPC). Proceedings of the National Academy of Sciences of the United States of America 107: 7395–7400. Available:http://www.pubmedcentral.nih.gov/articlerender.fcgi?artid=2867697&tool=pmcentrez&rendertype=abstract.

21. Fritsche LG, Freitag-Wolf S, Bettecken T, Meitinger T, Keilhauer CN, et al. (2009) Age-related macular degeneration and functional promoter and coding variants of the apolipoprotein E gene. Human mutation 30: 1048–1053. Available:http://www.ncbi.nlm.nih.gov/pubmed/19384966.

22. Klaver CCW, Kliffen M, Duijn CMV, Hofman A, Cruts M, et al. (1998) Genetic Association of Apolipoprotein E with Age-Related Macular Degeneration. Ophthalmic Research. pp 200–206.

23. Yu Y, Bhangale TR, Fagerness J, Ripke S, Thorleifsson G, et al. (2011) Common variants near FRK/COL10A1 and VEGFA are associated with advanced age-related macular degeneration. Human molecular genetics 20: 3699–3709. Available:http://www.ncbi.nlm.nih.gov/pubmed/21665990.

24. Janssens ACJW, Aulchenko YS, Elefante S, Borsboom GJJM (2006) Predictive testing for complex diseases using multiple genes: Fact or fiction? Genetics in Medicine 8: 395–400. doi:10.1097/01.gim.0000229689.18263.f4.

25. Meigs JB, Shrader P, Sullivan LM, McAteer JB, Fox CS, et al. (2008) Genotype score in addition to common risk factors for prediction of type 2 diabetes. The New England journal of medicine 359: 2208–2219. Available:http://www.pubmedcentral.nih.gov/articlerender.fcgi?artid=2746946&tool=pmcentrez&rendertype=abstract.

26. Seddon JM, Reynolds R, Maller J, Fagerness Ja, Daly MJ, et al. (2009) Prediction model for prevalence and incidence of advanced age-related macular degeneration based on genetic, demographic, and environmental variables. Investigative ophthalmology & visual science 50: 2044–2053. Available:http://www.ncbi.nlm.nih.gov/pubmed/19117936.

27. Johnson AD, Handsaker RE, Pulit SL, Nizzari MM, O'Donnell CJ, et al. (2008) SNAP: a web-based tool for identification and annotation of proxy SNPs using HapMap. Bioinformatics (Oxford, England) 24: 2938–2939. Available:http://www.pubmedcentral.nih.gov/articlerender.fcgi?artid=2720775&tool=pmcentrez&rendertype=abstract.

28. Friedrich U, Myers Ca, Fritsche LG, Milenkovich a, Wolf a, et al. (2011) Risk and non risk associated variants at the 10q26 AMD locus influence ARMS2 mRNA expression but exclude pathogenic effects due to protein deficiency. Human Molecular Genetics 20: 1387–1399. Available:http://www.hmg.oxfordjournals.org/cgi/doi/10.1093/hmg/ddr020. Accessed 2011 Jan 21.

29. Purcell S, Neale B, Todd-Brown K, Thomas L, Ferreira MAR, et al. (2007) PLINK: a tool set for whole-genome association and population-based linkage analyses. American journal of human genetics 81: 559–575. Available:http://www.pubmedcentral.nih.gov/articlerender.fcgi?artid=1950838&tool=pmcentrez&rendertype=abstract.

30. Augood Ca, Vingerling JR, de Jong PTVM, Chakravarthy U, Seland J, et al. (2006) Prevalence of age-related maculopathy in older Europeans: the European Eye Study (EUREYE). Archives of ophthalmology 124: 529–535. Available:http://www.ncbi.nlm.nih.gov/pubmed/16606879.

31. Friedman DS, O'Colmain BJ, Muñoz B, Tomany SC, McCarty C, et al. (2004) Prevalence of age-related macular degeneration in the United States. Archives of ophthalmology 122: 564–572. Available:http://www.ncbi.nlm.nih.gov/pubmed/15078675.

32. Jonasson F, Arnarsson A, Eiríksdottir G, Harris TB, Launer IJ, et al. (2011) Prevalence of age-related macular degeneration in old persons: Age, Gene/environment Susceptibility Reykjavik Study. Ophthalmology 118: 825–830. Available:http://www.pubmedcentral.nih.gov/articlerender.fcgi?artid=3087833&tool=pmcentrez&rendertype=abstract. Accessed 2011 Jul 25.

33. Gibson J, Cree A, Collins A, Lotery A, Ennis S (2010) Determination of a gene and environment risk model for age-related macular degeneration. The British journal of ophthalmology 94: 1382–1387. Available:http://www.ncbi.nlm.nih.gov/pubmed/20576771.

34. Jakobsdottir J, Gorin MB, Conley YP, Ferrell RE, Weeks DE (2009) Interpretation of genetic association studies: markers with replicated highly significant odds ratios may be poor classifiers. PLoS genetics 5: e1000337. Available:http://www.pubmedcentral.nih.gov/articlerender.fcgi?artid=2629574&tool=pmcentrez&rendertype=abstract.

Author Contributions

Conceived and designed the experiments: IMH BHFW. Performed the experiments: FG LGF. Analyzed the data: FG LGF IMH. Contributed reagents/materials/analysis tools: CNK. Wrote the paper: FG IMH BHFW. Provided clinical follow-ups: CNK.

35. Spencer KL, Olson LM, Schnetz-Boutaud N, Gallins P, Agarwal A, et al. (2011) Using genetic variation and environmental risk factor data to identify individuals at high risk for age-related macular degeneration. PloS one 6: e17784. Available:http://www.ncbi.nlm.nih.gov/pubmed/21455292. Accessed 2011 3 Apr 3.

36. Seddon JM, Reynolds R, Yu Y, Daly MJ, Rosner B (2011) Risk models for progression to advanced age-related macular degeneration using demographic, environmental, genetic, and ocular factors. Ophthalmology 118: 2203–2211. Available:http://www.ncbi.nlm.nih.gov/pubmed/21959373. Accessed 2012 Mar 2.

37. Mistry K, Cable G (2003) Meta-Analysis of Prostate-Specific Antigen and Digital Rectal Examination as Screening Tests for Prostate Carcinoma. The Journal of the American Board of Family Medicine 16: 95–101. Available:http://www.jabfm.org/cgi/doi/10.3122/jabfm.16.2.95. Accessed 2012 Feb 18.

38. Miller JW (2010) Treatment of age-related macular degeneration: beyond VEGF. Japanese journal of ophthalmology 54: 523–528. Available:http://www.ncbi.nlm.nih.gov/pubmed/21191711. Accessed 2011 Feb 7.

39. Age-Related Eye Disease Study Research Group (2001) A randomized, placebo-controlled, clinical trial of high-dose supplementation with vitamins C and E, beta carotene, and zinc for age-related macular degeneration and vision loss: AREDS report no. 8. Archives of ophthalmology 119: 1417–1436. Available:http://www.pubmedcentral.nih.gov/articlerender.fcgi?artid=1462955&tool=pmcentrez&rendertype=abstract.

40. SanGiovanni JP, Chew EY, Clemons TE, Davis MD, Ferris FL, et al. (2007) The relationship of dietary lipid intake and age-related macular degeneration in a case-control study: AREDS Report No. 20. Archives of ophthalmology 125: 671–679. Available:http://www.ncbi.nlm.nih.gov/pubmed/17502507. Accessed 28 September 2011.

41. SanGiovanni JP, Chew EY, Clemons TE, Ferris FL, Gensler G, et al. (2007) The relationship of dietary carotenoid and vitamin A, E, and C intake with age-related macular degeneration in a case-control study: AREDS Report No. 22. Archives of ophthalmology 125: 1225–1232. Available:http://www.ncbi.nlm.nih.gov/pubmed/17846363.

42. Klein R, Davis MD, Magli YL, Segal P, Klein BE, et al. (1991) The Wisconsin age-related maculopathy grading system. Ophthalmology 98: 1128–1134. Available:http://www.ncbi.nlm.nih.gov/pubmed/1843453. Accessed 2011 Sept 28.

43. Bird a C, Bressler NM, Bressler SB, Chisholm IH, Coscas G, et al. (1995) An international classification and grading system for age-related maculopathy and age-related macular degeneration. The International ARM Epidemiological Study Group. Survey of ophthalmology 39: 367–374. Available:http://www.ncbi.nlm.nih.gov/pubmed/7604360.

44. R Development Core Team (2010) R: A Language and Environment for Statistical Computing. R website. Available:http://www.r-project.org/. Accessed 2012 May 2.

45. McFadden D (1974) Conditional Logit Analysis of Qualitative Choice Behavior. FRONTIERS IN ECONOMETRICS. pp 105–142. Available:http://www.econ.berkeley.edu/reprints/mcfadden/zarembka.pdf. /. Accessed 2012 May 2.

46. Hu B, Shao J, Palta M (2006) PSEUDO-R 2 IN LOGISTIC REGRESSION MODEL. Statistica Sinica 16: 847–860.

47. Chongsuvivatwong V (2010) epicalc: Epidemiological calculator. R website. Available:http://cran.r-project.org/web/packages/epicalc/index.html. /. Accessed 2012 May 2.

48. Lumley T (2009) rmeta: Meta-analysis. R package version 2.16. R website. Available:http://cran.r-project.org/web/packages/rmeta/index.html. /. Accessed 2012 May 2.

49. Steyerberg EW, Harrell FE, Borsboom GJ, Eijkemans MJ, Vergouwe Y, et al. (2001) Internal validation of predictive models: efficiency of some procedures for logistic regression analysis. Journal of clinical epidemiology 54: 774–781. Available:http://www.ncbi.nlm.nih.gov/pubmed/11470385.

50. Liu Q, Sung AH, Chen Z, Liu J, Huang X, et al. (2009) Feature selection and classification of MAQC-II breast cancer and multiple myeloma microarray gene expression data. PloS one 4: e8250. Available:http://www.pubmedcentral.nih.gov/articlerender.fcgi?artid=2789385&tool=pmcentrez&rendertype=abstract. Accessed 2012 Feb 29.

15

Genetic and Functional Dissection of ARMS2 in Age-Related Macular Degeneration and Polypoidal Choroidal Vasculopathy

Yong Cheng[1,2,9], LvZhen Huang[1,2,9], Xiaoxin Li[1,2*], Peng Zhou[3], Wotan Zeng[4], ChunFang Zhang[5]

1 Department of Ophthalmology, People's Hospital, Peking University, Beijing, China, 2 Key Laboratory of Vision Loss and Restoration, Ministry of Education, Beijing, China, 3 Department of Ophthalmology, Eye and ENT Hospital of Fudan University, Shanghai, China, 4 Chinese National Human Genome Center, Beijing, China, 5 Department of Clinical Epidemiology, People's Hospital, Peking University, Beijing, China

Abstract

Age-related maculopathy susceptibility 2(ARMS2) was suggested to be associated with neovascular age-related macular degeneration (nAMD) and polypoidal choroidal vasculopathy (PCV) in multiple genetic studies in Caucasians and Japanese. To date, no biological properties have been attributed to the putative protein in nAMD and PCV. The complete genes of ARMS2 and HTRA1 including all exons and the promoter region were assessed using direct sequencing technology in 284 unrelated mainland northern Chinese individuals: 96 nAMD patients, 92 PCV patients and 96 controls. Significant associations with both nAMD and PCV were observed in 2 polymorphisms of ARMS2 and HTRA1 rs11200638, with different genotypic distributions between nAMD and PCV ($p<0.001$). After adjusting for rs11200638, ARMS2 rs10490924 remained significantly associated with nAMD and PCV ($p<0.001$). Then we overexpressed wild-type ARMS2 and ARMS2 A69S mutation (rs10490924) in RF/6A cells and RPE cells as in vitro study model. Cell proliferation, attachment, migration and tube formation were analyzed for the first time. Compare with wild-type ARMS2, A69S mutation resulted in a significant increase in proliferation and attachment but inhibited cell migration. Moreover, neither wild-type ARMS2 nor A69S mutation affected tube formation of RF/6A cells. There is a strong and consistent association of the ARMS2/HTRA1 locus with both nAMD and PCV, suggesting the two disorders share, at least partially, similar molecular mechanisms. Neither wild-type ARMS2 nor A69S mutation had direct association with neovascularisation in the pathogenesis of AMD.

Editor: Hoong-Chien Lee, National Central University, Taiwan

Funding: Research supported by the National Basic Research Program of China (973 Program; #2011CB510200). The funders had no role in study design, data collection and analysis, decision to publish, or preparation of the manuscript.

Competing Interests: The authors have declared that no competing interests exist.

* E-mail: drlixiaoxin@163.com

⑨ These authors contributed equally to this work.

Introduction

Age-related macular degeneration (AMD) causes irreversible central vision loss and is the leading cause of blindness in the elderly population, characterized as chronic and progressive degeneration of photoreceptors, the underlying retinal pigment epithelium (RPE), Bruch's membrane, and possibly, the choriocapillaris in the macula. [1,2,3,4,5] AMD is divided clinically into dry and wet AMD. The "wet" form of the disease or neovascular, characterized by the development of choroidal neovascular (CNV) membranes, is the main cause of visual impairment in macular degeneration. [6].

Polypoidal choroidal vasculopathy (PCV) is a macular disease found in the elderly that is as prevalent as exudative AMD in the Asian population, accounting for approximately 30% to 50% of the total number of eyes with senile macular diseases in elderly Asians [7,8]. It is characterized by an abnormal choroidal vascular network with characteristic aneurismal dilations at the border of the vascular network [9,10]. The incidence of PCV in the Chinese and Japanese populations with neovascular AMD has been reported to be 24.5% and 54.7% respectively, compared with a much lower incidence in Caucasians [10,11,12]. PCV has been described as a separate clinical entity differing from AMD and other disease associated with subretinal neovascularization and it remains controversial as to whether or not PCV represents a subtype of nAMD [10].

Initial efforts to investigate the genetic basis of AMD utilized family studies. A concordance for AMD phenotypes in twins, and a higher risk of siblings of individuals with AMD have been reported [13,14,15,16,17,18]. These early studies lead to genome-wide linkage analyses using microsatellite markers to search for chromosomal regions associated with affected individuals [19,20,21,22,23,24,25,26,27]. Several candidate regions including 1q32 and 10q26 were confirmed by a metaanalysis [28]. Progress in genotyping and sequencing technology extended detailed genetic association studies to the entire genome. Age-related eye disease studies (AREDS) of AMD case-control subjects using 100,000 SNPs resulted in the identification of four chromosomal regions significantly associated with the disease, namely complement factor H (CFH) (1q32), the age-related maculopathy susceptibility 2(ARMS2)/Htra serine peptidase 1 (HTRA1) (10q26), complement component 2/complement factor B (C2/BF, 6p21), and complement component 3 (C3, 19p13). Based on

Table 1. Characteristics of the study population.

	nAMD	PCV	Controls	P
Total	96	92	96	
Males.n(%)	62(64.6)	48(52.2)	43(44.8)	>0.05
Female.n(%)	34(35.4)	44(47.8)	53(55.2)	
Mean age (±SD)(yrs)	70.3±8.8	69.5±9.4	67±9.5	0.08

the reported AMD-associated genes, genetic studies have been initiated to investigate the molecular mechanisms underlying nAMD and PCV. Recently, numerous studies by direct examinations of single nucleotide polymorphism (SNP) in chromosomal regions identified by genome-wide linkage analysis have presented several genes have been reported to be strongly associated with these two diseases, including complement factor H [29,30,31,32], ARMS2 and HTRA1 genes [33,34,35,36,37,38]. The association between AMD,PCV and three SNPs in these gene regions, namely rs1061170 (CFH), rs10490924 (ARMS2), and rs11200638 (HTRA1), were verified by a number of research groups in Caucasians and Japanese [33,36,37,38,39,40,41,42,43].

There is strong linkage disequilibrium (LD) across the ARMS2-HTRA1 region, making genetic association studies alone insufficient to distinguish between the two candidates. Instead, a comprehensive characterization of AMD-associated variants in the region of high LD is warranted, closely accompanied by a sophisticated analysis of their possible functional relevance in the disease process. Nevertheless, reports of a causal variant in the promoter region of HTRA1 [33,34] could not be verified by others [37]. In contrast, ARMS2 is an evolutionarily recent gene within the primate lineage and, so far, no biological properties have been attributed to the putative protein.

In this study, we investigated the genetic determinants of nAMD and PCV to highlight their genetic differentiation. We sequenced the entire ARMS2 and HTRA1 gene including all exons and the promoter region. Our intention was to investigate whether these associations occur in Chinese patients with nAMD and PCV from Northern Chinese and second, sought to investigate the biological function of ARMS2.

Materials and Methods

Subjects

Two hundred and eighty-four unrelated northern Chinese were studied (Table 1); 96 patients had neovascular Age-Related Macular Degeneration (nAMD) (mean age ± standard deviation [SD], 70.3±8.8 years; ratio of men to woman, 64.6:35.4×) and 92 patients had Polypoidal Choroidal Vasculopathy (PCV) (mean age ± SD, 69.5±9.4 years; ratio of men to woman, 52.2:47.8). For controls, 96 individuals without age-related maculopathy (ARM) were studied (mean age ± SD, 67±9.5 years; ratio of men to woman, 44.8:55.2). They were recruited at the Department of Ophthalmology in the Peking University People's Hospital. The study was approved by the Ethnic Committee of Peking University People's Hospital. An informed consent process was established following the guidelines of the Helsinki Declaration, and consent forms were signed by all subjects. All subjects received a standard ophthalmic examination, including visual acuity measurement, slit-lamp biomicroscopy, and dilated fundus examination that performed by a retinal specialist. All cases with Age-Related Macular Degeneration (AMD) and Polypoidal Choroidal Vasculopathy (PCV) underwent fluorescein angiography, optic coherence tomography (OCT), and indocyanine green angiograms with HRA2 (Heidelberg Engineering, Heidelberg, Germany). Diagnosis of neovascular AMD (nAMD) or age related maculopathy (ARM) was defined by International Classification System for ARM. [44] The diagnosis of PCV was based on indocyanine green angiography (ICGA) results, which showed a branching vascular network that terminated in aneurysmal enlargements, that is, polypoidal lesions. Eyes with other macular abnormalities, such as pathologic myopia, idiopathic choroidal neovascularization (CNV), presumed ocular histoplasmosis, angioid streaks, and other secondary CNV, were excluded. Normal controls were defined as no clinical evidence of early or late AMD in either eye or any other eye diseases except mild age-related cataract. Subjects with severe cataracts were excluded from the study.

Genomic DNA Extraction and PCR Amplification

Genomic DNAs were extracted from venous blood leukocytes with a genomic extraction kit (Beijing eBios Biotechnology Co., Ltd). A PCR amplification kit was purchased from Dingguo Biotechnology (Beijing) Co., Ltd. The PCR primers were designed by using Primer 3 online design tool and synthesized by Invitrogen

Table 2. Polymorphisms in the ARMS2 gene lesion: Distribution and Genotypes in neovascular Age-Related Macular Degeneration (nAMD), Polypoidal Choroidal Vasculopathy, and Controls in the northern Chinese Population.

Marker	Relative Position	Risk Allele	WT Allele	Risk Allele Frequency				p value* & OR(95%CI)**		
				nAMD	PCV	Controls		nAMD-Control	PCV-Control	nAMD-PCV
c.147G>T	Exon 1	T	G	0.43	0.31	0.39	p values	0.425	0.099	0.016
							OR (95%CI)	1.18(0.78–1.78)	0.69(0.45–1.07)	0.59(0.38–0.91)
c.148T>A	Exon 1	A	T	0.43	0.31	0.49	p values	0.211	3.17×10⁻⁴	0.016
							OR (95%CI)	0.77(0.52–1.19)	0.45(0.29–0.70)	0.59(0.38–0.91)
rs10490924	Exon 1	T	G	0.71	0.69	0.25	p values	3.49×10⁻¹⁹	7.98×10⁻¹⁵	0.309
							OR (95%CI)	7.34(4.66–11.57)	5.81(3.67–9.20)	0.79(0.50–1.24)
EU 427528 (310–311)	Intron 1	TG	–	0.70	0.66	0.26	p values	1.31×10⁻¹⁷	4.22×10⁻¹⁴	0.419
							OR (95%CI)	6.61(4.22–10.37)	5.50(3.49–8.69)	0.83(0.53–1.30)

*: p-Value <0.05 is considered to be statistically significant and they are shown in bold.
**: OR(95%CI): Odds ratios are given for the risk allele compared with the wildtype allele.

Table 3. Polymorphisms in the *ARMS2* gene lesion: Distribution and Allele in neovascular Age-Related Macular Degeneration (nAMD), Polypoidal Choroidal Vasculopathy, and Controls in the northern Chinese Population.

SNP	Genotype Distribution (%)			nAMD Vs Controls			PCV Vs Controls			nAMD Vs PCV		
	nAMD	PCV	Controls	Genotypic	Homo*	Heter**	Genotypic	Homo*	Heter**	Genotypic	Homo*	Heter**
c.147G>T												
GG	13(13.8)	32(38.6)	21(21.9)	NA	NA	0.148	NA	NA	0.015	NA	NA	1.63×10^{-4}
GT	81(86.2)	51(61.4)	75(78.1)		NA	1.75	NA	NA	0.45	NA	NA	0.26
						(0.82–3.73)			(0.23–0.86)			(0.12–0.53)
TT^§	0	0	0									
c.148 T>A												
TT	13(13.8)	32(38.6)	1(1.0)	NA	NA	7.43×10^{-4}	NA	NA	1.09×10^{-10}	NA	NA	1.63×10^{-4}
TA	81(86.2)	51(61.4)	95(99.0)		NA	0.07	NA	NA	0.02	NA	NA	3.91
						(0.01–0.51)			(0.002–0.13)			(1.88–8.14)
AA^§	0	0	0									
rs 10490924												
GG	10(10.6)	13(15.7)	58(61.1)	9.94×10^{-14}	2.06×10^{-14}	6.11×10^{-7}	1.97×10^{-10}	3.90×10^{-11}	3.06×10^{-5}	0.585	0.3	0.427
GT	34(36.2)	30(36.1)	26(27.4)		26.36	7.59		16.22	5.15		1.63	1.47
					(10.34–67.23)	(3.24–17.63)		(6.61–39.84)	(2.32–11.44)		(0.65–4.09)	(0.56–3.85)
TT^§	50(53.2)	40(48.2)	11(11.5)									
EU427528												
NO^#	11(11.7)	13(15.7)	57(60.0)	9.57×10^{-13}	2.47×10^{-12}	1.61×10^{-6}	4.60×10^{-10}	9.59×10^{-10}	3.54×10^{-5}	0.719	0.417	0.546
HE^#	35(37.2)	31(37.3)	27(28.4)		17.77	6.72		12.21	5.03		0.69	0.75
(310–311)					(7.38–42.75)	(2.97–15.22)		(5.18–28.80)	(2.28–11.13)		(0.28–1.70)	(0.29–1.91)
HO^###	48(51.1)	39(47.0)	11(11.6)									

After Bonferroni correction the represent significance at $P<0.05/8 = 0.00625$.
*Homozygous;Comparing the likelihood of individuals with two copies of the risk allele versus individuals with no copies of the risk allele;
**Hetrozygous;Comparing the likelihood of individuals with one copy of the risk allele versus individuals with no copies of the risk allele;
§homozygous for the risk factor.
##HE: Hetrozygous insertion.
###HO: Homozygous insertion.

Table 4. Polymorphisms in the *HTRA1* gene lesion: Distribution and Genotypes in neovascular Age-Related Macular Degeneration (nAMD), Polypoidal Choroidal Vasculopathy, and Controls in the northern Chinese Population.

Marker	Relative Position	Risk Allele	WT Allele	Risk Allele Frequency					*p* value* & OR(95%CI)**		
				nAMD	PCV	Controls			nAMD-Control	PCV-Control	nAMD-PCV
rs11200638	Promoter	A	G	0.73	0.65	0.45		P values	1.42×10^{-7}	1.05×10^{-4}	0.157
								OR (95%CI)	3.13(2.03–4.82)	2.28(1.50–3.46)	0.73(0.47–1.13)
rs55928386	Promoter	T	C	0.03	0.05	0.07		P values	0.050	0.379	0.267
								OR (95%CI)	0.36(0.13–1.04)	0.68(0.28–1.62)	0.54(0.18–1.63)
rs2672598	Promoter	C	T	0.85	0.79	0.73		P values	0.004	0.177	0.121
								OR (95%CI)	2.14(1.27–3.61)	1.40(0.86–2.26)	1.53(0.89–2.64)
rs72171000	Promoter	–	TGTT	0.16	0.11	0.09		P values	0.064	0.655	0.162
								OR (95%CI)	1.79(0.96–3.34)	1.17(0.60–2.28)	0.65(0.36–1.19)

*p-Value <0.05 is considered to be statistically significant and they are shown in bold.
**OR(95%CI): Odds ratios are given for the risk allele compared with the wildtype allele.

Corporation Shanghai. A PCR amplification was performed in 50 µL reactions containing 50 ng genomic DNA, 20µM primers, 32 µL ddH$_2$O, 2.5 mM dNTPs, 2.0U Taq, and 5 µL 10×PCR Buffer. Thermo-cycling was carried out with an initial denaturation step of 94C for 5 min, followed by 10 cycles of 94 C for 30 s, 60 C for 1 min and 72C for 45 s; then 30 cycles of 94C for 30 sec, 55C for 1 min, and 72C for 45 s; and ended with a final single extension at 72C for 3 min. The PCR products were assessed by 1.0% agarose gel electrophoresis; then DNA bands with correct sizes were purified with a 96-well PCR purification kit (MILLIPORE, USA).

Genotyping by Sequencing

All above purified PCR products were directly sequenced with ABI 3730XL DNA sequencer. Variants in *ARMS2* and HTRA1 genes were identified by an ABI automatic allele calling software. Genotyping had 99% completeness and 99% accuracy as determined by random re-sequencing of 10% samples.

Plasmid Constructs

The entire open reading frame of the wild-type human ARMS2 gene (XM_001131263) was amplified from ARPE19 cells by RT-PCR using gene-specific primers (forward: CACACTCCATGATCCCAGCTTCTAAAATCCACACTGAGCTCTGC-3; reverse: GCAGAGCTCAGTGTGGATTTTAGAAGCTGGGATCATGGAGTGTG-3) and was subsequently cloned in pcDNA3.1-CT-GFP to construct a human wild-type ARMS2 expression vector using the pcDNATM3.1 Directional TOPO expression kit (Invitrogen, Carlsbad, CA, USA) according to the manufacturer's instructions. All constructs were verified before use by direct sequencing. Plasmid containing the ARMS2 A69S mutation (rs10490924, G270T in mRNA) was made by site-directed mutagenesis using oligonucleotides annealed to the target sequence and the QuikChange kit (Stratagene Santa Clara, CA, USA).

Cell Culture and Reagents

RF/6A cells (CRL-1780 cell line) and human RPE cells (ARPE-19 cell line) were obtained from the American Tissue Culture Collection (Manassas, VA) and were cultured in Dulbecco's Modified Eagle Media (DMEM) with 10% fetal bovine serum (FBS, Gibco, Invitrogen, Grand island, NY), 100 units/ml penicillin, 100 µg/ml streptomycin (Sigma, St. Louis, MO) at 37°C under 5% CO$_2$, and 95% humidified air. Before hypoxia, the media was replaced with DMEM free of serum. The cells were then incubated overnight and perfused with 1% O$_2$, 94% N^2, and 5% CO$_2$ in a CO$_2$ incubator for 24 h [45]. Cells were transfected with plasmid DNA (pcDNA3.1-CT-GFP–270G/T as test vectors and pReceiver-M29-Basic as a negative control). Transfections were performed using Lipofectamine 2000 reagent (Invitrogen) according to the manufacturer's protocol.

RT-PCR and Relative Quantitative Real-time PCR

Total RNA was isolated using a TRIzol reagent (Invitrogen). The first strand of cDNA was synthesized with 1 ug of total RNA, oligo(dT)$_{15}$ primer, and AMV reverse transcriptase (Promega). The primers used in RT-PCR were ARMS2: forward, 5′-GGTCTAGATAGTTATTAATAGTAATCAAT -3′; reverse, 5′- GAATTCACCTTGCTGCAGTGTGGATG -3′; and β-actin: forward, 5′-AGCGGGAAATCGTGCGTG-3′; reverse, 5′-CAGGGTACATGGTGGTGCC-3′ Real-time PCR reactions were performed with SYBR Green PCR master mix (Roche, Basel, Switzerland). The specificity of the PCR amplification products was checked by performing dissociation melting-curve analysis and by 1% agarose gel electrophoresis. Quantification analysis of BMP4 mRNA was normalized with a housekeeping gene, β-actin, as an internal control. Relative multiples of changes in mRNA expression were determined by calculating $2^{-\Delta\Delta ct.}$

Western Blot Analysis

Proteins were extracted from cultured RF/6A cells and ARPE-19 cells using T-PER tissue protein extraction reagent (Pierce, Rockford, IL, USA), and the protein concentration was measured using the Bio-Rad protein assay kit (Bio-Rad, Hercules, CA, USA). Equal amounts of protein lysate (20–60 ug) were resolved on 10% Tris-HCl polyacrylamide gels and then transferred to a PVDF blotting membrane (Millipore, Billerica, MA, USA). After blocking, each membrane was incubated with antibodies specific for human ARMS2 and β-actin (Abcam, Cambridge, MA, USA). After incubation with peroxidase-conjugated goat anti-rabbit secondary antibodies (ZSGB-Bio, Beijing, China), protein bands were detected by chemiluminescence (Pierce). Western blots were repeated three times and qualitatively similar results were obtained.

Table 5. Polymorphisms in the *HTRA1* gene lesion: Distribution and Allele in neovascular Age-Related Macular Degeneration (nAMD), Polypoidal Choroidal Vasculopathy, and Controls in the northern Chinese Population.

SNP		Genotype Distribution (%)			nAMD Vs Controls			PCV Vs Controls			nAMD Vs PCV		
		nAMD	PCV	Controls	Genotypic	Homo*	Heter**	Genotypic	Homo*	Heter**	Genotypic	Homo*	Heter**
rs11200638	GG	11(11.8)	9(9.8)	30(32.3)	6.24×10^{-6}	4.74×10^{-6}	0.115	3.53×10^{-4}	8.23×10^{-5}	2.19×10^{-3}	0.048	0.779	0.212
	GA	30(32.3)	46(50.0)	42(45.2)		6.75	1.95		5.87	3.65		0.87	1.87
						(2.87–15.91)	(0.85–4.49)		(2.35–14.70)	(1.55–8.58)		(0.33–2.31)	(0.69–5.06)
	AA$^\$$	52(55.9)	37(40.2)	21(22.5)	NA	NA		NA	NA		NA	NA	
rs55928386	CC	88(94.6)	84(91.3)	79(85.9)	NA	NA	0.045	NA	NA	0.163	0.491	NA	0.525
	CT	5(5.4)	7(7.6)	13(14.1)			0.35			0.51		NA	1.47
							(0.12–1.01)			(0.19–1.33)			(0.45–4.80)
	TT$^\$$	0	1(1.1)	0									
rs2672598	TT	3(3.2)	4(4.4)	4(4.4)	4.60×10^{-3}	0.386	0.636	0.24	0.774	0.675	0.262	0.553	0.933
	TC	21(22.6)	30(32.6)	41(44.6)		1.96	0.68		1.23	0.73		0.63	1.07
						(0.42–9.15)	(0.14–3.34)		(0.29–5.20)	(0.17–3.16)		(0.14–2.93)	(0.22–5.29)
	CC$^\$$	69(74.2)	58(63.0)	47(51.0)									
rs72171000	NO$^\#$	65(68.4)	73(79.3)	80(84.2)	2.17×10^{-3}	NA	0.002	0.29	0.369	0.218	0.11	NA	0.066
	HE$^{\#\#}$	30(31.6)	18(19.6)	12(12.6)		NA	3.08		0.37	1.64		NA	0.53
							(1.46–6.48)		(0.04–3.59)	(0.74–3.65)			(0.27–1.05)
	HO$^{\#\#\#}$	0	1(1.1)	3(3.2)									

After Bonferroni correction the represent significance at $P<0.05/8=0.00625$.
*Homozygous;Comparing the likelihood of individuals with two copies of the risk allele versus individuals with no copies of the risk allele;
**Hetrozygous;Comparing the likelihood of individuals with one copy of the risk allele versus individuals with no copies of the risk allele;
$^\$$homozygous for the risk factor.
$^{\#\#}$HE: Hetrozygous insertion.
$^{\#\#\#}$HO: Homozygous insertion.

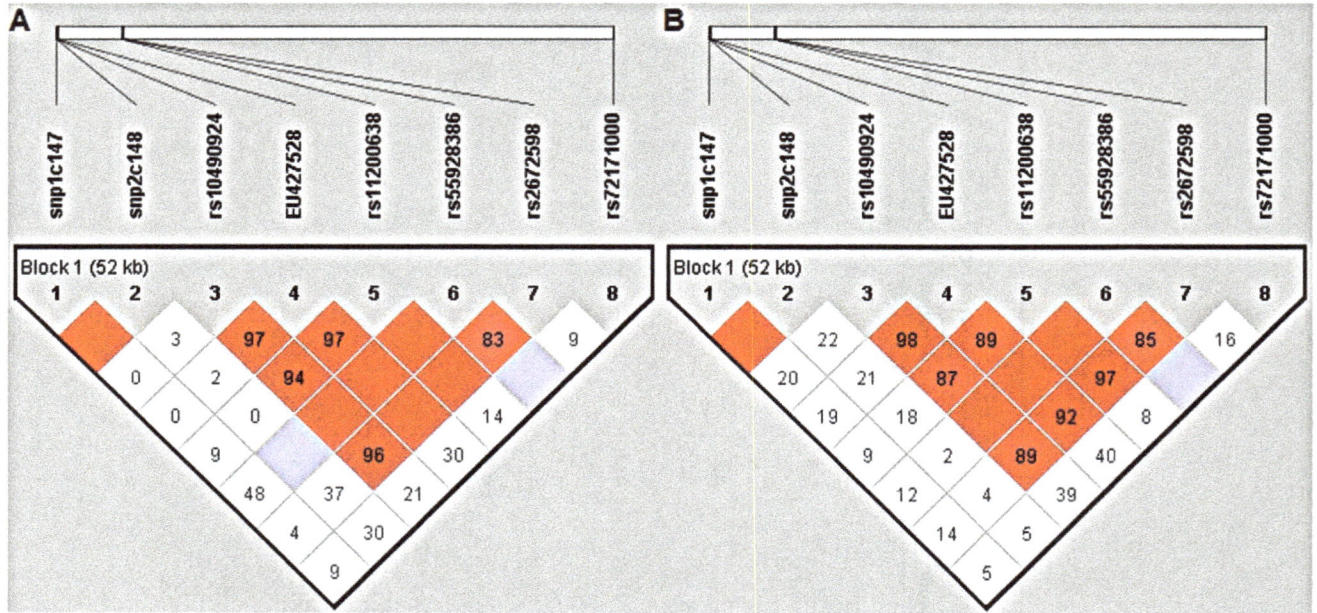

Figure 1. Analysis of pair-wise LD across *ARMS2* and *HTRA1* SNPs in northern Chinese PCV and nAMD cohort. A) Analysis of pair-wise LD across the eight *ARMS2* and *HTRA1* SNPs in northern Chinese PCV cohort. B) Analysis of pair-wise LD across the eight *ARMS2* and *HTRA1* SNPs in northern Chinese nAMD cohort. The relative physical position of each SNP is given in the upper diagram. The pairwise D′ between all SNPs is given below each SNP combination. And when D′ = 1.0, no number is given inside the square. Bright red squares indicate D′≥0.90 and LOD≥2. Bright red squares indicate D′<0.90 and LOD≥2. White squares indicate D′<0.90 and LOD<2.

Cell Proliferation Assay

To assess cell proliferation, a 3-[4,5-dimethylthiazol-2-yl]-2,5-diphenyltetrazolium bromide (MTT; Roche, Molecular Biochemicals, Mannheim, Germany) assay was used. Briefly, RF/6A cells and ARPE-19 cells were plated at a density of 2×10^3 cells per well in 96-well culture plates. After attachment, the culture medium was changed to DMEM containing 10% FBS, and the cells were incubated for 24 h. After reaching 80% confluence, the cells were starved with DMEM containing 1% FBS for 6 h and then were transfected with a mixture of Lipofectamine 2000 (Invitrogen) and plasmids pcDNA3.1-CT-GFP–270G/T, pReceiver-M29-Basic, respectively. After 24 h, MTT was added to the culture medium and the cells were incubated for an additional 4 h. Formazan crystals that formed were then dissolved by the addition of dimethyl sulfoxide (100 μl/well). Absorbance at 570 nm was measured using an ELISA plate reader (Dynatech Medica, Guernsey, UK) [46]. Cell proliferation was measured by a modified MTT assay on 24, 48, 72, and 96 h. Media were changed on day 3. Each experiment

Table 6. Haplotype analysis of *ARMS2* and *HTRA1* polymorphisms in exudative AMD and PCV.

No.	SNPs included	Haplotype	Frequency			AMD-Control		PCV-Control		AMD-PCV	
			AMD	PCV	Control	p	OR(95%CI)	p	OR(95%CI)	p	OR(95%CI)
1.	rs10490924	G1	0.287	0.337	0.742	8.89×10^{-19}	0.140	1.81×10^{-14}	0.177	0.3093	0.792
	EU 427528						(0.089–2.20)		(0.112–0.280)		(0.504–1.243)
	(310–311)	T2	0.697	0.657	0.247	2.08×10^{-18}	6.993	8.24×10^{-15}	5.818	0.4194	1.202
							(4.445–11.001)		(3.674–9.213)		(0.769–1.878)
2.	rs 10490924	TA	0.697	0.614	0.244	1.92×10^{-18}	6.953	2.37×10^{-12}	4.691	0.1038	1.452
							(4.436–10.904)		(3.015–7.299)		(0.946–2.227)
	rs 11200638	GG	0.269	0.298	0.544	2.47×10^{-8}	0.300	1.57×10^{-6}	0.361	0.4941	0.871
							(0.195–0.460)		(0.236–0.552)		(0.556–1.346)
3.	rs 11200638	ACC	0.720	0.651	0.452	1.42×10^{-7}	3.129	1.0×10^{-4}	2.277	0.1557	1.374
							(2.033–4.816)		(1.498–3.461)		(0.884–2.136)
	rs 55928386	GCC	0.134	0.142	0.269	9.0×10^{-4}	0.422	0.0019	0.436	0.842	0.944
	rs 2672598						(0.248–0.719)		(0.258–0.737)		(0.522–1.704)

*For the polymorphisms that were not a single nucleotide change, the wild type was denoted as 1 and the variant denoted as 2.

Table 7. Logistic regression analysis of SNPs in ARMS2 and HTRA1 between AMD and PCV.

	AMD				PCV			
	rs10490924		rs11200638		rs10490924		rs11200638	
	adjusted P	OR (95%CI)	adjusted P	OR (95%CI)	adjusted P	OR (95%CI)	adjusted P	OR (95%CI)
c.147G>T	4.980×10^{-11}	13.937 (6.352, 30.577)	0.002	3.354 (1.553, 7.244)	2.488×10^{-8}	7.912 (3.823, 16.373)	3.755×10^{-4}	5.096 (2.077, 12.501)
c.148 T>A	2.792×10^{-10}	14.712 (6.382, 33.912)	0.001	3.910 (1.724, 8.869)	5.568×10^{-7}	8.883 (3.777, 20.891)	0.004	4.219 (1.571, 11.327)
rs 10490924	–	–	0.043	0.114 (0.014, 0.931)	–	–	0.793	1.167 (0.367, 3.714)
EU427528 (310–311)	–	–	0.043	0.113 (0.014, 0.931)	–	–	0.751	1.207 (0.379, 3.845)
rs 11200638	5.926×10^{-5}	63.749 (8.390,484.385)	–	–	1.259×10^{-5}	7.752 (3.092, 19.436)	–	–
rs 55928386	5.097×10^{-10}	12.602 (5.668, 28.015)	0.005	3.192 (1.431, 7.119)	1.190×10^{-8}	9.241 (4.302, 19.848)	0.001	4.624 (1.932, 4.066)
rs 2672598	2.735×10^{-10}	17.192 (7.109, 41.576)	0.001	4.298 (1.822, 10.141)	6.003×10^{-9}	10.400 (4.724, 22.894)	1.715×10^{-4}	6.961 (2.530, 19.152)
rs 72171000	5.361×10^{-10}	23.736 (8.733, 64.512)	4.144×10^{-4}	4.301 (1.914, 9.666)	6.846×10^{-9}	9.549 (4.451, 20.483)	2.597×10^{-4}	4.622 (2.033, 10.510)

P value and OR (95%CI) of rs10490924 and rs11200638 after adjusting for the following SNPs.

ment was undertaken using three wells and was performed at least three times.

Cell Attachment Assay

Ninety-six-well plates coated with 1.25 µg/ml fibronectin in 100 µl of PBS were put into the incubator overnight at 4°C. Transfected cells (1×104) were trypsinized, added to each well, and allowed to attach for 6 h [47]. The cells were then washed gently twice with PBS, and 150 µl fresh medium was added to each well with MTT. The absorbance was measured with an ELISA plate reader at 570 nm. We used three different wells to detect the cell attachment and repeated all the experiments three times.

Cell Migration

Migration assay was performed as described before [48]. Briefly, 2×104 cells were placed in the upper chamber in a final volume of 200 µl of serum-free medium. Next 10% FBS was placed in the bottom chamber for a final volume of 600 µl. All migration assays were conducted for 6 h at 37°C. At the end of the assay, the cells were fixed in 4% PFA and stained with DAPI for 15 min. Remaining cells were wiped away with a cotton bud, and the membrane was imaged. The number of cells from five random fields of view was counted.

Tube Formation

The tube formation assay was conducted to investigate the effect of pcDNA3.1-CT-GFP–270G/T and pReceiver-M29-Basic on RF/6A in vitro. Aliquots (150 µl) of matrigel solution were poured into the 48 well plates (repeated 2 more times), and the plates were incubated at 37°C for 1 h in a 5% $CO2$ incubator to form a matrigel gel [49]. RF/6A cells (1×104 per well) treated with siRNA for 48 h were seeded on the matrigel and cultured in DMEM medium. The networks in matrigel from five randomly chosen fields were counted and photographed under a microscope.

Flow Cytometry

Apoptosis was measured with a FITC Annexin V Apoptosis Detection Kit (BD Science, US, Cat# 556547), according to the manufacturer's instructions. Briefly, ARPE-19 cells (1×10^5) after transfection were seeded in six-well plates and incubated for 24 h, 48 h, 72 h and 96 h. Then, the cells were detached with EDTA, washed in cold phosphate buffered saline (PBS), and stained with Annexin-V-FITC and propidium iodide (P.I.), according to the manufacturers' instructions. Flow cytometry analysis was immediately performed (ex/em = 488/530 nm). The samples were analyzed by flow cytometer (FACSCalibur; BD Biosciences, Franklin Lakes, NJ) with Cell Quest software (BD, Biosciences). Then, 10^4 cells were collected and divided into four groups: dead cells (Annexin V−/PI+, UL), late apoptotic cells (Annexin V+/PI+, UR), viable cells (Annexin V−/PI-, LL), and early apoptotic cells (Annexin V+/PI-, LR). The apoptotic rate was calculated as the percentage of early apoptotic cells (LR) plus late apoptotic cells (UR).

ARPE-19 cells (1×10^5) after transfection were seeded in six-well plates and incubated for 48 h. Cells were detached using ethylene diamine tetraacetic acid (EDTA), washed in ice-cold PBS (4°C), and treated with the BD Cycletest™ Plus DNA Reagent Kit (Becton Dickinson) according to the manufacturer's protocol. Samples were analyzed using a FACS Caliber cytometer (Becton Dickinson). Three samples were used per experiment, and each experiment was repeated.

Statistical Analysis

All the identified polymorphisms were assessed for Hardy-Weinberg equilibrium using χ^2 analysis. Allelic and genotypic distributions among different groups were compared using the χ^2

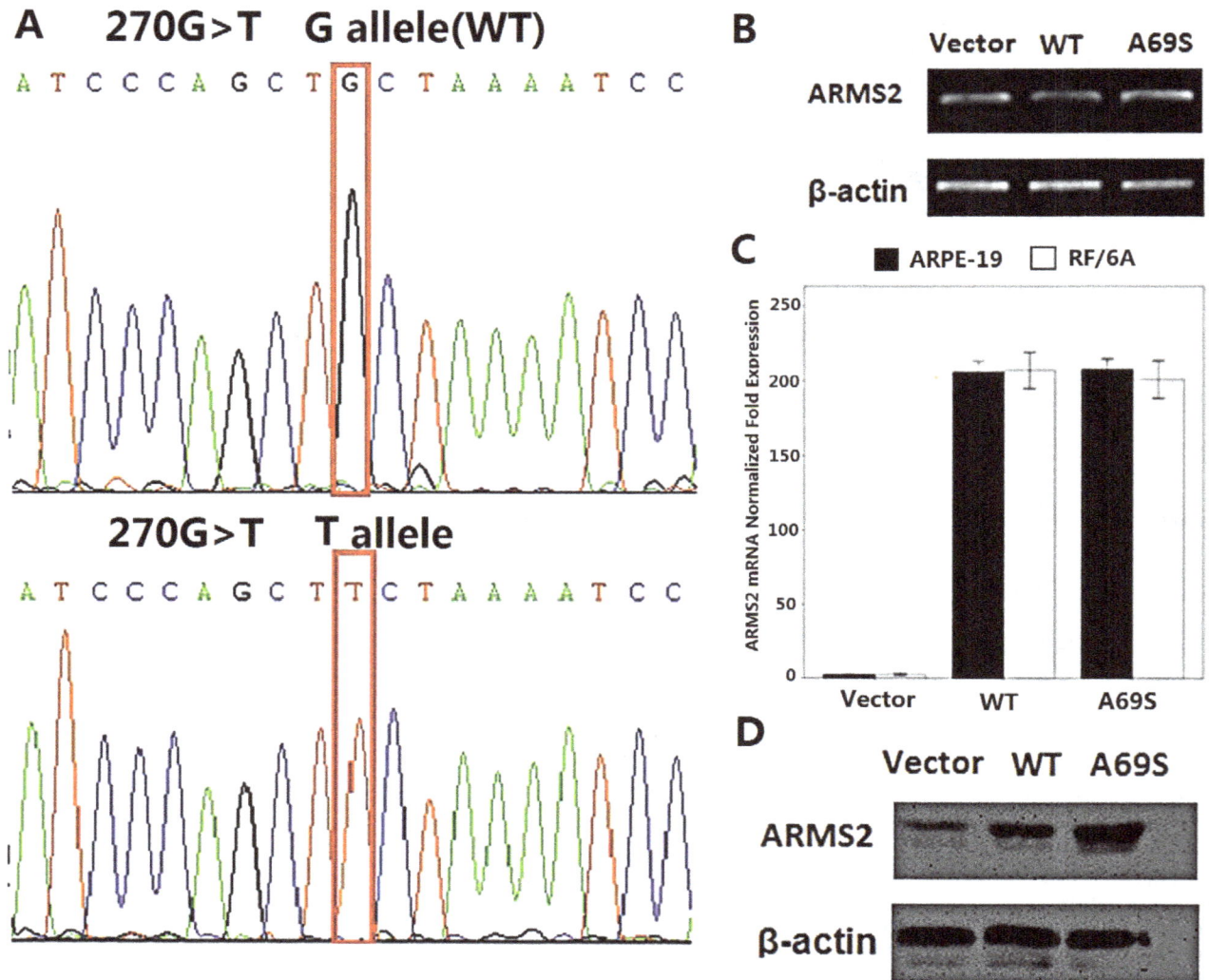

Figure 2. Rs10490924 (A69S in a coding change) does not affect mRNA, protein, or surface expression of ARMS2. A)Direct sequencing verified the wild-type (WT) and G270T ARMS2 plasmids. B) RT-PCR showed no significant difference between wild-type and G270T ARMS2 mRNA expression. C) Real-time RT-PCR confirmed the mRNA level finding. D) Western blot showed that the levels and migrations of the SNP mutant proteins were comparable with wild type. All experiments were repeated >3 times.

test or Fisher's exact test, and logistic regression analysis was performed to identify the strongest associated SNPs in the *ARMS2/HTRA1* locus (SPSS, version 16.0; SPSS Science, Chicago, IL). LD and haplotype-based association analyses were performed (Haploview, version 4.2). All experiments were repeated ≥3 times. Statistical analyses were performed with Student's *t* test. Values are expressed as mean±SD. Values of $P<0.05$ were considered statistically significant.

Results

SNP Analysis

The complete gene of *ARMS2* including all exons and the promoter region were sequenced. Four polymorphisms (three single nucleotide polymorphisms [SNPs] including two novel SNPs: c.147G>T & c.148T>A, and one insertion) in which there was statistically significant among AMD patients, PCV patients and control subjects were identified. The distributions of the

polymorphisms and genotypes of the *ARMS2* gene for the 284 participants were presented in Table 2 and 3.

There was no significant difference in c.147G>T both between AMD patients and controls ($p = 0.425$; OR [95%CI] = 1.18 [0.78–1.78]) and between PCV patients and controls ($p = 0.099$; OR [95%CI] = 0.69 [0.45–1.07]). However, there was statistical significance between AMD patients and PCV patients ($p = 0.016$; OR [95%CI] = 0.59 [0.38–0.91]). The frequency of risk T allele (AMD = 0.43, PCV = 0.31 & controls = 0.39) showed there was little difference among them. Therefore, the risk T allele had low association with AMD or PCV diseases. The similar results presented in c.148T>A. Comparing with c.147G>T, there was statistically significant difference between PCV patients and controls ($p = 3.17 \times 10^{-4}$) while the OR (95%CI) was 0.45 (0.29–0.70).

The significant association was found in rs10490924 and EU427528 (310–311). For rs10490924, there was a great difference both between AMD patients and controls

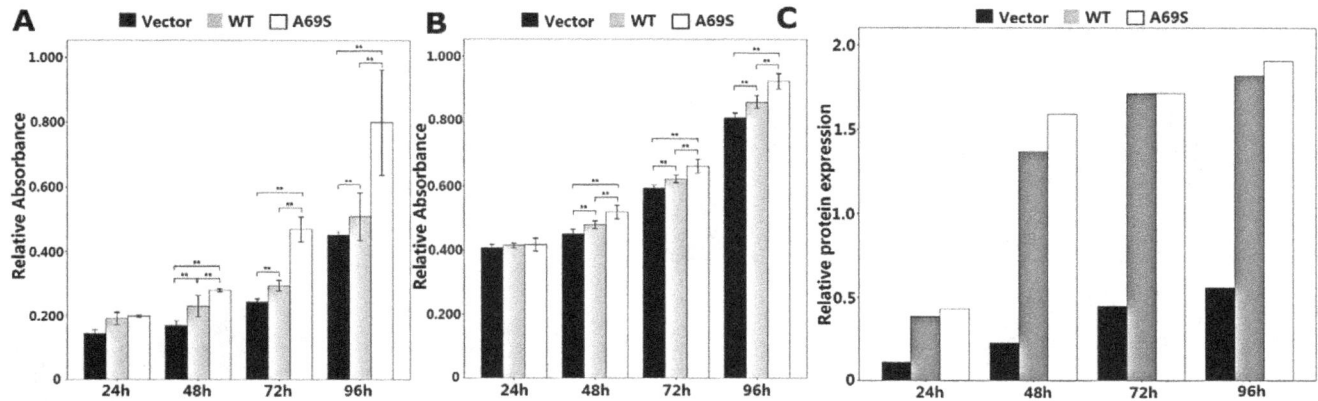

Figure 3. Effect of wild-type ARMS2 and rs10490924 on the proliferation of RF/6A and human RPE cells. RF/6A (**A**) and ARPE-19 (**B**) cell proliferation was measured with an MTT assay at 24 h, 48 h, 72 h, 96 h. Values are the means±SD of at least three independent experiments. Asterisks denote values significantly different from those of cells treated with wild-type ARMS2 and rs10490924 compared to negative control (p<0.01). (**C**)The time course of the ARMS2 protein expression profile mirrored that for ARMS2 protein expression levels after transfection in ARPE-19 cells. Abbreviations: wild-type ARMS2 plasmid-treated cells (WT); rs10490924 plasmid -treated cells (G270T); pReceiver-M29-Basic plasmid-treated cells (Vector) (*P<0.05, **P<0.01).

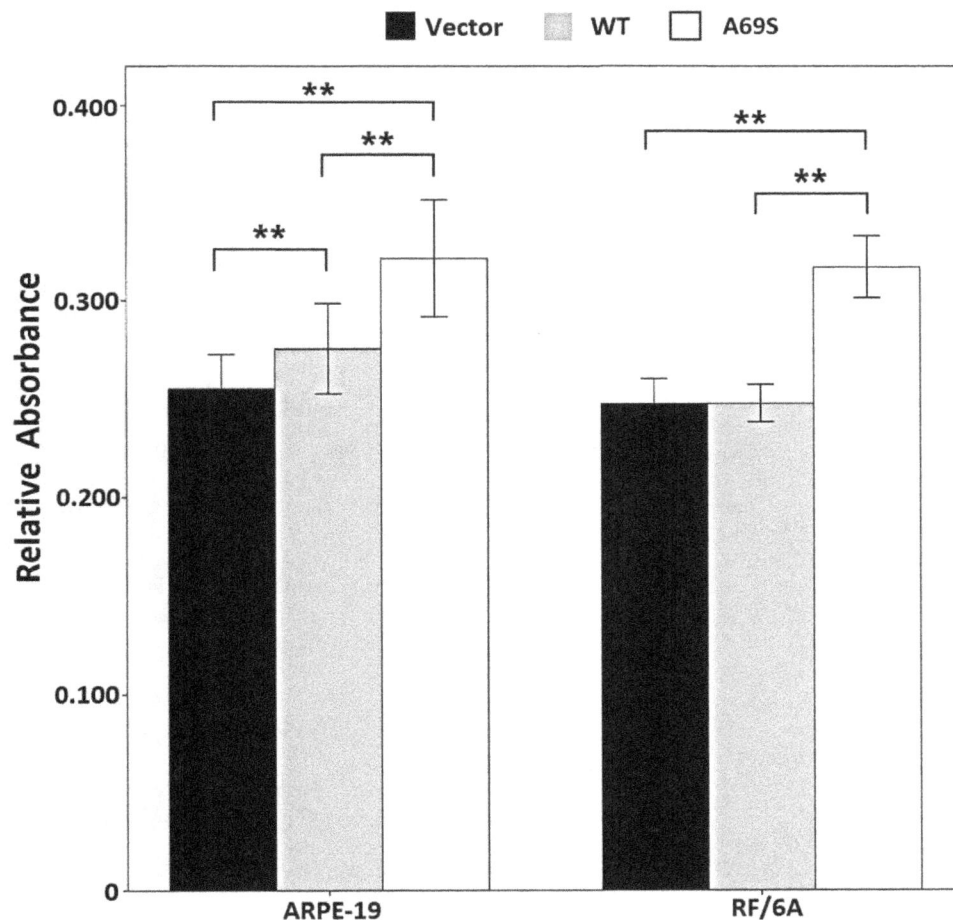

Figure 4. Effects of wild-type ARMS2 and rs10490924 on the attachment of RF/6A and RPE cells. Cell attachment was assessed after 6 h incubation and subsequent MTT assay. Values are the means±SD of at least three independent experiments. Asterisks denote values significantly different from those of cells treated with wild-type ARMS2 and rs10490924 compared to negative control (p<0.01). Abbreviations: wild-type ARMS2 plasmid-treated cells (WT); rs10490924 plasmid -treated cells (G270T); pReceiver-M29-Basic plasmid-treated cells (Vector) (*P<0.05, **P<0.01).

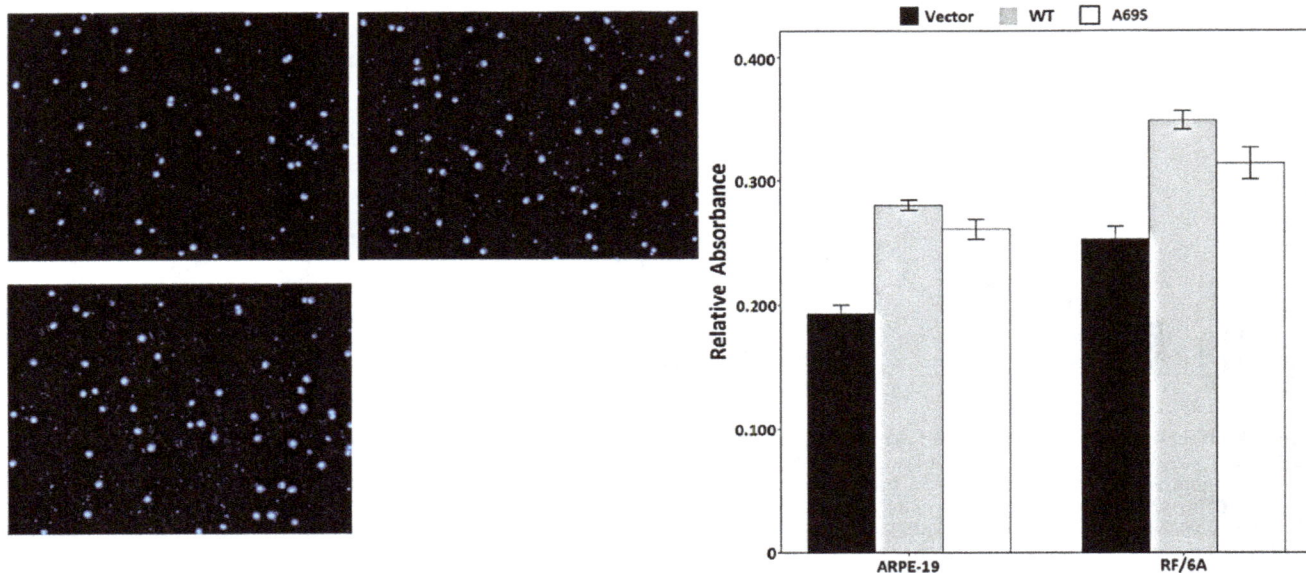

Figure 5. Effect of wild-type ARMS2 and rs10490924 on the migration of RF/6A and human RPE cells. The migratory activity of both cell lines was estimated based on the number of cells that had migrated through the filter of the chamber. A) Migrated cells of pReceiver-M29-Basic plasmid-treated RF/6A cells. B) Migrated cells of wild-type ARMS2 plasmid-treated RF/6A cells. C) Migrated cells of rs10490924 plasmid -treated RF/6A cells. Values are the means±SD of at least three independent experiments. D) The results showed that the number of migrating cells in the wild-type ARMS2 plasmid -treated group was the most during the three groups(p<0.01). Abbreviations: wild-type ARMS2 plasmid-treated cells (WT); rs10490924 plasmid -treated cells (G270T); pReceiver-M29-Basic plasmid-treated cells (Vector) (*P<0.05, **P<0.01).

$(p = 3.49 \times 10^{-19};$ OR [95%CI] = 7.34[4.66–11.57]) and between PCV patients and controls $(p = 7.98 \times 10^{-15};$ OR [95%CI] = 5.81[3.67–9.20]). The frequency of risk T allele was much higher in AMD patients (0.71) and in PCV patients (0.69) than in control subjects (0.25). It suggested that the risk allele was tightly associated with AMD and PCV in northern Chinese population. Meanwhile, the almost same results were presented in EU427528 (310–311). There was also a greatly significant difference both between AMD patients and controls $(p = 1.31 \times 10^{-17};$ OR [95%CI] = 6.61[4.22–10.37]) and between PCV patients and controls $(p = 4.22 \times 10^{-14};$ OR [95%CI] = 5.50[3.49–8.69]). The frequency of TG insertion in AMD patients and in PCV patients were 0.70 and 0.66, respectively, whereas the frequency in controls was 0.26. The risk allele of TG insertion had a strongly increased risk of developing AMD and PCV. However, between AMD patients and PCV patients, there was no statistical significance both in rs10490924 $(p = 0.309;$ OR [95%CI] = 0.79[0.50–1.24]) and in EU427528 (310–311) $(p = 0.419;$ OR [95%CI] = 0.83[0.53–1.30]).

The complete gene of *HTRA1* were also sequenced. Four polymorphisms in which there was statistically significant among AMD patients, PCV patients and control subjects were identified. The distributions of the polymorphisms and genotypes of the *HTRA1* gene for the 284 participants were presented in Table 4 and 5.

The significant association was found in rs11200638. For rs11200638, there was a great difference both between AMD patients and controls $(p = 1.42 \times 10^{-7};$ OR [95%CI] = 3.13[2.03–4.82]) and between PCV patients and controls $(p = 1.05 \times 10^{-4};$ OR [95%CI] = 2.28[1.50–3.46]). The frequency of risk G allele was much higher in AMD patients (0.73) and in PCV patients (0.65) than in control subjects (0.45). It suggested that the risk allele was tightly associated with AMD and PCV in northern Chinese population.

There was no significant difference in rs55928386 both between PCV patients and controls $(p = 0.379;$ OR [95%CI] = 0.68 [0.28–1.62]) and between AMD patients and PCV $(p = 0.267;$ OR [95%CI] = 0.54 [0.18–1.63]).However, there was statistical significance between AMD patients and controls $(p = 0.05;$ OR [95%CI] = 0.36 [0.13–1.04]). The frequency of risk T allele (AMD = 0.05, PCV = 0.379 & controls = 0.267) showed there was difference between AMD patients and controls and little difference between PCV patients and controls. Therefore, the risk T allele had association with AMD. The similar results presented in rs2672598.

There was no significant difference in rs72171000 both between AMD patients and controls $(p = 0.064;$ OR [95%CI] = 1.79 [0.96–3.34]) and between PCV patients and controls $(p = 0.655;$ OR [95%CI] = 1.17 [0.60–2.28]) and between AMD patients and PCV patients $(p = 0.162;$ OR [95%CI] = 0.65 [0.36–1.19]). The frequency of TGTT deletion (AMD = 0.064, PCV = 0.655 & controls = 0.162) showed there was little difference among them. Therefore, the TGTT deletion allele had low association with AMD or PCV diseases.

Linkage Disequilibrium (LD) and Haplotype Association Analysis

Haplotype analysis revealed an extensive LD across all the 8 common polymorphisms, except rs72171000, in AMD (Figure 1A) and in PCV (Figure 1B).

Within the ARMS2 gene, pair-wise LD analysis in AMD cases showed rs10490924 was in high LD with EU427528 (310–311) in AMD (D′ = 0.97, 95% CI: 4.445–11.001; Fig. 1A) and in PCV(D′ = 0.97, 95% CI: 3.674–9.213; Fig. 1B). One significant association was noted for the TTG haplotype (P = 2.08 × 10⁻¹⁸) that was present approximately three times higher frequency (69.7% vs. 24.7%) in controls than in AMD and (65.7% vs. 24.7%) in controls than in PCV, indicating that it was risky.

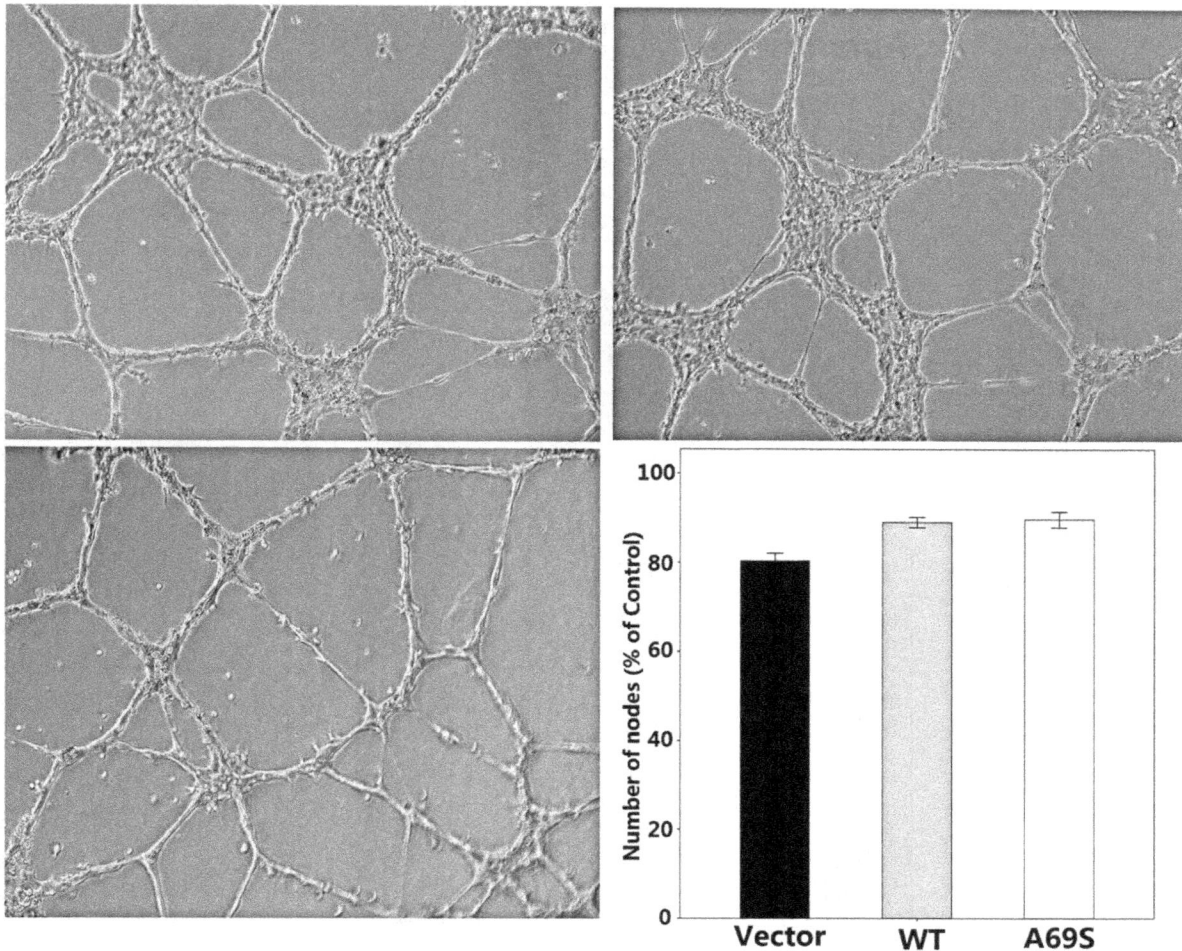

Figure 6. Effect of wild-type ARMS2 and rs10490924 on the tube formation of RF/6A cells. PReceiver-M29-Basic plasmid-treated RF/6A cells (A), wild-type ARMS2 plasmid-treated cells RF/6A cells (B) and rs10490924 plasmid -treated RF/6A cells (C) were plated on Matrigel as described in Methods. After 24 h of incubation, the three groups cells formed well organized capillary-like structures. Values are the means±SD of at least three independent experiments. There are no significant difference during the three groups (D, p>0.05). Abbreviations: wild-type ARMS2 plasmid-treated cells (WT); rs10490924 plasmid -treated cells (G270T); pReceiver-M29-Basic plasmid-treated cells (Vector).

Within HTRA1, among haplotypes defined by a risk SNPS(rs 11200638, rs 55928386, rs 2672598), a risk haplotype ACC and a non-risk haplotype GCC were significantly associated with both nAMD (p 1.42×10^{-7}; OR 3.129, 95% CI: 2.033–4.816 and p 9.0×10^{-4}; OR 0.422, 95% CI: 0.248–0.719, respectively) and PCV (p 1.0×10^{-4}, OR 2.277, 95% CI: 1.498–3.461 and p 0.0019, OR 0.436, 95% CI: 0.258–0.737, respectively; Table 6).

Moreover, haplotype analysis of rs10490924 and rs11200638 revealed that two haplotypes TA and GG were significantly associated with both nAMD (p 1.92×10^{-18}, OR 6.953, 95% CI: 4.436–10.904 and p 2.47×10^{-8}, OR 0.300, 95% CI: 0.195–0.460, respectively) and PCV (p 2.37×10^{-12}, OR 4.691, 95% CI: 3.015–7.299 and p 1.57×10^{-6}, OR 0.361, 95% CI: 0.236–0.552, respectively). There was no significant differences in haplotype frequencies between nAMD and PCV were also observed (p 0.1038, OR 1.452, 95% CI: 0.946–2.227 and p 0.4941, OR 0.871, 95% CI: 0.556–1.346, respectively).

We included the 8 polymorphisms used for haplotype analysis in logistic regression analysis. SNPs *ARMS2* rs10490924 and *HTRA1* rs11200638 were chosen for comparison since they showed strongest associations. Rs10490924 remained statistically signifi-

cant in AMD (p 5.926×10^{-5}) and in PCV (p 1.259×10^{-5}) after adjusting for other SNPs, including rs11200638 (Table 7).

SNP rs10490924 does not Affect mRNA, Protein, or Surface Expression of ARMS2

We next investigated the effect of the rs10490924 on ARMS2 expression. Wild-type ARMS2 and ARMS2 A69S mutation plasmids were verified before use by direct sequencing (Fig. 2*A*). Real-time PCR were performed to determine whether rs10490924 affected ARMS2 mRNA expression. No difference was found between ARMS2 wild-type and rs10490924 (Fig. 2*B*, *C*). To examine whether the rs10490924 affected protein expression, a Western blot was performed. β-Actin served as an internal loading control. The levels and migration of the mutant proteins were comparable with wild type (Fig. 2*D*).

Effects of Wild-type ARMS2 and rs10490924 on the Proliferation of RF/6A Cells and ARPE-19 Cells

The up-regulation of wild-type ARMS2 and rs10490924 both promoted cell proliferation in RF/6A cells and ARPE-19 cells at 48 compared with the proliferation of the pReceiver-M29-Basic

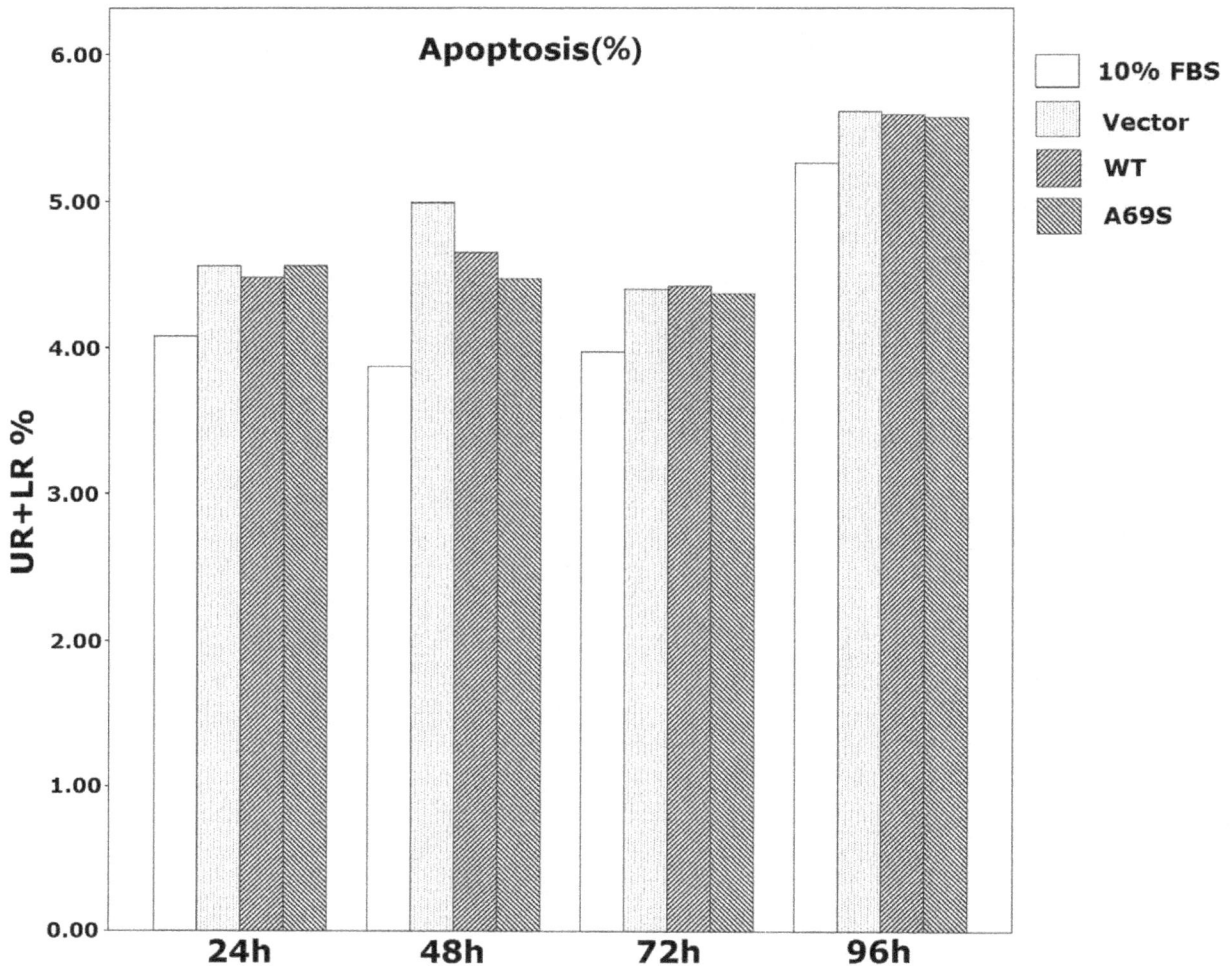

Figure 7. Effect of wild-type ARMS2 and rs10490924 on the apoptosis of human RPE cells. Apoptosis was quantified by flow cytometry measured by Annexin V and PI staining. Data are presented as mean±SEM.Each experiment was repeated at least three independent times. DMEM+10%FBS control was set to 100%.*P<0.05. UR: late apoptotic cells; LR: early apoptotic cells, UR+LR: apoptotic cells. Abbreviations: wild-type ARMS2 plasmid-treated cells (WT); rs10490924 plasmid -treated cells (G270T); pReceiver-M29-Basic plasmid-treated cells (Vector).

vectors as a negative control(p<0.01), and the up-regulation peaked on the fourth day (p<0.01). Compare with the wild-type, rs10490924 promoted cell proliferation more significantly (p<0.01; Figure 3A&B). The time course of the ARMS2 protein expression profile (Fig. 3C) mirrored that for ARMS2 protein expression levels after transfection in ARPE-19 cells.

Effects of Wild-type ARMS2 and rs10490924 on the Attachment and Migration of RF/6A Cells and ARPE-19 Cells

In the cell attachment assay, the rs10490924 increased the attachment capacity of RF/6A cells and of ARPE-19 cells (p<0.01; Figure 4) after 6h compared with that of the negative control. The negative control and wild-type ARMS2 groups were not significantly different in their capacities for cell attachment (p>0.05).

Next, we explored the role of wild-type ARMS2 and rs10490924 in the migration of RF/6A and RPE cells using a modified Boyden chamber in which the RF/6A and ARPE-19 cells migrated through a porous membrane. As shown in Figure 5,

the mean numbers of migrated cells among the wild-type ARMS2 and rs10490924-treated RF/6A and ARPE-19 cells were significantly higher than the number of migrated control cells (p<0.05), and then the mean numbers of migrated cells in the wild-type ARMS2 groups were highest during the three groups (p<0.05).

Effects of Wild-type ARMS2 and rs10490924 on the Tube Formation of RF/6A Cells

In a Matrigel assay, wild-type ARMS2 and rs10490924-treated RF/6A cells showed the same capacity to form a regular network compare with negative control. There was no significant difference during the three groups(p>0.05; Figure 6).

Effects of Wild-type ARMS2 and rs10490924 on ARPE-19 Apoptosis and Cell Cycle

FACS was used to evaluate early and late apoptosis effects. As shown in Table 8 and Figure 7, after transfection for 24, 48, 72 h and 96 h, the early and late apoptotic ARPE-19 cells showed no significant differences during the three groups, with the percentage of apoptotic cells (UR+LR%) (p>0.05).

Table 8. Summary of flow cytomery data of apoSptosis measured by Annexin V and PI.

Time point	%	10%FBS	Vector	WT	A69S
24 h	UL	0.93±0.13	2.18±0.15	2.27±0.07	2.13±0.18
	UR	2.07±0.03	2.47±0.11	2.15±0.03	2.33±0.21
	LL	94.99±0.28	93.26±0.36	93.25±0.38	93.31±0.20
	LR	2.01±0.21	2.09±0.43	2.33±0.36	2.23±0.27
	UR+LR	4.08±0.20	4.56±0.20	4.48±0.35	4.56±0.19
48 h	UL	1.43±0.13	1.85±0.03	2.31±0.08	2.16±0.19
	UR	1.15±0.02	1.24±0.08	1.27±0.07	1.29±0.13
	LL	94.6±0.13	93.16±0.32	93.04±0.69	93.37±0.38
	LR	2.82±0.16	3.75±0.38	3.38±0.61	3.18±0.38
	UR+LR	3.87±0.14	4.99±0.32	4.65±0.61	4.47±0.52
72 h	UL	1.62±0.19	2.15±0.13	2.31±0.11	2.36±0.21
	UR	1.25±0.02	1.23±0.09	1.34±0.10	1.39±0.15
	LL	94.41±0.13	93.45±0.25	93.27±0.63	93.37±0.40
	LR	2.72±0.16	3.17±0.31	3.08±0.54	2.88±0.36
	UR+LR	3.97±0.16	4.40±0.32	4.42±0.53	4.37±0.43
96 h	UL	2.10±0.28	1.90±0.08	1.57±0.09	2.27±0.14
	UR	1.96±0.05	1.97±0.06	1.84±0.13	2.25±0.11
	LL	92.64±0.41	92.49±0.23	92.84±0.40	92.16±0.33
	LR	3.30±0.13	3.64±0.28	3.75±0.38	3.32±0.21
	UR+LR	5.26±0.15	5.61±0.27	5.59±0.48	5.57±0.25

As shown in Figure 8, the wild-type ARMS2 and rs10490924 resulted in a significant reduction of ARPE-19 cells in the G0/G1 phase and promoted an accumulation of cells in the S phase compared to controls in 48 h. Of the cells treated, 60.20% and 57.6% were in the G1 phase when treated with the wild-type ARMS2 and rs10490924, respectively, compared to 69.62% of the control group in the G1 phase (p<0.01; Figure 8). Moreover, 29.12% and 38.01% were in the S phase of the cell cycle, respectively, compared to 19.62% of cells in the control group (p<0.01; Figure 8). 10.76% were in the G2/M phase treated with the rs10490924 in the G2/M phase, respectively, compared to 4.39% of the control group in the G2/M phase (p<0.05; Figure 8) and there was no significant difference between the wild-type ARMS2 and control groups in the number of cells in the G2/M phase (p>0.05; Figure 8).

Discussion

Neovascular AMD and PCV are important macular disorders sharing similar phenotypes and serious clinical complications, including hemorrhagic RPE detachment and vitreous hemorrhage [50], both of which have been used to classify PCV as a subtype of neovascular AMD [28]. However, there are discernable differences in their natural courses [51], responses to treatments and overall visual prognosis [52], indicating that PCV could be a type of macular disease that is different from AMD. Based on the reported AMD-associated genes [29,33,34,39], genetic studies have been initiated to investigate the molecular mechanisms underlying the two diseases. Results of genotype analysis, variants at 10q26,have indicated that neovascular AMD and PCV may share common genetic background [38,42,53]. The associated

variants at 10q26 overlap two known genes, *PLEKHA1*, *HTRA1*, and a predicted gene *ARMS2*. Each of these can have a plausible biological relationship to macular degeneration [28].

To clarify the genetic association and evaluate possible mechanism of disease susceptibility, we investigated the genetic profiles of nAMD and PCV through analysis of the *ARMS2/HTRA1* locus. A total of 8 polymorphisms in *ARMS2* and *HTRA1* were found to be associated with both diseases (Tables 2, 3, 4 and 5). Their genotype frequencies were all significantly different between nAMD and PCV (*p*<0.05). These results indicate resembling genetic effects in the *ARMS2/HTRA1* locus between the two diseases, but the size of the effects were different. Therefore, other genetic variations might also determine the development of exudative AMD and PCV. It is noted that, while the *p* values and ORs between the individual SNPs with AMD and with PCV may differ, the trend of associations remained the same (Tables 2, 3, 4 and 5). Therefore, the results showed that nAMD and PCV are subject to the same genetic influence as far as *ARMS2* and *HTRA1* SNPs are concerned.

In the study reported herein, the significant association was found in rs10490924 and EU427528 (310–311) in the ARMS2. For rs10490924, Our findings suggest risk allele is strongly associated with neovascular AMD and PCV, and with a stronger association in neovascular AMD than in PCV for northern Chinese population. This has been found in Janpanese and Caucasian [39,41,42,54,55]. Meanwhile, the almost same results were presented in EU427528 (310–311). a intron in ARMS2. Some reseaches have mentioned that this risk allele of TG insertion had a strongly increased risk of developing AMD and PCV [43,56]. Within HTRA1, there was statistical significance in rs55928386 and rs2672598 between AMD patients and controls, but not between PCV patients and controls. Therefore, the two allele had association with AMD, but not with PCV. Our findings also suggest that HTRA1 is involved in nAMD and in PCV for northern Chinese population. In the previous studies for the Japanese population, Kondo and Gotoh found that HTRA1 rs11200638 was significantly associated with PCV and nAMD although the odds ratios were higher for the nAMD cases than the PCV cases in Japanese [32,38]. Lee comparing PCV and controls in Chinese population in Singapore showed rs11200638 to be significantly associated with PCV [31] and Liang found ARMS2 in southern Chinese remained significantly associated with AMD but not with PCV [57]. However, in our study we found the risk allele was tightly associated with AMD and PCV in northern Chinese population. The different results may be due to the different genetic background between southern and northern Chinese population in mainland China.

Our data indicate that both rs11200638 and rs10490924 share the same LD block which contains ARMS2 and HTRA1. This result is consistent with previous Caucasian studies [34,39,54]. There is high linkage disequilibrium (LD) across the *ARMS2/HTRA1* region, adding to the difficulty in identifying true causal variant(s) by association mapping alone [36]. The association signal at 10q26 converges on a region of an extensive LD block spanning *ARMS2* and *HTRA1* [36,37]. This LD block harbors multiple susceptibility alleles of which the *ARMS2* rs10490924 has been reported to show the strongest evidence for association [37]. Two variants within this LD block that were correlated with A69S through strong LD–SNP rs11200638 in the promoter of HTRA1 [33,34] and the insertion/deletion polymorphism (c.(*)372_815de-l443ins54) in the 3'-UTR region of *ARMS2* [36] –have recently been proposed as causal variants based on mechanistic functional evidence, but there is no agreement across studies

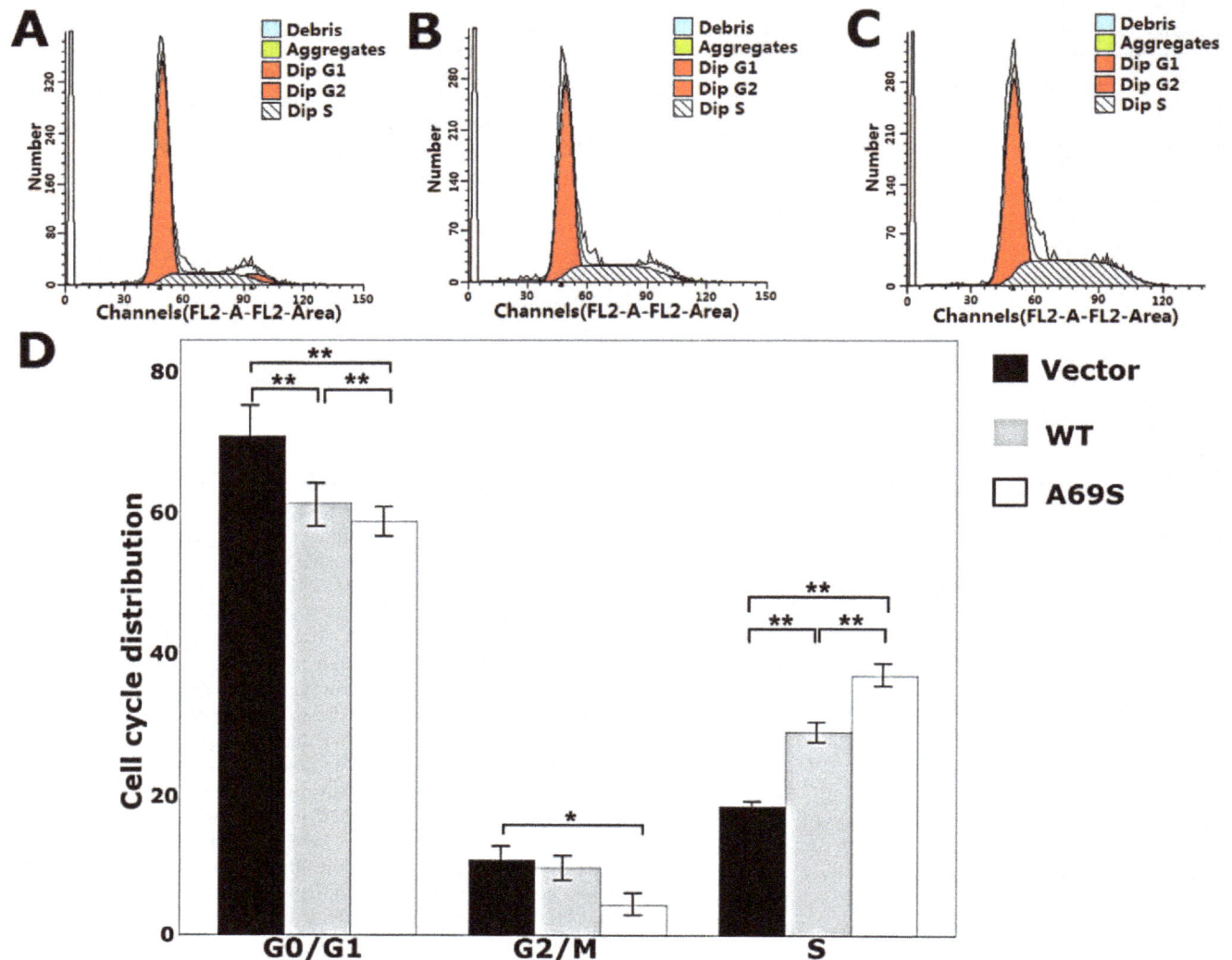

Figure 8. Effects of wild-type ARMS2 and rs10490924 on the cell cycles of human RPE cells. A) Cell cycle of pReceiver-M29-Basic plasmid-treated ARPE-19 cells. B) Cell cycle of wild-type ARMS2 plasmid-treated ARPE-19 cells. C) Cell cycle of rs10490924 plasmid-treated ARPE-19 cells. D) Data from the ARPE-19 cell cycle distribution of the control group, wild-type ARMS2 and rs10490924 group. Flow cytometric analysis demonstrates the effects of wild-type ARMS2 and rs10490924 on the human RPE cell cycle. The x-axis represents fluorescence intensity on a logarithmic scale and the y-axis represents the number of events. The results show that the fraction of cells in the G1 phase has decreased and the proportion of cells in the S phase has increased in the presence of wild-type ARMS2 and rs10490924-treated cells(*P<0.05, **P<0.01). Values are the mean±SD from three independent experiments. Abbreviations: wild-type ARMS2 plasmid-treated cells (WT); rs10490924 plasmid -treated cells (G270T); pReceiver-M29-Basic plasmid-treated cells (Vector).

[33,34,36,37,56,58,59]. Thus, the molecular basis of the susceptibility remains obscure.

To clarify the plausible biological function of wild-type ARMS2 and ARMS2 A69S mutation in AMD and PCV, we overexpressed these two genes in RF/6A cells and RPE cells as in vitro study model. Our findings showed that compare with wild-type ARMS2, A69S mutation resulted in a significant increase in proliferation and attachment but inhibited cell migration. However, neither wild-type ARMS2 nor A69S mutation affected cell apoptosis. Moreover, we found that neither wild-type ARMS2 nor A69S mutation affected tube formation of RF/6A cells. Tube formation is one of the main characteristics of retinal and choroid vascular endothelial cells, however, A69S mutation overexpressed RF/6A cells showed no significant difference with wild-type ARMS2

overexpressed ones on tubule formation. Therefore, neither wild-type ARMS2 nor A69S mutation might play a role in maintaining the tube-forming properties of RF/6A cells. Therefore, we thought neither wild-type ARMS2 nor A69S mutation had direct association with neovascularisation in the pathogenesis of AMD, which can explained ARMS2 has a significant association with pure dry AMD [60,61]. Although we cannot formally reject the hypothesis that loss of LOC387715 is irrelevant to the disease, the spatiotemporal expression pattern of this gene and its exclusive emergence with the evolution of the macula in non-human primates, provide partial evidence for its role in AMD pathogenesis. We must note that AMD is a multifactorial disease with numerous susceptibility loci, therefore, the altered ARMS2 expression or function alone will not be sufficient to cause AMD.

Acknowledgments

The authors thank Dr. Liyun Jia for kindly analyzing the data of SNP analysis.

Author Contributions

Conceived and designed the experiments: XL YC LH PZ. Performed the experiments: YC LH. Analyzed the data: YC LH XL CZ. Contributed reagents/materials/analysis tools: XL YC LH WZ. Wrote the paper: YC LH.

References

1. Congdon N, O'Colmain B, Klaver CC, Klein R, Munoz B, et al. (2004) Causes and prevalence of visual impairment among adults in the United States. Arch Ophthalmol. 2004/04/14 ed. 477–485.
2. Fine SL, Berger JW, Maguire MG, Ho AC (2000) Age-related macular degeneration. N Engl J Med 342: 483–492.
3. Jager RD, Mieler WF, Miller JW (2008) Age-related macular degeneration. N Engl J Med 358: 2606–2617.
4. Liu NP (2009) [Characteristics of age-related macular degeneration in Chinese population]. Zhonghua Yan Ke Za Zhi 45: 393–395.
5. Pascolini D, Mariotti SP, Pokharel GP, Pararajasegaram R, Etya'ale D, et al. (2004) 2002 global update of available data on visual impairment: a compilation of population-based prevalence studies. Ophthalmic Epidemiol 11: 67–115.
6. Sayen A, Hubert I, Berrod JP (2011) [Age related macular degeneration]. Rev Prat 61: 159–164.
7. Hauswirth WW, Beaufrere L (2000) Ocular gene therapy: quo vadis? Invest Ophthalmol Vis Sci 41: 2821–2826.
8. Shen WY, Lai CM, Lai YK, Zhang D, Zaknich T, et al. (2003) Practical considerations of recombinant adeno-associated virus-mediated gene transfer for treatment of retinal degenerations. J Gene Med 5: 576–587.
9. Yannuzzi LA, Sorenson J, Spaide RF, Lipson B (2012) Idiopathic polypoidal choroidal vasculopathy (IPCV). Retina 32 Suppl 1: 1–8.
10. Ciardella AP, Donsoff IM, Huang SJ, Costa DL, Yannuzzi LA (2004) Polypoidal choroidal vasculopathy. Surv Ophthalmol 49: 25–37.
11. Maruko I, Iida T, Saito M, Nagayama D, Saito K (2007) Clinical characteristics of exudative age-related macular degeneration in Japanese patients. Am J Ophthalmol 144: 15–22.
12. Liu Y, Wen F, Huang S, Luo G, Yan H, et al. (2007) Subtype lesions of neovascular age-related macular degeneration in Chinese patients. Graefes Arch Clin Exp Ophthalmol 245: 1441–1445.
13. Meyers SM (1994) A twin study on age-related macular degeneration. Trans Am Ophthalmol Soc 92: 775–843.
14. Hammond CJ, Webster AR, Snieder H, Bird AC, Gilbert CE, et al. (2002) Genetic influence on early age-related maculopathy: a twin study. Ophthalmology 109: 730–736.
15. Seddon JM, Cote J, Page WF, Aggen SH, Neale MC (2005) The US twin study of age-related macular degeneration: relative roles of genetic and environmental influences. Arch Ophthalmol 123: 321–327.
16. Heiba IM, Elston RC, Klein BE, Klein R (1994) Sibling correlations and segregation analysis of age-related maculopathy: the Beaver Dam Eye Study. Genet Epidemiol 11: 51–67.
17. Seddon JM, Ajani UA, Mitchell BD (1997) Familial aggregation of age-related maculopathy. Am J Ophthalmol 123: 199–206.
18. Klaver CC, Wolfs RC, Assink JJ, van Duijn CM, Hofman A, et al. (1998) Genetic risk of age-related maculopathy. Population-based familial aggregation study. Arch Ophthalmol 116: 1646–1651.
19. Abecasis GR, Yashar BM, Zhao Y, Ghiasvand NM, Zareparsi S, et al. (2004) Age-related macular degeneration: a high-resolution genome scan for susceptibility loci in a population enriched for late-stage disease. Am J Hum Genet 74: 482–494.
20. Barral S, Francis PJ, Schultz DW, Schain MB, Haynes C, et al. (2006) Expanded genome scan in extended families with age-related macular degeneration. Invest Ophthalmol Vis Sci 47: 5453–5459.
21. Iyengar SK, Song D, Klein BE, Klein R, Schick JH, et al. (2004) Dissection of genomewide-scan data in extended families reveals a major locus and oligogenic susceptibility for age-related macular degeneration. Am J Hum Genet 74: 20–39.
22. Kenealy SJ, Schmidt S, Agarwal A, Postel EA, De La Paz MA, et al. (2004) Linkage analysis for age-related macular degeneration supports a gene on chromosome 10q26. Mol Vis 10: 57–61.
23. Majewski J, Schultz DW, Weleber RG, Schain MB, Edwards AO, et al. (2003) Age-related macular degeneration–a genome scan in extended families. Am J Hum Genet 73: 540–550.
24. Schick JH, Iyengar SK, Klein BE, Klein R, Reading K, et al. (2003) A whole-genome screen of a quantitative trait of age-related maculopathy in sibships from the Beaver Dam Eye Study. Am J Hum Genet 72: 1412–1424.
25. Schmidt S, Scott WK, Postel EA, Agarwal A, Hauser ER, et al. (2004) Ordered subset linkage analysis supports a susceptibility locus for age-related macular degeneration on chromosome 16p12. BMC Genet 5: 18.
26. Seddon JM, Santangelo SL, Book K, Chong S, Cote J (2003) A genomewide scan for age-related macular degeneration provides evidence for linkage to several chromosomal regions. Am J Hum Genet 73: 780–790.
27. Weeks DE, Conley YP, Tsai HJ, Mah TS, Schmidt S, et al. (2004) Age-related maculopathy: a genomewide scan with continued evidence of susceptibility loci within the 1q31, 10q26, and 17q25 regions. Am J Hum Genet 75: 174–189.
28. Fisher SA, Abecasis GR, Yashar BM, Zareparsi S, Swaroop A, et al. (2005) Meta-analysis of genome scans of age-related macular degeneration. Hum Mol Genet 14: 2257–2264.
29. Klein RJ, Zeiss C, Chew EY, Tsai JY, Sackler RS, et al. (2005) Complement factor H polymorphism in age-related macular degeneration. Science 308: 385–389.
30. Narayanan R, Butani V, Boyer DS, Atilano SR, Resende GP, et al. (2007) Complement factor H polymorphism in age-related macular degeneration. Ophthalmology 114: 1327–1331.
31. Lee KY, Vithana EN, Mathur R, Yong VH, Yeo IY, et al. (2008) Association analysis of CFH, C2, BF, and HTRA1 gene polymorphisms in Chinese patients with polypoidal choroidal vasculopathy. Invest Ophthalmol Vis Sci 49: 2613–2619.
32. Gotoh N, Yamada R, Nakanishi H, Saito M, Iida T, et al. (2008) Correlation between CFH Y402H and HTRA1 rs11200638 genotype to typical exudative age-related macular degeneration and polypoidal choroidal vasculopathy phenotype in the Japanese population. Clin Experiment Ophthalmol 36: 437–442.
33. Yang Z, Camp NJ, Sun H, Tong Z, Gibbs D, et al. (2006) A variant of the HTRA1 gene increases susceptibility to age-related macular degeneration. Science 314: 992–993.
34. Dewan A, Liu M, Hartman S, Zhang SS, Liu DT, et al. (2006) HTRA1 promoter polymorphism in wet age-related macular degeneration. Science 314: 989–992.
35. Wang G, Spencer KL, Scott WK, Whitehead P, Court BL, et al. (2010) Analysis of the indel at the ARMS2 3'UTR in age-related macular degeneration. Hum Genet 127: 595–602.
36. Fritsche LG, Loenhardt T, Janssen A, Fisher SA, Rivera A, et al. (2008) Age-related macular degeneration is associated with an unstable ARMS2 (LOC387715) mRNA. Nat Genet 40: 892–896.
37. Kanda A, Chen W, Othman M, Branham KE, Brooks M, et al. (2007) A variant of mitochondrial protein LOC387715/ARMS2, not HTRA1, is strongly associated with age-related macular degeneration. Proc Natl Acad Sci U S A 104: 16227–16232.
38. Kondo N, Honda S, Ishibashi K, Tsukahara Y, Negi A (2007) LOC387715/HTRA1 variants in polypoidal choroidal vasculopathy and age-related macular degeneration in a Japanese population. Am J Ophthalmol 144: 608–612.
39. Rivera A, Fisher SA, Fritsche LG, Keilhauer CN, Lichtner P, et al. (2005) Hypothetical LOC387715 is a second major susceptibility gene for age-related macular degeneration, contributing independently of complement factor H to disease risk. Hum Mol Genet 14: 3227–3236.
40. Hadley D, Orlin A, Brown G, Brucker AJ, Ho AC, et al. (2010) Analysis of six genetic risk factors highly associated with AMD in the region surrounding ARMS2 and HTRA1 on chromosome 10, region q26. Invest Ophthalmol Vis Sci 51: 2191–2196.
41. Lima LH, Schubert C, Ferrara DC, Merriam JE, Imamura Y, et al. (2010) Three major loci involved in age-related macular degeneration are also associated with polypoidal choroidal vasculopathy. Ophthalmology 117: 1567–1570.
42. Goto A, Akahori M, Okamoto H, Minami M, Terauchi N, et al. (2009) Genetic analysis of typical wet-type age-related macular degeneration and polypoidal choroidal vasculopathy in Japanese population. J Ocul Biol Dis Infor 2: 164–175.
43. Gotoh N, Nakanishi H, Hayashi H, Yamada R, Otani A, et al. (2009) ARMS2 (LOC387715) variants in Japanese patients with exudative age-related macular degeneration and polypoidal choroidal vasculopathy. Am J Ophthalmol 147: 1037–1041, 1041 e1031–1032.
44. Bird AC, Bressler NM, Bressler SB, Chisholm IH, Coscas G, et al. (1995) An international classification and grading system for age-related maculopathy and age-related macular degeneration. The International ARM Epidemiological Study Group. Surv Ophthalmol 39: 367–374.
45. Zhang T, Li X, Yu W, Yan Z, Zou H, et al. (2009) Overexpression of thymosin beta-10 inhibits VEGF mRNA expression, autocrine VEGF protein production, and tube formation in hypoxia-induced monkey choroid-retinal endothelial cells. Ophthalmic Res 41: 36–43.
46. Huang L, Yu W, Li X, Xu Y, Niu L, et al. (2009) Expression of Robo4 in the fibrovascular membranes from patients with proliferative diabetic retinopathy and its role in RF/6A and RPE cells. Mol Vis 15: 1057–1069.
47. Lu X, Le Noble F, Yuan L, Jiang Q, De Lafarge B, et al. (2004) The netrin receptor UNC5B mediates guidance events controlling morphogenesis of the vascular system. Nature 432: 179–186.
48. Zhou P, Zhao MW, Li XX, Yu WZ, Bian ZM (2007) siRNA targeting mammalian target of rapamycin (mTOR) attenuates experimental proliferative vitreoretinopathy. Curr Eye Res 32: 973–984.

49. Chen Y, Li XX, Xing NZ, Cao XG (2008) Quercetin inhibits choroidal and retinal angiogenesis in vitro. Graefes Arch Clin Exp Ophthalmol 246: 373–378.
50. Yannuzzi LA, Wong DW, Sforzolini BS, Goldbaum M, Tang KC, et al. (1999) Polypoidal choroidal vasculopathy and neovascularized age-related macular degeneration. Arch Ophthalmol 117: 1503–1510.
51. Laude A, Cackett PD, Vithana EN, Yeo IY, Wong D, et al. (2010) Polypoidal choroidal vasculopathy and neovascular age-related macular degeneration: same or different disease? Prog Retin Eye Res 29: 19–29.
52. Chan WM, Lam DS, Lai TY, Liu DT, Li KK, et al. (2004) Photodynamic therapy with verteporfin for symptomatic polypoidal choroidal vasculopathy: one-year results of a prospective case series. Ophthalmology 111: 1576–1584.
53. Hayashi H, Yamashiro K, Gotoh N, Nakanishi H, Nakata I, et al. (2010) CFH and ARMS2 variations in age-related macular degeneration, polypoidal choroidal vasculopathy, and retinal angiomatous proliferation. Invest Ophthalmol Vis Sci 51: 5914–5919.
54. Jakobsdottir J, Conley YP, Weeks DE, Mah TS, Ferrell RE, et al. (2005) Susceptibility genes for age-related maculopathy on chromosome 10q26. Am J Hum Genet 77: 389–407.
55. Yu Y, Bhangale TR, Fagerness J, Ripke S, Thorleifsson G, et al. (2011) Common variants near FRK/COL10A1 and VEGFA are associated with advanced age-related macular degeneration. Hum Mol Genet 20: 3699–3709.
56. Friedrich U, Myers CA, Fritsche LG, Milenkovich A, Wolf A, et al. (2011) Risk- and non-risk-associated variants at the 10q26 AMD locus influence ARMS2 mRNA expression but exclude pathogenic effects due to protein deficiency. Hum Mol Genet 20: 1387–1399.
57. Liang XY, Lai TY, Liu DT, Fan AH, Chen LJ, et al. (2012) Differentiation of Exudative Age-Related Macular Degeneration and Polypoidal Choroidal Vasculopathy in the ARMS2/HTRA1 Locus. Invest Ophthalmol Vis Sci 53: 3175–3182.
58. Kanda A, Stambolian D, Chen W, Curcio CA, Abecasis GR, et al. (2010) Age-related macular degeneration-associated variants at chromosome 10q26 do not significantly alter ARMS2 and HTRA1 transcript levels in the human retina. Mol Vis 16: 1317–1323.
59. Yang Z, Tong Z, Chen Y, Zeng J, Lu F, et al. (2010) Genetic and functional dissection of HTRA1 and LOC387715 in age-related macular degeneration. PLoS Genet 6: e1000836.
60. Scholl HP, Fleckenstein M, Fritsche LG, Schmitz-Valckenberg S, Gobel A, et al. (2009) CFH, C3 and ARMS2 are significant risk loci for susceptibility but not for disease progression of geographic atrophy due to AMD. PLoS One 4: e7418.
61. Klein ML, Ferris FL, 3rd, Francis PJ, Lindblad AS, Chew EY, et al. (2010) Progression of geographic atrophy and genotype in age-related macular degeneration. Ophthalmology 117: 1554–1559, 1559 e1551.

16

A Novel Source of Methylglyoxal and Glyoxal in Retina: Implications for Age-Related Macular Degeneration

Kee Dong Yoon[1], Kazunori Yamamoto[1], Keiko Ueda[1], Jilin Zhou[1], Janet R. Sparrow[1,2]*

1 Department of Ophthalmology, Columbia University, New York, New York, United States of America, 2 Department of Pathology and Cell Biology, Columbia University, New York, New York, United States of America

Abstract

Aging of retinal pigment epithelial (RPE) cells of the eye is marked by accumulations of bisretinoid fluorophores; two of the compounds within this lipofuscin mixture are A2E and all-*trans*-retinal dimer. These pigments are implicated in pathological mechanisms involved in some vision-threatening disorders including age-related macular degeneration (AMD). Studies have shown that bisretinoids are photosensitive compounds that undergo photooxidation and photodegradation when irradiated with short wavelength visible light. Utilizing ultra performance liquid chromatography (UPLC) with electrospray ionization mass spectrometry (ESI-MS) we demonstrate that photodegradation of A2E and all-*trans*-retinal dimer generates the dicarbonyls glyoxal (GO) and methylglyoxal (MG), that are known to modify proteins by advanced glycation endproduct (AGE) formation. By extracellular trapping with aminoguanidine, we established that these oxo-aldehydes are released from irradiated A2E-containing RPE cells. Enzyme-linked immunosorbant assays (ELISA) revealed that the substrate underlying A2E-containing RPE was AGE-modified after irradiation. This AGE deposition was suppressed by prior treatment of the cells with aminoguanidine. AGE-modification causes structural and functional impairment of proteins. In chronic diseases such as diabetes and atherosclerosis, MG and GO modify proteins by non-enzymatic glycation and oxidation reactions. AGE-modified proteins are also components of drusen, the sub-RPE deposits that confer increased risk of AMD onset. These results indicate that photodegraded RPE bisretinoid is likely to be a previously unknown source of MG and GO in the eye.

Editor: Alfred Lewin, University of Florida, United States of America

Funding: Supported by National Institutes of Health grants EY12951 (JRS) and P30EY019007; and a grant from Research to Prevent Blindness to the Department of Ophthalmology. KDY was supported in part by National Research Foundation of Korea (NRF-2009-352-E00060). KDY is currently at the Catholic University of Korea. The funders had no role in study design, data collection and analysis, decision to publish, or preparation of the manuscript.

Competing Interests: The authors have declared that no competing interests exist.

* E-mail: jrs88@columbia.edu

Introduction

Several histopathological changes in the retinal pigment epithelial cell (RPE) and in its underlying basement membrane (Bruch's membrane), are distinctly characteristic of aging and may contribute to sight-threatening age-related macular degeneration (AMD). For instance, aging of RPE is associated with a progressive accumulation of autofluorescent pigments (lipofuscin) consisting of photo-sensitive bisretinoid compounds [1]. In Bruch's membrane, there is a build-up of esterified cholesterol-rich apolipoprotein B-containing lipoprotein that originates from RPE cells [2]. Bruch's membrane also undergoes thickening, diffusional rates across this layer are diminished [3], the integrity of the elastic lamina of Bruch's membrane is compromised [4] and collagens in this layer become cross-linked and less soluble [5]. Histologically visible dome-shaped extracellular deposits (drusen) that can be detected as yellow-white lesions in a retinal fundus image, are also common in older individuals. Drusen size and area within the macula are factors considered in the clinical characterization of age-related macular degeneration [6]. Besides containing neutral lipid, drusen house a number of proteins which function within the complement system [7]. This feature is of interest since genetic studies demonstrate that sequence variants in some complement related proteins confer increased risk or protection against age-related macular degeneration (AMD) [8–13].

As part of the pathological process, resident proteins within drusen accumulate non-enzymatic modifications in the form of advanced glycation end-products (AGEs). AGE-modified proteins have been detected in drusen by immunocytochemistry, by Raman confocal microscopy and by chromatography [14–18]. AGE formation is pronounced in diabetes and several disorders of aging such as atherosclerosis. In diabetes, AGE modification is a product of autooxidation and decomposition of carbohydrates and is considered to be a major pathogenic link between hyperglycemia and the onset and progression of disease [19]. Conversely, the origin of AGEs such as carboxymethyllysine (CML) and carboxyethyllysine (CEL) in ocular drusen is not known. Here we have demonstrated that methylglyoxal (MG) and glyoxal (GO) (Figure 1), two agents known to form AGEs, are released upon photodegradation of A2E and all-*trans*-retinal dimer, two bisretinoids that accumulate as lipofuscin in RPE. Bisretinoid cleavage, upon exposure to wavelengths of light that reach the retina, represents a previously unrecognized source of these dicarbonyls. While various processes play a role in Bruch's membrane changes and drusen formation, these findings are indicative of a contribution from lipofuscin photooxidation and cleavage in RPE.

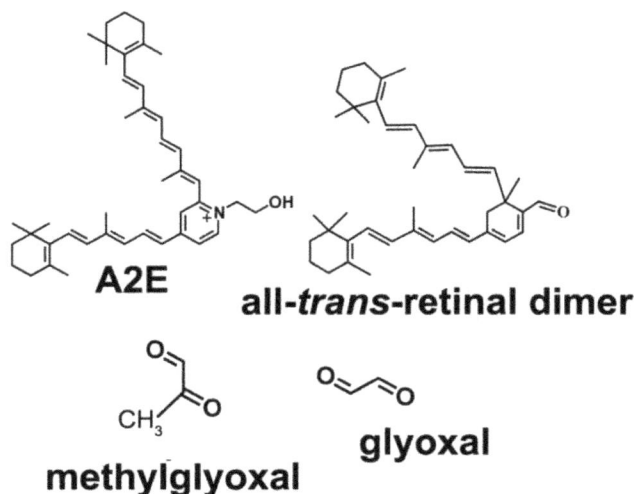

Figure 1. Structures of the bisretinoids A2E and all-*trans*-retinal dimer; and the oxo-aldehydes, methylglyoxal and glyoxal.

Results

Detection of MG and GO as Photodegradation Products of A2E and all-*trans*-retinal Dimer. Reaction with 4NPH

To acquire evidence for the liberation of GO and MG when the bisretinoids A2E and all-*trans*-retinal dimer undergo photooxidation-elicited photodegradation, we trapped these volatile dicarbonyl fragments with 4NPH, a compound known to readily react with carbonyl moieties. As demonstrated in Figure 2, reaction of 4NPH with commercially available MG (m/z 72) and GO (m/z 58) generated the expected products at m/z 327 ([GO/4NPH-H]$^-$) ([M-H]$^-$) and m/z 341 ([MG/4NPH-H]$^-$) ([M-H]$^-$) [2-(4-nitrophenyl)hydrazone], respectively. Subsequently, samples of A2E and all-*trans*-retinal dimer were irradiated (430 nm) under conditions known to result in their photooxidation and photodegradation [20–22]. The samples were then incubated with 4NPH and analyzed by negative mode ESI-MS. The reaction yielded peaks at m/z 327 and m/z 341 (Figure 2 C, E) that were considerably magnified relative to non-irradiated samples (Figure 2, B and D) and that were indicative of the presence of GO and MG, respectively, in the photodegradative mixtures. These adducts were generated when assaying at both 60°C and room temperature. The generation of these peaks could be explained by the facile reaction of 4NPH with the photo-products GO and MG, that were released after photooxidation and photodegradation of the bisretinoids. Since we employed a cell-free assay, the MG and GO detected was not attributable to the degradation of other organic compounds such as glyceraldehyde-3-phosphate [23].

MG and GO Released upon Bisretinoid Photodegradation Form Adducts with Aminoguanidine

Another compound with MG and GO scavenging capability is aminoguanidine (m/z 74), a small molecule that was initially designed to therapeutically inhibit AGE-modification of proteins [24]. Thus to further test for release of MG (m/z 72) and GO (m/z 58) upon photodegradation of A2E and all-*trans*-retinal dimer, we also incubated aminoguanidine with irradiated A2E and all-*trans*-retinal dimer. Reaction of aminoguanidine with commercially obtained GO and MG demonstrated production of the expected

adducts at m/z 97 ([M+H]$^+$; GO-derivatized aminoguanidine) and m/z 111 ([M+H]$^+$; MG-derivatized aminoguanidine, 3-amino-5/6-methyl-1,2,4-triazine) (Figure 3A) [24]. The GO-AG adduct that we detected had the same molecular weight as authentic 3-amino-1,2,4-triazine (Figure S1). These m/z species were negligible in samples of aminoguanidine alone (Figure 3B) and when non-irradiated A2E (Figure 3C) or non-irradiated all-*trans*-retinal dimer (Figure 3D) were analyzed. However, incubation of aminoguanidine with A2E (Figure 3, E and G) and all-*trans*-retinal dimer (Figure 3, F and H) during irradiation (Figure 3, E and F) or after irradiation (Figure 3, G and H) resulted in marked m/z 97 and m/z 111 ([M+H]$^+$; MG-derivatized aminoguanidine, 3-amino-5/6-methyl-1,2,4-triazine) signals. These results were indicative of the release of GO and MG upon photooxidation-associated degradation of the bisretinoids. Again, since we utilized a cell-free assay, the MG and GO detected was not attributable to the degradation of other organic compounds [23].

AGE Formation on Extracellular Fibronectin

We next sought to determine whether GO or MG released from photodegraded intracellular A2E could lead to extracellular AGE formation, in this case AGE-modification of a fibronectin substrate on which cultured cells were grown [25]. To that end, we used a culture model wherein the bisretinoid A2E is allowed to accumulate in ARPE-19 cells. We have previously shown that in this model, A2E accumulates in the lysosomal compartment of the cells just as *in vivo* [26]. ARPE-19 cells are preferable for these experiments since in primary cultures of RPE, bisretinoid levels vary. The A2E-containing cells were irradiated at 430 nm and fibronectin was immunoprecipitated from the recovered cells and substrate. The protein samples were adsorbed onto 96-well ELISA plates and the AGE-adducts were probed with an anti-AGE antibody. Conditions included A2E-ARPE19 cells pre-treated with aminoguanidine to allow for intracellular accumulation [27]. As shown in Figure 4, irradiation of A2E-ARPE19 cells resulted in consumption of A2E reflecting A2E photooxidation and photodegradation [22,28]. The magnitude of the decrease was similar with and without aminoguanidine pre-treatment (Figure 4A). Irradiation of A2E-ARPE19 overlying the fibronectin substrate resulted in substantial AGE-deposition within the extracellular fibronectin when compared to A2E-containing cells that were not irradiated (Figure 4B). Note that the anti-AGE antibody used in the ELISA reacted with both CML-bovine serum albumin (BSA) and CEL-BSA (Figure 4B), indicating an ability of the antibody to recognize forms of AGE produced by both GO and MG, respectively. In the case of A2E-ARPE19 cells that had accumulated aminoguanidine, AGE-fibronectin adduct formation was reduced. The perturbation of AGE-modification could be explained by the ability of intracellular aminoguanidine to scavenge GO and MG as it was generated during photodegradation of A2E within the cells, thus reducing its release into the extracellular milieu. To test for this possibility, we analyzed the cell homogenates for GO- and MG-aminoguanidine adducts. Accordingly, UPLC chromatographic separation (Figure 5A) with MS detection demonstrated a pronounced species at m/z 97 indicative of the GO-aminoguanidine adduct (Figure 5B). However we did not detect a compound at mz 111 as would be expected for an MG-aminoguanidine conjugate (Figure 5C). Triosephosphates (e.g. glyceraldehyde-3-phosphate) are known to be a cellular source of MG, particularly under conditions of hyperglycemia wherein triosephosphates accumulate [23]. However, in these experiments we negated the latter source as an explanation for the dicarbonyl release by comparison to control nonirradiated A2E-ARPE19 cells.

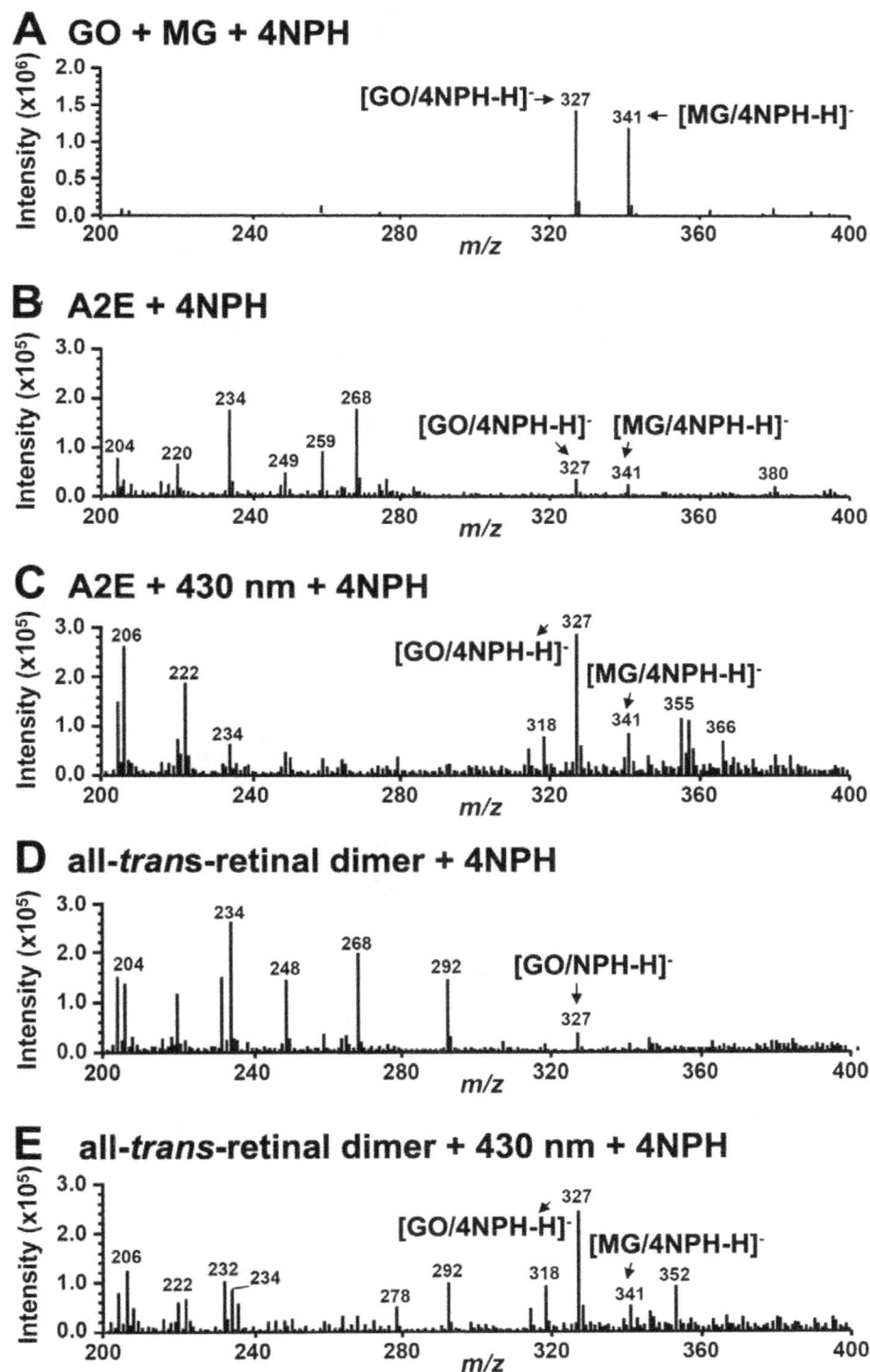

Figure 2. Irradiation (430 nm) of A2E and all-*trans*-retinal dimer leads to production of glyoxal (GO) and methylglyoxal (MG). **Negative ESI-MS spectra in the range *m/z* 200–400. Detection of GO and MG by reaction with 4NPH.** (*A*) Authentic standards. Incubation of 4NPH with GO and MG (obtained commercially) yielded products at *m/z* 327 ([GO/4NPH-H]⁻) and *m/z* 341 ([MG/4NPH-H]⁻), respectively. (*B*) Incubation of 4NPH with A2E. (*C*) Incubation of 4NPH with irradiated A2E. (*D*) Incubation of 4NPH with all-*trans*-retinal dimer. (*E*) Incubation of 4NPH with irradiated all-*trans*-retinal dimer. Augmentation of the *m/z* 327 and *m/z* 341 peaks in the irradiated samples is indicative of photodegradation-associated release of GO and MG.

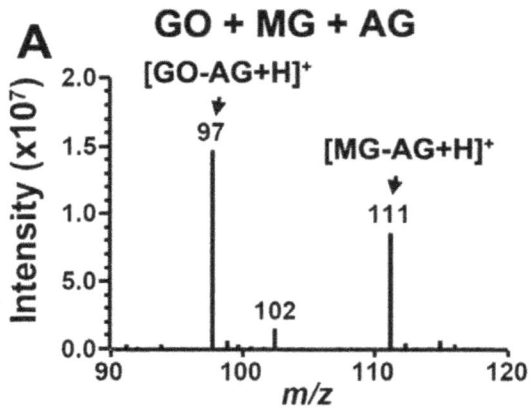

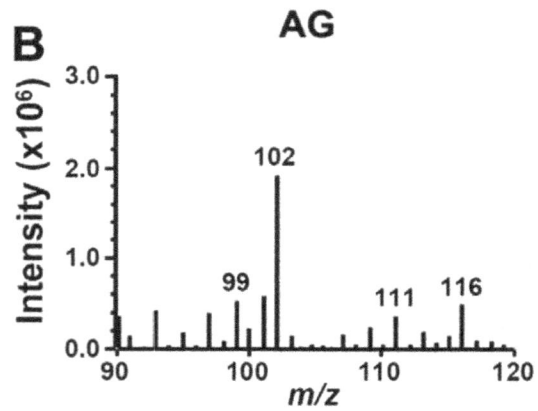

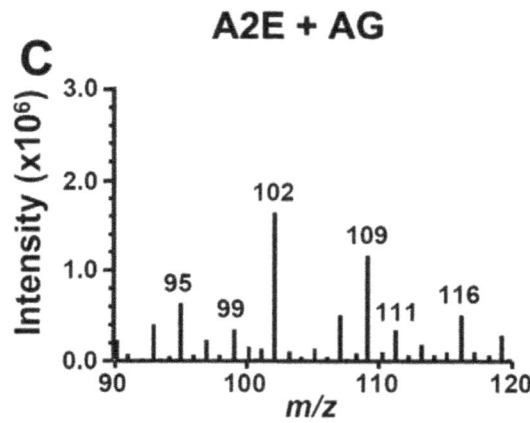

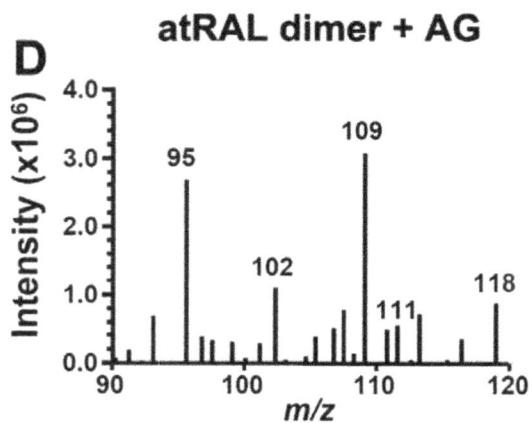

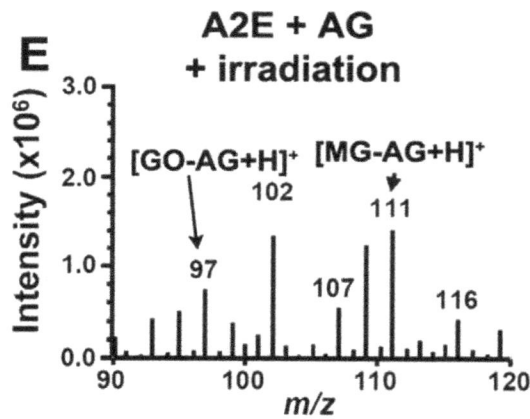

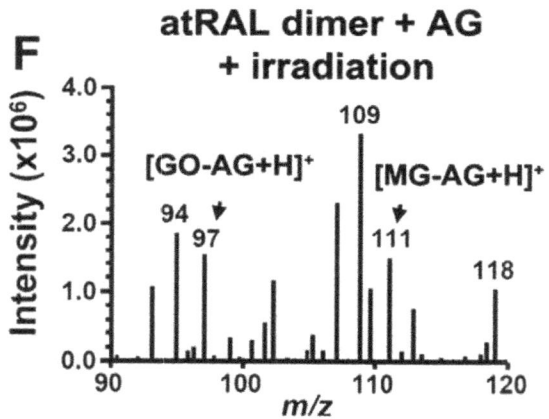

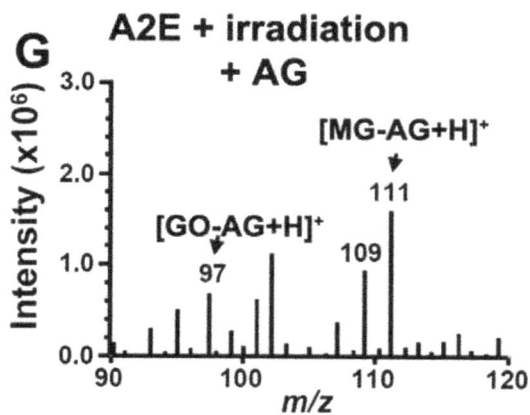

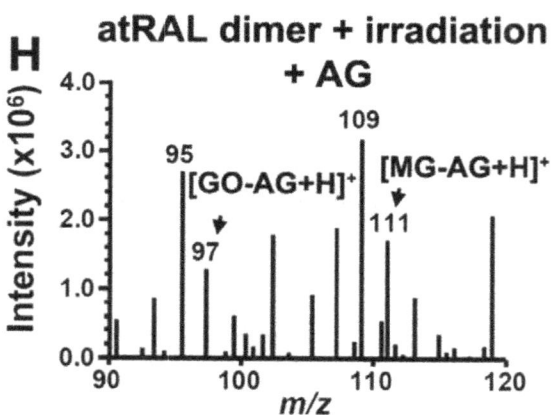

Figure 3. Methylglyoxal (MG) and glyoxal (GO) released by photodegradation of A2E and all-*trans*-retinal dimer (atRAL dimer) forms adducts with aminoguanidine (AG). Positive ESI-MS spectra in the range m/z 90–120 to detect GO-AG adduct (m/z 97; [M+H]$^+$) and MG-AG adduct (m/z 111; [M+H]$^+$). (*A*) AG reaction with commercial glyoxal (GO) and methylglyoxal (MG). (*B*) AG alone. Note the absence of m/z 97 and m/z 111. (*C*) A2E and AG (no irradiation). (*D*) atRAL dimer and AG (no irradiation). (*E*) Irradiation of a mixture of A2E and AG. (*F*) Irradiation of a mixture of atRAL dimer and AG. (*G*) Incubation of photooxidized A2E (A2E + irradiation) and AG. (*H*) Incubation of photooxidized all-*trans*-retinal dimer (atRAL dimer + irradiation) and AG.

Trapping of GO and MG Released into the Extracellular Milieu Following Photodegradation of Intracellular A2E

AGE-modification of fibronectin under conditions in which intracellular A2E photodegrades, suggests that AGE-eliciting photoproducts such as MG and GO, are liberated from the cells. Thus we next designed experiments to trap MG and GO by aminoguanidine if the dicarbonyls were released from cells upon irradiation of A2E-ARPE19 cells. By positive mode ESI, MG- and GO-aminoguanidine adducts were expected to yield peaks at m/z 111 and m/z 97 ([M+H]$^+$), respectively. As shown in Figure 6, aminoguanidine-containing PBS that had been incubated with non-irradiated A2E-ARPE19 cells exhibited MS signals indicative of background levels of MG-aminoguanidine and GO-aminoguanidine adducts (Figure 6A). The signal for the MG-aminoguanidine adduct (m/z 111) was increased within PBS-aminoguanidine that had been incubated with A2E-ARPE19 cells during irradiation (Figure 6B). Intracellular accumulation of aminoguanidine 48 hours prior to irradiation, reduced the external MG-aminoguanidine signal (Figure 6C). We interpret the latter decrease as intracellular scavenging of MG by aminoguanidine as it was generated during photodegradation of A2E within the cells. Aminoguanidine-mediated scavenging would reduce MG release into the extracellular milieu. Note that the m/z 102 signal present in all of the MS spectra originates from ethylacetate (Figure 6B, inset) and does not vary in intensity. All samples were reconstituted in ethylacetate before injection into the MS detector; thus this peak served as an internal standard controlling for run-to-run variability in sample injection or instrument response. The GO-aminoguanidine adduct peak (m/z 97) was of low intensity and exhibited little change, perhaps due to insufficient detection sensitivity. It is of interest however, that in these experiments, the adduct we detected intracellularly was GO-aminoguanidine (Figure 5), while MG-aminoguanidine was measurable extracellu-

larly. Whether or not these findings reflect differences in the properties of GO and MG (e.g. membrane permeability) remains to be determined.

Discussion

The bisretinoid compounds that accumulate as autofluorescent lipofuscin in RPE cells originate in photoreceptors cells from inadvertent reactions of all-*trans*-retinal, the latter being generated when photons are absorbed by visual pigment [1]. These photoactive compounds are transferred secondarily to the RPE. All of these compounds are bestowed with two side-arms, each of which bears systems of alternating single and double carbon-carbon bonds. As a consequence, the pigments in this group absorb in both the UV and visible range of the spectrum. These diretinal pigments include but are not limited to the pyridinium bisretinoid A2E, all-*trans*-retinal dimer and its conjugated family members, A2-DHP-PE and glycerophosphoethanolamine (A2-GPE) [1,29].

RPE bisretinoid pigments are well known to be both photogenerators and quenchers of reactive forms of oxygen [1]. Specifically, the singlet oxygen that is generated when the bisretinoids are excited with short wavelength light, adds to the bisretinoid, oxidizing at carbon-carbon double bonds. Oxidized forms of A2E and all-*trans*-retinal dimer have been identified *in vivo* [30–32]. It is at sites of singlet oxygen addition that photocleavage occurs. We have recently demonstrated that photodegradation of bisretinoid produces a complex mixture of aldehyde-bearing fragments of varying molecular size [22]. In the work we currently discuss, we have shown that both A2E and all-*trans*-retinal dimer undergo photodegradation leading to the release of the oxo-aldehydes GO and MG, the latter being major players in AGE-adduct formation. Unlike reactive forms of molecular oxygen, these small aldehydes are rather long lived and can diffuse from

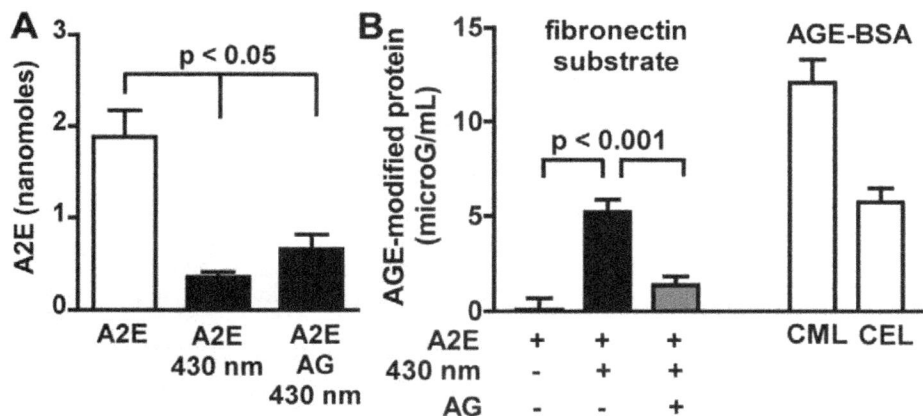

Figure 4. AGE-modification of a fibronectin substrate accompanies photooxidation/photodegradation of intracellular A2E. (*A*) A2E content of ARPE19 is diminished by irradiation (430 nm) in the presence/absence of aminoguanidine (AG). UPLC quantitation; Mean ± SEM of 3 experiments. (*B*) AGE-modification of fibronectin substrate underlying irradiated A2E-containing ARPE19 cells. Prior accumulation of aminoguanidine within the cells reduced AGE-formation. ELISA quantitation as AGE-BSA equivalent units. The anti-AGE antibody recognized both carboxymethyllysine (CML)-BSA and carboxyethyllysine (CEL)-BSA. + presence of condition. Mean ± SEM of 7 experiments.

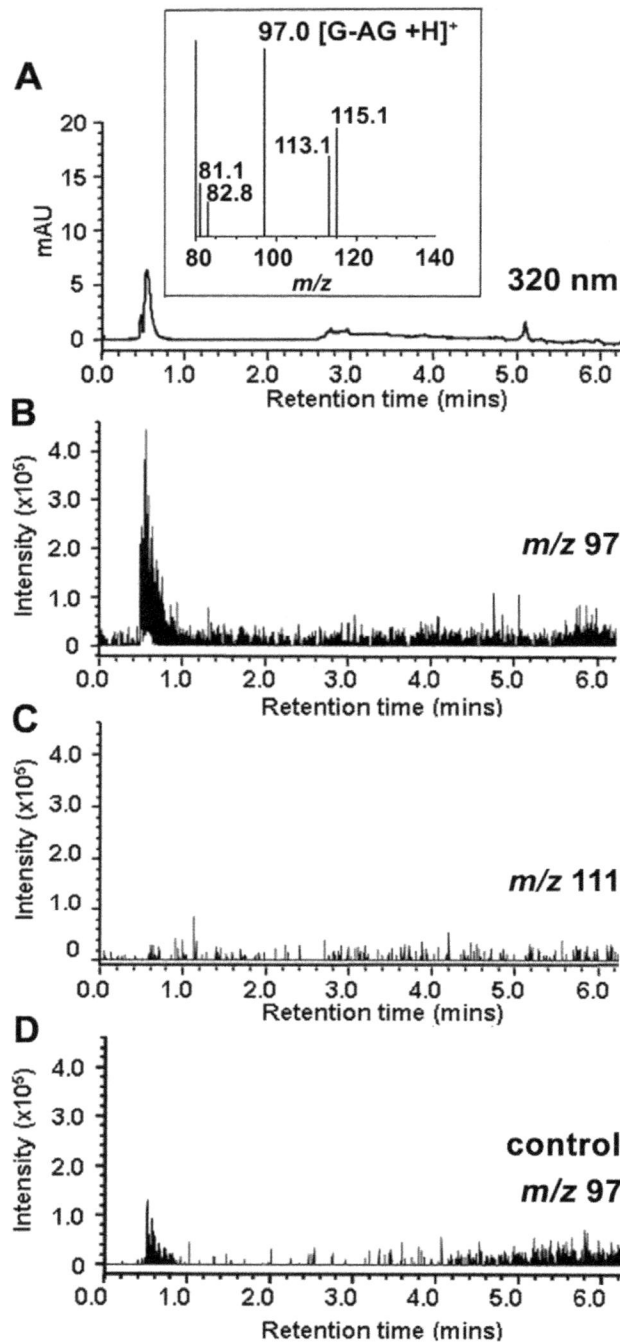

Figure 5. UPLC-MS detection of aminoguanidine (AG)-adducts in extracts of 430 nm irradiated A2E-ARPE19 cells. (A) Chromatogram with UV detection at 320 nm. Irradiated A2E-ARPE19 cells. Inset, mass spectrum of peak eluting at retention time 0.6 mins. (B,C) Selected ion monitoring chromatograms at m/z 97 (GO-AG adduct) and m/z 111 (MG-AG adduct). Irradiated A2E-ARPE19 cells. (D) Selected ion monitoring chromatogram at m/z 97. Control nonirradiated A2E-ARPE19 cells.

Figure 6. Positive ESI-MS spectra indicating release of methylglyoxal (MG) into the extracellular milieu following photodegradation of intracellular A2E. Pretreatment of the cells with aminoguanidine (RPE-AG) reduces this release. Extracellular trapping by aminoguanidine in PBS (PBS-AG). (A) PBS-AG recovered from ARPE19 cells that had accumulated A2E (A2E-ARPE19) and were not irradiated. (B) Recovered PBS-AG that had overlaid A2E-ARPE19 cells during irradiation. Note increase in MG-AG adduct (m/z 111; [M+H]$^+$). Inset, ESI-spectra (direct injection) obtained with ethylacetate only. The prominent m/z 102 peak attributable to ethylacetate serves as an internal control (C) Aminoguanidine-containing PBS that had overlaid irradiated A2E-ARPE19 cells pre-treated with aminoguanidine. GO-AG adduct, m/z 97; [M+H]$^+$; MG-AG adduct, (m/z 111; [M+H]$^+$.

their site of origin [33]. Accordingly, in an *in vitro* assay we have detected the liberation of dicarbonyl from the cells and AGE-adduct formation on extracellular fibronectin. The latter AGE-modification was reduced by aminoguanidine-mediated intracel-

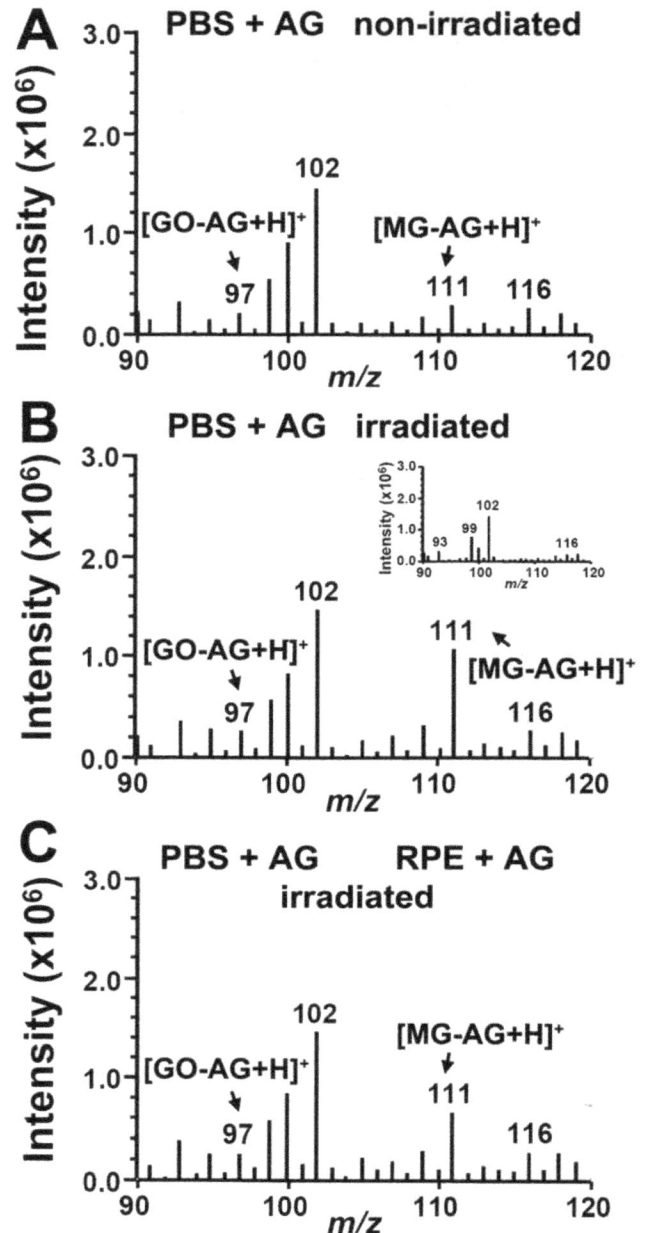

lular scavenging. AGE-modification of the fibronectin substrate indicated that MG and GO can be released from the basal surface of the cells, however apical release cannot be excluded. Taken together, these studies implicate RPE bisretinoids as an important source of MG and GO (Figure 1). To the extent that RPE bisretinoids are specific to the latter cell, this source of MG and GO is likely to be unique to the retina.

For some time, glycolysis has been recognized as the major source of MG and GO and under both physiological and hyperglycemic conditions, MG and GO are endogenously produced within cells. MG and GO can exit cells across the plasma membrane, as evidenced for instance, by cross-linking of extracellular proteins such as collagen IV [34–36]. In diabetic retinopathy, AGE-modification of extracellular matrix proteins such as fibronectin and laminin, has been shown to lead to over-expression of the proteins, with the resulting basement membrane thickening promoting the progression to acellular capillaries and vascular leakage that is typical of long-term diabetic complications [37,38]. As compared to oxidative degradation of glucose, direct AGE formation by MG or GO is more efficient, by several orders of magnitude [39]. Reaction of MG and GO with nucleophilic groups in proteins leads to structurally diverse AGE-modifications. The adducts form primarily on arginine and lysine residues and the major products are nonfluorescent hydroimidazolones; the blue fluorescent argpyrimidine; N^ϵ-CEL and N^ϵ-CML that form by reaction of MG and GO, respectively, with lysine residues of proteins; methylglyoxal-lysine dimer (MOLD), a cross-linking adduct between two lysine residues; and methyl glyoxal-derived imidazolium cross-link (MODIC), a lysine-arginine cross-linking structure. Other uncharacterized AGE adducts are also known to exist [40]. That MG and GO can partake in covalent cross-linking of extracellular proteins is significant, since the collagen of Bruch's membrane is increasingly cross-linked with age [5]. This change in the extracellular matrix is thought to explain altered properties of Bruch's membrane such as reduced hydraulic conductivity and permeability, enhanced rigidity and thickening [41]. Cultured RPE grown on an AGE-modified basement membrane substrate exhibits reduced tight junctions and changes in mRNA expression including mRNA that encodes proteins involved in cell attachment and immune responses [42]. Protein cross-linking by AGE-modification can also confer resistance to proteolysis, including that mediated by matrix metalloproteinases [35]. CEL and CML along with pentosidine have all been shown to increase with age in human Bruch's membrane [14,15,17,18] and are reported to be prominent in both neovascular and atrophic AMD [16,43].

Does bisretinoid photooxidation and photodegradation occur in vivo? Some lines of evidence indicate that indeed these processes occur in the eye. For instance, mono- and bis-peroxy-A2E, mono- and bis-furano-A2E, mono- and bis-peroxy-all-transretinal dimer and mono- and bis-furano-all-trans-retinal dimer are detected in extracts from human and mouse eyes [28,31]. The photolysis of bisretinoid at sites of photooxidation could also explain the observation that photooxidized forms of A2E do not accumulate with age [44]. Nevertheless, this is a question that should be addressed in future studies.

Some currently ongoing clinical trials aim to develop treatments for age-related macular degeneration based on limiting RPE bisretinoid lipofuscin formation [45]. The results reported here indicate that therapies such as these may have benefits that extend beyond effects on RPE bisretinoid accumulation alone and that could include preservation of Bruch's membrane integrity.

Materials and Methods

Cells

Confluent human RPE cells (ARPE19; American Type Culture Collection, Manassas, VA) devoid of bisretinoid lipofuscin [26] were allowed to accumulate synthesized A2E [46] into the lysosomal compartment [26] from a 10 microM concentration in media (A2E-ARPE19) [25]. The cells subsequently remained quiescent for 1 week. For some experiments the dishes were coated with fibronectin (10 microG/cm^2; Invitrogen, Carlsbad, CA) before cell plating. After incubating for 5 days in A2E-free medium, the cells were treated/not treated with aminoguanidine (100 microM in culture medium; 48 hrs; Cayman, Ann Arbor, MI). Transport of aminoguanidine into cells is evidenced by its ability to interrupt intracellular signaling pathways [27,47]. Before light exposure, culture medium was replaced with phosphate-buffered saline (PBS; with calcium, magnesium and glucose) that contained/did not contain aminoguanidine (100 microM; PBS-AG). Irradiation at 430 ± 30 nm was delivered to the entire area of a 35 mm dish (1 mW/cm^2, 20 min). PBS- aminoguanidine samples were recovered, concentrated, re-dissolved in ethylacetate (5 microL) and subjected to ultra performance liquid chromatography/mass spectrometry (UPLC/MS) as described below.

Reaction with 4-nitrophenylhydrazine (4NPH)

Authentic samples of MG and GO (Sigma-Aldrich, St. Louis MO) derivatized with 4NPH (Sigma-Aldrich) were generated as described [22]. After dilution in methanol the sample was subjected to electrospray ionization-mass spectrometry (ESI-MS) analysis. In addition, A2E or all-trans-retinal dimer (200 microM in 200 microL water with 1% DMSO) were irradiated (430 ± 20 nm, 1.3 mW/cm^2; 30 min for A2E and 15 min for all-trans-retinal dimer). Samples were dried under argon and pooled, dissolved in 200 microL ethanol, and then mixed with 200 microL of 200 μM 4NPH with 400 microL of glacial acetic acid and stirred for 2 hours at 60°C. Aliquots (10 microL) of the latter mixture were added to acetonitrile (100 microL) and 5 microL samples were analyzed by negative ESI-MS using a Waters Acquity Quadrupole (SQD) mass spectrometer (MS). The capillary voltage was set to 3.0 KV and the cone voltage was set to -30 V.

Reaction with Aminoguanidine

Authentic MG- and GO-aminoguanidine adducts were generated by incubating aminoguanidine (6 mM; Sigma-Aldrich) with MG and GO (0.14 mmol in PBS) at 37°C for 10 min. A2E or all-trans-retinal dimer (200 microM in DBPS with 1% DMSO) were irradiated (430 ± 20 nm, 1.3 mW/cm^2; 30 min for A2E and 15 min for all-trans-retinal dimer) and then incubated (1 hour, 37°C, with stirring) with aminoguanidine (3 mM). Alternatively, A2E or all-trans-retinal dimer were first combined with amino-guanidine then irradiated and the mixture was stirred for 30 minutes (37°C). All samples were concentrated and re-dissolved in ethylacetate and prepared in 50% acetonitrile/methanol (1:1 v/v, with 0.1% formic acid) with 50% water (with 0.1% formic acid) for direct injection positive ESI-MS (capillary voltage, 3.0 KV; cone voltage, 30 V). Authentic 3-amino 1,2,4-triazine (1 mM in ethylacetate; Sigma-Aldrich), the product of reaction of AG and GO [24], was also analyzed by direct injection ESI-MS.

Detection of A2E and Aminoguanidine-adducts in RPE

A Waters Acquity ultra performance liquid chromatography (UPLC) system (Waters, New Jersey, USA) was operated with a Waters SQD single quadrupole mass spectrometer (electrospray ionization mode, ESI). PDA detection at 320 nm; and an Xbridge® C18 column (2.5 μm, 3.0×50 mm I.D.) were used. Chromatographic separation was performed using a gradient of acetonitrile/methanol (1:1) in water with 0.1% formic acid and flow rate of 0.5 mL/min. For aminoguanidine-adduct detection, a concentrated extract in 100% methanol was delivered as a 5 microL injectant and the gradient used was 0% (0–1 min) acetonitrile/methanol; 0–98% (1–10 min) acetonitrile/methanol; 98% (10–12 min) acetonitrile/methanol. To quantify A2E, the gradient was 70–85% acetonitrile/methanol (0–60 min).

ELISA

The cells and substrate were harvested by scraping and fibronectin was immunoprecipitated from the lysate using rabbit polyclonal antibody to fibronection (ABCAM Inc, Cambridge, MA) and protein A-Agarose (Roche Diagnostics GmbH, Germany). Protein concentrations were measured with Bio-Rad protein assay kit (Bio-Rad Laboratories, Hercules, CA) and samples were adjusted to 10 microG/mL total protein with PBS. Advanced glycation end product (AGE) was measured using the AGE ELISA kit (Cell Biolabs, Inc. San Diego, CA). Unknown samples (10 microG/mL), CML-modified bovine serum albumin (BSA) (10 microG/mL; CycLex Ltd, Nagana Japan), CEL-

modified BSA (10 microG/mL; CycLex Ltd) and AGE-BSA standards (Cell Biolabs) were loaded into 96-well protein binding plate in duplicate and incubated at 4°C overnight. After incubating in the diluent buffer followed by anti-AGE antibody and HRP-conjugated second antibody, absorbance was read at 450 nm and background values (BSA or stock fibronectin, as appropriate) were subtracted to control for extraneous sources of AGE in the analyte. Absorbance readings were converted to microG/ml by comparison to a standard curve constructed from known amounts of AGE-BSA.

Author Contributions

Conceived and designed the experiments: KDY JRS. Performed the experiments: KDY KY KU JZ JRS. Analyzed the data: KDY KY KU JZ JRS. Wrote the paper: KDY JRS.

References

1. Sparrow JR, Wu Y, Kim CY, Zhou J (2010) Phospholipid meets all-*trans*-retinal: the making of RPE bisretinoids. J Lipid Res 51: 247–261.
2. Curcio CA, Johnson M, Huang JD, Rudolf M (2009) Aging, age-related macular degeneration, and the response-to-retention of apolipoprotein B-containing lipoproteins. Prog Retin Eye Res 28: 393–422.
3. Hussain AA, Starita C, Hodgetts A, Marshall J (2010) Macromolecular diffusion characteristics of ageing human Bruch's membrane: implications for age-related macular degeneration (AMD). Exp Eye Res 90: 703–710.
4. Chong NH, Keonin J, Luthert PJ, Frennesson CI, Weingeist DM, et al. (2005) Decreased Thickness and Integrity of the Macular Elastic Layer of Bruch's Membrane Correspond to the Distribution of Lesions Associated with Age-Related Macular Degeneration. Am J Pathol 166: 241–251.
5. Booij JC, Baas DC, Beisekeeva J, Gorgels TG, Bergen AA (2010) The dynamic nature of Bruch's membrane. Prog Retin Eye Res 29: 1–18.
6. Ferris FL, Davis MD, Clemons TE, Lee LY, Chew EY, et al. (2005) A simplified severity scale for age-related macular degeneration: AREDS Report No. 18. Arch Ophthalmol 123: 1570–1574.
7. Anderson DH, Radeke MJ, Gallo NB, Chapin EA, Johnson PT, et al. (2010) The pivotal role of the complement system in aging and age-related macular degeneration: hypothesis re-visited. Prog Retin Eye Res 29: 95–112.
8. Gold B, Merriam JE, Zernant J, Hancox LS, Taiber AJ, et al. (2006) Variation in factor B (BF) and complement component 2 (C2) genes is associated with age-related macular degeneration. Nat Genet 38: 458–462.
9. Hageman GS, Anderson DH, Johnson LV, Hancox LS, Taiber AJ, et al. (2005) A common haplotype in the complement regulatory gene factor H (HF1/CFH) predisposes individuals to age-related macular degeneration. Proc Natl Acad Sci U S A 102: 7227–7232.
10. Edwards AO, Ritter R, Abel KJ, Manning A, Panhuysen C, et al. (2005) Complement factor H polymorphism and age-related macular degeneration. Science 308: 421–424.
11. Haines JL, Hauser MA, Schmidt S, Scott WK, Olson LM, et al. (2005) Complement factor H variant increases the risk of age-related macular degeneration. Science 308: 419–421.
12. Klein RJ, Zeiss C, Chew EY, Tsai JY, Sackler RS, et al. (2005) Complement factor H polymorphism in age-related macular degeneration. Science 308: 385–389.
13. Yates JR, Sepp T, Matharu BK, Khan JC, Thurlby DA, et al. (2007) Complement C3 variant and the risk of age-related macular degeneration. N Engl J Med 357: 553–561.
14. Handa JT, Verzijl N, Matsunaga H, Aotaki-Keen A, Lutty GA, et al. (1999) Increase in advanced glycation end product pentosidine in Bruch's membrane with age. Invest Ophthalmol Vis Sci 40: 775–779.
15. Farboud B, Aotaki-Keen A, Miyata T, Hjelmeland LM, Handa JT (1999) Development of a polyclonal antibody with broad epitope specificity for advanced glycation endproducts and localization of these epitopes in Bruch's membrane of the aging eye. Mol Vision 5: 11.
16. Ishibashi T, Murata T, Hangai M, Nagai R, Horiuchi S, et al. (1998) Advanced glycation end products in age-related macular degeneration. Arch Ophthalmol 116: 1629–1632.
17. Crabb JW, Miyagi M, Gu X, Shadrach K, West KA, et al. (2002) Drusen proteome analysis: an approach to the etiology of age-related macular degeneration. Proc Natl Acad Sci U S A 99: 14682–14687.
18. Glenn JV, Beattie JR, Barrett L, Frizzell N, Thorpe SR, et al. (2007) Confocal raman microscopy can quantify advanced glycation end product (AGE) modification in Bruch's membrane leading to accurate nondestructive prediction of ocular aging. FASEB J 21: 3542–3552.

19. Price CL, Knight SC (2009) Methylglyoxal: possible link between hyperglycaemia and immune suppression? Trends Endocrinol Metab 20: 312–317.
20. Ben-Shabat S, Itagaki Y, Jockusch S, Sparrow JR, Turro NJ, et al. (2002) Formation of a nona-oxirane from A2E, a lipofuscin fluorophore related to macular degeneration, and evidence of singlet oxygen involvement. Angew Chem Int Ed 41: 814–817.
21. Sparrow JR, Zhou J, Ben-Shabat S, Vollmer H, Itagaki Y, et al. (2002) Involvement of oxidative mechanisms in blue light induced damage to A2E-laden RPE. Invest Ophthalmol Vis Sci 43: 1222–1227.
22. Wu Y, Yanase E, Feng X, Siegel MM, Sparrow JR (2010) Structural characterization of bisretinoid A2E photocleavage products and implications for age-related macular degeneration. Proc Natl Acad Sci 107: 7275–7280.
23. Phillips SA, Thornalley PJ (1993) The formation of methylglyoxal from triose phosphates. Investigation using a specific assay for methylglyoxal. Eur J Biochem 212: 101–105.
24. Thornalley PJ, Yurek-George A, Argirov OK (2000) Kinetics and mechanism of the reaction of aminoguanidine with the alpha-oxoaldehydes glyoxal, methylglyoxal, and 3-deoxyglucosone under physiological conditions. Biochem Pharmacol 60: 55–65.
25. Zhou J, Cai B, Jang YP, Pachydaki S, Schmidt AM, et al. (2005) Mechanisms for the induction of HNE- MDA- and AGE-adducts, RAGE and VEGF in retinal pigment epithelial cells. Exp Eye Res 80: 567–580.
26. Sparrow JR, Parish CA, Hashimoto M, Nakanishi K (1999) A2E, a lipofuscin fluorophore, in human retinal pigmented epithelial cells in culture. Invest Ophthalmol Vis Sci 40: 2988–2995.
27. Wolff DJ, Lubeskie A, Li C (1997) Inactivation and recovery of nitric oxide synthetic capability in cytokine-induced RAW 264.7 cell treated with "irreversible NO synthase inhibitors. Arch Biochem Biophys 338: 73–82.
28. Jang YP, Matsuda H, Itagaki Y, Nakanishi K, Sparrow JR (2005) Characterization of peroxy-A2E and furan-A2E photooxidation products and detection in human and mouse retinal pigment epithelial cells lipofuscin. J Biol Chem 280: 39732–39739.
29. Yamamoto K, Yoon KD, Ueda K, Hashimoto M, Sparrow JR (2011) A novel bisretinoid of retina is an adduct on glycerophosphoethanolamine. Invest Ophthalmol Vis Sci 52: 9084–9090.
30. Radu RA, Mata NL, Bagla A, Travis GH (2004) Light exposure stimulates formation of A2E oxiranes in a mouse model of Stargardt's macular degeneration. Proc Natl Acad Sci U S A 101: 5928–5933.
31. Kim SR, Jang YP, Jockusch S, Fishkin NE, Turro NJ, et al. (2007) The all-trans-retinal dimer series of lipofuscin pigments in retinal pigment epithelial cells in a recessive Stargardt disease model. Proc Natl Acad Sci U S A 104: 19273–19278.
32. Kim SR, Jang Y, Sparrow JR (2010) Photooxidation of RPE Lipofuscin bisretinoids enhanced fluorescence intensity. Vision Res 50: 729–736.
33. Wang W, Ballatori N (1998) Endogenous glutathione conjugates: occurrence and biological functions. Pharmacol Rev 50: 335–355.
34. Dobler D, Ahmed N, Song L, Eboigbodin KE, Thornalley PJ (2006) Increased dicarbonyl metabolism in endothelial cells in hyperglycemia Induces anoikis and impairs angiogenesis by RGD and GFOGER motif modification. Diabetes 55: 1961–1969.
35. Rabbani N, Thornalley PJ (2008) The dicarbonyl proteome. Proteins susceptible to dicarbonyl glycation at functional sites in health, aging and disease. Ann NY Acad Sci 1126: 124–127.
36. Abordo EA, Minhas HS, Thornalley PJ (1999) Accumulation of alpha-oxoaldehydes during oxidative stress: a role in cytotoxicity. Biochem Pharmacol 58: 641–648.

37. Alderson NL, Chachich ME, Frizzell N, Canning P, Metz TO, et al. (2004) Effect of antioxidants and ACE inhibition on chemical modification of proteins and progression of nephropathy in the streptozotocin diabetic rat. Diabetologia 47: 1385–1395.

38. Roy S, Nasser S, Yee M, Graves DT, Roy S (2011) A long-term siRNA strategy regulates fibronectin overexpression and improves vascular lesions in retinas of diabetic rats. Mol Vis 17: 3166–3174.

39. Rabbani N, Thornalley PJ (2008) Dicarbonyls linked to damage in the powerhouse: glycation of mitochondrial proteins and oxidative stress. Biochem Soc Trans 36: 1045–1050.

40. Ahmed N, Thornalley PJ (2002) Chromatographic assay of glycation adducts in human serum albumin glycated *in vitro* by derivatization with 6-aminoquinolyl-*N*-hydroxysuccinimidyl-carbamate and intrinsic fluorescence. Biochem J 364: 15–24.

41. Moore DJ, Hussain AA, Marshall J (1995) Age-related variation in the hydraulic conductivity of Bruch's membrane. Invest Ophthalmol Vis Sci 36: 1290–1297.

42. Glenn JV, Mahaffy H, Wu K, Smith G, Nagai R, et al. (2009) Advanced glycation end product (AGE) accumulation on Bruch's membrane: links to age-related RPE dysfunction. Invest Ophthalmol Vis Sci 50: 441–451.

43. Howes KA, Liu Y, Dunaief JL, Milam AH, Frederick JM, et al. (2004) Receptor for advanced glycation end products and age-related macular degeneration. Invest Ophthalmol Vis Sci 45: 3713–3720.

44. Grey AC, Crouch RK, Koutalos Y, Schey KL, Ablonczy Z (2011) Spatial localization of A2E in the retinal pigment epithelium. Invest Ophthalmol Vis Sci 52: 3926–3933.

45. Zarbin MA, Rosenfeld PJ (2010) Pathway-based therapies for age-related macular degeneration. An integrated survey of emerging treatment alternatives. Retina 30: 1350–1367.

46. Parish CA, Hashimoto M, Nakanishi K, Dillon J, Sparrow JR (1998) Isolation and one-step preparation of A2E and iso-A2E, fluorophores from human retinal pigment epithelium. Proc Natl Acad Sci U S A 95: 14609–14613.

47. Nawa A, Fujita HW, Tokuyama S (2010) Inducible nitric oxide synthase-mediated decrease of intestinal P-glycoprotein expression under streptozotocin-induced diabetic conditions. LIfe Sci 86: 402–409.

17

Fucoidan Reduces Secretion and Expression of Vascular Endothelial Growth Factor in the Retinal Pigment Epithelium and Reduces Angiogenesis In Vitro

Michaela Dithmer[1], Sabine Fuchs[2], Yang Shi[2], Harald Schmidt[3], Elisabeth Richert[1], Johann Roider[1], Alexa Klettner[1]*

1 University of Kiel, University Medical Center, Department of Ophthalmology, Kiel, Germany, **2** University of Kiel, University Medical Center, Experimental Trauma Surgery, Kiel, Germany, **3** MetaPhysiol, Essenheim, Germany

Abstract

Fucoidan is a polysaccharide isolated from brown algae which is of current interest for anti-tumor therapy. In this study, we investigated the effect of fucoidan on the retinal pigment epithelium (RPE), looking at physiology, vascular endothelial growth factor (VEGF) secretion, and angiogenesis, thus investigating a potential use of fucoidan for the treatment of exudative age-related macular degeneration. For this study, human RPE cell line ARPE-19 and primary porcine RPE cells were used, as well as RPE/choroid perfusion organ cultures. The effect of fucoidan on RPE cells was investigated with methyl thiazolyl tetrazolium – assay, trypan blue exclusion assay, phagocytosis assay and a wound healing assay. VEGF expression was evaluated in immunocytochemistry and Western blot, VEGF secretion was evaluated in ELISA. The effect of fucoidan on angiogenesis was tested in a Matrigel assay using calcein-AM vital staining, evaluated by confocal laser scanning microcopy and quantitative image analysis. Fucoidan displays no toxicity and does not diminish proliferation or phagocytosis, but reduces wound healing in RPE cells. Fucoidan decreases VEGF secretion in RPE/choroid explants and RPE cells. Furthermore, it diminishes VEGF expression in RPE cells even when co-applied with bevacizumab. Furthermore, fucoidan reduces RPE-supernatant- and VEGF-induced angiogenesis of peripheral endothelial cells. In conclusion, fucoidan is a non-toxic agent that reduces VEGF expression and angiogenesis in vitro and may be of interest for further studies as a potential therapy against exudative age-related macular degeneration.

Editor: Ted S. Acott, Casey Eye Institute, United States of America

Funding: This study has been partly supported by a DFG research grand (KL2425) and the Hermann Wacker Fond. The funders had no role in study design, data collection and analysis, decision to publish, or preparation of the manuscript.

Competing Interests: Regarding the subject of this paper, the authors declare that no competing interest exist. Independent of this study, AK has been a consultant for and received lecture fees and research funding from Novartis.

* E-mail: aklettner@auge.uni-kiel.de

Introduction

Age-related macular degeneration (AMD) is the leading cause for legal blindness in the industrialized countries and, due to demographic developments, the burden of AMD will increase both as a clinical and as a socio-economical problem [1]. Factors discussed to contribute to AMD development are oxidative stress, chronic inflammation and complement activation [2–4]. In exudative, or wet, AMD, which is responsible for the majority of vision loss in AMD, choroidal neovascularizations (CNV) occur, in which vessels grow from the choroid into the subretinal and retinal space. These immature vessels leak into the retina, leading to vision loss or blindness [5]. For the development of CNV, the presence of vascular endothelial growth factor (VEGF) is vital [6]. Currently, no cure for wet AMD is available, but a deceleration of the disease and even moderate vision improvement can be achieved by anti-VEGF therapies [7]. The antagonist, either ranibizumab, aflibercept or the off-label used bevacizumab, is intravitreally injected. For best therapeutic outcome, injections need to be repeated on a monthly base [8]. Monthly intravitreal

injections are a considerable burden for the patient and the executive clinics [9].

An important source for VEGF in the retina is the retinal pigment epithelium (RPE) [10,11]. The RPE is an epithelial monolayer situated between the choroid and the photoreceptors. It has many functions which are necessary for upholding vision, such as nutrient supply, phagocytosis of shed photoreceptor fragments, recycling of visual pigment or the secretion of growth factors [12]. The RPE constitutively secretes VEGF towards the choroid as a protective factor and to uphold the fenestration of the choriocapillaries [11,13,14]. The secretion of VEGF can be elevated by many factors, such as oxidative stress or hypoxia [15]. The upregulation of VEGF by the RPE due to age-dependent or pathological alterations is considered an important factor in the development of wet AMD [16,17].

Fucoidan is a complex sulfated polysaccharide extracted from brown algae which has been implicated to have anti-tumor, antioxidant and anti-inflammatory effects [18–22]. It is easily available from several marine algae species and is considered as functional food, which may exert systemic effects after oral administration. It has an excellent oral safety profile in animals and humans.

Recently, it has been investigated in a clinical phase I and II study for the treatment of osteoarthritis [23–26]. Its anti-tumor properties have been suggested to be mediated by anti-angiogenic effects, which may be facilitated by interference of fucoidan with VEGF signaling [27,28]. As these properties of fucoidan could also be beneficial in age-related macular degeneration, we were interested in the effects of fucoidan on RPE cells. In this study, we investigated the effects of fucoidan on RPE cells physiology, RPE- derived VEGF and RPE-induced angiogenesis.

Material and Methods

Primary RPE isolation and culture

Porcine eyes were obtained with permission from the local abattoir (Fleischerei Loepthin, Jevenstedt, Germany), where the animals are killed for the purpose of food production and the eyes are regularly removed from the slaughtered animals due to legal regulations (Tier-LMHV (Anlage 5 zu §7 Satz 2, Kapitel III, Nr. 2.4). The usage of the eyes for experimental purposes was conducted in agreement with the animal welfare officer of the University of Kiel. According to the German animal welfare act (TierSchG), it is not considered to be animal research, but an alternative to the use of animals in research.

Primary porcine RPE cells are an established model and were isolated as previously described [29,30]. The eyes were cleaned of adjacent tissue and immersed briefly in antiseptic solution. The anterior part of the eye was removed, as well as lens, vitreous and retina. In each eye cup, trypsin was added, and incubated for 5 min at 37°C. Trypsin solution was removed and substituted with trypsin-EDTA for 45 min at 37°C. RPE cells were gently pipetted off the choroid, collected in medium and washed. Cells were cultivated in Dulbecco's modified Eagle's medium (DMEM, PAA, Cölbe, Germany) supplemented with penicillin/streptomycin (1%), HEPES (25 mM), sodium-pyruvate (110 mg/ml) and 10% fetal calf serum (Linaris GmbH, Wertheim-Bettingen, Germany).

ARPE-19 cell culture

ARPE-19 cells, an immortal human RPE cell line, were purchased from ATCC (Wesel, Germany) and cultivated in Dulbecco's modified Eagle's medium (DMEM; PAA,), supplemented with penicillin/streptomycin (1%), non-essential amino acids (1%), and 10% fetal calf serum (Linaris GmbH).

Perfusion organ culture

Organ culture was prepared as previously described [31]. In brief, freshly slaughtered pig eyes were cleaned of adjacent tissue and immersed briefly in antiseptic solution. The anterior part of the eye was removed, RPE/choroid sheet were separated from sclera and the prepared tissue was fixed between the lower and upper part of a fixation ring. Organ sheets were cultivated in a perfusion chamber (Minucells & Minutissue, Bad Abbach, Germany). The chamber was placed on a heating plate and perfused with medium, (DMEM and Ham F12 medium (PAA) (1:1) supplemented with penicillin/streptomycin (1%), HEPES (25 mM), sodium-pyruvate (110 mg/ml) and 10% porcine serum (PAA). The flow rate was 2 ml/hour. The gas exchange in this system takes place via silicone tubes; the pH and CO_2 content of the media were stabilized by HEPES. The perfusion of the tissue allows a steady-state equilibrium of the tissue [32]. On the second day of cultivation, RPE/choroid sheets were exposed to fucoidan from *Fucus vesiculosus* (Sigma-Aldrich, Steinheim, Germany, Cat-Nr: F5631) (100 µg/ml) and the experiment was conducted as described elsewhere with modification [33]. In brief, supernatant was collected for one hour before treatment. Perfusion of the tissue

was interrupted and the medium was transferred to a falcon tube where fucoidan was added. Additionally, fucoidan was added to the medium reservoir. The medium was transferred back into the chamber and the perfusion was restarted. For untreated cultures, the same procedure was conducted without addition of any substance. The supernatant was collected at designated time points (6 hours, 24 hours and 3 days) for one hour, centrifuged for 5 minutes at 13.000 rpm and stored at −20°C until further evaluation.

MTT - assay

Cell viability in cell culture was tested on confluent cells with methyl thiazolyl tetrazolium (MTT) assay as described elsewhere [34] with modifications. In brief, MTT was solved 0.5 mg/ml in DMEM without phenol red (PAA). The cells were washed three times with PBS and incubated with MTT at 37°C for 2 hours. MTT was discarded and dimethyl sulfoxide (DMSO) was added to the cells. The tissue plates were shaken for 5 minutes, the DMSO collected and the absorption was measured at 550 nm with Elx800 (BioTek, Bad Friedrichshall, Germany).

Trypan-blue exclusion assay (proliferation assay)

To determine the influence of fucoidan on proliferation, a defined number of ARPE-19 (500,000 cells) or primary porcine RPE cells (600,000 cells) were seeded on a 60 mm cell culture dish (Nunc, Roskilde, Denmark). One day after seeding, the cells were stimulated with 100 µg/ml fucoidan for 3 or 7 days. Cells were detached using trypsin/EDTA, centrifuged and resuspended in PBS. To determine the cell number, a trypan-blue exclusion assay was conducted as previously described [35].

Scratch-assay

ARPE-19 cells, or porcine RPE-cells, were seeded in a 12-well-plate. Three wounds were scratched in the confluent cell layer with a toothpick and the cells were washed with PBS to remove detached cells. DMEM without phenolred supplemented with penicillin/streptomycin (1%), HEPES (25 mM), sodium-pyruvate (110 mg/ml), and 10% fetal calf serum was added, microscopic bright field pictures of three precise spots were taken and the coordinates were noted (Zeiss, Jena, Germany). Fucoidan (100 µg/ml) was added to the wells. 24 hours after application, another picture was taken at the same coordinates. To analyze the wound healing capability of the cells, application was conducted in duplicates and three pictures per well were taken. The gap size of the wound was measured with AxioVision Rel.4.8. (Zeiss, Jena, Germany), and the percentage of coverage of the wound was evaluated. Complete coverage was defined as 100%.

Phagocytosis assay

Phagocytosis was assessed as previously described [36]. In brief, photoreceptor outer segments were prepared from porcine retina and used to opsonize FITC-labeled latex beads (diameter 1 µm). Opsonized beads were added to confluent primary RPE cells of 2nd passage, treated with 100 µg/ml fucoidan for 1 hour, and incubated for 4 hour at 37°C. Cells were fixed and prepared for fluorescence microscopy. Eight pictures per slide were taken, beads and nuclei were counted, and the ratio determined.

Treatment of cells for VEGF secretion

Confluent ARPE-19 cells were cultured with addition of 100 µg/ml fucoidan for 1, 3 and five days. Medium was changed and fucoidan added again at day 3 and 4 hours before collection

Supernatant was collected, centrifuged for 5 minutes at 13.000 rpm and stored at $-20°C$ until further evaluation.

VEGF-ELISA

The VEGF-content of the supernatant of cell and organ cultures was measured by a VEGF-ELISA (R&D Systems, Wiesbaden, Germany) following the manufacturer's instructions. The range of detection of the ELISA was between 15 pg/ml and 1046 pg/ml. The ELISA detects all isoforms of VEGF-A, and readily detects porcine VEGF-A [29] as well as human VEGF-A.

Immunocytochemistry

ARPE-19 or porcine RPE-cells, were seeded on coverslips (TH. Geyer, Hamburg, Germany), coated with Collagen A (Biochrom, Berlin, Germany). Confluent cells were exposed to fucoidan (100 µg/ml) for different time intervals. After incubation, cells were washed with PBS and fixed first in 6% PFA (Merck, Darmstadt, Germany), diluted in 2 x PEM-buffer (200 mM PIPES (Carl Roth GmbH, Karlsruhe, Germany), 2 mM magnesium chloride (Merck), 2 mM EGTA (Merck), pH 6.5) for 5 minutes. They were fixed in 6% PFA, diluted in 2 x borate-buffer (200 mM di-sodium tetraborate (Merck), 1.97 mM magnesium chloride, pH 11) for 10 minutes. The cells were permeabilized with 1% Triton X (Carl Roth GmbH) for 15 minutes and borohydride-solution was added to each well. After twofold washing with PBS, binding sites were blocked with Roti Immunoblock (Carl Roth GmbH) for at least one hour. Anti-VEGF (A-20) (Santa Cruz Biotechnology, Heidelberg, Germany, sc-152) as first antibody was dissolved in Roti Immunoblock, added and incubated over night at 4°C. Cells were washed with PBS three times, and the second antibody (Alexa Fluor 488 donkey anti-rabbit IgG (Invitrogen, Darmstadt, Germany)) with 0.4 µM bisbenzimide H in Roti Immunoblock was added. After washing with PBS and aqua dest., cover slides were mounted. As mounting medium, Slowfade gold antifade reagent (Invitrogen) was used. For analyzing, stained cells were visualized with Axio Imager Z1 (Zeiss, Jena, Germany).

Treatment of cells for Western blotting

In order to determine the influence of fucoidan on VEGF in the presence of bevacizumab, confluent ARPE-19 cells were stimulated with 250 µg/ml bevacizumab and 100 µg/ml fucoidan for 1 day, 5 days and 7 days.

Whole cell lysate

Whole cell lysates of ARPE-19 cells after treatment were prepared in an NP-40 buffer. For this, cells were scraped off in PBS, centrifuged, and the pellet was resuspended in in NP-40 buffer (1% Nonidet P40 Substitute (Fluka, Steinheim, Germany), 150 mM NaCl (Carl Roth GmbH), 50 mM Tris (Sigma-Aldrich), pH 8,0) and lysed on ice for at least 30 minutes. Samples were centrifuged at 13.000 rpm for 15 minutes. The protein concentration of the supernatant was determined by BioRad protein assay with BSA as standard.

Western blot

Western blot to detect VEGF expression was conducted as described elsewhere with modifications [30]. To separate proteins with SDS-PAGE, a resolving gel with 12% acrylamide was used. After blotting the gel, the PVDF-membrane (Carl Roth GmbH) was blocked with 4% skim milk in Tris buffered saline with 0.1% Tween for 1 hour at room temperature. The blot was treated with the first antibodies, against beta-actin (Cell Signaling Technologies) or VEGF (A-20) (Santa Cruz Biotechnology), overnight at 4°C in 2% skim milk in Tris buffered saline with 0.1% Tween.

The VEGF antibody used detects intracellular VEGF containing a signal peptide which initiates export across the endoplasmic reticulum; this signal peptide is cleaved before secretion. After washing, the blot was incubated with anti-rabbit IgG, HRP-linked Antibody (Cell Signaling Technologies) in 2% skim milk in Tris buffered saline with 0.1% Tween. Following the final washing, the blot was incubated with Immobilon chemiluminescence reagent (Millipore, Schwalbach, Germany) and the signal was detected with MF-ChemiBis 1.6 (Biostep, Jahnsdorf, Germany). The density of the bands was evaluated using Total lab software (Biostep) and the signal was normalized for β-actin.

Isolation of outgrowth endothelial cells from the peripheral blood

Outgrowth endothelial cells are endothelial cells which can be isolated from peripheral blood in high purity in terms of endothelial cell markers. These cells were isolated from buffy coats and characterized as previously described [37,38]. In brief, blood mononuclear cells were isolated by Biocoll (Biochrom, Berlin, Germany) density centrifugation. Mononuclear cells were seeded onto collagen coated 24-well plates in a density of 5×10^6 cells/well in EGM-2 (Lonza, Belgium) with full supplements from the kit, 5% FBS (PAA Laboratories, Pasching, Austria), and 1% penicillin/streptomycin (PAA Laboratories). After one week, adherent cells were collected by trypsin and reseeded on collagen coated 24-well plates in a density of 0.6×10^6 cells/well. After 2–3 weeks, colonies of endothelial cells (OEC) were harvested and further expanded over several passages using EGM-2 in a splitting ratio of 1:2.

Matrigel angiogenese assay and viability assessment

Angiogenesis experiments were performed on Ibidi Angiogenesis slides by placing 10 µl of matrigel diluted 1:1 in EGM-2 without VEGF in the inner well of the IBIDI slide. After gelation at 37°C for 30 minutes, 10.000 cell OEC/well were seeded in volume of 50 µl EGM-2 (without VEGF) containing the following factors: a) 50 ng/ml VEGF b) 50 ng/ml VEGF plus 100 µg/ml fucoidan c) 100 µg/ml fucoidan d) conditioned medium from retinal pigment epithelial cells donor 1 (RPE1) e) conditioned medium from retinal pigment epithelial cells donor 2 (RPE2) f) conditioned medium from RPE1 plus fucoidan (100 µg/ml), e) conditioned medium from RPE2 plus fucoidan (100 µg/ml) and g) EGM-2 containing all supplements from the kit besides VEGF.

After 1 day of culture, cells were analysed for angiogenic activity after the treatment with respective substances as described above. In addition, the cellular viability was assessed using calcein-AM. For this purpose, cells were treated with 0.2 µg/ml calcein-AM (BD, Heidelberg, Germany) in cell culture medium for 10 minutes. After medium exchange, cells grown on the matrigel substrate were visualized on a confocal laser scanning microscope (Zeiss LSM 510 Meta, Jena, Germany). For each treatment, at least 3 pictures were taken from two technical replicates. These experiments and the picture analysis were performed with endothelial cells from three different donors.

Image Analysis

The microscopic images were analyzed using the image processing program ImageJ Vers. 1.47 [39]. In brief, tube-like structures were extracted from the background by automatic segmentation after background correction. The binaries of the tube-like structures were further processed, including smoothing and a final manual correction. The resulting binaries were processed in several steps, yielding a skeleton as previously

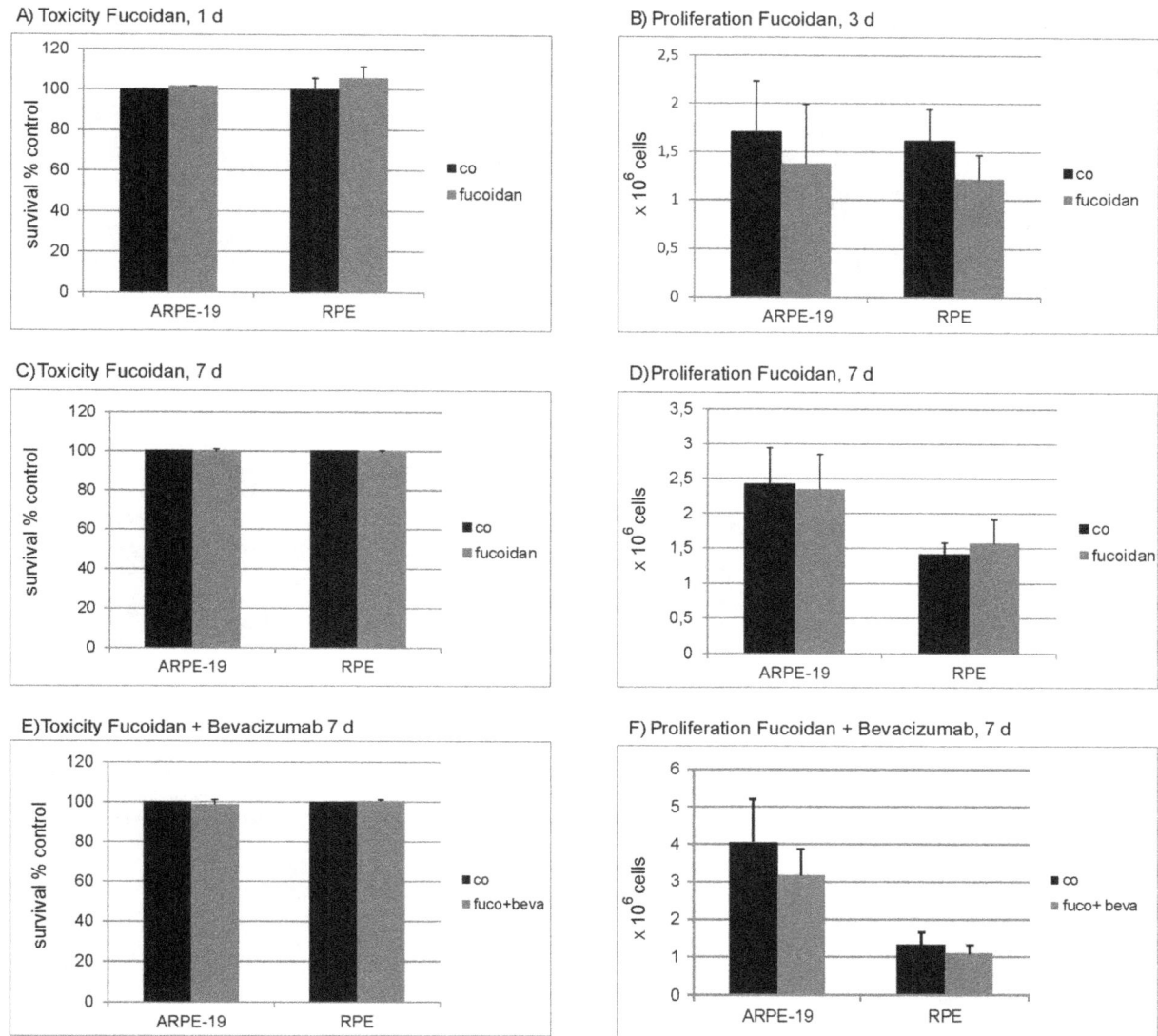

Figure 1. Toxicity and proliferation. To investigate toxicity, RPE or ARPE-19 cells were treated with 100 μg/ml fucoidan for 24 hours (A) or 7 days (C). In addition, cells were treated with a combination of fucoidan (100 μg/ml) and bevacizumab (250 μg/ml) for 7 days (E). Toxicity was measured with MTT test. Fucoidan did not exert toxic effects on RPE or ARPE-19 cells at any tested application (A,C,E). To investigate proliferation, a defined number of cells were seeded, cells were treated with fucoidan (100 μg/ml) and cell number was assessed after 3 days (B) and 7 days (D). In addition, cells were treated with a combination of fucoidan (100 μg/ml) and bevacizumab (250 μg/ml) and cell number was assessed after 7 days (F). No significant influence on proliferation was found. Significance was determined with student's t-test. Co = untreated control, fuco = fucoidan, beva = bevacizumab.

described [40] and the quantitative analysis of skeleton-length was used to characterize the tubular structures.

Statistics

Statistical analysis was performed with MS-Excel. Means ± standard deviation (s.d.) was calculated for at least 3 independent sets of experiments. Significant differences between means were calculated by an unpaired t-test. A p-value of 0.05 or less was considered significant. For angiogenesis assay, images from 3 donors were quantified and means ± s.d. were calculated for each treatment (n = 9 to 14). Significant differences between means were calculated by an unpaired t-test for either homoscedastic or heteroscedastic variances according to the results of a previous variance ratio analysis (F-test, p<0.05).

Results

Toxicity of fucoidan

Toxicity of fucoidan was tested in MTT assay. No toxicity of fucoidan (100 μg/ml) applied for 24 hours could be detected in ARPE-19 (101.5% (±5.52)) or in porcine primary RPE cells (105.6% (±5.50)) (Fig. 1A). Similar results were obtained after 7 days, with no toxicity detected in ARPE-19 cells (99.72% (±1.36)) and in primary porcine RPE cells (99.38% (± 0.93)) (Fig. 1C). Additionally, the toxicity of a combined treatment with fucoidan and bevacizumab after seven days was assessed. No toxicity could be observed (ARPE-19: 98.7% (±2.25); RPE: 100.47% (±0.55)) (Fig. 1E).

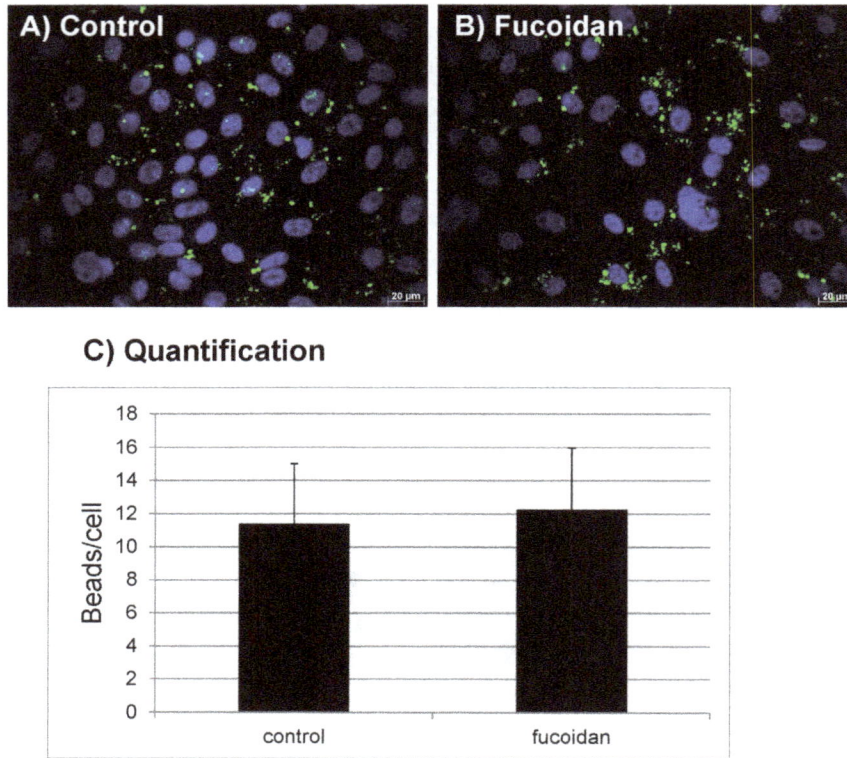

Figure 2. Phagocytosis. Primary RPE cells were stimulated with 100 µg/ml fucoidan for 1 hour. RPE cells were exposed to FITC-labeled, photoreceptor outer segment opsonized beads for 4 hours and uptake of the beads was evaluated in fluorescence microscope. No influence of fucoidan on RPE phagocytosis was found. A) control, B) fucoidan, C) quantification of uptaken beads. Significance was determined with student's t-test.

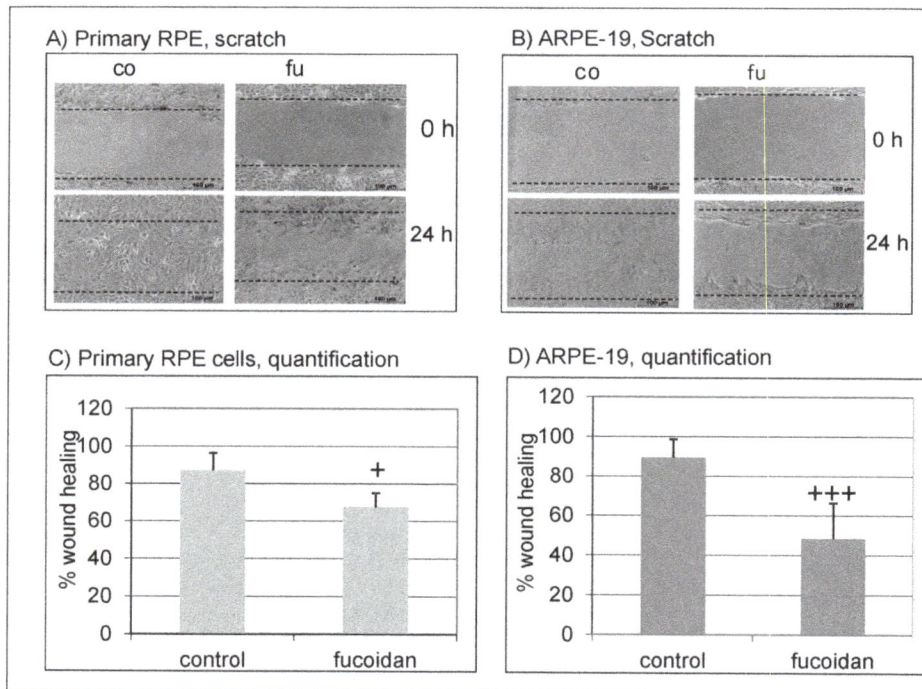

Figure 3. Wound healing. A wound was scratched in a confluent cell layer of primary porcine RPE cells and ARPE-19 cells. Cells were either untreated (control) or exposed to fucoidan (100 µg/ml) for 24 hours. Exemplary pictures of wound healing are depicted for primary RPE cells (A) and ARPE-19 cells (B). The percentage of coverage after 24 hours of wound healing is depicted in the graphs for primary RPE cells (C) and ARPE-19 cells (D). Fucoidan significantly reduces wound healing in both RPE and ARPE-19 cells. Significance was determined with student's t-test, + $p<0.05$; +++ $p<0.001$.

A) RPE/choroid organ culture

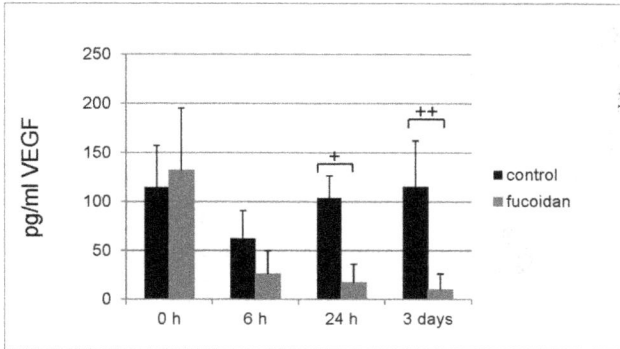

B) ARPE-19

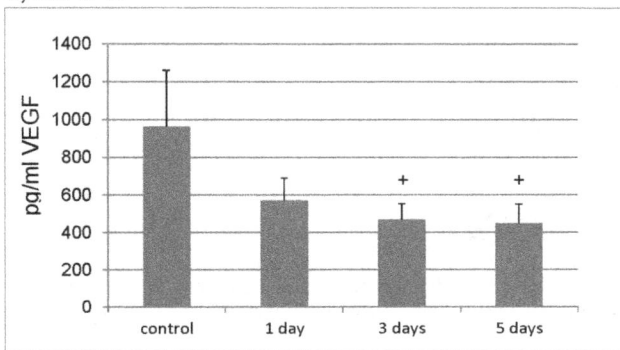

Figure 4. VEGF secretion. VEGF secretion was investigated in RPE/choroid organ culture (A) and ARPE-19 cell culture (B). RPE/choroid perfusion organ cultures were treated with 100 μg/ml fucoidan for 3 days and supernatant was collected at 6 hours, 24 hours and 3 days for one hour. ARPE-19 cells were treated with 100 μg/ml fucoidan for five days, and medium was collected after 1 day, 3 days and 5 days. VEGF content was evaluated with ELISA. Fucoidan reduced VEGF content compared to control in organ culture after 24 hours and 3 days (A). In cell culture, a reduction of VEGF secretion can be found after 3 days and 5 days (B). Significance was determined with student's t-test, + p<0.05; ++ p<0.01.

Influence of fucoidan on proliferation

To analyze the effect of fucoidan on proliferation, definite cell numbers of ARPE-19, or porcine RPE cells, were seeded and the cell number was assessed with a trypan blue exclusion assay after 3 days or 7 days of incubation. No statistical significant effect on proliferation was found for either cell type after 3 days (ARPE-19: control 1.46×10^6 cells (± 0.77); fucoidan 1.44×10^6 cells (± 0.25); RPE: control 1.61×10^6 cells (± 0.32); fucoidan 1.21×10^6 cells (± 0.28)) (Fig. 1B), or after 7 days (ARPE-19: control 2.42×10^6 cells (± 0.52); fucoidan 2.35×10^6 cells (± 0.50); RPE: control 1.41×10^6 cells (± 0.17); fucoidan 1.57×10^6 cells (± 0.34)) (Fig. 1D). In addition, the effect of a combined treatment with fucoidan and bevacizumab on proliferation was assessed. After 7 days of combined treatment, no statistical significant effect on proliferation was found for either cell type (ARPE-19: control 4.05×10^6 cells (± 1.17), fucoidan and bevacizumab: 3.16×10^6 cells (± 0.72); RPE: control 1.32×10^6 cells (± 0.32), fucoidan and bevacizumab 1.09×10^6 cells (± 0.21)) (Fig. 1F).

Influence of fucoidan on phagocytosis

To analyze the effect of fucoidan on the phagocytosis of photoreceptor outer segments by primary RPE, a phagocytosis assay using POS-opsonized beads was conducted, which detects bound and internalized beads. No influence of fucoidan on the phagocytosis by the RPE could be found (control: 11.38 ± 3.63 beads/cells; 100 μg/ml fucoidan: 12.24 ± 3.72 beads/cell) (Fig. 2).

Influence of fucoidan on wound healing

To analyze the effect of fucoidan on wound healing, a scratch assay was performed with ARPE-19 and primary porcine RPE cells. In untreated primary RPE cells, 87.30% (± 9.05) of the wound was closed after 24 hours. In contrast, in primary RPE cells treated with fucoidan, only 67.47% (± 7.56) of the wound was closed. Similar results were obtained in ARPE-19 cells, where in the untreated control, 87.23% (± 8.7) of the wound was covered in contrast to fucoidan stimulated cells, where only 41.24% (± 9.54) of the area was covered (Fig. 3).

Influence of fucoidan on VEGF secretion

The effect of fucoidan on the secretion of VEGF was tested in ARPE-19 cells and RPE/choroid perfusion organ culture. Supernatant of cell and organ cultures was evaluated for VEGF content in VEGF ELISA. In RPE/choroid organ culture, VEGF reduction was found after 6 hours, and reduction reached significance 1 day and 3 days post stimulus compared to untreated control (6 hours: control 62.40 ± 28.29 pg/ml, fucoidan $25.90\% \pm 24.00$, p=0.16; 1 day: control 103.76 ± 22.80 pg/ml, fucoidan 16.91 ± 19.09), p<0.01; 3 days: control 115.35 ± 47.00 pg/ml, fucoidan 9.53 ± 16.51, p<0.05) (Fig. 4A). In ARPE-19 cell culture, the secretion of VEGF was reduced compared to control after 1 day (earliest time point tested), and the reduction was significant at day 3 and day 5 (control: 965.45 ± 295.21 pg/ml VEGF; 1 day: 571.26. ± 118.52, p=0.098; 3 days: 469.48, $\pm 82.83.$, p<0.05; 5 days: 447.92 ± 102.02, p<0.05)) (Fig. 4B).

Influence of fucoidan on VEGF expression

Confluent ARPE-19 or primary RPE cells were exposed to fucoidan (100 μg/ml) for 3 days, and the expression of intracellular VEGF was detected in immunohistochemistry. A clear reduction of the intracellular VEGF signal is seen in cells stimulated with fucoidan (Fig. 5).

Influence of fucoidan on VEGF expression in the presence of bevacizumab

Bevacizumab is an anti-VEGF antibody commonly used in anti-VEGF therapy. In order to evaluate whether fucoidan also exerts effects on VEGF expression in cells treated with a VEGF antagonist, ARPE-19 cells were stimulated with the clinically relevant concentration of bevacizumab (250 μg/ml) and fucoidan (100 μg/ml) for 1 day, 5 days and 7 days, evaluating the effect on VEGF expression in Western blot. After one day of application, a slight reduction of VEGF165 expression can be found (Fig. 6A). After 5 and 7 days of incubation, a strong reduction was seen (Fig. 6A) that reached significance in densitometric evaluation (day 1: 0.544 ± 0.39; day 5: 0.085 ± 0.036, p<0.001; day 7: 0.256 ± 0.16, p<0.05) (Fig. 6B).

Influence of fucoidan on angiogenesis

On the matrigel matrix outgrowth, endothelial cells formed interconnected vascular networks. These networks were increased in the presence of conditioned medium from the retinal pigment epithelium cells (Fig. 7A), RPE1 and RPE 2, in comparison to the positive control for angiogenesis including a concentration of

A) primary RPE

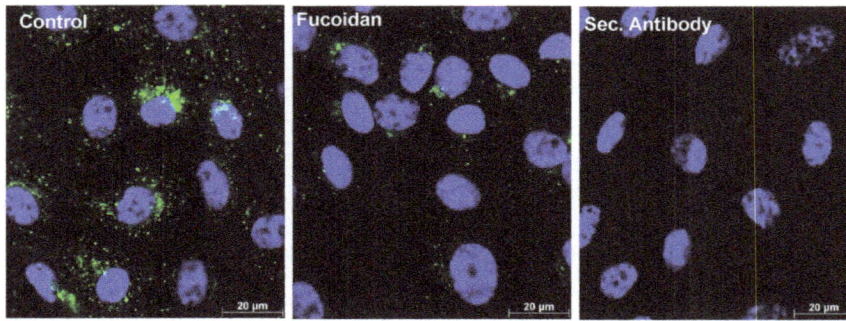

B) ARPE-19

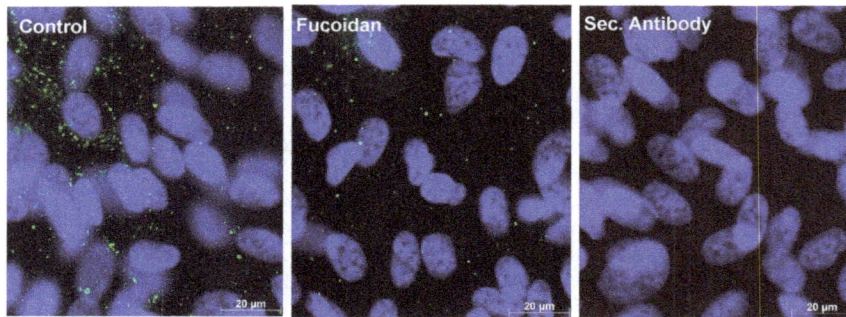

Figure 5. VEGF165 expression. Primary RPE cells (A) and ARPE-19 cells (B) were treated with 100 µg/ml fucoidan for 24 hours and the expression of intracellular VEGF (still containing signal peptide) was evaluated using immunocytochemistry. Cells treated with fucoidan exhibited a substantial decrease in intracellular VEGF expression.

A) Exemplary Western blot

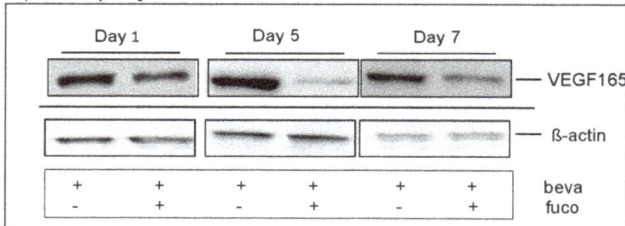

B) Densitometric evaluation

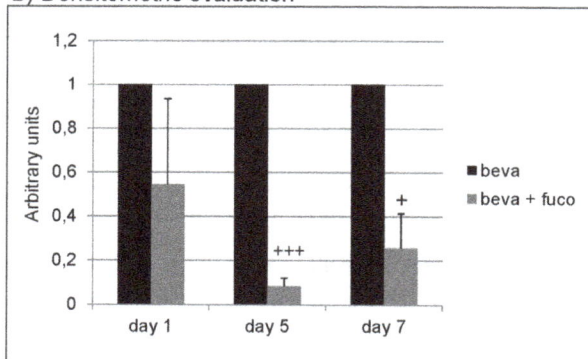

Figure 6. VEGF expression in presence of bevacizumab. ARPE-19 cells were treated with 250 µg/ml bevacizumab and 100 µg/ml fucoidan for 1 day, 5 days and 7 days. Controls cells were treated with bevacizumab only. Western blot for intracellular VEGF (still containing signal peptide) depicted a reduction of VEGF165 in Western blot at day 5 and day 7 (A), which was significant in densitrometric evaluation (B). Significance was determined with student's t-test, + $p < 0.05$; +++ $p < 0.001$. beva = bevacizumab, fuco = fucoidan.

50 ng/ml VEGF. In EGM-2, which contained all growth factors provided by the bullet kit with the exception of VEGF, OEC showed some angiogenic structures. Nevertheless, in all approaches, the addition of fucoidan resulted in a reduction of angiogenic structures, whereas the cells were still viable as indicated by the staining for the viability marker calcein-AM. According to these morphological observations, images derived from experiments of three different donors of OEC were analysed by quantitative image analysis to quantify the anti-angiogenic effect of fucoidan. The results are depicted in Fig. 7B using the skeleton length of vascular structures as indicator for the angiogenic activity. Quantitative evaluation indicated a statistical significant reduction of the skeleton length in the presence of fucoidan in all groups tested.

Discussion

In our study, we investigated the effects of fucoidan on RPE cells, utilizing three different models of RPE cells: ARPE-19 cells, primary porcine cells of second and third passage, and RPE/ choroid organ culture. While the use of ARPE-19 cells as a model of RPE cells is under debate [41], it is still considered a valuable tool in RPE research. However, data obtained with ARPE-19 cells should be confirmed using models which resemble natural RPE cells more closely. In our study, we have used primary RPE cells of second and third passage, which display a cobble-stone morphology and are still pigmented, indicating a high differentiation. Moreover, in RPE/choroid organ cultures, RPE cells are cultured on their natural substrate, the Bruch's membrane, with connections to the choroid. A constant perfusion generates a steady state equilibrium. RPE cells in this culture maintain their morphology and differentiation for the time period investigated [31].

A) Vascular networks

B) Quantification

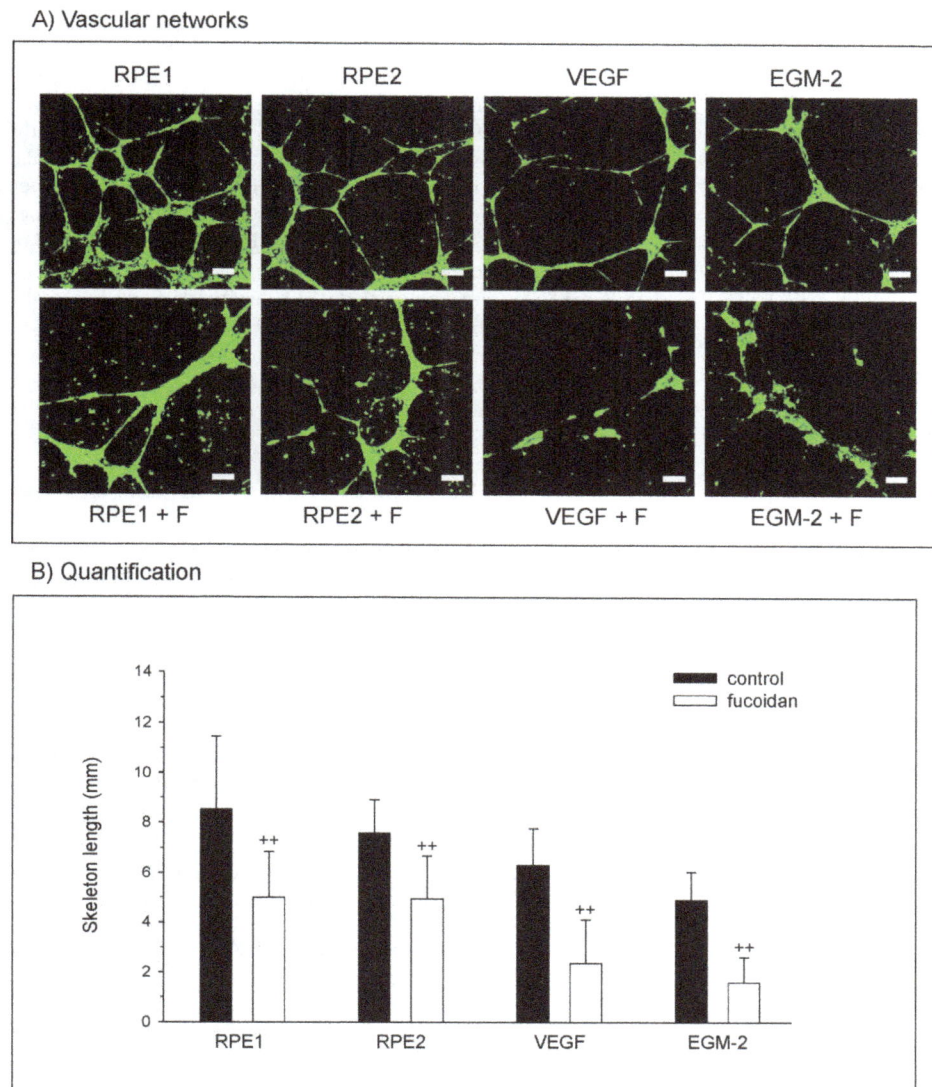

Figure 7. Angiogenesis. (A) Morphological appearance of OEC grown on Matrigel and stained with Calcein-AM which is converted to a green fluorescence by viable cells. Results indicated angiogenic structures in OEC treated with conditioned medium from RPE cells from different donors, VEGF and the EGM-2 (no VEGF). Additional treatment with fucoidan resulted in the reduction of vascular structures. (B) Quantitative image analysis depicting the skeleton length of angiogenic structures. Significance was determined with student's t-test, ++ p<0.01.

The rationale of this study was to conduct first line in vitro experiments to test whether fucoidan might be a possible candidate for further investigation for the treatment of AMD. Fucoidan is a complex, heterogeneous mixture of branched, sulfated polysaccharides found in brown algae and marine organisms [18]. Many studies have shown a variety of beneficial effects of this polysaccharide, such as anti-inflammatory, anti-tumor, anti-oxidative and even complement inhibiting properties [18–22]. As the current concepts of AMD development include oxidative stress, complement activation and inflammatory events, fucoidan may be an interesting molecule to be studied for possible AMD intervention. Furthermore, fucoidan has been described to be anti-angiogenic, possibly by inhibiting VEGFR-2 signal transduction [27,28]. As VEGF is the current treatment target for the therapy of AMD, we focused on its effects on VEGF derived from the retinal pigment epithelium.

First, we assessed the effect of fucoidan on the physiology of RPE cells. We tested toxicity, proliferation, wound healing and phagocytosis. Fucoidan has been described to exert apoptotic effects on neoplastic cells [42,43], but no general toxicity has been found so far [23–26]. In accordance with this, no toxicity of fucoidan on RPE cells, both primary and cell line, could be detected in our study. In addition, no toxicity on endothelial cells could be detected at the investigated time points. Furthermore, RPE cell proliferation was not altered, in contrast to the effect of fucoidan on neoplastic cells [42,44]. An important task of RPE cells is the phagocytosis of photoreceptor outer segment. Fucoidan has previously been shown to interfere with phagocytotic functions [45]. However, we did not find any reduction of phagocytosis of photoreceptor outer segments in fucoidan treated cells, suggesting that no interference with this function occurred. The only effect of fucoidan on RPE cell physiology found in our study was a decline in wound healing ability assessed by scratch assay. As we did not find any influence of RPE cell proliferation, this reduction is most likely due to an impairment of migration. Fucoidan is the binding partner of several extracellular matrix interacting molecules such as integrins [46], which may provide an explanation for a reduced migratory ability. As RPE cells are generally post mitotic and do not migrate in a physiological situation, this property of fucoidan should not be of further consequence in the retina. However, therapeutic laser burns in the retina may be covered by migrating RPE cells [47], so fucoidan may interfere with wound healing after laser treatment. Furthermore, coverage of small RPE lesions or small RPE tears may be disturbed when migration is inhibited by fucoidan [48,49]. In dry AMD, however, RPE migration in the retina has been observed in a high percentage of patients, which is found especially over drusen [50]. This might also be suppressed by fucoidan, thus possibly reducing AMD-related anatomical changes. Taken together, a general excellent toxicity profile can be confirmed for RPE cells.

The main topic of this study was the effect of fucoidan on RPE derived VEGF. We were able to show that fucoidan reduces VEGF secretion in RPE cells and RPE/choroid organ cultures. In addition, fucoidan reduces intracellular VEGF expression in RPE cells. These data indicate a possible use as a VEGF-antagonist. Moreover, even when bevacizumab is present, fucoidan further reduces VEGF expression, indicating that fucoidan may exert additional beneficial effects even under anti-VEGF treatment and may be useful as an additive therapy. Finally, we were able to show that fucoidan reduces angiogenesis induced by RPE supernatant as well as by VEGF alone, which is in concordance with the published anti-angiogenic effects of fucoidan [27,51]. This shows that the anti-angiogenic effect is not only found in a neoplastic context but is also valid for RPE-induced angiogenesis.

The pathways through which fucoidan reduces VEGF expression and secretion are not known. Fucoidan is able to bind to VEGF165 and reduce VEGFR-2 signaling [27,28]. In previous studies, we could show that extracellular inhibition of VEGF reduces VEGF expression in RPE cells [30] and that inhibition of VEGFR-2 reduces VEGF secretion in RPE organ culture [33],

indicating positive autocrine regulatory effects of VEGF. Thus, a possible pathway through which fucoidan reduces VEGF expression may be the inhibition of autocrine VEGFR-2 signaling. However, fucoidan reduces VEGF expression even at a concomitant application with bevacizumab. As bevacizumab at the concentrations used is able to bind to all available extracellular VEGF [30], the inhibition of an autocrine positive feedback loop cannot be the only mechanism of VEGF reduction. The exact pathways of fucoidan mediated VEGF reduction needs to be further elucidated.

Fucoidan is currently considered a functional food, but is also investigated in clinical trials [23,52]. Its effects have been studied not only in vitro, but also in animal and human studies, were it exhibits an excellent toxic profile [23–26]. While its oral availability is under debate [22], recent studies indicate a possible absorption of fucoidan by the gastrointestinal tract [18,26], which would render an oral application an attractive alternative to intravitreal injections. However, our data, obtained in vitro, need to be confirmed in vivo in order to elucidate its possible transferability into the living organism.

In conclusion, we show that fucoidan is safe for RPE cells and reduces VEGF expression and secretion in RPE cells, as well as VEGF-induced angiogenesis, making it an interesting molecule for further studies for the use in AMD.

Acknowledgments

Parts of the data presented here were presented at the ARVO meeting 2013, the DOG meeting 2013 and the VNA meeting 2013.

Author Contributions

Conceived and designed the experiments: MD SF YS HS AK JR. Performed the experiments: MD SF YS HS ER AK. Analyzed the data: MD SF YS HS ER JR AK. Contributed reagents/materials/analysis tools: MD SF HS JR AK. Wrote the paper: MD SF AK. Revision: MD SF YS HS ER JR AK.

References

1. Schrader WF (2006) Age-related macular degeneration: a socioeconomic time bomb in our aging society. Ophthalmologe 103: 742–748.
2. Zarbin M (2004) Current concepts in the pathogenesis of age-related macular degeneration. Arch Ophthalmol 122: 598–614.
3. Sparrow JR, Ueda K, Zhou J (2012) Complement dysregulation in AMD: RPE-Bruch's membrane-choroid. Mol Aspects Med 33: 436–445.
4. Parmeggiani F, Romano MR, Costagliola C, Semeraro F, Incorvaia C, et al. (2012) Mechanism of inflammation in age-related macular degeneration. Mediators Inflamm 2012: 546786.
5. Miller DW, Joussen AM, Holz FG (2003) The molecular mechanisms of age-related macular degeneration. Ophthalmologe 100: 92–96.
6. Lu M, Adamis AP (2006) Molecular biology of choroidal neovascularization. Ophthalmol Clin North Am 19: 323–334.
7. Miller JW, Le Couter J, Strauss EC, Ferrara N (2013) Vascular endothelial growth factor a in intraocular vascular disease. Ophthalmology 120: 106–114.
8. Rosenfeld PJ, Rich RM, Lalwani GA (2006) Ranibizumab: Phase III clinical trial results. Ophthalmol Clin North Am 19: 361–372.
9. Hodge W, Brown A, Kymes S, Cruess A, Blackhouse G, et al. (2010) Pharmacologic management of neovascular age-related macular degeneration: systematic review of economic evidence and primary economic evaluation. Can J Ophthalmol 45: 223–230.
10. Saint-Geniez M, Maldonado AE, D'Amore PA (2006) VEGF expression and receptor activation in the choroid during development and in the adult. Invest Ophthalmol Vis Sci 47: 3135–3142.
11. Blaauwgeers HGT, Holtkamp GM, Rutten H, Witmer AN, Koolwijk P, et al. (1999) Polarized vascular endothelial growth factor secretion by human retinal pigment epithelium and localization of vascular endothelial growth factor receptors on the inner choriocapillaris. Evidence for a trophic paracrine relation. Am J Pathol 155: 421–428.
12. Strauss O (2005) The retinal pigment epithelium in visual function. Physiol Rev 85: 845–881.
13. Peters S, Heiduschka P, Julien S, Ziemssen F, Fietz H, et al. (2007) Ultrastructural findings in the primate eye after intravitreal injection of bevacizumab. Am J Ophthalmol 143: 995–1002.
14. Gerber HP, McMurtrey A, Kowalski J, Yan M, Keyt BA, et al. (1998) Vascular endothelial growth factor regulates endothelial cell survival through the phosphatidylinositol 3'-kinase/Akt signal transduction pathway. Requirement for Flk-1/KDR activation. J Biol Chem 273: 30336–30343.
15. Klettner A, Roider J (2012) Mechanisms of Pathological VEGF Production in the Retina and Modification with VEGF-Antagonists. In: Stratton R, Hauswirth W, Gardner T, editors. Oxidative Stress in Applied Basic Research and Clinical Practise: Studies on Retinal and Choroidal Disorders. Humana Press. pp. 277–307.
16. Campochiaro P, Soloway P, Ryan SJ, Miller JW (1999) The pathogenesis of choroidal neovascularization in patients with age-related macular degeneration. Mol Vis 5: 34–38.
17. Schlingemann RO (2004) The role of growth factors and the wound healing response in age-related macular degeneration. Graefes Arch Clin Exp Ophthalmol 242: 91–101.
18. Fitton JH (2011) Therapies from fucoidan; multifunctional marine polymers. Mar Drugs 9: 1731–1760.
19. Tissot B, Montdargent B, Chevolot L, Varenne A, Descroix S, et al. (2003) Interaction of fucoidan with the protein of the complement classical pathway. Biochim Biophys Acta 1651: 5–16.
20. Rocha de Souza MC, Marques CT, Guerra Dore CM, Ferreira da Silva FR, Oliveira Rocha HA, et al. (2007) Antioxidant activities of sulfated polysaccharides form brown and red seaweeds. J Appl Phycol 19: 153–160.
21. Cumashi A, Ushakova N, Preobrazhenskaya ME, D'Incecco A, Piccoli A, et al. (2007) A comparative study of the anti-inflammatory, anticoagulant, antiangiogenic, and antiadhesive activities of the nine different fucoidans from brown seaweed. Glycobiology 17: 541–552.
22. Azuma K, Ishihara T, Nakamoto H, Amaha T, Osaki T, et al. (2012) Effects of oral administration of fucoidan extracted from Cladosiphon okamuranus on

tumor growth and survival time in a tumor bearing mouse model. Mar Drugs 10: 2337–2348.

23. Myers SP, O'Connor J, Fitton JH, Brooks L, Rolfe M, et al. (2010) A combined phase I and phase II open label study on the effects of a seaweed extract nutrient complex on osteoarthritis. Biologics 4: 33–44.

24. Irhimeh MR, Fitton JH, Lowenthal RM (2007) Fucoidan ingestion increases the expression of CXCR4 on human CD34+ cells. Exp Hematol 35: 989–994.

25. Li N, Zhang Q, Song J (2005) Toxicological evaluation of fucoidan extracted from Laminaria japonica in Wistar rats. Food Chem Toxicol 43: 421–426.

26. Abe S, Hiramatsu K, Ichikawa O, Kawamoto H, Kasagi T, et al. (2013) Safety evaluation of excessive ingestion of mozuku fucoidan in human. J Food Sci 78: T648–T651.

27. Koyanagi S, Tanigawa N, Nakagawa H, Soeda S, Shimeno H (2003) Oversulfation of fucoidan enhances its anti-angiogenic and antitumor activities. Biochem Pharmacol 65: 173–179.

28. Narazaki M, Segarra M, Tosato G (2008) Sulfated polysaccharides identified as inducers of neuropilin-1 internalization and functional inhibition of VEGF165 and semaphorin3A. Blood 111: 4126–4136.

29. Wiencke AK, Kiilgaard JF, Nicolini J, Bundgaard M, Röpke C, et al. (2003) Growth of cultured porcine retinal pigment epithelial cells. Acta Ophthalmol Scand 81: 170–176.

30. Klettner A, Roider J (2008) Comparison of bevacizumab, ranibizumab and pegaptanib in vitro: efficiency and possible additional pathways. Invest Ophthalmol Vis Sci 49: 4523–4527.

31. Miura Y, Klettner A, Noelle B, Hasselbach H, Roider J (2010) Change of morphological and functional characteristics of retinal pigment epithelium cells during cultivation of retinal pigment epithelium-choroid perfusion tissue culture. Ophthalmic Res 43: 122–133.

32. Minuth WW, Steiner P, Strehl R, Schumacher K, de Vries U, et al. (1999) Modulation of cell differentiation in perfusion culture. Exp Nephrol 7: 394–406.

33. Klettner A, Westhues D, Lassen J, Bartsch S, Roider J (2013) Regulation of constitutive vascular endothelial growth factor secretion in retinal pigment epithelium/choroid organ cultures: p38, nuclear factor κB, and the vascular endothelial growth factor receptor-2/phosphatidylinositol 3 kinase pathway. Mol Vis 19: 281–291.

34. Klettner AK, Kruse ML, Meyer T, Wesch D, Kabelitz D, et al (2009) Different properties of VEGF-antagonists: Bevacizumab but not Ranibizumab accumulates in RPE cells. Graefes Arch Clin Exp Ophthalmol 247: 1601–1608.

35. Klettner A, Koinzer S, Waetzig V, Herdegen T, Roider J (2010) Deferoxamine mesylate is toxic for retinal pigment epithelium cells, and its toxicity is mediated by p38. Cutan Ocul Toxicol 29:122–129.

36. Klettner A, Möhle F, Lucius R, Roider J (2011) Quantifiying FITC-labeled latex beads opsonized with photoreceptor outer segment fragments: an easy and inexpensive method of investigating phagocytosis in retinal pigment epithelium cells. Ophthalmic Res 46: 88–91.

37. Fuchs S, Motta A, Migliaresi C, Kirkpatrick CJ (2006) Outgrowth endothelial cells isolated and expanded from human peripheral blood progenitor cells as a

potential source of autologous cells for endothelialization of silk fibroin biomaterials. Biomaterials 27: 5399–5408.

38. Fuchs S, Hofmann A, Kirkpartrick C (2007) Microvessel-like structures from outgrowth endothelial cells from human peripheral blood in 2-dimensional and 3-dimensional co-cultures with osteoblastic lineage cells. Tissue Eng 13: 2577–2588.

39. Rasband WS (1997–2012) ImageJ, U. S. National Institutes of Health, Bethesda, Maryland, USA, http://imagej.nih.gov/ij/.

40. Fuchs S, Jiang X, Schmidt H, Dohle E, Ghanaati S, et al. (2009) Dynamic processes involved in the pre-vascularization of silk fibroin constructs for bone regeneration using outgrowth endothelial cells. Biomaterials 30: 1329–1338.

41. Cai H, Del Priore LV (2006) Gene expression profile of cultured adult compared to immortalized human RPE. Mol Vis 12:1–14.

42. Aisa Y, Miyakawa Y, Nakazato T, Shibata H, Saito K, et al. (2005) Fucoidan induces apoptosis of human HS-Sultan cells accompanied by activation of caspase-3 and down-regulation of ERK pathways. Am J Hematol 78: 7–14.

43. Kim EJ, Park SY, Lee JY, Park JH (2010) Fucoidan present in brown algae induces apoptosis of human colon cancer cells. BMC Gastroenterology 10: 96–107.

44. Riou D, Colliec-Jouault S, Pinczon du Sel D, Bosch S, Siavoshian S, et al. (1996) Antitumor and antiproliferative effects of a fucan extracted from ascophyllum nodosum against a non-small-cell bronchopulmonary carcinoma line. Anticancer Res 16: 1213–1218.

45. Johnson JD, Hess KL, Cook-Mills JM (2003) CD44, α_4 integrin, and fucoidin receptor-mediated phagocytosis of apoptotic leukocytes. J Leukoc Biol 74: 810–820.

46. Liu JM, Bignon J, Haroun-Bouhedja F, Bittoun P, Vassy J, et al. (2005) Inhibitory effect of fucoidan on the adhesion of adenocarcinoma cells to fibronectin. Anticancer Res 25: 2129–2134.

47. Roider J, Michaud NA, Flotte TJ, Birngruber R (1992) Response of the retinal pigment epithelium to selective photocoagulation. Arch Ophthalmol 110: 1786–1792.

48. Caramoy A, Fauser S, Kirchhof B (2012) Fundus autofluorescence and spectral-domain optical coherence tomography findings suggesting tissue remodelling in retinal pigment epithelium tear. Br J Ophthalmol 96: 1211–1216.

49. Lopez PF, Yan Q, Kohen L, Rao NA, Spee C, et al. (1995) Retinal pigment epithelial wound healing in vivo. Arch Ophthalmol 113: 1437–1446.

50. Ho J, Witkin AJ, Liu J, Chen Y, Fujimoto JG, et al. (2011) Documentation of intraretinal retinal pigment epithelium migration via high-speed ultrahigh-resolution optical coherence tomography. Ophthalmology 118: 687–693.

51. Matou S, Helley D, Chabut D, Bros A, Fischer AM (2002) Effect of fucoidan on fibroblast growth factor-2-induced angiogenesis in vitro. Thromb Res 106: 213–221.

52. Araya N, Takahashi K, Sato T, Nakamura T, Sawa C, et al. (2011) Fucoidan therapy decreases the proviral load in patients with human T-lymphotropic virus type-1-associated neurological disease. Antivir Ther 16: 89–98.

Outcomes in Cochrane Systematic Reviews Addressing Four Common Eye Conditions: An Evaluation of Completeness and Comparability

Ian J. Saldanha*, Kay Dickersin, Xue Wang, Tianjing Li

Department of Epidemiology, Johns Hopkins Bloomberg School of Public Health, Baltimore, Maryland, United States of America

Abstract

Introduction: Choice of outcomes is critical for clinical trialists and systematic reviewers. It is currently unclear how systematic reviewers choose and pre-specify outcomes for systematic reviews. Our objective was to assess the completeness of pre-specification and comparability of outcomes in all Cochrane reviews addressing four common eye conditions.

Methods: We examined protocols for all Cochrane reviews as of June 2013 that addressed glaucoma, cataract, age-related macular degeneration (AMD), and diabetic retinopathy (DR). We assessed completeness and comparability for each outcome that was named in ≥25% of protocols on those topics. We defined a completely-specified outcome as including information about five elements: *domain, specific measurement, specific metric, method of aggregation,* and *time-points.* For each domain, we assessed comparability in how individual elements were specified across protocols.

Results: We identified 57 protocols addressing glaucoma (22), cataract (16), AMD (15), and DR (4). We assessed completeness and comparability for five outcome domains: quality-of-life, visual acuity, intraocular pressure, disease progression, and contrast sensitivity. Overall, these five outcome domains appeared 145 times (instances). Only 15/145 instances (10.3%) were completely specified (all five elements) (median = three elements per outcome). Primary outcomes were more completely specified than non-primary (median = four versus two elements). Quality-of-life was least completely specified (median = one element). Due to largely incomplete outcome pre-specification, conclusive assessment of comparability in outcome usage across the various protocols per condition was not possible.

Discussion: Outcome pre-specification was largely incomplete; we encourage systematic reviewers to consider all five elements. This will indicate the importance of complete specification to clinical trialists, on whose work systematic reviewers depend, and will indirectly encourage comparable outcome choice to reviewers undertaking related research questions. Complete pre-specification could improve efficiency and reduce bias in data abstraction and analysis during a systematic review. Ultimately, more completely specified and comparable outcomes could make systematic reviews more useful to decision-makers.

Editor: Kypros Kypri, University of Newcastle, Australia, Australia

Funding: This project was funded by the National Eye Institute, grant number 1U01EY020522 (http://www.nei.nih.gov/). The funder had no role in study design, data collection and analysis, decision to publish, or preparation of the manuscript.

Competing Interests: All authors are affiliated with the US Satellite of the Cochrane Eyes and Vision Group (the group responsible for producing the Cochrane Reviews evaluated as part of this work): Drs. Kay Dickersin and Tianjing Li are Faculty members; Dr. Xue Wang is a Methodologist; and Dr. Ian Saldanha is a Research Assistant. Drs. Kay Dickersin, Tianjing Li, and Xue Wang have authored several Cochrane systematic reviews that are assessed as part of this study.

* Email: isaldan1@jhmi.edu

Introduction

In clinical trials, an outcome is an event or measure in study participants that is used to assess the effectiveness and/or safety of the intervention being studied [1]. Choosing relevant outcomes is a critical early step in the design of clinical trials and systematic reviews for a number of reasons [2]. In clinical trials, expected effect sizes on critical outcomes are used to determine sample size [3]. In addition, there is general agreement that by pre-specifying the primary and secondary outcomes and limiting the number of

statistical analyses, clinical trialists reduce the likelihood of Type I error (i.e., finding a statistically significant treatment effect just by chance, in the absence of a true treatment effect) and outcome reporting bias (i.e., selectively reporting outcomes based on the strength and/or direction of the findings). Although satisfactory solutions have not yet been developed, there is growing recognition that these issues also apply to systematic reviews [4]–[5]. Indeed, the Cochrane Collaboration recommends that systematic reviewers limit the number of and pre-specify all outcomes for their systematic review [6]–[7].

The process of conducting a systematic review of intervention effectiveness begins with formulating a research question, and then, finding and synthesizing the evidence from studies that address the question. In formulating the question, the systematic reviewer defines the population, intervention, comparison, and outcomes (PICO) to be examined. Studies that address the review question, typically clinical trials, should be broadly similar on the population, intervention and comparison groups, but frequently report different outcomes from those chosen by the systematic reviewer. Clinical trialists typically measure numerous outcomes, sometimes in the hundreds [8]. It is likely that these outcomes are different from those chosen by the systematic reviewer; overlap of the chosen outcomes can vary from none to complete (Figure 1). In many cases, the primary outcome of interest to the systematic reviewers may not have been an outcome of interest to the clinical trialists [9], or may not be reported clearly or consistently in the clinical trial reports or associated documents [10]. Systematic reviewers thus face an important decision: should they choose outcomes to be examined based on what they believe to be important outcomes ("systematic review author judgment") or based on what they know is reported in the relevant clinical trials ("clinical trialist judgment")?

How systematic reviewers choose outcomes and pre-specify them in systematic review protocols is currently unclear. One view is that, unlike clinical trialists, systematic reviewers should not base outcome choice on sample size/power calculations and Type I error rates. Instead, the objective of medical research should be to draw conclusions based on all sources of available evidence [11]. Systematic reviews, which are often used to inform clinical practice guidelines and policy, could and even should include all the outcomes that patients, clinicians, and policy-makers need to know about. Systematic reviews also allow elucidation of existing research gaps in a given field [12], for example, when outcomes are not examined in trials and should be.

In our view, regardless of who chooses the outcomes to be assessed in a systematic review and how those outcomes are chosen, all outcomes need to be specified completely and clearly if they are to be of use to decision-makers.

The objective of our study was to assess the completeness of pre-specification and comparability of outcomes in all Cochrane reviews addressing four common eye conditions. Our purpose is not to hold systematic review protocols to a standard that may not

have been described at the time they were published, rather it is to initiate a discussion on important questions for systematic reviewers: how should systematic reviewers choose outcomes to address in the review; how should these outcomes be reported (i.e., which elements are necessary for complete reporting) by systematic reviewers; and if outcomes are pre-specified in systematic review protocols, should these protocols be formally updated with amendments to reflect changing outcome specification?

Methods

Review protocols examined

The Cochrane Collaboration publishes and archives all its systematic review protocols, completed reviews, and updates in *The Cochrane Database of Systematic Reviews*. Protocols for systematic reviews, hereafter referred to as 'protocols', were eligible for our study if they were published by the Cochrane Eyes and Vision Group (CEVG) in *The Cochrane Database of Systematic Reviews* in or before June 2013 (Issue 6), and if they addressed any of the following four eye conditions: glaucoma, age-related macular degeneration (AMD), cataract, and diabetic retinopathy (DR). We selected these four conditions because of their high disease burden across populations and the range of interventions addressing them [13]. For each eligible review, we identified the oldest available protocol and, when no protocol could be found for a review, we contacted CEVG editors and review authors via email to ask whether they had a copy. When these efforts were not successful, we used the most recent version of the completed review in place of the protocol.

Five elements of a completely specified outcome

We used an outcome definition that includes five elements: (1) the *domain* or outcome title (e.g., visual acuity); (2) the *specific measurement* or technique/instrument used to make the measurement (e.g., Snellen chart); (3) the *specific metric* or format of the outcome data from each participant that will be used for analysis (e.g., value at a time-point, change from baseline); (4) the *method of aggregation* or how data from each group will be summarized (e.g., mean, percent/proportion); and (5) the *time-points* that will be used for analysis (e.g., 3 months) (Figure 2). Whereas Zarin et al. specify these same elements [8], they define the first four elements and consider time-points related to each of those four.

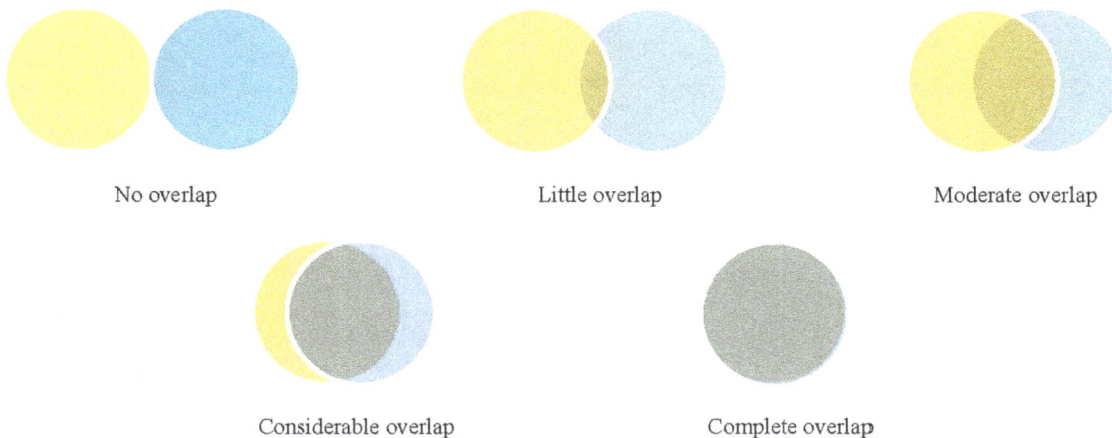

No overlap   Little overlap   Moderate overlap

Considerable overlap   Complete overlap

Figure 1. Examples of extent of overlap of possible outcome domains chosen by clinical trialists and systematic reviewers. Yellow - Outcomes chosen by clinical trialists. Blue - Outcomes chosen by systematic reviewers. Grey - Outcomes chosen by BOTH clinical trialists and systematic reviewers.

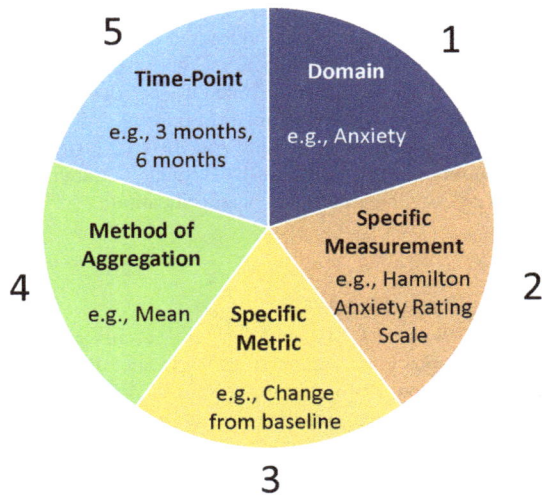

Figure 2. Five elements of a completely specified outcome, with anxiety as an example.

Selecting outcome domains for data extraction

Before beginning data extraction, one investigator (IS) identified all outcome domains in the Methods sections of included protocols. We then selected for data extraction those outcome domains appearing in at least 25% of eligible protocols. Then, for those eligible protocols with published completed reviews, we compared the Methods section of the protocol with the Methods section of the most recent version of the corresponding completed review, noting any differences in the specified outcome domains. We did this step to evaluate whether focusing on the protocols, some of which were published a while ago, would mean that we were assessing a different set of outcome domains than those currently being evaluated by the review authors.

Data extraction

We designed, tested, and finalized a data extraction form using Google Forms©. Two investigators (IS and XW) extracted data independently and resolved discrepancies through consensus or discussion with a third author (TL). We extracted data about the eye condition and year of publication of each protocol. We extracted from the Methods section the following data pertaining to each eligible outcome: type of outcome (primary, non-primary, or unclear [if not specified]) and each of the five outcome elements described earlier. For element 2, we extracted all specific measurements that were specified, or classified the specific measurement as unclear (if not specified). We classified element 3 (specific metric) into one or more of the following categories: (i) value at a time-point, (ii) time-to-event, (iii) change from baseline, and (iv) unclear (if not specified). We classified element 4 (method of aggregation) into one or more of the following categories: (i) mean, (ii) median, (iii) percent/proportion, (iv) absolute number, and (v) unclear (if not specified). For element 5, we extracted all time-points that were specified, or classified the time-points as unclear (if not specified).

Data analysis

We assessed the extent of completeness using the number of elements specified out of five possible, and considered an outcome specified in the Methods section as "complete" if all five elements were specified. For each outcome, we calculated median,

interquartile range (IQR), and proportion of outcome elements specified. We performed Kruskal-Wallis tests for nonparametric comparisons of medians and distributions of extent of completeness by condition addressed, year of protocol publication, type of outcome, and outcome domain.

We assessed the frequency and comparability of outcome elements (i.e., similarity of categories for each element) for elements 3 and 4 across protocols addressing each of the four eye conditions. Protocols could specify more than one category for a given element. Comparability was therefore assessed as the distribution of those categories across protocols. As an example, if one protocol specified visual acuity at a time-point as well as change in visual acuity from baseline, we counted both categories for specific metric (element 3). In another example, protocols addressing cataract and assessing the outcome of visual acuity were considered to be comparable in method of aggregation (element 4) if they all specified mean or all specified median or both. However, they would not be comparable in element 4 if some specified mean and others specified median.

Statistical significance was defined at the 5% level. All data were analyzed using STATA© version 12 (College Station, TX).

Results

Characteristics of protocols examined

Our search identified 57 eligible systematic reviews (Table 1). We were able to find protocols for 54 reviews (94.7%), and used the Methods section of completed reviews for the remaining three (5.3%). An updated protocol was published for one of the 54 protocols. Glaucoma was the most frequently addressed condition (22 protocols), followed by cataract (16 protocols), AMD (15 protocols), and DR (4 protocols). Approximately half of the protocols (29/57; 50.9%) were published between 2006 and 2010. Thirty-four protocols were associated with a completed review, the most recent version of which was published a median of five (IQR 4–8, range 0–15) years after publication of the protocol.

Outcome domains used in protocols

We examined five outcome domains named in at least 25% of the eligible protocols (Table 2): quality-of-life (47/57 protocols; 82.5%), visual acuity (47/57; 82.5%), intraocular pressure (21/57; 36.8%), disease progression (15/57; 26.3%), and contrast sensitivity (15/57; 26.3%). One protocol did not name any of these five outcome domains. For most completed systematic reviews (30/34; 88.2%), these five outcome domains were similar to what was named in their corresponding protocols. Compared to their protocols, two completed systematic reviews dropped quality-of-life while one completed review added it. One completed systematic review dropped contrast sensitivity.

Completeness of outcome pre-specification

Across the 57 protocols, the five most frequent outcome domains appeared 145 times ('instances'); however, only 15/145 instances (10.3%) involved complete pre-specification (i.e., where all five elements of the outcome were specified). Overall, a median of three (IQR 2–4) elements were specified per outcome (Table 3). Extent of completeness was not statistically significantly different by condition. Completeness of outcome specification may be better in protocols published later compared to earlier, (median of three [IQR 2–4] elements specified in 2006–2010 versus one [IQR 1–3] in 2000 or earlier), although the difference was not statistically significant (p = 0.1635).

Fifty-four of 57 protocols (94.7%) specified at least one primary outcome. Among the five outcome domains evaluated in our

Table 1. Number of protocols and outcome domains by condition, year published, and whether specified as primary outcome.

Characteristic	Number (%) of protocols	Number (%) of outcomes
All	57[1] (100)	145[2] (100)
Condition addressed		
Glaucoma	22 (38.6)	51 (35.2)
Cataract	16 (28.1)	35 (24.1)
Age-related macular degeneration (AMD)	15 (26.3)	47 (32.4)
Diabetic retinopathy (DR)	4 (7.0)	12 (8.3)
Year of protocol publication		
2000 or earlier	6 (10.5)	13 (9.0)
2001 to 2005	15 (26.3)	37 (25.5)
2006 to 2010	29 (50.9)	76 (52.4)
2011 or later	7 (12.3)	19 (13.1)
Type of outcomes domain specified	Not applicable	
Outcomes specified as primary		48 (33.1)
Outcomes specified as non-primary		88 (60.7)
Type of outcome unclear		9 (6.2)

[1] 54 protocols and 3 completed reviews; One protocol did not include any of the outcome domains selected for detailed data extraction.
[2] 139/145 of the outcomes were described in the 54 protocols.

study, at least one was a primary outcome in 48/57 (84.2%) protocols. Extent of completeness appeared to differ by outcome type, with primary outcomes being most completely specified and outcomes with type unclear being least completely specified (median four versus one respectively, p = 0.0001). Intraocular pressure was the most completely specified outcome in our sample, with a median of four (IQR 3–4) elements specified (Table 2). Quality-of-life was least completely specified, with a median of one (IQR 1–2) element specified. The patterns of completeness of individual elements were similar across outcomes (Figure 3). Method of aggregation was specified least often, while domain and time-points were specified more often than other elements. The completeness of individual elements for the quality-of-life outcome was less than for other outcomes, overall. Although intraocular pressure was the most completely specified outcome, only 24% of protocols assessing it specified the specific measurement. Patterns of completeness of individual outcome elements also appeared to be similar across conditions, except for outcomes in DR protocols, where there were only four protocols and so the percentages are unlikely to be reliable (Figure 4).

Table 4 provides some examples of incomplete specification of outcomes in our sample of systematic reviews.

Comparability of outcome elements

Table 5 shows the distribution of specific metrics (element 3) and methods of aggregation (element 4) across instances of usage of outcome domain, by condition. The specific metric was unclear for large proportions of individual instances (often as high as 100% for the 16 instances of usage of quality-of-life in protocols addressing glaucoma and for the four instances of usage of contrast sensitivity in protocols addressing cataract). For instances where the specific metric was specified, the most frequent specific metrics were 'value at a time-point' and 'change from baseline'.

The method of aggregation was unclear for large proportions of individual instances (often as high as 100% for the 16 instances of usage of quality-of-life in protocols addressing glaucoma and for the four instances of usage of visual acuity in protocols addressing DR). For instances where the method of aggregation was specified, the most frequent methods of aggregation were 'mean' and 'percent/proportion'.

Table 2. Completeness (number of completely-specified elements out of five possible) by outcome domain.

Characteristic	Number (%) of protocols	Median (IQR) number of completely-specified elements per outcome	p-value
All	57[1] (100)	3.0 (2.0–4.0)	-
Outcome domain			
Quality-of-life	47 (82.5)	1.0 (1.0–2.0)	0.0001
Visual acuity	47 (82.5)	3.0 (2.0–4.0)	
Intraocular pressure	21 (36.8)	4.0 (3.0–4.0)	
Disease progression	15 (26.3)	3.0 (2.0–4.0)	
Contrast sensitivity	15 (26.3)	2.0 (1.0–3.0)	

[1] One protocol did not include any of the outcome domains selected for detailed data extraction.

Table 3. Completeness (number of completely-specified elements out of five possible) by type of protocol/outcome.

Characteristic	Median (IQR) number of completely specified elements per outcome	p-value
All[1]	3.0 (2.0–4.0)	NA
Condition addressed		
Glaucoma	3.0 (2.0–4.0)	0.1218
Cataract	3.0 (2.0–4.0)	
Age-related macular degeneration (AMD)	2.0 (1.0–3.0)	
Diabetic retinopathy (DR)	3.0 (1.5–4.0)	
Year of protocol publication		
2000 or earlier	1.0 (1.0–3.0)	0.1635
2001 to 2005	2.0 (2.0–4.0)	
2006 to 2010	3.0 (2.0–4.0)	
2011 or later	2.0 (2.0–3.0)	
Type of outcome domain specified		
Outcomes specified as primary	4.0 (3.0–4.0)	0.0001
Outcomes specified as non-primary	2.0 (1.0–3.0)	
Type of outcome not specified	1.0 (1.0–2.0)	

[1] 54 protocols and 3 completed reviews; Median 3.0 (2.0–4.0) for outcomes in the 54 protocols and 1.5 (1.0–2.0) for outcomes in the 3 reviews (p = 0.0627); One protocol did not include any of the outcome domains selected for detailed data extraction.

Discussion

Summary of main findings

We have shown that, if outcome pre-specification in systematic review protocols is judged using recommended standards for clinical trials, then it is largely incomplete. Although completeness appears to have improved somewhat over time, on average, only three of five standard elements of an outcome were pre-specified. Due to largely incomplete outcome pre-specification, a conclusive assessment of comparability in outcome elements across the various protocols per condition was not possible. However, we observed variation in specific metrics and methods of aggregation.

Completeness of outcome pre-specification

There are some reasons that might explain why outcomes were not completely specified in our study of systematic review protocols. First, although we believe complete specification of all five elements is necessary for a number of reasons, the idea is new to the systematic review community. This is demonstrated by the fact that the Cochrane Handbook states only that the name of the

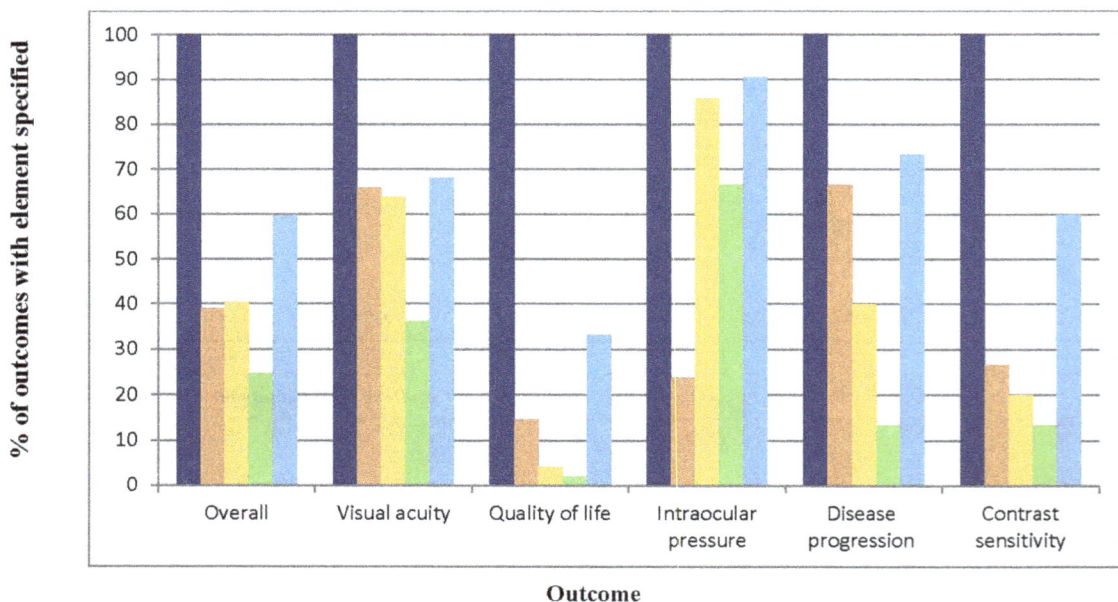

Figure 3. Completeness of specification of outcome elements, by outcome. Navy blue - Domain. Orange – Specific measurement. Yellow – Specific metric. Green – Method of aggregation. Blue – Time-point(s).

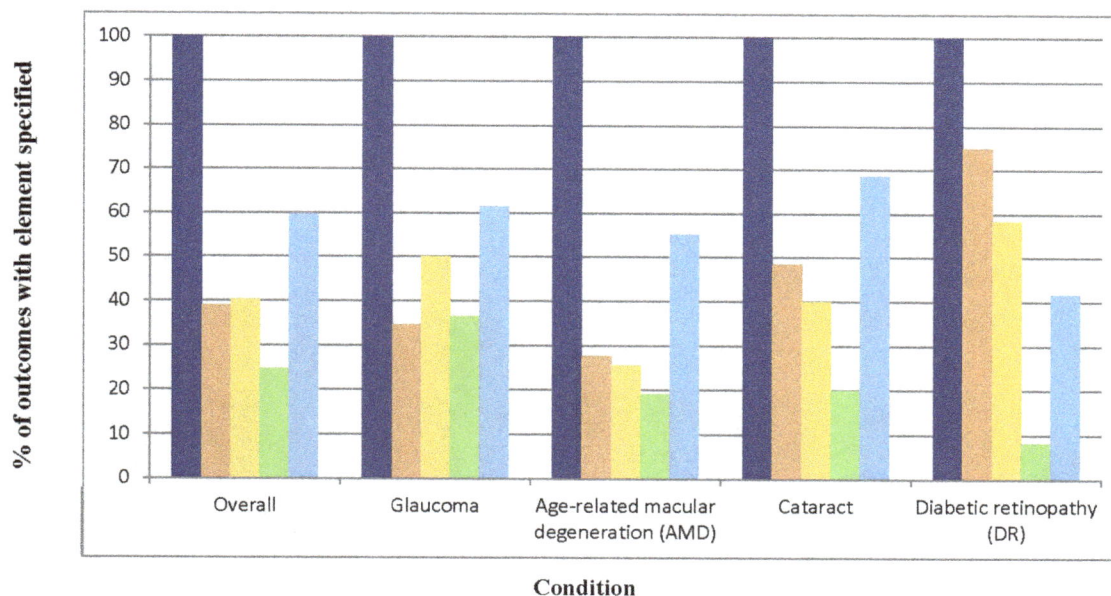

Figure 4. Completeness of specification of outcome elements, by condition. Navy blue - Domain. Orange – Specific measurement. Yellow – Specific metric. Green – Method of aggregation. Sky blue – Time-point(s).

outcome (equivalent to *domain* [element 1]), type of scale (equivalent to *specific measurement* [element 2]), and timing of measurement (equivalent to *time-points* [element 5]) must be pre-specified[6]; and there is no explicit mention of pre-specification of *specific metric* (element 3) or *method of aggregation* (element 4). Indeed, elements 1 and 5 were the most often-specified elements in our sample of protocols, though element 2 was frequently not specified (70% of the time) (Figure 3).

Another possible explanation for incomplete pre-specification of outcomes is that choice of outcomes could be influenced by the findings of (and outcomes examined in) the clinical trials that would be included in the review. We did not assess the outcomes examined at the level of the clinical trials to determine the likelihood that this occurred, but suggest that doing so may contribute to a better understanding of how review outcomes are chosen. Are they chosen because systematic reviewers consider them the most important outcomes to examine, because they are the outcomes that have been examined in clinical trials, or both? If the review outcomes were chosen purely because they were the outcomes that have been reported in clinical trials, this is troubling because of the possibility of "meta-bias". We know, for example,

that outcomes reported in clinical trials could have been selectively reported because of desirable or undesirable findings [14]–[15]. By pre-specifying in the protocol the outcomes to be examined in the review, systematic reviewers minimize the potential for bias [5], [16], and reassure readers that the choice of outcomes was not influenced by the results of individual clinical trials. That said, systematic reviewers are usually familiar with their field and *a priori* aware of potentially eligible clinical trials and/or how the outcome in question is frequently measured. Complete pre-specification also could improve efficiency in data abstraction and analysis during a systematic review.

Systematic reviewers may also anticipate potential variation in outcomes across included clinical trials, and may allow for this by pre-specifying the elements of the outcome domain of interest in broad rather than specific terms (e.g., "visual acuity" versus "change in visual acuity from baseline to 1 year, as measured using a Snellen chart"). If such variation is suspected, systematic reviewers could explicitly state that all variations of a given element(s) will be included. This could minimize the occurrence of what Page et al. refer to as "selective inclusion" in systematic reviews [5].

Table 4. Examples of incomplete outcome pre-specification.

Exact text from methods section of protocol	Number of completely-specified elements (out of five possible)
"The primary outcome for the review will be visual acuity."	1
"When available quality of life data will be described for those with operated and unoperated cataract."	1
"Postoperative visual acuity"	1
"Quality of life"	1
"Contrast sensitivity"	1
"Vision-related quality of life at one year"	2
"Mean IOP"	2

Table 5. Frequency of categories of specific metric (element 3) and method of aggregation (element 4) across instances of usage of outcome domains by condition.

Condition/Outcome domain (Number of protocols/Number of instances)	Categories of specific metric (element 3) (% of instances)				Categories of method of aggregation (element 4) (% of instances)			
	Value at a time-point	Time-to-event	Change from baseline	Unclear	Mean	Percent/proportion	Absolute number	Unclear
Glaucoma (22 protocols)								
Quality-of-life (16 instances)	-	-	-	100	-	-	-	100
Visual acuity (13 instances)	31	-	31	46	8	39	-	54
Intraocular pressure (20 instances)	55	10	25	15	50	10	-	40
Disease progression (2 instances)	-	50	50	-	-	-	-	100
Cataract (16 protocols)								
Quality-of-life (12 instances)	17	-	-	83	-	8	-	92
Visual acuity (15 instances)	53	-	20	33	-	33	-	67
Intraocular pressure (1 instance)	100	-	-	-	100	100	-	-
Disease progression (3 instances)	-	-	33	67	-	-	-	100
Contrast sensitivity (4 instances)	-	-	-	100	-	-	-	100
Age-related macular degeneration (15 protocols)								
Quality-of-life (15 instances)	-	-	-	100	-	-	-	100
Visual acuity (15 instances)	47	-	33	40	20	13	13	60
Disease progression (6 instances)	-	-	-	100	-	-	17	83
Contrast sensitivity (11 instances)	18	-	9	73	18	18	-	82
Diabetic retinopathy (4 protocols)								
Quality-of-life (4 instances)	-	-	-	100	-	-	-	100
Visual acuity (4 instances)	100	-	25	-	-	-	-	100
Disease progression (4 instances)	50	25	-	25	25	-	-	75

Notes:
• If there was no instance of usage of a certain outcome domain across all reviews addressing a given condition, the above table does not include a row for that outcome domain for that condition.
• Percentages are row percentages (adding up individual categories within an element). Percentages sometimes total more than 100% for an element because some protocols used more than one category for that element.
• No reviews used "median" as a method of aggregation (element 4).

We assume that primary outcomes for both clinical trials and systematic reviews are chosen based on perceived clinical importance and/or importance to patients; and that they are usually measured and reported more thoroughly than non-primary outcomes [17]. Not surprisingly, in our study, primary outcomes were more completely specified than other outcome types. Our estimate of 94.7% protocols pre-specifying a primary outcome is somewhat higher than the 88% that has been reported as pre-specified in clinical trial protocols [18], and this could be related to the fact that we were examining protocols entered into software that requests the domain names of the pre-specified outcomes.

In our study, the most incompletely pre-specified outcome was quality-of-life, a key patient-important outcome. This finding is concordant with other studies that have found that outcome reporting in clinical trials is a bigger problem for patient-important outcomes than other types of outcomes [19]–[20]. Further, when patient-important outcomes are not primary outcomes in clinical trials, the likelihood that reporting is complete is further reduced [20]. Our study aimed to evaluate the completeness and comparability of all outcomes, both patient-important and not.

Our recommendation is that systematic reviewers should engage in discussion about and strongly consider pre-specifying all five elements of each outcome they wish to examine. When explicit pre-specification of all five elements of a given outcome is not possible, for example when all possible options for a given outcome element are not known or are too numerous, the systematic reviewers should enumerate all known acceptable options for each element and explicitly state that all options for that element would be accepted, or provide rationale for why it is impossible to completely pre-specify an element.

The Preferred Reporting Items for Systematic Reviews and Meta-analyses Protocols (PRISMA-P) is currently under development [21]. We hope that the availability of reporting guidelines (including details about outcome specification) will improve the completeness of specification of outcomes. Assuming that the Cochrane Collaboration recognizes the importance of completeness of pre-specification, there are some possible ways to ensure that review authors are aware of the five elements of a completely specified outcome. First, editorial teams at Cochrane Review Groups (CRGs) should make all review authors aware of the five outcome elements early in the process (no later than the protocol development stage). Second, peer reviewers should be directed to consider whether the outcomes are completely pre-specified and not likely to have been chosen based on the strength and direction of the findings for those outcomes. Third, the Cochrane Handbook and other systematic review guidance materials, in addition to training workshops and other educational avenues, should incorporate explicit descriptions of all five outcome elements. Other organizations producing guidance on systematic review methodology (e.g., Agency for Healthcare Research and Quality [AHRQ], the Centre for Reviews and Dissemination [CRD]) should also incorporate descriptions of the five outcome elements in their guidance materials.

Organizations such as the Cochrane Collaboration suggest limiting the number of outcomes examined in a systematic review [6]. However, in order to evaluate whether the effect of an intervention persists over time, an otherwise identical outcome (i.e., identical in the other four elements) is often measured at a number of time-points. For the purpose of counting the number of outcomes measured, we recommend that these repeated measurements be counted as one outcome regardless of the number of time-points at which the outcome is assessed.

Comparability of outcome elements

In the era of evidence-based medicine, decision-makers in healthcare (e.g., patients, clinicians, and policy-makers) increasingly rely on systematic reviews. It is important that decision-makers have access to high quality and up-to-date individual systematic reviews as well as are able to compare results across systematic reviews. Cochrane "overviews" (Cochrane reviews which compile evidence from related reviews of interventions into a single accessible and usable document) [6], and network meta-analyses (analyses of three or more interventions for a given condition in one meta-analysis) [22]–[23] are examples of formal comparisons across systematic reviews. To better feed into these formal comparisons and clinical practice guidelines, the elements of outcomes used in the various systematic reviews addressing a given condition should be comparable. In our study, the largely incomplete pre-specification of outcomes in protocols restricted our ability to assess comparability in outcome elements across protocols. In cases where the various elements were specified, however, we observed variation in specific metrics and methods of aggregation. An example of such variation is: one protocol pre-specified that the outcome domain of visual acuity would be measured as mean change in visual acuity (number of letters) from baseline to one year, while another protocol pre-specified that visual acuity would be measured as percent of participants with improvement in visual acuity of at least three letters at one year. While both protocols specified the same outcome domain at the same time-point, differences in the specific metric (mean change versus value at a time-point) and method of aggregation (mean versus percent) would preclude a direct comparison of the visual acuity results.

Efforts to promote comparability of outcomes across related clinical trials have led to the creation of core outcome measures within research fields [24]–[26]. One such effort is the Core Outcome Measures in Effectiveness Trials (COMET) Initiative [27], whose investigators have produced guidance on methods for identifying core outcome sets [28]. Because the issue of comparability of outcomes across systematic reviews is complex, we recommend that researchers within a field (e.g., systematic reviewers, Cochrane review group editors, clinical trialists) and patients consider developing comparable outcomes across systematic reviews, adding to a core list over time as appropriate.

There are pros and cons of establishing comparability in outcomes across reviews, however. Increased comparability will likely facilitate formal comparisons across systematic reviews and development of clinical practice guidelines. In addition, decision-makers would be better able to compare more directly the effectiveness of treatment options. For example, hundreds of measurement scales (*specific measurements*) have been used to assess mental status in schizophrenia [29] and quality-of-life [30], making comparability across clinical trials very challenging. Finally, use of comparable outcomes could discourage authors from 'cherry-picking' outcomes to be used in their studies [31].

On the other hand, comparability across reviews is not always possible or desirable. Limiting outcomes to those used by previous researchers risks excluding an outcome that is in fact important, or authors may be compelled to include an outcome that they do not consider important. Additionally, it might not be possible to identify *a priori* all relevant outcomes and outcome elements for a rapidly evolving field or for a field with a large number of relevant outcomes.

Availability of protocols and amendments to protocols

We were unable to obtain 3/57 (5.3%) protocols associated with our sample of Cochrane reviews. This poses a concern for investigators conducting methodological research in systematic reviews, and for users of systematic reviews generally. Although we do not believe that relying on the Methods sections of three completed Cochrane reviews in the cases where we could not find the protocols is likely to have influenced our findings, we believe that all protocols and previous versions of completed systematic reviews should be made available to researchers. Furthermore, an updated protocol was published for only one of the protocols we examined. The Cochrane Collaboration should consider keeping all protocols up-to-date by publishing updated versions of protocols or publishing protocol amendments for all its reviews. In this way, Cochrane review protocols would be formally amended in the same way that clinical trial protocols are amended and made available, providing an accessible audit trail. This practice will facilitate Cochrane's contribution of its protocols and updates to PROSPERO [32]–[33], an international database of prospectively registered systematic reviews.

Our focus on Cochrane reviews is both a strength and a limitation. Assuming that Cochrane reviews are among the most rigorously conducted and reported systematic reviews [34]–[35], it is likely that completeness and comparability of outcomes are higher in our sample of reviews than in other reviews. It would be useful to know how others producing systematic reviews (e.g., AHRQ, CRD, independent authors) choose and describe outcomes in their systematic reviews.

As discussed, we did not examine the individual clinical trials examined by each Cochrane review in our sample to learn more about the source of non-comparability in outcome elements. Nor did we test for empirical evidence of outcome reporting bias on the part of the systematic reviewers. Because our assessments of completeness and comparability were based on what was reported in the protocols (and some completed reviews), it is possible that our findings were a consequence of unsatisfactory reporting and that the rationale for the outcomes chosen could not be determined without asking the systematic review authors directly.

Our study should be replicated in other disease areas and on a larger scale to assess the applicability of our findings to other fields.

Although we have compared the outcomes pre-specified in the protocol with what is in the corresponding completed review's Methods section, a next step would be to compare the outcomes in the Methods with those in the Results section. This would allow a confirmation of the potential bias by systematic reviewers that has been demonstrated by Kirkham et al. using a cohort of Cochrane reviews [36] and by various investigators studying this issue in clinical trials [14], [17], [37]–[38].

Conclusions

We recommend that systematic review authors strongly consider pre-specifying all outcomes of interest using the five elements of a completely specified outcome (domain, specific measurement, specific metric, method of aggregation, and time-points), amending the protocol formally, as needed. We further suggest that researchers and other stakeholders, such as patients, carefully consider the pros and cons of establishing comparability in outcomes across systematic reviews addressing a given condition.

Acknowledgments

We acknowledge the contributions of Deborah Zarin, MD; Karen Robinson, MA, PhD; Swaroop Vedula, MD, MPH, PhD; and Evan Mayo-Wilson, MSc, MPA, DPhil for their comments on previous versions of this manuscript. We also acknowledge the contributions of Michael Marrone, MPH, Kristina Lindsley, MS, and James Heyward, BA for their help with data abstraction and locating systematic review protocols for this study.

Author Contributions

Conceived and designed the experiments: IJS KD XW TL. Performed the experiments: IJS KD XW TL. Analyzed the data: IJS KD XW TL. Contributed reagents/materials/analysis tools: IJS KD XW TL. Wrote the paper: IJS KD XW TL.

References

1. Meinert CL (2012) Clinical trials dictionary: Terminology and usage recommendations. 2nd edition. Wiley. Hoboken, NJ.
2. Institute of Medicine (2011) Finding what works in health care: standards for systematic reviews. Available: http://www.iom.edu/Reports/2011/Finding-What-Works-in-Health-Care-Standards-for-Systematic-Reviews.aspx. Accessed 2014 September 12.
3. Campbell MJ, Julious SA, Altman DG (1995) Estimating sample sizes for binary, ordered categorical, and continuous outcomes in two group comparisons. BMJ 311(7013): 1145–1148.
4. Bender R, Bunce C, Clarke M, Gates S, Lange S, et al. (2008) Attention should be given to multiplicity issues in systematic reviews. J Clin Epidemiol 61(9): 857–865.
5. Page MJ, McKenzie JE, Forbes A (2013) Many scenarios exist for selective inclusion and reporting of results in randomized trials and systematic reviews. J Clin Epidemiol 66(5): 524–537.
6. Higgins JPTGreen S, (editors) (2011) Cochrane Handbook for Systematic Reviews of Interventions Version 5.1.0 [updated March 2011]. The Cochrane Collaboration. Available: www.cochrane-handbook.org. Accessed 2014 September 12.
7. Chandler J, Churchill R, Higgins J, Tovey D (2012) Methodological standards for the conduct of new Cochrane Intervention Reviews. Version 2.2. 17, December 2012. Available: http://www.editorial-unit.cochrane.org/sites/editorial-unit.cochrane.org/files/uploads/MECIR_conduct_standards%202.2%2017122012.pdf. Accessed 2014 September 12.
8. Zarin DA, Tse T, Williams RJ, Califf RM, Ide NC (2011) The ClinicalTrials.gov results database–update and key issues. N Engl J Med 364(9): 852–860.
9. Singh S, Loke YK, Enright PL, Furberg CD (2011) Mortality associated with tiotropium mist inhaler in patients with chronic obstructive pulmonary disease: systematic review and meta-analysis of randomised controlled trials. BMJ 14; 342:d3215. doi: 10.1136/bmj.d3215

10. Jefferson T, Jones MA, Doshi P, Del Mar CB, Heneghan CJ, et al. (2012) Neuraminidase inhibitors for preventing and treating influenza in healthy adults and children. Cochrane Database Syst Rev (1):CD008965.
11. Goodman SN (1989) Meta-analysis and evidence. http://www.ncbi.nlm.nih.gov/pubmed/2666026Control Clin Trials 10(2): 188–204.
12. Robinson KA, Saldanha IJ, Mckoy NA (2011) Development of a framework to identify research gaps from systematic reviews. J Clin Epidemiol 64(12): 1325–1330.
13. National Eye Institute (2010) Statistics and Data Available: http://www.nei.nih.gov/eyedata. Accessed 2014 September 12.
14. Vedula SS, Bero L, Scherer RW, Dickersin K (2009) Outcome reporting in industry-sponsored trials of gabapentin for off-label use. N Engl J Med 361(20): 1963–1971.
15. Dwan K, Altman DG, Cresswell L, Blundell M, Gamble CL, et al. (2011) Comparison of protocols and registry entries to published reports for randomised controlled trials. Cochrane Database Syst Rev Issue 1. Art. No.: MR000031. doi: 10.1002/14651858.MR000031.pub2
16. Stewart L, Moher D, Shekelle P (2012) Why prospective registration of systematic reviews makes sense. Syst Rev 1: 7. doi:10.1186/2046-4053-1-7
17. Kirkham JJ, Dwan KM, Altman DG, Gamble C, Dodd S, et al. (2010) The impact of outcome reporting bias in randomised controlled trials on a cohort of systematic reviews. BMJ 340: c365. doi: 10.1136/bmj.c365
18. Mathieu S, Boutron I, Moher D, Altman DG, Ravaud P (2009) Comparison of registered and published primary outcomes in randomized controlled trials. JAMA 302(9): 977–984.
19. Wieseler B, Kerekes MF, Vervolgyi V, Kohlepp P, McGauran N, et al. (2012) Impact of document type on reporting quality of clinical drug trials: a comparison registry reports, clinical study reports, and journal publications. BMJ 344 d8141 doi: 10.1136/bmj.d8141
20. Wieseler B, Wolfram N, McGauran N, Kerekes MF, Vervolgyi V, et al. (2013) Completeness of reporting of patient-relevant clinical trial outcomes: comparison

of unpublished clinical study reports with publicly available data. PLOS Med 10 (10) e1001526. doi: 10.1371/journal.pmed.1001526

21. EQUATOR Network (2014) Reporting Guidelines under development. Available: http://www.equator-network.org/library/reporting-guidelines-under-development/#99. Accessed 2014 September 12.

22. Caldwell DM, Ades AE, Higgins JP (2005) Simultaneous comparison of multiple treatments: combining direct and indirect evidence. BMJ 331(7521): 897–900.

23. Li T, Puhan M, Vedula SS, Singh S, Dickersin K for the Ad Hoc Network Meta-analysis Methods Meeting Working Group (2011) Network meta-analysis – highly attractive and more methodological research is needed. BMC Medicine 9(1): 79. doi:10.1186/1741-7015-9-79

24. Miller AB, Hoogstraten B, Staquet M, Winkler A (1981) Reporting results of cancer treatment. Cancer 47(1): 207–214.

25. Tugwell P, Boers M, Brooks P, Simon LS, Strand V (2007) OMERACT: An international initiative to improve outcome measures in rheumatology. Trials 8: 38.

26. Dworkin RH, Turk DC, Farrar JT, Haythornthwaite JA, Jensen MP, et al. (2005) Core outcome measures for chronic pain trials: IMMPACT recommendations. Pain 113(1–2): 9–19.

27. COMET Initiative (2014) Overview. Available: http://www.comet-initiative.org/about/overview. Accessed 2014 September 12.

28. Williamson PR, Altman DG, Blazeby JM, Clarke M, Devane D, et al. (2012) Developing core outcome sets for clinical trials: issues to consider. Trials 13(132). doi: 10.1186/1745-6215-13-132

29. Thornley B, Adams C (1998) Content and quality of 2000 controlled trials in schizophrenia over 50 years. BMJ 317(7167): 1181–1184.

30. Salek S (1999) Compendium of Quality of Life Instruments. Wiley. ISBN: 0-471-98145-1.

31. Clarke M (2007) Standardising outcomes for clinical trials and systematic reviews. Trials 8: 39.

32. Booth A, Clarke M, Dooley G, Ghersi D, Moher D, et al. (2012) The nuts and bolts of PROSPERO: an international prospective register of systematic reviews. Sys Rev 1: 2. doi: 10.1186/2046-4053-1-2

33. Booth A, Clarke M, Dooley G, Ghersi D, Moher D, et al. (2013) PROSPERO at one year: an evaluation of its utility. Sys Rev 2: 4. doi: 10.1186/2046-4053-2-4

34. Jadad AR, Cook DJ, Jones A, Klassen TP, Tugwell P, et al. (1998) Methodology and reports of systematic reviews and meta-analyses: A comparison of Cochrane reviews with articles published in paper-based journals. JAMA 280(3): 278–280.

35. Moher D, Tetzlaff J, Tricco AC, Sampson M, Altman DG (2007) Epidemiology and reporting characteristics of systematic reviews. PLoS Med 4(3): e78.

36. Kirkham JJ, Altman DG, Williamson PR (2010) Bias due to changes in prespecified outcomes during the systematic review process. PLoS One 5(3): e9810. doi: 10.1371/journal.pone.0009810

37. Chan AW, Altman D (2005) Identifying outcome reporting bias in randomized trials on PubMed: review of publications and survey of authors. BMJ 330(7494): 753.

38. Chan AW, Hrobjartsson A, Haahr MT, Gøtzsche PC, Altman DG (2004) Empirical evidence for selective reporting of outcomes in randomized trials: comparison of protocols to published articles. JAMA 291(20): 2457–2465.

19

The Effect of Modified Eggs and an Egg-Yolk Based Beverage on Serum Lutein and Zeaxanthin Concentrations and Macular Pigment Optical Density: Results from a Randomized Trial

Elton R. Kelly[1], Jogchum Plat[2], Guido R. M. M. Haenen[3], Aize Kijlstra[1], Tos T. J. M. Berendschot[1]*

1 University Eye Clinic Maastricht, Maastricht University, Maastricht, the Netherlands, 2 Department of Human Biology, Maastricht University, Maastricht, the Netherlands, 3 Department of Pharmacology and Toxicology, Maastricht University, Maastricht, the Netherlands

Abstract

Increasing evidence suggests a beneficial effect of lutein and zeaxanthin on the progression of age-related macular degeneration. The aim of this study was to investigate the effect of lutein or zeaxanthin enriched eggs or a lutein enriched egg-yolk based buttermilk beverage on serum lutein and zeaxanthin concentrations and macular pigment levels. Naturally enriched eggs were made by increasing the levels of the xanthophylls lutein and zeaxanthin in the feed given to laying hens. One hundred healthy volunteers were recruited and randomized into 5 groups for 90 days. Group one added one normal egg to their daily diet and group two received a lutein enriched egg-yolk based beverage. Group three added one lutein enriched egg and group four one zeaxanthin enriched egg to their diet. Group five was the control group and individuals in this group did not modify their daily diet. Serum lutein and zeaxanthin concentrations and macular pigment densities were obtained at baseline, day 45 and day 90. Macular pigment density was measured by heterochromatic flicker photometry. Serum lutein concentration in the lutein enriched egg and egg yolk-based beverage groups increased significantly ($p<0.001$, 76% and 77%). A strong increase in the serum zeaxanthin concentration was observed in individuals receiving zeaxanthin enriched eggs ($P< 0.001$, 430%). No changes were observed in macular pigment density in the various groups tested. The results indicate that daily consumption of lutein or zeaxanthin enriched egg yolks as well as an egg yolk-based beverage show increases in serum lutein and zeaxanthin levels that are comparable with a daily use of 5 mg supplements.

Editor: Robert K. Hills, Cardiff University, United Kingdom

Funding: The study was financially supported by Newtricious (Oirlo, The Netherlands) and an OP-Zuid grant. The funders had no role in study design, data collection and analysis, decision to publish, or preparation of the manuscript.

Competing Interests: The study was financially supported by Newtricious (Oirlo, The Netherlands) and an OP-Zuid grant. Two of the authors, Tos TJM Berendschot and Jogchum Plat, are co-inventors and co-applicant of the patent "Method of producing egg yolk based functional food product and products obtainable thereby" (published as WO2009078716 A1, NZ585997 A, JP2011505870 A, EP2219478 A1, EA201001023 A, EA017773 B1, CA2708258 A1 and AU2008339158 A1).

* E-mail: t.berendschot@maastrichtuniversity.nl

Introduction

As the world's population ages, more and more people are affected by age-related macular degeneration (AMD), leading to an increased awareness and interest in the prevention and treatment of this blinding disease [1,2].

The xanthophylls lutein and zeaxanthin are not endogenously synthesized by the human body and tissue levels therefore depend on dietary intake. These natural compounds found in the bodies of animals, and in dietary animal products, are ultimately derived from plant sources in the diet, mainly from dark green leafy plants. The xanthophylls lutein, zeaxanthin and meso-zeaxanthin are naturally occurring macular pigments, giving the fovea its' yellowish color [3]. These specific xanthophylls do not function in the mechanism of sight, since they cannot be converted to retinal. These xanthophylls have anti-oxidative and blue-light filtering properties [4–6]. Recent evidence suggests that they also have anti-inflammatory properties thereby reducing immune-mediated damage to the macula [7,8].

It has been shown that increased consumption of lutein and zeaxanthin markedly increases the concentration in blood, which can subsequently lead to an increase in macular pigment levels [9–12]. Accumulation of these xanthophylls in the retina is considered to play a role in the prevention of age-related macular degeneration. In line with these assumptions, epidemiological studies have indeed shown that subjects with the highest dietary intake of lutein and zeaxanthin have a lower prevalence and incidence of age-related macular degeneration [13,14]. Lower macular xanthophyll levels have been associated with an increased risk of AMD progression [15,16]. Altogether, these findings have prompted many individuals to take supplements containing both lutein and zeaxanthin as a preventive strategy against AMD.

Egg yolks are an important natural dietary source of lutein and zeaxanthin and their concentration can easily be enhanced via the feed given to laying hens [17–19].Within eggs, lutein and zeaxanthin are packed into lipid matrixes. Studies in humans have shown that these lipid-rich matrixes result in a relatively higher xanthophyll bioavailability as compared to other dietary sources such as spinach [20].

In this study we investigated whether daily intake of lutein or zeaxanthin enriched eggs could lead to increased serum values, to provide an alternative to the daily consumption of supplements. We also included an egg-yolk based beverage, that was developed from a practical point of view in terms of providing possibilities to maintain compliance. Furthermore, an advantage of a beverage over eggs is the fact that it is much better suited for future double blind, placebo controlled studies since color and taste of such beverages can be adjusted. Our study shows that intake of lutein enriched eggs can raise circulating lutein and zeaxanthin levels to values that are comparable with taking 5 mg (pill) supplements.

Subjects and Methods

The protocol for this trial and supporting CONSORT checklist are available as supporting information; see Checklist S1 and Protocol S1.

Ethics statement

This study was conducted according to the declarations of Helsinki and was approved by the Medical Ethical Committee of the University Hospital of Maastricht. Written informed consent was obtained from all participants.

Subjects

For this study one hundred subjects were recruited through local newspapers and posters at the university and hospital buildings. Healthy individuals, 18 years and older were eligible for participation. Exclusion criteria were diabetes, having heart disease, lipid metabolic diseases, AMD in both eyes (at least the eye studied in the trial had to be healthy), ocular media opacity or other ocular diseases. Most studies that have investigated the relationship between macular pigment optical density and cigarette smoking have reported an inverse association between these two. In order to avoid possible confounding we therefore chose not to include smokers. Furthermore, individuals taking supplements containing lutein and/or zeaxanthin in the past six months, and those with a body mass index > 30 kg/m^2 were excluded. Finally, only subjects with a macular pigment optical density (MPOD) score below 0.55 were included. Recruitment started September 2007. Data collection ended February 2008.

Diet and design

Lutein and zeaxanthin enriched eggs as well as the lutein egg yolk beverage were obtained from Newtricious (Oirlo, The Netherlands). These eggs were produced by feeding laying hens with feed enriched with natural sources of lutein and or zeaxanthin. The exact composition of the feed cannot be provided due to proprietary reasons of the manufacturer but did not exceed the EU regulation concerning the maximal xanthophyll level of 80 ppm. The lutein egg yolk beverage was based on traditionally prepared buttermilk drink, indicating that it consisted of the liquid remaining after the manufacturing of cheese and butter (churning) [21]. Vanilla sugar was added to increase palatability (5.0 g per 100 mL). All appropriate food safety standards were applied to the ingredients, the processing and the packaging of the investigational products.

Subjects were randomly allocated into one of five groups. Group one received 1 normal egg a day, group two received a beverage prepared from a lutein enriched egg yolk (one yolk per day), group three received one lutein enriched egg per day, and group four consumed a zeaxanthin enriched egg a day. Finally, group five was the control group, whereby individuals did not modify their daily diet. The egg groups were double blinded; this was for obvious reasons not possible for the egg beverage group. Eggs were analyzed on carotenoid content throughout the study to ensure consistency. Table 1 shows lutein and zeaxanthin concentration of the different egg/egg products used in this study. Subjects were tested on day one when they started with the trial, at day 45 and at the end of the study on day 90. They were asked not to make any major modifications to their diet except for the addition of the egg/egg yolk containing beverage to their daily lunch or dinner for the duration of the study.

Serum analysis

Fasting blood samples were taken using 10 mL serum tubes (Becton, Dickinson and Company, Franklin Lakes, NY, USA). These were left for at least 30 minutes before they were centrifuged for 30 minutes at 4°C and 2.000 g, divided into 500 μL portions, snap frozen and stored at −80°C for later analysis as a single batch. Lutein and zeaxanthin concentrations were analyzed using high performance liquid chromatography (HPLC) [22]. Briefly, on the day of analysis, the samples were thawed and mixed well. Samples were deproteinized by adding a 500 μL sample to 500 μL ethanol. The samples were mixed and allowed to stand for 15 minutes at room temperature to complete the precipitation of proteins. The carotenoids were subsequently extracted by adding 1.0 mL n-hexane. After centrifugation for 10 minutes at 4°C and 3.000 g, 0.5 mL of the upper hexane layer was evaporated to dryness under a stream of nitrogen. The residue was dissolved in 0.5 mL of a mixture of methanol, acetonitril (1:1) and dichloromethane and subsequently analyzed by HPLC. Separation was obtained on a C18 reversed-phase column, thermostatically controlled at 30°C. The samples were eluted by use of a mobile phase consisting of methanol, acetonitril, 2-propanol and water at a flow rate of 1.5 mL/min. Detection was performed with a diode array UV detector at 450 nm. Quantification was carried out by including commercially available lutein and zeaxanthin as a standard (Sigma-Aldrich, St Louis, USA).

Macular pigment

The amount of macular pigment is determined by measuring its absorbance, the macular pigment optical density (MPOD). This dimensionless parameter is defined as the logarithmic ratio of the light falling upon a material, to the light transmitted through a material.

MPOD was determined using the principle of heterochromatic flicker photometry (QuantifEYE; Topcon, Newbury, UK) [23]. In short, observers view a target composed of two light emitting diodes (blue, 470 nm and green, 540 nm) flickering in counterphase. Initially the luminance of the green light is higher than that of the blue. The initial temporal frequency is above the normal critical flicker fusion frequency (60 Hz) and is reduced at 6 Hz/sec. The subject fixates on the target and presses a button when flicker is detected. The luminance ratio of blue and green is then changed, incrementing blue and decrementing green. The temporal frequency is re-set to 60 Hz and again ramped down at 6 Hz/sec, until the subject detects flicker and presses the response button. This cycle continues for a series of blue-green luminance ratios until a V shaped function is obtained with a clear minimum that corresponds to the equalization of the blue and

Table 1. Lutein and zeaxanthin content of egg yolks (mean ± standard deviation).

Egg type	Egg yolk concentration	
	Lutein	Zeaxanthin
Non enriched	167.8±8.7 µg/yolk	85.0±1.7 µg/yolk
Lutein enriched	921.4±105 µg/yolk	137.3±14.0 µg/yolk
Zeaxanthin enriched	174.3±14.5 µg/yolk	487.3±31.0 µg/yolk
Lutein beverage[1]	970	340

[1]Based on one egg yolk. Data are from a homogenized sample. Measurement error was 5.7 µg for lutein and 2 µg for zeaxanthin.

green luminance. This process of detecting flicker for a series of blue-green luminance ratios is then repeated for peripheral viewing at 6 degrees eccentricity, and again a V shaped curve is obtained which provides a minimum for the periphery. The MPOD is then calculated according to the formula MPOD = Log[Lc/Lp], where Lc and Lp are the luminances of the blue light at the minimum for central and peripheral viewing, respectively.

Power calculation and randomization

Intake of 10 mg lutein from supplements induces a 5% monthly increase in MPOD [9]. Although the amount of lutein per egg is much less, the bioavailability is higher [20]. We therefore anticipated a 3% monthly increase in MPOD, resulting in a 9% MPOD increase over the study period. The repeatability of the QuantifEYE is 11.7% [23]. With $\alpha = 0.05$ and $\beta = 0.1$ this yielded 18 subjects per group [24]. Taking into account a 10% dropout we included 20 subjects per group. The random allocation sequence was generated by AK using Research Randomizer [25].

Statistical analyses

Statistical analysis was performed using SPSS 21.0.0.1. Differences in gender distribution over the experimental groups were tested using the Pearson Chi-square test, while differences in age and serum concentrations between groups was evaluated using ANOVA. To analyze serum lutein/zeaxanthin and MPOD, i.e. changes in time and possible differences between groups, we performed a Linear Mixed Models analysis (LMM) with subject as grouping factor, and gender, diet, time and the interaction term of the latter two as covariates. The LMM procedure expands the general linear model so that the data are permitted to exhibit correlated and non-constant variability. The LMM analysis, therefore, provides the flexibility of modeling not only the means of the data but their variances and covariances as well. LMM handle data where observations are not independent. That is, LMM correctly models correlated errors, whereas procedures in the general linear model family usually do not. Since we used subject as grouping factor, we take into account individual differences in baseline values. The model does assume similar linear changes in time for all subjects. P-values were considered significant if P<0.05. For post-hoc test we applied the Bonferroni correction. Results are shown as mean ± standard deviation.

Results

In total, 97 subjects completed the entire study. Two dropped out because they moved out of the area and one for unknown reasons (see Figure 1). Table 2 presents baseline characteristics of the participants. There were no statistically significant differences between the five groups for age (P = 0.34), gender (P = 0.99), serum zeaxanthin (P = 0.48) and MPOD (P = 0.60). There was a

significant difference between the groups for serum lutein at baseline (P = 0.030). A post-hoc analysis showed that the lutein egg group had significantly higher serum baseline levels. All other groups were comparable.

Supplementation with lutein enriched eggs caused a 76% increase in serum lutein concentrations while the egg-yolk based beverage caused a comparable increase of 77% (P<0.001, paired T-test, Table 3). Daily consumption of a normal egg or a zeaxanthin enriched egg also led to an increase of the serum lutein levels of 16 and 18% respectively, but these changes did not reach significance (P>0.29). This was confirmed by an LMM analysis using the serum lutein levels as dependent, and with diets, gender and time and their interaction terms as covariate. A significant effect was observed for time (P<0.001), gender (P = 0.012, women having on average 61 ng/ml higher lutein level than men) as well as an interaction between diet and time on serum lutein level (P< 0.001). This interaction was seen for both the lutein enriched eggs as for the lutein enriched egg-yolk based beverage groups as compared to the control group. Table 4 shows the β-coefficients of the LMM analysis and their P-values, with the control group as the reference. No difference was observed concerning the increase in serum lutein level between the lutein enriched egg and the lutein enriched egg-yolk based beverage group.

The serum zeaxanthin level increased markedly (430%) following consumption of zeaxanthin enriched eggs, whereas no significant changes were observed in the other four groups (Table 5). A LMM analysis with serum zeaxanthin levels as dependent, and with diets and gender as factor and time, and the interaction between diet and time as covariates revealed a significant effect for time (P<0.001) and the interaction term diets and time (P<0.001). This interaction was seen for the zeaxanthin enriched egg group (P<0.001) as compared to the control groups (see Table 4). A gender effect could not be detected.

No MPOD changes could be detected over time during the 90 day's trial period (Table 4 and 6).

Discussion

Daily consumption of lutein enriched eggs caused a 76% increase in serum lutein concentration. A similar increase of 77% was observed in the group taking a lutein enriched egg beverage. Consumption of zeaxanthin enriched eggs caused a marked 430% increase in serum zeaxanthin concentration. Our data are in agreement with earlier studies that showed that the daily consumption of eggs results in significantly increased serum xanthophyll levels [18,20,26–28].However, consumption of lutein or zeaxanthin enriched egg yolks led to a higher increase in xanthophylls blood levels compared to studies using "normal" eggs. Goodrow et al. for instance found a 26% and 38% increase in serum lutein and zeaxanthin concentrations following consump-

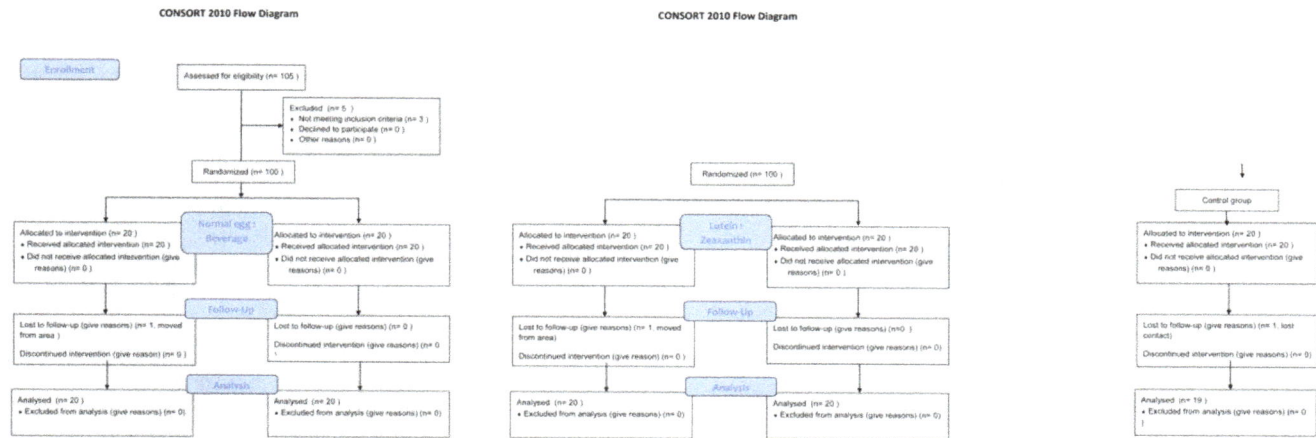

Figure 1. Flow diagram of the participants in the study.

tion of normal non-enriched eggs, that contain less lutein and zeaxanthin (143±28 and 94±18 μg/yolk) as compared to the enriched eggs used in our study [18]. In our non-enriched egg group (Table 3 and 5) we observed an increase of 16% in serum lutein and a 100% increase in serum zeaxanthin concentrations. Handelman et al. found a 28% and 142% increase using 1.3 egg yolk containing 292±117 μg/yolk of lutein and 213±85 μg/yolk of zeaxanthin for 4.5 weeks [26].

Most interest concerning xanthophylls in eggs in the past was related to consumer's wishes concerning egg yolk color. This can be achieved by raising the amount of natural or synthetic xanthophylls in chicken feed. It should be noted that the enriched eggs used in our study were obtained by providing the laying hens with a feed containing a higher amount of natural sources of xanthophylls derived from maize and marigold sources.

There is a growing awareness that individuals can modulate their risk of developing AMD by enhancing their intake of xanthophylls like lutein and zeaxanthin. They can either chose to do so by taking lutein and/or zeaxanthin containing supplements (pills) or by changing their diet, including functional foods. Lutein or zeaxanthin enriched eggs can be seen as a functional food to improve the xanthophyll status of an individual. In Europe, many elderly would chose to not take pills but to improve their lifestyle. Our investigations are aimed at proving the feasibility of such an approach, whereby we argued that consumption of xanthophyll enriched eggs could be a natural alternative for a pill. Xanthophyll content of eggs not only depends on the feed given to laying hens, but is also dependent on the husbandry system [29,30]. Organic

eggs were shown to have the highest lutein content (mean: 1,764 ug/100 g egg yolk), whereas caged eggs have the lowest level (mean: 410 ug/100 g egg yolk) [30]. Organic chickens obtain their xanthophylls from the grass and herbs in the outdoor run and due to the fact that outdoor run coverage and the outdoor run use by the hens is extremely variable, the xanthophyll content in eggs from this husbandry system has a wide range. The amount of lutein in the eggs used in our study can be maintained fairly constant due to the use of a well-defined feed. The obtained lutein content in the eggs used in our study contained approximately 4,600 ug of lutein per 100 g of egg yolk, which is almost threefold higher than the levels present in organic eggs. The zeaxanthin levels reached in our eggs (2,435 ug/ 100 g egg yolk) was also much higher than observed in organic eggs (1,021 ug/100 g egg yolk).

An important aspect of using eggs or egg yolks as a lutein source relates to the suggested elevated bioavailability [20]. It is well known that lutein depends on a lipophilic environment for optimal gastrointestinal uptake [31]. The change in serum lutein concentrations we observed following daily consumption of an egg yolk containing one mg of lutein per day, was comparable to the increase observed in a study using a five mg lutein supplement [32]. The finding that the zeaxanthin supplemented group had a 430% increase in serum zeaxanthin concentration compared to the lutein supplemented group which had a 76% increase in serum lutein concentration may be due to the fact that the zeaxanthin enriched egg had a relatively high zeaxanthin level as compared to the other dietary sources taken by our participants. This is evident

Table 2. Baseline characteristics of study subjects (mean ± standard deviation).

	Age	Gender (m/f)	Lutein (ng/ml)	Zeaxanthin (ng/ml)	MPOD[1]
Normal Egg	53±12	9/11	216±106	27.8±19.3	0.31±0.14
Lutein beverage	43±16	8/12	174±69	23.5±14.5	0.38±0.12
Lutein Egg	45±19	8/12	290±213	27.5±16.4	0.32±0.12
Zeaxanthin Egg	48±17	9/11	217±104	29.2±23.2	0.35±0.14
Control	44±16	9/11	180±51	20.4±10.2	0.34±0.15
P-value	0.34	0.99	0.030	0.48	0.60

[1]MPOD Macular Pigment Optical Density.
P-values are from an ANOVA analysis comparing the different groups.

Table 3. Serum lutein concentrations (ng/ml, mean ± standard deviation) during study follow up in males and females separately and combined.

Lutein	Baseline				Midpoint				Endpoint			
	Both	Male	Female	p²	Both	Male	Female	p²	Both	Male	Female	p²
Normal Egg	216±106	193±76	235±126	0.40	239±111	205±79	266±129	0.23	235±93	212±54	255±117	0.33
Lutein beverage	174±69	137±40	198±75	0.048	284±126	210±85	334±126	0.026	310±135	219±75	371±133	0.009
Lutein Egg	290±213	213±96	334±251	0.24	438±196	336±114	497±212	0.082	465±201	389±125	509±227	0.22
Zeaxanthin Egg	217±104	215±112	219±102	0.93	232±125	234±155	230±99	0.95	248±118	235±130	260±112	0.67
Control	180±51	174±48	185±56	0.66	188±72	190±75	186±72	0.91	177±55	169±59	184±53	0.55
P-value[1]	0.030	0.27	0.11		<0.001	0.082	<0.001		<0.001	0.001	<0.001	

[1]P-values are from an ANOVA analysis comparing the different groups at each time point.
[2]P-values for the difference between male and female subjects.

in view of the fact that baseline blood levels of zeaxanthin were much lower as compared to the lutein blood level. We did not asses the diets taken by our participants and further studies are needed to address this issue.

Safety issues of this study included the fact that an increased egg consumption can alter circulating lipoprotein levels and that the use of xanthophyll enriched eggs could result in a higher circulating level of lutein and zeaxanthin in our volunteers. Eggs are a concentrated source of cholesterol [33] and dietary cholesterol increases low-density lipoprotein cholesterol (LDL-C) concentrations [34]. To address these possible adverse side effects we compared serum lipoprotein levels between the different groups. None of the individuals participating in the study attained a lipoprotein level that was considered as abnormal. The data that are presented in a separate paper showed that the rise in serum LDL-C concentrations was less pronounced when egg yolk was incorporated into the buttermilk drink, suggesting that fractions in the buttermilk may influence dietary cholesterol absorption [35].

We did not perform any additional tests to address possible safety issues related to an increased lutein or zeaxanthin level associated with the consumption of the enriched eggs used in our project since this has been covered in detail in earlier studies [36,37]. Short-term and long-term toxicity profile of lutein was studied in young adult Wistar rats [38]. Administration of up to 400 mg/kg body weight of lutein did not produce any mortality, change in body weight, food consumption pattern, organ weight, and other adverse side reactions. It also did not alter hepatic or renal function, and did not produce any change in the hematological parameters or lipid profile. Histopathological analysis of the organs supported the absence of toxicity of lutein. A similar study was undertaken by Ravikrishnan *et al.* [36]. In comparison with a control group, they also found no treatment-related changes in clinical observations, ophthalmic examinations, body weights, body weight gains, feed consumption, and organ weights. No toxicologically relevant findings were noted in urinalysis, hematology or clinical biochemistry parameters. Terminal necropsy did not reveal any treatment-related gross or histopathology findings. The no observed-adverse-effect level for their lutein/zeaxanthin concentrate was determined as 400 mg/kg bw/day, the highest dose tested. These levels are far higher than the dose used in our study which is equivalent to a 5 mg lutein containing daily supplement per individual.

Others studied acute and subacute toxicity of lutein in lutein-deficient mice [39]. Compared to a control (peanut oil without lutein) group, they found no treatment-related toxicologically significant effects of lutein in clinical observation, ophthalmic examinations, body, and organ weights. Further, no toxicologically significant findings were eminent in hematological, histopathological, and other clinical chemistry parameters. Further, in an oral sub acute toxicity study, the no-observed-adverse-effect level for lutein was determined as 1000 mg/kg/day, the highest dose tested, which as mentioned above is several orders of magnitude higher than our doses.

Various independent clinical studies assessing retinal electrophysiological functions following the intake of lutein or zeaxanthin containing supplements did not show adverse effects and even reported an improved retinal function [40–43].

We could not detect a significant change in the macular pigment optical density during our trial among the various groups tested. We believe that this is an absence of evidence instead of evidence of absence of an effect. It is probably due to the fact that our study was carried out during a relatively short time period. Xanthophyll supplementation leads to a rapid response in circulating blood levels and a subsequent slow increase in macular

Table 4. β-coefficients of the Linear Mixed Model (LMM) analyses, their P-values and confidence intervals.

	Lutein			Zeaxanthin			MPOD		
	β	P-Value	CI	β	P-Value	CI	β	P-Value	CI
Intercept	149.5	<0.001	89.1 – 210.0	25.0	<0.001	11.3 – 38.6	0.32	<0.001	0.25 – 0.38
Diet:Normal Egg	36.5	0.35	-40.5 – 78.6	7.0	0.44	-10.8 – 24.7	-0.021	0.62	-0.10 – 0.06
Diet:Lutein beverage	1.5	0.97	-75.6 – 78.6	2.8	0.76	15.0 – 20.6	0.003	0.93	-0.08 – 0.08
Diet:Lutein Egg	121.6	0.003	43.4 – 199.7	7.7	0.4	-10.4 – 25.7	-0.017	0.68	-0.99 – 0.06
Diet:Zeaxanthin Egg	35.4	0.37	-42.7 – 113.4	23.4	0.011	5.4 – 41.4	-0.006	0.89	-0.09 – 0.08
Diet:Control	0			0			0		
Gender:Female	61.3	0.012	13.6 – 109.0	-5.1	0.3	-14.8 – 4.6	0.022	0.36	-0.03 – 0.07
Gender:Male	0			0			0		
Time	-0.23	0.87	-2.9 – 2.5	0.53	0.36	-0.6 – 1.7	0.002	0.47	-0.003 – 0.007
Time*Diet:Normal Egg	2.2	0.26	-1.6 – 6.1	1	0.23	-0.6 – 2.6	0.002	0.58	-0.006 – 0.010
Time*Diet:Lutein beverage	11.6	<0.001	7.8 – 15.4	1.29	0.12	-0.3 – 2.0	-0.004	0.34	-0.011 – 0.004
Time*Diet:Lutein Egg	14.9	<0.001	11.0 – 18.7	1.58	0.059	-0.05 – 3.2	0.004	0.3	-0.004 – 0.012
Time*Diet:Zeaxanthin Egg	2.8	0.16	-1.1 –6.7	7.65	<0.001	6.0 –9.3	0	0.94	-0.008 – 0.007
Time*Diet:Control	0			0			0		

Table 5. Serum zeaxanthin concentrations (ng/ml, mean ± standard deviation) during study follow up.

Zeaxanthin	Baseline				Midpoint				Endpoint			
	Both	Male	Female	P^2	Both	Male	Female	P^2	Both	Male	Female	P^2
Normal Egg	27.8±19.3	37.2±23.4	20.1±11.1	0.45	40.9±23.4	51.5±27.1	32.2±16.4	0.63	45.6±25.3	53.7±30.6	38.4±18.1	0.20
Lutein beverage	23.5±14.5	20.3±7.4	25.7±17.8	0.42	37.8±19.8	28.1±8.9	44.3±22.6	0.07	45.4±18.1	37.6±11.4	50.6±20.3	0.12
Lutein Egg	27.5±16.4	31.3±18.2	25.3±15.7	0.45	45.9±16.2	52.4±16.7	42.1±15.3	0.19	52.8±23.3	62.4±27.5	47.3±19.6	0.18
Zeaxanthin Egg	29.2±23.2	31.0±29.3	27.7±17.6	0.77	127.8±65.3	129.9±77.1	125.8±56.2	0.89	127.5±54.3	125.8±77.1	128.9±24.8	0.91
Control	20.4±10.2	23.7±10.3	17.75±9.9	0.21	28.8±22.4	36.1±31.1	22.8±9.8	0.20	26.8±10.6	29.9±13.5	24.18±7.2	0.24
P-value[1]	0.48	0.43	0.49		<0.001	<0.001	<0.001		<0.001	<0.001	<0.001	

[1]P-values are from an ANOVA analysis comparing the different groups at each time point.
[2]P-values for the difference between male and female subjects.

Table 6. Macular pigment optical density (MPOD) during study follow up.

MPOD	Baseline				Midpoint				Endpoint			
	Both	Male	Female	P^2	Both	Male	Female	P^2	Both	Male	Female	P^2
Normal Egg	0.31±0.14	0.27±0.09	0.34±0.17	0.25	0.35±0.18	0.30±0.11	0.40±0.22	0.25	0.35±0.22	0.25±0.13	0.45±0.25	0.04
Lutein beverage	0.38±0.12	0.37±0.14	0.38±0.11	0.96	0.32±0.15	0.34±0.15	0.30±0.15	0.54	0.32±0.16	0.33±0.20	0.32±0.14	0.96
Lutein Egg	0.32±0.12	0.27±0.11	0.35±0.12	0.18	0.42±0.23	0.33±0.06	0.48±0.27	0.18	0.36±0.16	0.32±0.16	0.38±0.17	0.44
Zeaxanthin Egg	0.35±0.14	0.29±0.12	0.40±0.13	0.07	0.31±0.16	0.25±0.15	0.37±0.15	0.81	0.36±0.21	0.42±0.27	0.31±0.14	0.33
Control	0.34±0.15	0.41±0.16	0.28±0.14	0.08	0.36±0.22	0.38±0.18	0.35±0.26	0.78	0.35±0.17	0.41±0.17	0.29±0.15	0.11
P-value[1]	0.60	0.37	0.08		0.38	0.37	0.35		0.96	0.24	0.31	

[1]P-values are from an ANOVA analysis comparing the different groups at each time point.
[2]P-values for the difference between male and female subjects.

pigment levels. Bone and Landrum showed that with supplementation MPOD tends to exhibit a linear increase in time [32], in particular in subjects proficient in heterochromatic flicker photometry. However, they also showed a great variation in the standard error of the slope of this linear increase, which implies that the fact that we did not achieve a measurable increase in the MPOD values is due to a small sample size and that a longer intervention period is needed to reach significance.

Participants were asked not to change their habitual diet, level of physical exercise, or use of alcohol throughout the study, although we did not assess their diet. On the other hand, participants were aware of the nature and background of the study and it cannot be excluded that this may have inadvertently affected their behavior. However, due to the strictly randomized placebo controlled nature of the trial this should have affected all groups. Medical ethical committees insist that subjects are adequately informed about the nature of clinical trials and one should be aware of the fact that this may introduce confounding circumstances. In the study we did not address possible confounders and to rule this out a larger sample size will be needed.

Using supplements varying from five to twenty mg of lutein, others have shown that serum lutein concentration increased rapidly during the first two–three weeks of supplementation, whereafter it reached a plateau up to the end of the supplementation period [32]. Although we only included three time points in our study, it appears that consumption of lutein enriched eggs causes a continuous increase in serum lutein levels during the whole trial period of 90 days, although less fast in the second half of the study. On the other hand, the changes in serum zeaxanthin levels following the daily consumption of a zeaxanthin enriched egg were more in line with results as shown earlier by others [32]. Serum zeaxanthin levels in our study leveled after week six. Since our first measurement was at week six, it is possible that maximum levels were already reached at an earlier time point.

It should be kept in mind that the present study does not provide evidence to support the fact that modified eggs or egg-yolk based beverages constitute a preventive or curative treatment of any form of age related macular degeneration or maculopathy.

In summary, we found significant increases in serum lutein and zeaxanthin concentration following consumption of enriched eggs providing one mg lutein/day, which was comparable with a daily use of five mg supplements. An egg yolk-based beverage showed similar results. Our study provides support for the concept that an adequate xanthophyll status can be achieved by the intake of naturally enriched functional foods.

Author Contributions

Conceived and designed the experiments: JP AK TB. Performed the experiments: EK. Analyzed the data: EK TB. Contributed reagents/materials/analysis tools: GH. Wrote the paper: EK AK TB. Revising the manuscript critically for important intellectual content: JP.

References

1. Hyman L (1987) Epidemiology of eye disease in the elderly. Eye (Lond) 1 (Pt 2): 330–341.
2. Kahn HA, Leibowitz HM, Ganley JP, Kini MM, Colton T, et al. (1977) The Framingham Eye Study. I. Outline and major prevalence findings. Am J Epidemiol 106: 17–32.
3. Snodderly DM, Auran JD, Delori FC (1984) The macular pigment. II. Spatial distribution in primate retinas. Invest Ophthalmol Vis Sc 25: 674–685.
4. Stahl W, Sies H (2003) Antioxidant activity of carotenoids. Mol Aspects Med 24: 345–351.
5. Junghans A, Sies H, Stahl W (2001) Macular pigments lutein and zeaxanthin as blue light filters studied in liposomes. Arch Biochem Biophys 391: 160–164.
6. Sujak A, Gabrielska J, Grudzinski W, Borc R, Mazurek P, et al. (1999) Lutein and zeaxanthin as protectors of lipid membranes against oxidative damage: the structural aspects. Arch Biochem Biophys 371: 301–307.
7. Izumi-Nagai K, Nagai N, Ohgami K, Satofuka S, Ozawa Y, et al. (2007) Macular Pigment Lutein Is Antiinflammatory in Preventing Choroidal Neovascularization. Arteriosclerosis Thrombosis and Vascular Biology 27: 2555–2562.
8. Kijlstra A, Tian Y, Kelly ER, Berendschot TTJM (2012) Lutein: more than just a filter for blue light. Prog Retin Eye Res 31: 303–315.
9. Berendschot TTJM, Goldbohm RA, Klöpping WA, van de Kraats J, van Norel J, et al. (2000) Influence of lutein supplementation on macular pigment, assessed with two objective techniques. Invest Ophthalmol Vis Sc 41: 3322–3326.
10. Landrum JT, Bone RA, Joa H, Kilburn MD, Moore LL, et al. (1997) A one year study of the macular pigment: the effect of 140 days of a lutein supplement. Exp Eye Res 65: 57–62.
11. Hammond BR, Johnson EJ, Russell RM, Krinsky NI, Yeum KJ, et al. (1997) Dietary modification of human macular pigment density. Invest Ophthalmol Vis Sc 38: 1795–1801.
12. Trieschmann M, Beatty S, Nolan JM, Hense HW, Heimes B, et al. (2007) Changes in macular pigment optical density and serum concentrations of its constituent carotenoids following supplemental lutein and zeaxanthin: the LUNA study. Exp Eye Res 84: 718–728.
13. Tan JS, Wang JJ, Flood V, Rochtchina E, Smith W, et al. (2008) Dietary antioxidants and the long-term incidence of age-related macular degeneration: the Blue Mountains Eye Study. Ophthalmol 115: 334–341.
14. SanGiovanni JP, Chew EY, Clemons TE, Ferris FL III, Gensler G, et al. (2007) The relationship of dietary carotenoid and vitamin A, E, and C intake with age-related macular degeneration in a case-control study: AREDS Report No. 22. Arch Ophthalmol 125: 1225–1232.
15. Obana A, Hiramitsu T, Gohto Y, Ohira A, Mizuno S, et al. (2008) Macular Carotenoid Levels of Normal Subjects and Age-Related Maculopathy Patients in a Japanese Population. Ophthalmol 115: 147–157.
16. The Age-Related Eye Disease Study 2 Research Group (2013) Lutein + Zeaxanthin and Omega-3 Fatty Acids for Age-Related Macular Degeneration: The Age-Related Eye Disease Study 2 (AREDS2) Randomized Clinical Trial. JAMA 1–11.
17. Wenzel AJ, Gerweck C, Barbato D, Nicolosi RJ, Handelman GJ, et al. (2006) A 12-Wk Egg Intervention Increases Serum Zeaxanthin and Macular Pigment Optical Density in Women. J Nutr 136: 2568–2573.
18. Goodrow EF, Wilson TA, Houde SC, Vishwanathan R, Scollin PA et al. (2006) Consumption of One Egg Per Day Increases Serum Lutein and Zeaxanthin Concentrations in Older Adults without Altering Serum Lipid and Lipoprotein Cholesterol Concentrations. J Nutr 136: 2519–2524.
19. Vishwanathan R, Goodrow-Kotyla EF, Wooten BR, Wilson TA, Nicolosi RJ (2009) Consumption of 2 and 4 egg yolks/d for 5 wk increases macular pigment concentrations in older adults with low macular pigment taking cholesterol-lowering statins. The American Journal of Clinical Nutrition 90: 1272–1279.
20. Chung HY, Rasmussen HM, Johnson EJ (2004) Lutein bioavailability is higher from lutein-enriched eggs than from supplements and spinach in men. J Nutr 134: 1887–1893.
21. Thompson AK, Singh H (2006) Preparation of liposomes from milk fat globule membrane phospholipids using a microfluidizer. J Dairy Sci 89: 410–419.
22. Vaisman N, Haenen GR, Zaruk Y, Verduyn C, Bindels JG, et al. (2006) Enteral feeding enriched with carotenoids normalizes the carotenoid status and reduces oxidative stress in long-term enterally fed patients. Clin Nutr 25: 897–905.
23. van der Veen RLP, Berendschot TTJM, Hendrikse F, Carden D, Makridaki M, et al. (2009) A new desktop instrument for measuring macular pigment optical density based on a novel technique for setting flicker thresholds. Ophthalmic Physiol Opt 29: 127–137.
24. Dupont WD, Plummer J (1997) PS power and sample size program available for free on the internet. Controlled Clinical Trials 18: 274.
25. Urbaniak GC, Plous S (2007) Research Randomizer, retrieved from Research Randomizer website, http://www.randomizer.org/, accessed September 2007
26. Handelman GJ, Nightingale ZD, Lichtenstein AH, Schaefer EJ, Blumberg JB (1999) Lutein and zeaxanthin concentrations in plasma after dietary supplementation with egg yolk. Am J Clin Nutr 70: 247–251.
27. Surai PF, MacPherson A, Speake BK, Sparks NHC (2000) Designer egg evaluation in a controlled trial. Eur J Clin Nutr 54: 298–305.

28. Clark RM, Herron KL, Waters D, Fernandez ML (2006) Hypo- and hyperresponse to egg cholesterol predicts plasma lutein and β-carotene concentrations in men and women. J Nutr 136: 601–607.

29. Hesterberg K, Schanzer S, Patzelt A, Sterry W, Fluhr JW, et al. (2012) Raman spectroscopic analysis of the carotenoid concentration in egg yolks depending on the feeding and housing conditions of the laying hens. J Biophotonics 5: 33–39.

30. Schlatterer J, Breithaupt DE (2006) Xanthophylls in commercial egg yolks: quantification and identification by HPLC and LC-(APCI)MS using a C30 phase. J Agric Food Chem 54: 2267–2273.

31. Roodenburg AJ, Leenen R, van het Hof KH, Weststrate JA, Tijburg LB (2000) Amount of fat in the diet affects bioavailability of lutein esters but not of alpha-carotene, beta-carotene, and vitamin E in humans. Am J Clin Nutr 71: 1187–1193.

32. Bone RA, Landrum JT (2010) Dose-dependent response of serum lutein and macular pigment optical density to supplementation with lutein esters. Arch Biochem Biophys 504: 50–55.

33. Applegate E (2000) Introduction: nutritional and functional roles of eggs in the diet. J Am Coll Nutr 19: 495S–498S.

34. Weggemans RM, Zock PL, Katan MB (2001) Dietary cholesterol from eggs increases the ratio of total cholesterol to high-density lipoprotein cholesterol in humans: a meta-analysis. Am J Clin Nutr 73: 885–891.

35. Baumgartner S, Kelly ER, van de Made S, Berendschot TTJM, Husche C, et al. (2013) The influence of consuming an egg or an egg-yolk buttermilk drink for 12 wk on serum lipids, inflammation, and liver function markers in human volunteers. Nutrition 29: 1237–1244.

36. Ravikrishnan R, Rusia S, Ilamurugan G, Salunkhe U, Deshpande J, et al. (2011) Safety assessment of lutein and zeaxanthin (Lutemax 2020): subchronic toxicity and mutagenicity studies. Food Chem Toxicol 49: 2841–2848.

37. Connolly EE, Beatty S, Loughman J, Howard AN, Louw MS, et al. (2011) Supplementation with all three macular carotenoids: response, stability, and safety. Invest Ophthalmol Vis Sci 52: 9207–9217.

38. Harikumar KB, Nimita CV, Preethi KC, Kuttan R, Shankaranarayana ML, et al. (2008) Toxicity Profile of Lutein and Lutein Ester Isolated From Marigold Flowers (Tagetes erecta). International Journal of Toxicology 27: 1–9.

39. Nidhi B, Baskaran V (2013) Acute and subacute toxicity assessment of lutein in lutein-deficient mice. J Food Sci 78: T1636–T1642.

40. Falsini B, Piccardi M, Iarossi G, Fadda A, Merendino E, et al. (2003) Influence of short-term antioxidant supplementation on macular function in age-related maculopathy: a pilot study including electrophysiologic assessment. Ophthalmol 110: 51–60.

41. Ma L, Dou HL, Huang YM, Lu XR, Xu XR, et al. (2012) Improvement of retinal function in early age-related macular degeneration after lutein and zeaxanthin supplementation: a randomized, double-masked, placebo-controlled trial. Am J Ophthalmol 154: 625–634.

42. Berrow EJ, Bartlett HE, Eperjesi F, Gibson JM (2013) The effects of a lutein-based supplement on objective and subjective measures of retinal and visual function in eyes with age-related maculopathy — a randomised controlled trial. Br J Nutr 109: 2008–2014.

43. Parisi V, Tedeschi M, Gallinaro G, Varano M, Saviano S, et al. (2008) Carotenoids and Antioxidants in Age-Related Maculopathy Italian Study: Multifocal Electroretinogram Modifications after 1 Year. Ophthalmol 115: 324–333.

20

Proteomics of Vitreous Humor of Patients with Exudative Age-Related Macular Degeneration

Michael Janusz Koss[1,2,3]*, Janosch Hoffmann[4], Nauke Nguyen[1], Marcel Pfister[2], Harald Mischak[4,5], William Mullen[5], Holger Husi[5], Robert Rejdak[6], Frank Koch[1], Joachim Jankowski[7], Katharina Krueger[7], Thomas Bertelmann[8], Julie Klein[4], Joost P. Schanstra[4,9,10], Justyna Siwy[4,7]

1 Department of Ophthalmology, Goethe University, Frankfurt am Main, Germany, 2 Doheny Eye Institute, Los Angeles, California, United States of America, 3 Department of Ophthalmology, Ruprecht Karls University, Heidelberg, Germany, 4 Mosaiques Diagnostics, Hannover, Germany, 5 BHF Glasgow Cardiovascular Research Centre, University of Glasgow, Glasgow, United Kingdom, 6 Department of General Ophthalmology, Lublin University, Poland, 7 Department of Nephrology, Endocrinology, and Transplantation Medicine Charité-Universitaetsmedizin, Berlin, Germany, 8 Department of Ophthalmology, Philipps University, Marburg, Germany, 9 Institut National de la Santé et de la Recherche Médicale (INSERM), U1048, Institut of Cardiovascular and Metabolic Disease, Toulouse, France, 10 Université Toulouse III Paul-Sabatier, Toulouse, France

Abstract

Background: There is absence of specific biomarkers and an incomplete understanding of the pathophysiology of exudative age-related macular degeneration (AMD).

Methods and Findings: Eighty-eight vitreous samples (73 from patients with treatment naïve AMD and 15 control samples from patients with idiopathic floaters) were analyzed with capillary electrophoresis coupled to mass spectrometry in this retrospective case series to define potential candidate protein markers of AMD. Nineteen proteins were found to be upregulated in vitreous of AMD patients. Most of the proteins were plasma derived and involved in biological (ion) transport, acute phase inflammatory reaction, and blood coagulation. A number of proteins have not been previously associated to AMD including alpha-1-antitrypsin, fibrinogen alpha chain and prostaglandin H2-D isomerase. Alpha-1-antitrypsin was validated in vitreous of an independent set of AMD patients using Western blot analysis. Further systems biology analysis of the data indicated that the observed proteomic changes may reflect upregulation of immune response and complement activity.

Conclusions: Proteome analysis of vitreous samples from patients with AMD, which underwent an intravitreal combination therapy including a core vitrectomy, steroids and bevacizumab, revealed apparent AMD-specific proteomic changes. The identified AMD-associated proteins provide some insight into the pathophysiological changes associated with AMD.

Editor: Sanjoy Bhattacharya, Bascom Palmer Eye Institute, University of Miami School of Medicine, United States of America

Funding: The study was financed in part by the Adolf Messer Stiftung in Königstein, Hessen, Germany; No additional external funding was received for this study. http://www.adolf-messer-stiftung.de/. The funders had no role in study design, data collection and analysis, decision to publish, or preparation of the manuscript.

Competing Interests: The authors have declared that no competing interests exist.

* E-mail: Michael.koss@me.com

Introduction

Age dependent alterations of the retinal pigment epithelium (RPE) and its basal membrane, called Bruchs membrane, are widely accepted as the main pathophysiological reason for age-related macular degeneration (AMD) and is thus the leading cause of blindness in people over the age of 60 years in industrialized countries [1]. The upregulation of vascular endothelial growth factor (VEGF) and the development of a choroidal neovascularization (CNV) are the blueprint for the conversion to the exudative or wet AMD form. Our understanding today of the disease and the interaction of intravitreal anti-VEGF treatment is thereby coined and determined by clinical diagnostics, mainly optical coherence tomography and fluorescein angiography. Since AMD is a pure retinochoroidal disease, circulating *in vivo* biomarkers such as HbA1c in the diagnosis and treatment of diabetes are still absent for AMD. Samples from the human vitreous might best qualify as a source of biomarkers for AMD due to the proximity to the retina and the efflux of cytokines into the vitreous cavity [2]. However, most published protein analyses in exudative AMD derive from experimental animal models, *ex vivo* samples or *in vivo* from ocular anterior chamber aspirates (AC) with the incorporated flaws [3,4,5,6]. Ecker et al. demonstrated, that cytokine and growth factor levels from the AC do not reliably reflect those levels found in the vitreous and thus it is questionable to assess the activity of a purely retinochoroidal disease by examining an AC aspirate [2,7,8]. But results from vitreous samples in AMD are scarce and published data differs on patient selection, sampling technique and analysis method [7,9,10,11,12,13,14,15].

Proteome analysis allows the simultaneous assessment of a large number of proteins in a sample. Proteome analyses have been performed in a variety of ocular diseases, including primary open-angle glaucoma and cataract [16,17,18]. Further exploration of vitreous protein profiles was performed even tough clinical factors, like consistency of the vitreous, length of the eye, attachment of the posterior hyaloid are to date neglected in the literature [19]. Especially in the context of wet AMD the current proteomic data on vitreous or aqueous humor are incomplete.

Capillary electrophoresis coupled to mass spectrometry (CE-MS) is a powerful and very reproducible technology platform with known performance characteristics [20]. This automated, sensitive, fast proteome analysis technique [21] using CE as a front-end fractionation coupled to mass spectrometry, separates peptides and small proteins (<20 kDa) based on migration in the electrical field with high resolution in a single step. It enables analysis of thousands of peptides per sample using a sub-microliter sample volume and it has been used in numerous clinical biomarker studies, mostly examining urine as the specimen of interest [22,23].

In this pilot study, we performed a bottom-up analysis combing the reproducibility of CE-MS for selection of candidate marker proteins, and LC-MS/MS for sequence identification of these markers in vitreous of 73 AMD patients and controls. This led to the identification of a number of candidate proteins not previously shown to be involved in AMD. Systems biology analysis of the data suggested an increase in immune response, complement activation and protease activity to be involved in the pathophysiology of AMD.

Material and Methods

Sampling and patient characteristics

Vitreous samples were acquired at the beginning of an intravitreal combination treatment for wet AMD, which involved a 23-gauge core vitrectomy of at least 4 cc vitreous, before the application of bevacizumab, triamcinolone, and dexamethasone [22]. The same surgical technique was applied for the removal of idiopathic vitreous floaters, substituting balanced salt solution (BSS Plus, Alcon, Freiburg, Germany). This study adhered to the Declaration of Helsinki and was approved by the Investigational Review Board of the Goethe University. Written informed consent was obtained from all participants, explaining the risks and benefits of the treatment (the advantage of a combination treatment for wet AMD rather than with anti-VEGF monotherapy is summarized here [24,25,26]; the vitreous samples would otherwise have been disposed).

A total of 88 undiluted and previously untreated (any intraviteal drug application) samples were analyzed (**Table 1**). The 73 AMD samples came from 73 patients (50 women 23 men) with a mean age 77.8 ± 8.9 years (standard deviation). Sixteen of the 73 patients had a hemorrhagic CNV; 37 had an active CNV (10 with signs accompanying bleeding); 13 had a CNV and greater than 80% fibrous staining in the fluorescein angiography (FA); and 7 had a CNV-associated RPE detachment and no intraretinal fluid. These classifications were assigned after a complete ocular examination, which included a slit-lamp biomicroscopy, indirect ophthalmoscopy, color fundus photography, spectral domain optical coherence tomography (3D-OCT 2000, Topcon, Willich, Germany), and FA. Patients with previous intravitreal anti-VEGF treatment, including intraocular steroids, or systemic diabetes, nephropathy or uncontrolled hypertension were excluded. Patients with any other compromising ocular condition, such as diabetic retinopathy or uveitis, were also considered ineligible for this study.

All patients were recruited from the retina clinic of the department of ophthalmology from the Goethe University in Frankfurt am Main in Germany. Vitreous samples from 15 patients with idiopathic floaters (8 women, 7 men; mean age 60 ±

Table 1. Epidemiology of the samples.

		Number	Age (± SD)	Sex		Eye	
				F	M	RE	LE
AMD	Hemorrhagic CNV Bleeding	16	80.8 ± 9.0	15	1	6	10
	CNV With blood signs	10	77.7 ± 10.5	4	6	8	2
	Without blood signs	27	77.2 ± 7.4	17	10	12	15
	Fibrous	13	75.4 ± 8.1	9	4	8	5
	RPE-Detachment	7	78.3 ± 12.9	5	2	4	3
Control		15	60.0 ± 16.0	8	7	6	9

SD = standard deviation, F = female, M = male, RE/LE = right/left eye, CNV = choroidal neovascularization, AMD = age related macular degeneration, RPE = retinal pigment epithelium.

16 years) served as controls. All vitreous samples were stored at $-80°C$.

Tryptic digestion of vitreous

A 10-μL portion of the thawed sample was diluted with 90 μL 0.1% SDS, 20 mM DTT, and 0.1 M TrisHCl (pH = 7.6). The sample was sonicated at room temperature for 30 minutes to decrease viscosity and break up hyaluronic polymers contained in the vitreous humor. This was followed by denaturation at 95°C for 3 min. Samples were subsequently incubated with 80 mM Iodoacetamide at room temperature for 30 min in the absence of light, followed by the addition of ammonium bicarbonate buffer solution (300 μL, 50 mM) and applied to NAP-5 columns equilibrated in 50 mM ammonium bicarbonate buffer solution.

Twenty μg of Lyophilized trypsin was dissolved in 50 μL of buffer solution provided with the lypholized product. Two μL of this solution was added to the desalted sample. Trypsin digestion was carried out overnight at a temperature of 37°C. Subsequently the samples were lyophilized, stored at 4°C and resuspendend in HPLC-grade H_2O shortly before mass spectrometry analysis.

CE-MS analysis

CE-MS analysis was performed as described by Theodorescu et al [27]. A P/ACE MDQ capillary electrophoresis system (Beckman Coulter, Brea, CA) was linked online to a micro-TOF MS (Bruker Daltonik, Leipzig, Germany). The sprayer (Agilent Technologies, Santa Clara, CA) interfacing the CE and MS was grounded and the interface potential was adjusted to -4.5 kV. Signals were recorded at an m/z range of 350–3000. The detection limit of the TOF-Analyzer is in the range of 1 fmol [27].

Data processing

Analysis of raw CE-MS data was carried out using Mosaiques-Visu [28]. MosaiquesVisu uses isotope identification and conjugated mass detection for mass deconvolution. Signals with a signal-to-random noise ratio >4 and charge >1 were used. Mass spectral ion peaks from the same molecule at different charge states were deconvoluted into a single mass.

In total, 292 signals for mass and CE-time with a frequency ≥ 35% could be determined that served as reference signals for normalization of peptide CE-time and mass using linear regression. For signal intensity normalization, 22 internal standards were selected that were consistently detected in vitreous samples (average frequency 83%) and that did not appear to be significantly associated with the disease. This signal intensity normalization using internal standards has been shown to be a reliable method to address both analytical and biological variances in biological samples [29].

The normalized peptides were deposited, matched, and annotated in a Microsoft SQL database. Peptides were considered identical when deviation of mass was < ±50 ppm for an 800 Da peptide. The mass deviation was adjusted by an increase in size of up to ±75 ppm for 15 kDa. Peptides were considered identical if the CE-migration time window did not exceed 2–5%, continuously increasing between 19 and 50 min. A number of peptides were only sporadically observed. To eliminate such low relevance peptides, all peptides that appeared only once were removed and were not considered for further analysis.

Tandem mass spectrometry (MS/MS) sequencing

For MS/MS analysis five lyophilized, tryptic-digested randomly selected vitreous samples were dissolved in 15 μL distilled water. Fractionation was carried out according to Metzger et al. [30]

using a Dionex Ultimate 3000 Nano LC System (Dionex, Camberly, UK). After loading (5 μl) onto a Dionex 0.1×20 mm 5 μm C18 nano trap column at a flowrate of 5 μl/min in 98% 0.1% formic acid and 2% acetonitrile, sample was eluted onto an Acclaim PepMap C18 nano column 75 μm×15 cm, 2 μm 100 Å at a flow rate of 0.3 μl/min. The trap and nano flow column were maintained at 35°C. The samples were eluted with a gradient of solvent A:98% 0.1% formic acid, 2% acetonitrile verses solvent B: 80% acetonitrile, 20% 0.1% formic acid starting at 1% B for 5 minutes rising to 20% B after 90 min and finally to 40%B after 120 min. The column was then washed and re-equilibrated prior to the next injection. The eluant was ionized using a Proxeon nano spray ESI source operating in positive ion mode into an Orbitrap Velos FTMS (Thermo Finnigan, Bremen, Germany). Ionization voltage was 2.6 kV and the capillary temperature was 200°C. The mass spectrometer was operated in MS/MS mode scanning from 380 to 2000 amu. The top 20 multiply charged ions were selected from each scan for MS/MS analysis using HCD at 40% collision energy. The resolution of ions in MS1 was 60,000 and 7,500 for HCD MS2. The MS data and the human, non redundant database IPI were matched using the SEQUEST software. Trypsin was used as the enzyme while screening for proteins. Hydroxylated proline from collagen fragments and oxidation of methionine were accepted as variable modifications and carbamidomethylated cystein as fixed modification. A maximal mass deviation of 10 ppm for MS and 0.8 Da for MS/MS was accepted. Only proteins represented by a minimum two peptides were accepted in LC-MS/MS analysis. The sequences were matched to the detected CE-MS data as described by Zürbig et al [19]. Although in this matching procedure the LC retention time can not be used, CE-MS data generate an additional parameter that can be used in this matching procedure, which is the charge of the peptides (at low pH, the condition in which peptides are analysed by CE-MS). Therefore, even when having identical or very close masses in the LC-MS/MS analysis, discrimination between peptides with similar masses can be performed on the basis of their charge. This is due to the fact that the number of basic and neutral polar amino acids of peptide sequences distinctly correlates with their CE-MS migration time/molecular weight coordinates. In nearly all cases this allows linking a unique LC-MS/MS peptide to a CE-MS peptide as shown previously [19].

CE-MS peptides with sequencing information were combined for each protein. Protein abundance was calculated as the average of all normalized CE-MS peptide intensities for the given protein. Mean protein abundance in the case group was compared to the mean protein abundance in the control group. Protein entries were mapped to the SwissProt database using either the mapping service provided by UniProt or via Blast searching (web.expasy.org/blast/) and merged according to the SwissProt names.

Biomarker definition

Candidate AMD biomarkers were defined by examination of differences in frequency and signal intensity of the proteins between the AMD patients and controls. Mean CE-MS based protein signal intensity was used as a measure for relative abundance. Statistical analysis was performed using Graph Pad Prism 5.0 software. A F-test was performed to test for data distribution. When data were normally distributed, a parametric t-test was performed; otherwise, the statistical analysis was performed using a Mann-Whitney test or Wilcoxon signed rank test. Multiple hypotheses testing correction was performed using the Benjamini-Hochberg test for false discovery rate [31].

Bioinformatics analysis

Gene ontology (GO) keyword-cluster analysis was done using CytoScape (www.cytoscape.org) and the ClueGO plug-in, where statistically significant molecules with p-values of less than 0.05 were compared. The interactome analysis was performed using CytoScape and the Michigan Molecular Interactor plug-in (mimi.ncibi.org). Full interactome analysis was carried out by connecting molecules through neighboring proteins, whereas the condensed protein-protein interaction analysis was performed by searching for direct associations. The paradigm of this analysis is that molecules with similar cellular involvement tend to cluster together through physical interactions, such as molecular machines. The disease analysis is based on known or inferred genetic disorders associated with mutations of specific genes using the Online Mendelian Inheritance in Man database for data mining. An additional pathway analysis was carried out using the Kyoto encyclopedia of genes and genomes (KEGG) database, where KEGG accession numbers of the statistically significant molecules were used for mapping-queries. Additionally, disease-specific descriptions were retrieved from the Online Mendelian Inheritance in Man (OMIM) database as well as the UniProt database. Cellular expression data was also obtained from the latter resource.

Western blot analysis

To determine the protein levels of Transthyretin, Apolipoprotein A 1, Alpha-1 Antitrypsin, Serotransferrin and Retinol-binding protein 3 we obtained vitreous fluid as described above. The extracted proteins (20 µl/5 µg protein) were loaded and subjected to 12.5% sodium dodecyl sulfate-polyacrylamide gel electrophoresis (SDS-PAGE) for 30 min at 100 V and then 90 min at 150 V and subsequently transferred onto nitrocellulose membranes using Trans-Blot Turbo Transfer System (Bio-Rad, Hercules, CA, USA). The membranes were blocked for 1 h at room temperature in blocking buffer consisting of 5% BSA in PBS and 0.1% Tween. This was followed by a 4×5 min washing procedure in Wash Buffer (PBS + 0.1% Tween). Blots were incubated with primary antibodies (Santa Cruz Biotechnology) for 2 h at 4°C followed by incubation with secondary antibodies conjugated to horseradish peroxidase (Santa Cruz Biotechnology) for 2 h at 4°C. Blots were visualized with enhanced chemiluminescence (Amersham Biosciences, Piscataway, NJ, USA).

Results

Sequencing of tryptic peptides

Using LC-MS/MS, 622 of the tryptic peptides detected with CE-MS could be identified. The mass of sequenced peptides ranged between 804 and 3953 Da. These tryptic peptides corresponded to 97 different proteins in vitreous humor (**Table 2**).

Definition of AMD-specific proteins

Figure 1 is a descriptive presentation of the study setup and findings. All samples were analysed by CE-MS. Next, for statistical analysis, CE-MS detected tryptic peptides were matched to the sequences identified by LC-MS/MS. 622 of the CE-MS detected peptides could be identified by their amino acid sequence. These peptides were combined to 97 proteins as described [29] and this protein distribution was statistically analysed. 19 proteins displayed significant differential abundance in vitreous (**Table 3**). All proteins with a p-value of <0.05 were found to be upregulated in the AMD population.

Validation using Western blot analysis

Western blot analysis was used to verify the findings in **table 3** on 5 randomly selected proteins for which antibodies were readily available, using a new but small set of AMD and control samples (n = 4/group). Four out of the 5 proteins analyzed did not display a significant variation, but the fold increases for apolipoprotein A1 and transthyretin suggested increased expression in vitreous of AMD patients similarly to what observed in the intial CE-MS experiments. The absence of significance is most probably due to the small patient population used for in the validation experiments (**Table 4** and **Figure 2**). However, we validated increased alpha-1-antitrypsin abundance in vitreous of AMD patients (p = 0.02).

Gene enrichment and pathway analysis

The 19 proteins with differential abundance in AMD were analyzed for their biological process, molecular function and the cellular component. GO cluster analysis using ClueGO showed that these proteins are primarily involved in biological (ion) transport and secretion/exocytosis (platelet degranulation (ALB, TF, APOA1, SERPINA1, HRG, FGA) and fatty acid binding (RBP3, ALB, PTGDS)), protease inhibitor activity (ITIH1, SERPINA1, SERPINC1, HRG), and processes involving hydrogen peroxide (GPX3, HP). These molecules consist mostly of secreted proteins (**Figure 3A**).

A global interactome analysis of the statistically relevant proteins using the Michigan Molecular Interactor plug-in, which mines data from protein-protein, protein-gene, gene-gene, molecule-pathway, and molecule-keyword associations, resulted in a densely interconnected network (**Figure 3B**). This expanded network of 54 proteins, including molecules known to be associated with the query molecules, consists of an immunoglobulin-cluster and complement activation (containing IGHA1, IGKC, IGHG1, IGLC2, AHSG, ITIH1, and FGA), suggesting inflammation and acute phase response processes being activated in the original source tissue, and processes including cell adhesion, lipid metabolism (RBP3, PTGDS), transport (APOA1, ALB, TTR, TF), anti-apoptosis (GPX3), and proteolysis (proteases (HP) and protease inhibitors (HRG, SERPINA1 and SERPINC1)). Inter-linking molecules suggest an involvement of transcriptional elements such as ONECUT and HNF1A/4A, which are modulators of genes involved in lipid metabolic processes, blood coagulation

Analysis of the condensed network of direct interactions between the 19 proteins shows the immunoglobulin cluster containing IGLC2, IGKC, and IGHG1, binary interactions between ALB and ITIH1, and between HRG and FGA, as well as a binary cluster of APOA1 and TTR. The latter suggests that the peroxisome proliferator-activated receptor (PPAR) signaling pathway is perturbed in AMD through an association with TTR and fibrils (**Figure 3B**).

Data mining of the Online Mendelian Inheritance in Man database by associated disease clustering showed one relevant cluster consisting of APOA1 (cataract formation) and TTR (fibril formation (neurodegenerative)). The same components were also found by association using a similar approach to mine the disease entries in the KEGG database, where the common denominator was found as familial amyloidosis (KEGG disease entry H00845), linking it to the complement and coagulation cascade (**Figure 3C**). Furthermore KEGG pathway analysis also suggested an involvement of arachidonic acid metabolism to be modulated in AMD. Literature mining also revealed a semantic link between cataract formation and up-regulated levels of GPX3 in the lens.

Table 2. Proteins in vitreous humor detected by CE-MS and identified by LC-MS/MS analysis.

Protein	UniProt*	Peptide number**	Coverage*** (%)	Peptide number control****	Peptide number case****
Actin, aortic smooth muscle	P62736	1	3	0	1
Afamin	P43652	2	4	2	2
Angiotensinogen	P01019	1	2	1	1
Alpha-1-acid glycoprotein 1	P02763	7	27	7	7
Alpha-1-acid glycoprotein 2	P19652	3	15	3	3
Alpha-1-antitrypsin	P01009	20	52	20	20
Alpha-1B-glycoprotein	P04217	5	11	5	5
Alpha-2-HS-glycoprotein	P02765	4	16	4	4
Alpha-2-macroglobulin	P01023	13	10	9	13
Alpha-crystallin B chain	P02511	2	14	1	2
Amyloid-like protein 2	Q06481	2	4	2	2
Antithrombin-III	P01008	10	23	4	10
Apolipoprotein E	P02649	13	43	12	13
Apolipoprotein A-I	P02647	18	63	16	18
Apolipoprotein A-II	P02652	4	41	4	4
Apolipoprotein A-IV	P06727	10	30	5	10
Beta-2-microglobulin	P61769	2	17	1	2
Beta-crystallin B2	P43320	11	50	11	11
Chitinase-3-like protein 1	P36222	1	3	1	1
Ceruloplasmin	P00450	14	20	12	14
Clusterin	P10909	12	31	11	12
Collagen alpha-1(I) chain	P02452	2	1	2	2
Collagen alpha-1(II) chain	P02458	38	27	35	36
Collagen alpha-1(III) chain	P02461	1	2	1	1
Collagen alpha-1(IX) chain	P20849	5	9	4	5
Collagen alpha-1(V) chain	P20908	4	1	2	3
Collagen alpha-1(XI) chain	P12107	5	3	5	5
Collagen alpha-1(XII) chain	Q99715	1	1	1	1
Collagen alpha-1(XXII) chain	Q8NFW1	1	1	1	1
Collagen alpha-1(XXIII) chain	Q86Y22	1	3	1	1
Collagen alpha-1(XXVIII) chain	Q2UY09	1	2	0	1
Collagen alpha-2(IX) chain	Q14055	4	6	4	4
Collagen alpha-2(XI) chain	P13942	1	2	1	1
Collagen alpha-3(IX) chain	Q14050	5	7	5	5
Complement C3	P01024	32	23	23	32
Complement C4-B	P0C0L5	11	7	10	11
Complement factor B	P00751	5	7	3	5
Alpha-crystallin A chain	P02489	3	19	3	3
Cathepsin D	P07339	3	11	3	3
Cystatin-C	P01034	2	18	2	2
Dermcidin	P81605	3	23	1	3
Dickkopf-related protein 3	Q9UBP4	6	22	6	6
Double-strand break repair protein MRE11A	P49959	1	2	0	1
Fibrinogen alpha chain	P02671	4	6	3	4
Fibrinogen beta chain	P02675	1	3	1	1
Gelsolin	P06396	1	2	0	1
Glutathione peroxidase 3	P22352	4	23	3	4
Haptoglobin	P00738	13	24	10	13

Table 2. Cont.

Protein	UniProt*	Peptide number**	Coverage*** (%)	Peptide number control****	Peptide number case****
Hemoglobin subunit beta	P68871	1	9	1	1
Hemopexin	P02790	14	29	12	14
Heparin cofactor 2	P05546	1	2	1	1
Histidine-rich glycoprotein	P04196	2	4	2	2
Ig alpha-1 chain C region	P01876	3	8	3	3
Ig alpha-2 chain C region	P01877	4	8	2	2
Ig gamma-1 chain C region	P01857	11	37	11	11
Ig gamma-3 chain C region	P01860	4	12	3	4
Ig heavy chain V-III region GAL	P01781	2	8	1	2
Ig heavy chain V-III region TRO	P01762	1	6	1	1
Ig kappa chain V-I region EU	P01598	1	17	1	1
Ig kappa chain V-III region SIE	P01620	1	17	1	1
Ig kappa chain C region	P01834	5	80	4	5
Ig lambda-2 chain C regions	P0CG05	3	42	3	3
IgGFc-binding protein	Q9Y6R7	4	1	4	4
Immunoglobulin lambda-like polypeptide 5	B9A064	1	9	1	1
Inter-alpha-trypsin inhibitor heavy chain H1	P19827	3	4	3	3
Inter-alpha-trypsin inhibitor heavy chain H4	Q14624	2	2	1	2
Keratin, type I cytoskeletal 10	P13645	18	34	16	18
Keratin, type I cytoskeletal 14	P02533	3	7	2	3
Keratin, type I cytoskeletal 9	P35527	7	14	6	7
Keratin, type II cytoskeletal 1	P04264	18	26	17	17
Keratin, type II cytoskeletal 2 epidermal	P35908	3	6	3	3
Keratin, type II cytoskeletal 5	P13647	1	2	1	1
Keratin, type II cytoskeletal 6A	P02538	1	2	1	1
Keratin, type II cytoskeletal 6B	P04259	2	4	2	2
Kininogen-1	P01042	4	5	2	4
Leucine-rich alpha-2-glycoprotein	P02750	1	3	0	1
Opticin	Q9UBM4	3	9	2	3
Osteopontin	P10451	7	34	7	7
Pigment epithelium-derived factor	P36955	12	31	11	12
Plasminogen	P00747	1	1	0	1
Prostaglandin-H2 D-isomerase	P41222	4	21	4	4
Protein Jade-2	Q9NQC1	1	1	1	1
Protein S100-A7	P31151	1	11	1	1
Protein S100-A9	P06702	2	18	2	2
Prothrombin	P00734	2	4	2	2
Retinol-binding protein 3	P10745	15	18	14	15
Ig kappa chain V-III region VG	P04433	2	23	1	2
Plasma protease C1 inhibitor	P05155	5	12	5	5
Serotransferrin	P02787	44	55	43	44
Alpha-1-antichymotrypsin	P01011	15	36	12	15
Serum albumin	P02768	55	75	51	55
Complement C4-A	P0C0L4	1	1	1	1
Titin	Q8WZ42	1	0	0	1
Transthyretin	P02766	7	63	7	7
Vitamin D-binding protein	P02774	5	9	4	5
Vitronectin	P04004	3	9	2	3

Table 2. Cont.

Protein	UniProt*	Peptide number**	Coverage*** (%)	Peptide number control****	Peptide number case****
Zinc-alpha-2-glycoprotein	P25311	2	9	2	2

*Uniprot accession numbers that can be found on www.uniprot.org; ** Number of peptides observed by CE-MS analysis and sequenced by LC-MS/MS for each identified protein; *** Percentage of peptide coverage of the protein sequence; ****, Number of peptides observed by CE-MS and sequenced by LC-MS/MS in controls or cases.

Discussion

The aim of this pilot study was to test the hypothesis that specific proteins in vitreous samples of patients with exudative AMD are significantly associated with the disease and may lead to a better understanding of the pathophysiology of the disease.

We initially set out to analyze native peptides from vitreous (top-down strategy) with a mass of up to 20 kDa using CE-MS analysis. However, this strategy did not result in satisfactory data, as a result of high variability (Koss M et al. Proteomics in AMD; Poster 2927/A327 at the annual meeting of the Assiciation for Research in Vision and Ophtalmology (AVRO), Ft.Lauderdale, USA in 2012). A possible reason for the large variation between the measurements could be the presence of hyaluronic acid. Because of the highly negative charge of its monomers, hyaluronic acid reacts with positively charged proteins such as albumin to build up polyelectrolyte complexes displaying low solubility [32]. Since the top-down strategy failed to give the expected results, we changed the strategy and in the current study employed trypsin digested samples for proteome analysis of vitreous.

Using this bottom-up approach we could successfully analyze the vitreous humor samples with CE-MS, including fragments of proteins with molecular masses above 20 kDa. We identified a total of 97 proteins, 19 of those significantly increased in AMD patients. We selected 5 random proteins among these 19 for validation by Western blot analysis. One protein (alpha-1-antitrypsin) reached statistical significance while two others (transthyretin and apoliprotein A1) displayed a non-significant but increased abundance in AMD. The latter is most likely due to the low number of patients in the validation set (n = 4/group) and needs validation.

Most of the upregulated proteins in AMD patients are plasma proteins. Our findings therefore may, to some degree, be

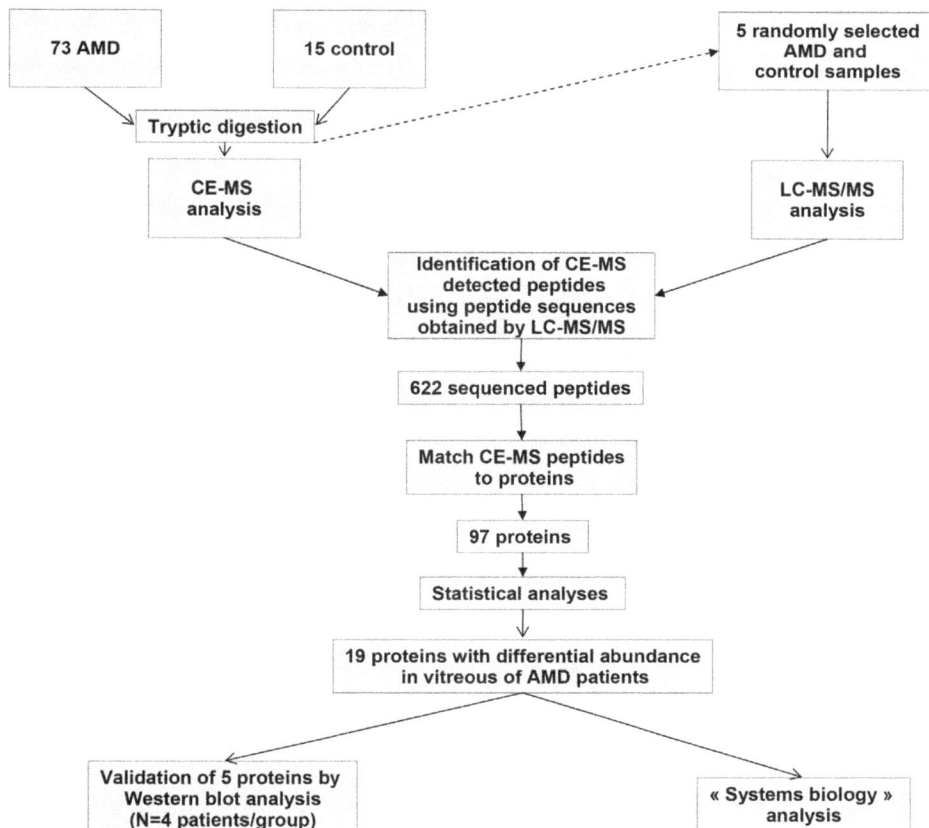

Figure 1. Study design and results.

Table 3. List of significant regulated proteins.

Protein name	Fold change AMD/control	Standard deviation for fold change	p-value	adjusted p-value
Ig kappa/lambda chain C region	6.56	13.27	**4.58E-06**	**4.45E-04**
Serum albumin	1.91	1.49	**3.27E-05**	**1.58E-03**
Ig gamma-1 chain C region	3.14	4.70	**6.54E-05**	**1.74E-03**
Antithrombin-III	5.50	12.29	**7.16E-05**	**1.74E-03**
Ig lambda-2 chain C regions	4.55	9.94	**1.30E-04**	**2.51E-03**
Serotransferrin*	1.74	1.52	**3.99E-04**	**6.45E-03**
Afamin	3.28	6.58	**1.93E-03**	**2.16E-02**
Histidine-rich glycoprotein	10.85	49.18	**2.45E-03**	**2.16E-02**
Retinol-binding protein 3*	2.78	5.51	**2.72E-03**	**2.20E-02**
Apolipoprotein A-I*	2.30	3.62	**3.88E-03**	**2.73E-02**
Fibrinogen alpha chain	2.90	6.30	**3.94E-03**	**2.73E-02**
Ig alpha-1 chain C region	35.34	147.90	**2.32E-03**	**2.16E-02**
Alpha-2-HS-glycoprotein	2.58	5.78	**1.55E-02**	8.70E-02
Transthyretin*	1.74	2.11	**1.61E-02**	8.70E-02
Prostaglandin-H2 D-isomerase	1.65	1.97	**2.33E-02**	1.19E-01
Haptoglobin	2.92	7.89	**3.34E-02**	1.46E-01
Glutathione peroxidase 3	4.26	18.42	**3.79E-02**	1.51E-01
Alpha-1-antitrypsin*	1.73	2.56	**4.04E-02**	1.51E-01
Inter-alpha-trypsin inhibitor heavy chain H1	2.34	5.84	**4.82E-02**	1.67E-01

Legend: Fold change AMD/control. Fold increase or decrease observed in AMD patients compared to controls; p-value - unadjusted p-value (Wilcoxon signed-rank test); adjusted p-value - p-value corrected for multiple testing (Benjamini and Hochberg method) and expressed in bold, when statistically significant. * proteins selected for western-blot analysis.

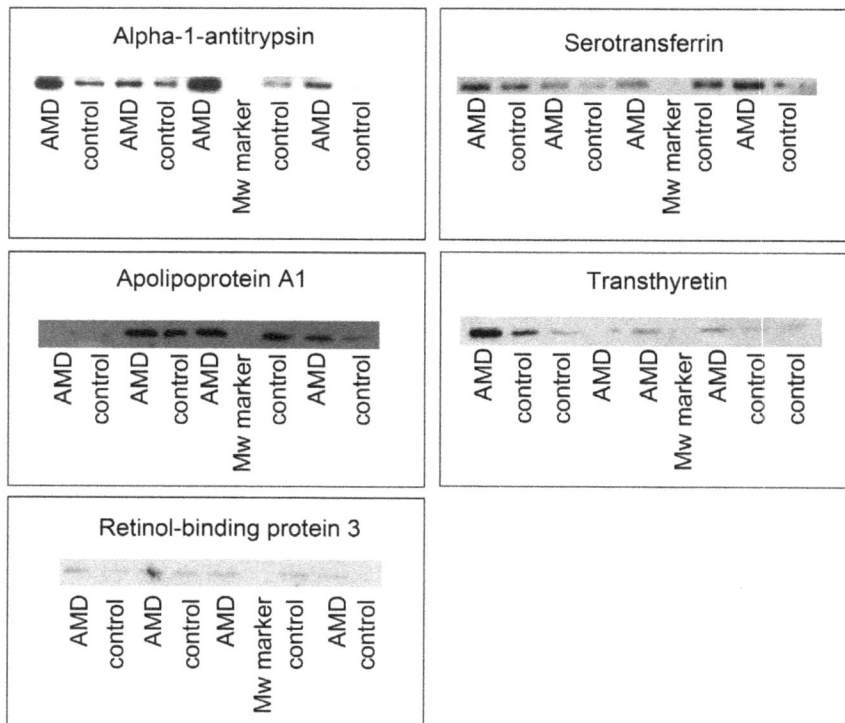

Figure 2. Western blot validation of candidate markers for AMD. Representative Western blots of analysis of expression of selected vitreous proteins.

Table 4. Western blot analysis of selected proteins found upregulated in vitreous of AMD patients by CE-MS.

Protein name	AMD	control	P-value	Fold change	Regulation in proteome analysis
Alpha-1-Antitrypsin	1618.6±610.2	689.5±174.1	p = 0.02	2.35	↑
Apolipoprotein A 1	1925.3±404.9	1463.2±360.4	p = 0.27	1.32	↑
Retinol-binding protein 3	471.9±50.9	427.3±53.9	p = 0.28	1.10	↑
Serotransferrin	1224.1±231.1	1059.6±247.7	p = 0.25	1.16	↑
Transthyretin	1169.8±592.8	747.4±143.8	p = 0.15	1.57	↑

Presented are the results of intensities measured by enhanced chemiluminescence from SDS PAGE Western blots. The mean ± standard deviation from 4 independent undiluted vitreous AMD and 4 independent undiluted vitreous control samples is given. P-values were calculated by the Mann-Whitney statistical test.

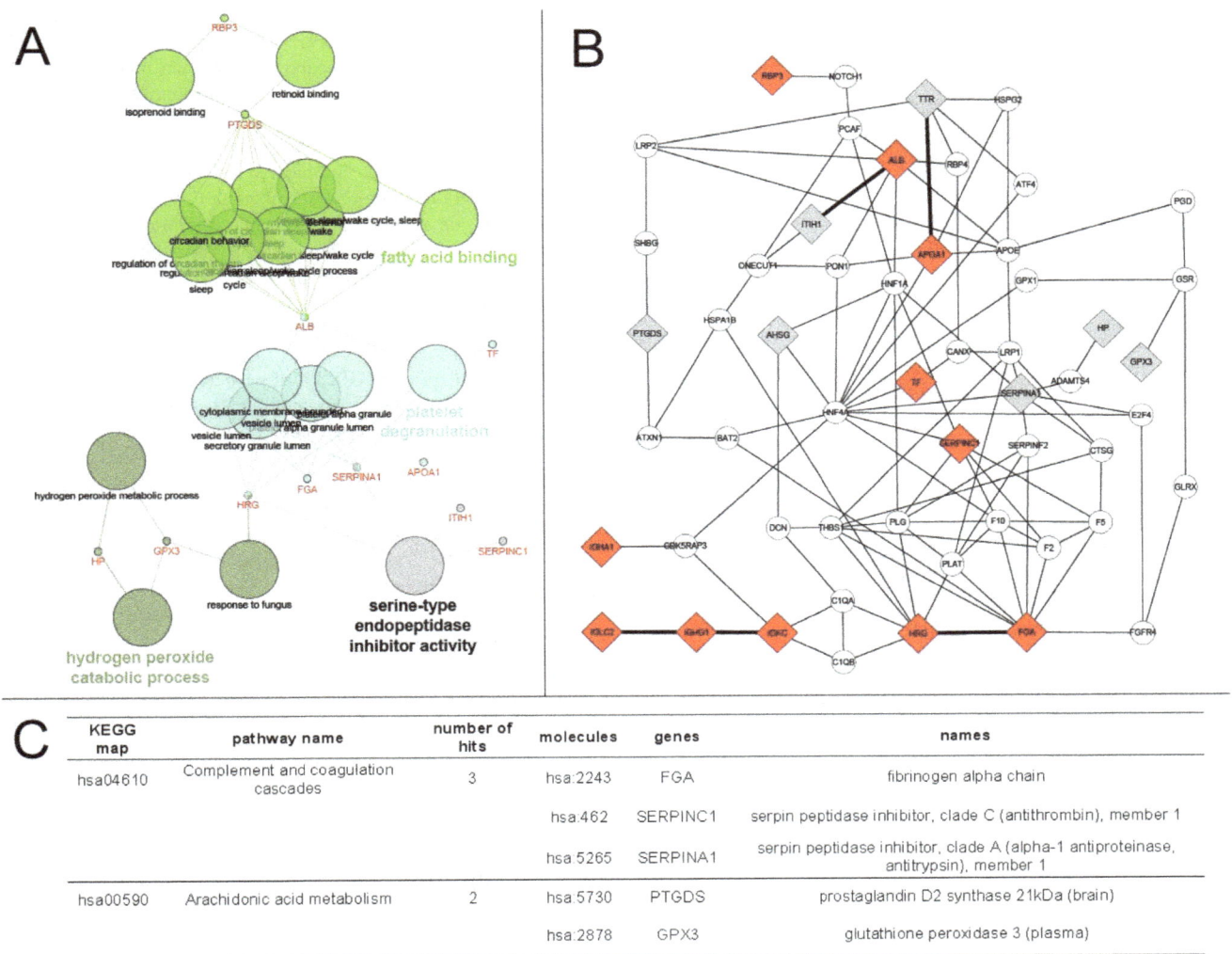

Figure 3. Bioinformatic analysis of identified biomarkers. A. Gene ontology analysis shows proteins involved in fatty acid binding. platelet degranulation. serine protease inhibitor activity and hydrogen peroxide catabolic processes. **B** Interaction network of identified biomarker candidates involving 18 out of the 19 proteins. Proteins involved in inflammation. acute phase response (including cellular adhesion). signaling via lipid-mediated pathways (including transport) and activation of proteolytic cascades. as well as transcriptional activity are indicated. Red diamonds indicate proteins which are significant after correction for multiple testing. and grey ones are the remainder of the query set. Circles indicate gap-fillers which were added to connect proteins via protein-protein interactions. Direct association between the significant biomarker set are indicated by a bold line. and relate to immune response (immunoglobulin cluster). protease inhibitor activity. and an activation of the peroxisome proliferator-activated receptor signaling pathway/CDC42 signal transduction pathway. as suggested through APOA1 interactions. **C.** Kyoto encyclopedia of genes and genomes pathway analysis. Statistically relevant biomarker proteins were mapped onto KEGG pathway maps and showed an involvement of fibril formation and inhibition of fibrinolysis in the coagulation cascade and association with arachidonic acid metabolism.

representative of the leakage from exudative CNV into the vitreous. Even though plasma proteins might not be responsible for the onset of an exudative AMD, their levels might be of diagnostic value for disease and represent the underlying pathophysiology of AMD. Future studies are important to identify which of these proteins are secreted from the abnormal CNV tissue.

The observed upregulation of a number of proteins in vitreous of AMD patients provides further insights into the pathophysiology of AMD:

Transport proteins

Upregulation of transport proteins such as albumin and serotransferrin in AMD patients confirms the findings from previous proteome analyses of anterior chamber fluids [5]. In addition, further transport proteins like transthyretin and apolipoprotein A-I were identified. All of these were upregulated in the AMD group; all are biologically essential for cell homeostasis (albumin) and are carriers of hormones like retinol (albumin and transthyretin) or ions (serotransferrin). It is important to stress that in chronic diseases, such as AMD, the dysregulation of these abundant proteins has been observed in serum [33,34], but so far, their presence in the vitreous has received little attention.

Inflammatory proteins

Immunoglobulin heavy chains and alpha-1-antitrypsin were upregulated in the AMD samples. Alpha-1-antitrypsin is an acute phase protein member of the serpin family that inhibits a wide variety of proteases and thereby protects tissues from enzymes of inflammatory cells, especially neutrophil elastase. This is the first time that increased alpha-1-antitrypsin abundance in vitreous has been associated with AMD. However alpha-1-antitrypsin does not seem specific for AMD since upregulation of alpha-1-antitrypsin was observed in both aqueous and blood of patients with glaucoma [35].

Mediators of coagulation

Fibrinogen is essential during coagulation as it is converted by plasmin into fibrin, and higher blood levels have been associated with AMD [36]. Rheopheresis, a treatment that microfilters fibrinogen from the blood of AMD patients, seems to be protective in the progression of AMD, however, the approach is controversial discussed [37]. In this study, we demonstrated that the fibrinogen alpha chain was upregulated in the AMD group. As for alpha-1-antitrypsin, although potentially involved in the pathophysiology of AMD, increased fibrinogen abundance in vitreous is not specific for AMD since such upregulation was previously also observed in vitreous samples of patients with diabetic retinopathy [38].

Specific ocular markers

In humans, prostaglandin H2-D isomerase catalyzes the conversion of prostaglandin H2 to prostaglandin D2, which functions as a neuromodulator and as a trophic factor in the central nervous system for fatty acid biosynthesis. Its occurrence has been described in proliferative diabetic retinopathy; but it has not been previously associated with AMD [39]. The inter-photoreceptor retinol binding protein is a large glycoprotein, located in the extracellular matrix between the RPE and the photoreceptors. It is known to bind retinoids and is thought to transport retinoids between the retinal pigment epithelium and the photoreceptors. Its potential involvement in AMD has recently been described based on the analysis of blood samples [40,41] and is confirmed by our findings.

The bioinformatic analyses using GO-term clustering, physical interaction module assembly, and KEGG pathway data mapping have shown an involvement of pathways consisting of fatty acid binding and transport, exocytosis, and protease inhibitory activity, which are also partially involved in Complement and coagulation cascades. However, more importantly is the notion that there appears to be an up-regulation of hydrogen peroxide catabolic processes, which suggest that oxidative stress is exerted in AMD.

The interactome analysis surprisingly showed a highly interconnected network of 18 of the 19 relevant proteins, where only 36 additional molecules were needed to generate a specific molecular network, suggesting that the up-regulated proteins form a potential dysregulated functional cluster encompassing immune responses and complement cascade proteins, protease cascades maybe linked to the membrane attack complex or possibly to counteract the enzymatic effect of up-regulated molecules such as GPX3, RBP3 and PTGDS, or as modulators of gene activation cascades. This unusually high selectivity also argues against the hypothesis that these proteins are observed in increased abundance merely as a result of unspecific leakage of plasma proteins, and support the hypothesis that the increase in these proteins is specifically linked to AMD.

The up-regulation of GPX3 is of particular interest, since it was shown previously that cataracts contain elevated levels of oxidants such as dehydroascorbic acid (DHA), indicative of oxidative stress, linked to a potentially elevated level of extracellular glutathione peroxidase GPX3 [42]. Mechanistically, the over-expression is suggested to result in accumulated oxidants in the glutathion/ascorbic acid homeostasis cycle, leading to DHA-polymer crystal formation in the lens as well as potentially toxic breakdown products of ascorbic acid.

In conclusion, in this study we could demonstrate that a bottom-up approach combining CE-MS (for protein selection) and LC-MS/MS (for protein identification) led to the identification of 19 candidate proteins in undiluted vitreous of AMD patients. Even with the limitations of this study (e.g., demographic matching, demand for validation in a larger cohort with a wider set of clinical parameters), the novel information gained from this study of a high number of undiluted vitreous samples provides additional insight into the pathophysiology of wet AMD.

Author Contributions

Conceived and designed the experiments: MK HM JH JPS FK. Performed the experiments: MK JH NN HM HH JJ FK. Analyzed the data: MK JH RR WM JK JS WM JPS. Contributed reagents/materials/analysis tools: JH MK NN JS KK HM JJ. Wrote the paper: MK JH TB JS MP JPS.

References

1. Evans JR (2001) Risk factors for age-related macular degeneration. Progress in retinal and eye research 20: 227–253.

2. Stefansson E (2009) Physiology of vitreous surgery. Graefes Arch Clin Exp Ophthalmol 247: 147–163.

3. Adamis AP, Shima DT, Tolentino MJ, Gragoudas ES, Ferrara N, et al. (1996) Inhibition of vascular endothelial growth factor prevents retinal ischemia-associated iris neovascularization in a nonhuman primate. Archives of ophthalmology 114: 66–71.

4. Funk M, Karl D, Georgopoulos M, Benesch T, Sacu S, et al. (2009) Neovascular age-related macular degeneration: intraocular cytokines and growth factors and the influence of therapy with ranibizumab. Ophthalmology 116: 2393–2399.

5. Grossniklaus HE, Green WR (2004) Choroidal neovascularization. Am J Ophthalmol 137: 496–503.

6. Kim TW, Kang JW, Ahn J, Lee EK, Cho KC, et al. (2012) Proteomic analysis of the aqueous humor in age-related macular degeneration (AMD) patients. Journal of proteome research 11: 4034–4043.

7. Ecker SM, Hines JC, Pfahler SM, Glaser BM (2011) Aqueous cytokine and growth factor levels do not reliably reflect those levels found in the vitreous. Molecular vision 17: 2856–2863.

8. Stefansson E, Loftsson T (2006) The Stokes-Einstein equation and the physiological effects of vitreous surgery. Acta Ophthalmol Scand 84: 718–719.

9. Angi M, Kalirai H, Coupland SE, Damato BE, Semeraro F, et al. (2012) Proteomic analyses of the vitreous humour. Mediators of inflammation 2012: 148039.

10. Ecker SM, Pfahler SM, Hines JC, Lovelace AS, Glaser BM (2012) Sequential in-office vitreous aspirates demonstrate vitreous matrix metalloproteinase 9 levels correlate with the amount of subretinal fluid in eyes with wet age-related macular degeneration. Molecular vision 18: 1658–1667.

11. Grus FH, Joachim SC, Pfeiffer N (2007) Proteomics in ocular fluids. Proteomics Clinical applications 1: 876–888.

12. Noma H, Funatsu H, Yamasaki M, Tsukamoto H, Mimura T, et al. (2008) Aqueous humour levels of cytokines are correlated to vitreous levels and severity of macular oedema in branch retinal vein occlusion. Eye 22: 42–48.

13. Pfister M, Koch FH, Cinatl J, Rothweiler F, Schubert R, et al. (2012) [Cytokine determination from vitreous samples in retinal vascular diseases.]. Der Ophthalmologe: Zeitschrift der Deutschen Ophthalmologischen Gesellschaft.

14. Walia S, Clermont AC, Gao BB, Aiello LP, Feener EP (2010) Vitreous proteomics and diabetic retinopathy. Seminars in ophthalmology 25: 289–294.

15. Yamane K, Minamoto A, Yamashita H, Takamura H, Miyamoto-Myoken Y, et al. (2003) Proteome analysis of human vitreous proteins. Molecular & cellular proteomics: MCP 2: 1177–1187.

16. Bennett KL, Funk M, Tschernutter M, Breitwieser FP, Planyavsky M, et al. (2011) Proteomic analysis of human cataract aqueous humour: Comparison of one-dimensional gel LCMS with two-dimensional LCMS of unlabelled and iTRAQ(R)-labelled specimens. Journal of proteomics 74: 151–166.

17. Chowdhury UR, Jea SY, Oh DJ, Rhee DJ, Fautsch MP (2011) Expression profile of the matricellular protein osteopontin in primary open-angle glaucoma and the normal human eye. Investigative ophthalmology & visual science 52: 6443–6451.

18. Cryan LM, O'Brien C (2008) Proteomics as a research tool in clinical and experimental ophthalmology. Proteomics Clinical applications 2: 762–775.

19. Zurbig P, Renfrow MB, Schiffer E, Novak J, Walden M, et al. (2006) Biomarker discovery by CE-MS enables sequence analysis via MS/MS with platform-independent separation. Electrophoresis 27: 2111–2125.

20. Mischak H, Vlahou A, Ioannidis JP (2013) Technical aspects and inter-laboratory variability in native peptide profiling: the CE-MS experience. Clinical biochemistry 46: 432–443.

21. Mischak H, Julian BA, Novak J (2007) High-resolution proteome/peptidome analysis of peptides and low-molecular-weight proteins in urine. Proteomics Clinical applications 1: 792.

22. Koss MJ, Scholtz S, Haeussler-Sinangin Y, Singh P, Koch FH (2009) Combined Intravitreal Pharmacosurgery in Patients with Occult Choroidal Neovascularization Secondary to Wet Age-Related Macular Degeneration. Ophthalmologica 224: 72–78.

23. Mischak H, Schanstra JP (2011) CE-MS in biomarker discovery, validation, and clinical application. Proteomics Clinical applications 5: 9–23.

24. Augustin AJ, Puls S, Offermann I (2007) Triple therapy for choroidal neovascularization due to age-related macular degeneration: verteporfin PDT, bevacizumab, and dexamethasone. Retina 27: 133–140.

25. Koch FH, Koss MJ (2011) Microincision vitrectomy procedure using Intrector technology. Archives of ophthalmology 129: 1599–1604.

26. Spaide RF (2006) Rationale for combination therapies for choroidal neovascularization. Am J Ophthalmol 141: 149–156.

27. Theodorescu D, Wittke S, Ross MM, Walden M, Conaway M, et al. (2006) Discovery and validation of new protein biomarkers for urothelial cancer: a prospective analysis. The lancet oncology 7: 230–240.

28. Neuhoff N, Kaiser T, Wittke S, Krebs R, Pitt A, et al. (2004) Mass spectrometry for the detection of differentially expressed proteins: a comparison of surface-enhanced laser desorption/ionization and capillary electrophoresis/mass spectrometry. Rapid communications in mass spectrometry: RCM 18: 149–156.

29. Jantos-Siwy J, Schiffer E, Brand K, Schumann G, Rossing K, et al. (2009) Quantitative urinary proteome analysis for biomarker evaluation in chronic kidney disease. Journal of proteome research 8: 268–281.

30. Metzger J, Negm AA, Plentz RR, Weismuller TJ, Wedemeyer J, et al. (2013) Urine proteomic analysis differentiates cholangiocarcinoma from primary sclerosing cholangitis and other benign biliary disorders. Gut 62: 122–130.

31. Benjamini Y, Hochberg Y (1995) Controlling the false discovery rate: a practical and powerful approach to multiple testing. J Royal Stat Soc B (Methodological): 125–133.

32. Wohlrab W, Neubert RRH, Wohlraub J (2004) Hyaluronsaeure und Haut. Aachen: Shaker. 384 p.

33. Chowers I, Wong R, Dentchev T, Farkas RH, Iacovelli J, et al. (2006) The iron carrier transferrin is upregulated in retinas from patients with age-related macular degeneration. Investigative ophthalmology & visual science 47: 2135–2140.

34. Wysokinski D, Danisz K, Blasiak J, Dorecka M, Romaniuk D, et al. (2013) An association of transferrin gene polymorphism and serum transferrin levels with age-related macular degeneration. Experimental eye research 1: 14–23.

35. Boehm N, Wolters D, Thiel U, Lossbrand U, Wiegel N, et al. (2012) New insights into autoantibody profiles from immune privileged sites in the eye: a glaucoma study. Brain, behavior, and immunity 26: 96–102.

36. Klingel R, Fassbender C, Fischer I, Hattenbach L, Gumbel H, et al. (2002) Rheopheresis for age-related macular degeneration: a novel indication for therapeutic apheresis in ophthalmology. Therapeutic apheresis: official journal of the International Society for Apheresis and the Japanese Society for Apheresis 6: 271–281.

37. Klingel R, Fassbender C, Heibges A, Koch F, Nasemann J, et al. (2010) RheoNet registry analysis of rheopheresis for microcirculatory disorders with a focus on age-related macular degeneration. Therapeutic apheresis and dialysis: official peer-reviewed journal of the International Society for Apheresis, the Japanese Society for Apheresis, the Japanese Society for Dialysis Therapy 14: 276–286.

38. Garcia-Ramirez M, Canals F, Hernandez C, Colome N, Ferrer C, et al. (2007) Proteomic analysis of human vitreous fluid by fluorescence-based difference gel electrophoresis (DIGE): a new strategy for identifying potential candidates in the pathogenesis of proliferative diabetic retinopathy. Diabetologia 50: 1294–1303.

39. Kim SJ, Kim S, Park J, Lee HK, Park KS, et al. (2006) Differential expression of vitreous proteins in proliferative diabetic retinopathy. Current eye research 31: 231–240.

40. Morohoshi K, Ohbayashi M, Patel N, Chong V, Bird AC, et al. (2012) Identification of anti-retinal antibodies in patients with age-related macular degeneration. Experimental and molecular pathology 93: 193–199.

41. Morohoshi K, Patel N, Ohbayashi M, Chong V, Grossniklaus HE, et al. (2012) Serum autoantibody biomarkers for age-related macular degeneration and possible regulators of neovascularization. Experimental and molecular pathology 92: 64–73.

42. Kisic B, Miric D, Zoric L, Ilic A, Dragojevic I (2012) Antioxidant capacity of lenses with age-related cataract. Oxidative medicine and cellular longevity 2012: 467130.

21

Diabetes Mellitus and Risk of Age-Related Macular Degeneration: A Systematic Review and Meta-Analysis

Xue Chen[1,2], Shi Song Rong[2], Qihua Xu[1,3], Fang Yao Tang[2], Yuan Liu[1], Hong Gu[2,4], Pancy O. S. Tam[2], Li Jia Chen[2], Mårten E. Brelén[2], Chi Pui Pang[2]*, Chen Zhao[1]*

1 Department of Ophthalmology, The First Affiliated Hospital of Nanjing Medical University and State Key Laboratory of Reproductive Medicine, Nanjing Medical University, Nanjing, China, 2 Department of Ophthalmology & Visual Sciences, The Chinese University of Hong Kong, Hong Kong, China, 3 Department of Ophthalmology, The Affiliated Jiangyin Hospital of Southeast University Medical College, Jiangyin, China, 4 Department of Ophthalmology, Ningbo Medical Treatment Center Lihuili Hospital, Ningbo, China

Abstract

Age-related macular degeneration (AMD) is a major cause of severe vision loss in elderly people. Diabetes mellitus is a common endocrine disorder with serious consequences, and diabetic retinopathy (DR) is the main ophthalmic complication. DR and AMD are different diseases and we seek to explore the relationship between diabetes and AMD. MEDLINE, EMBASE, and the Cochrane Library were searched for potentially eligible studies. Studies based on longitudinal cohort, cross-sectional, and case-control associations, reporting evaluation data of diabetes as an independent factor for AMD were included. Reports of relative risks (RRs), hazard ratios (HRs), odds ratio (ORs), or evaluation data of diabetes as an independent factor for AMD were included. Review Manager and STATA were used for the meta-analysis. Twenty four articles involving 27 study populations were included for meta-analysis. In 7 cohort studies, diabetes was shown to be a risk factor for AMD (OR, 1.05; 95% CI, 1.00–1.14). Results of 9 cross-sectional studies revealed consistent association of diabetes with AMD (OR, 1.21; 95% CI, 1.00–1.45), especially for late AMD (OR, 1.48; 95% CI, 1.44–1.51). Similar association was also detected for AMD (OR, 1.29; 95% CI, 1.13–1.49) and late AMD (OR, 1.16; 95% CI, 1.11–1.21) in 11 case-control studies. The pooled ORs for risk of neovascular AMD (nAMD) were 1.10 (95% CI, 0.96–1.26), 1.48 (95% CI, 1.44–1.51), and 1.15 (95% CI, 1.11–1.21) from cohort, cross-sectional and case-control studies, respectively. No obvious divergence existed among different ethnic groups. Therefore, we find diabetes a risk factor for AMD, stronger for late AMD than earlier stages. However, most of the included studies only adjusted for age and sex; we thus cannot rule out confounding as a potential explanation for the association. More well-designed prospective cohort studies are still warranted to further examine the association.

Editor: Yuk Fai Leung, Purdue University, United States of America

Funding: This work was supported by National Key Basic Research Program of China (2013CB967500); National Natural Science Foundation of China (No. 81222009 and 81170856); Thousand Youth Talents Program of China (to C.Z.); Jiangsu Outstanding Young Investigator Program (BK2012046); Jiangsu Province's Key Provincial Talents Program (RC201149); Jiangsu Province's Scientific Research Innovation Program for Postgraduates (CXZZ13_0590 to X.C.); an Endowment Fund for the Lim Por-Yen Eye Genetics Research Centre; the General Research Fund from the Research Grants Council of Hong Kong (No. 473410); and A Project Funded by the Priority Academic Program Development of Jiangsu Higher Education Institutions (PAPD). The sponsor or funding organization had no role in the design or conduct of this research.

Competing Interests: The authors have declared that no competing interests exist.

* Email: dr.zhaochen@gmail.com (CZ); cppang@cuhk.edu.hk (CP)

Background

Age-related macular degeneration (AMD) has become a major cause of irreversible visual impairments in elderly people around the world, casting a heavy socio-economic burden on eye care [1,2,3]. AMD can be classified into the early and late stages. Patients with early AMD are usually asymptomatic, while severe vision loss frequently occurs in its late stage. Late AMD can be further categorized into two main subtypes: neovascular AMD (nAMD) and geographic atrophy (GA) [3]. The estimated prevalence is 6.8% for early AMD and 1.5% for late AMD in Caucasians over the age of 40 years [3]. It is estimated that 5% of early AMD patients will progress to late AMD over a 5-year period, increasing to nearly 15% over a 15-year period [4,5].

Similar prevalence has been identified in Asians but not in the black population [6,7].

The pathogenesis of AMD is complicated with multiple risk factors, including age, ocular dysfunctions, systemic diseases, diet, smoking, genetic, and environmental factors [8]. As a modifiable personal factor, whether diabetes play a role in the development and progression of AMD has been vigorously studied. While several reports presented positive correlations between diabetes and AMD [9,10,11,12,13,14], some other reports showed no such effect [15,16]. Even inversed relationship has been reported [17]. To gain a clear insight into the relationship between AMD and diabetes, we conducted a meta-analysis to assess whether diabetes is a risk factor for AMD.

Methods

Eligibility Criteria for Considering Studies for This Review

Included studies were: (1) studies evaluating diabetes as an individual risk factor for AMD; (2) prospective or retrospective cohort study, or study of cross-sectional or case-control design; (3) studies using predefined criteria and procedures for diabetes diagnosis and AMD grading; and (4) relative risks (RRs), hazard ratios (HRs), and odds ratio (ORs) have been reported, or data provided that enabled calculations of these outcomes. Case reports, reviews, abstracts, conference proceedings, editorials, reports with incomplete data, and non-English articles were excluded. For serial publications from the same research team using overlapped subjects, we included those: (1) with the latest follow-up information; and (2) providing adjusted RRs, HRs, or ORs with 95% CIs. To come up with a more precise insight into whether diabetes is an independent risk factor for AMD, only studies investigating diabetes as the main exposure, or provides adjusted RRs, HRs, or ORs with 95% CIs were included. This study was approved and reviewed by the institutional ethics committee of The First Affiliated Hospital of Nanjing Medical University and adhered to the tenets of the Declaration of Helsinki.

Search Methods for Identifying Studies

We searched MEDLINE, EMBASE, and the Cochrane Library for all relevant articles starting from year 1946 to March 18, 2014. We followed the Cochrane Handbook for Systematic Reviews of Interventions [18] and Meta-analysis of Observational Studies in Epidemiology (MOOSE) guideline [19] in designing and reporting the current study. Our search strategies were detailed in **Appendix S1**. No language filters was applied. Additional studies were identified from reference lists of the retrieved reports. Retrieved records and eligibility status were managed using EndNote X5 software (http://endnote.com/).

Study Selection

Two investigators (X.C. and S.S.R.) independently screened all retrieved citations based on title, abstract, and complete document if necessary. All relevant full-text articles were obtained and reviewed to determine the eligibility of each study. Disagreements were resolved via consensus with a senior reviewer (C.Z.).

Data Collection and Risk of Bias Assessment

The two reviewers (X.C. and S.S.R.) extracted outcomes from each study separately with a customized datasheet. Data obtained included: first author, year of publication, title of the study (if any), duration of the study, country or region, races, study design, sample size, estimated ORs, RRs, or HRs, adjusted factors in multiple regression analysis, and clinical examinations and diagnostic criteria for AMD and diabetes. We used the Newcastle Ottawa Scale (NOS, accessed via http://www.ncbi.nlm.nih.gov/books/NBK35156/) [20] and the criteria recommended by Agency for Healthcare Research and Quality (AHRQ, accessed via http://www.ncbi.nlm.nih.gov/books/NBK35156/) [21] to evaluate the risk of biases for prospective cohorts or case-control studies, and cross-sectional studies, respectively. All data from these two reviewers were compared. Agreement among the reviewers was sought after completion of grading.

Data Synthesis and Analysis

We assessed the association between diabetes and AMD by combining ORs from case-control and cross-sectional studies, and RRs or HRs from cohort studies. Heterogeneity between studies were tested by Cochran's Q statistic, and evaluated by the proportion of variation attributable to among-study heterogeneity, I^2. Heterogeneity among studies was considered no, low, moderate, and high when I^2 equals to 0% to 24%, 25% to 49%, 50% to 74%, and more than 75%, respectively. If p for Q< 0.1 or $I^2 > 50\%$, a random-effects model (the DerSimonian and Laird method) was used [22], otherwise we used a fixed-effects model(the Mantel-Haenszel method) [23]. Subgroup analysis was conducted by the study designs, AMD stages and clinical subtypes, and ethnic groups. The Asians were further divided into subgroups, including the East Asians (Japan, China, Taiwan, and Korea), Southeast Asians (Singapore), West Asians (Israel, Iran, and Turkey), and South Asians (Nepal, and India). As to the subgroup analysis concerning different AMD stages, we applied the widely accepted clinical classification system as described by the Age-Related Eye Disease Study Research Group [24,25]. Briefly, early AMD was defined by the appearance of drusen and pigmentary alterations within 2 disc diameters of the fovea. Late AMD was featured by the presence of large drusen (soft and/or indistinct) together with pigmentary abnormalities, or can be generally recognized as nAMD and/or GA. Moreover, sensitivity analysis was conducted to affirm the estimated association by removing studies with poor quality or prone to introducing biases. Publication bias and small-study effects were assessed with funnel plots [26] and Egger's test [27]. All analyses were conducted with Review Manager version 5.2 (Cochrane Collaboration, Oxford, UK; http://ims.cochrane.org/revman) and STATA software (version 12.0; StataCorp LP, College Station, TX). Alpha was set to 0.05 for two-sided test.

Results

Literature

A total of 3205 records were yielded from digital search and manual screen of reference list. Thirty-eight articles, published from 1986 to 2013, were included for the systematic review. Workflow of literature screen and review was shown in **Figure 1**. In addition, to provide a better understanding in diabetes as an independent risk factor for AMD, fourteen studies that presented diabetes as a covariate and provided ORs/RRs/HRs from baseline data without any adjustment were excluded, involving 12 cross-sectional [11,15,17,28,29,30,31,32,33,34,35,36] and 2 case-control studies [37,38]. The 24 articles included 1858350 participants in 27 independent study populations, comprising 7 cohort studies [39,40,41,42,43], 9 cross-sectional studies [9,14,16,44,45,46,47,48], and 11 case-control studies [12,13,36,49,50,51,52,53,54,55,56]. Among the 27 study populations, 10 were in Asia, 9 in North America (United States), 6 in Europe, 1 in Oceania (Australia), and 1 in South America (Barbados). Most studies used predefined criteria for AMD diagnosis and adopted standard grading system [57,58]. Samples sizes varied widely, from less than 50 to over 1.5 million (**Table 1**). Only two of the earliest studies, in 1986 [49] and 1998 [50], had sample sizes less than 100. Risk of bias assessments for cohort, cross-sectional, and case-control studies has been performed (**Tables S1–S3**). Tan et al [59] and Tomany et al [42] both involved the Blue Mountain Eye Study cohort, we included latter one in the analysis. The ORs/RRs/HRs with 95% CI and the corresponding adjusted variables for each study were listed in overall AMD, early AMD or late AMD (**Table 2**).

Meta-Analysis

The effects of diabetes on the risk of AMD in all these studies were found to be essentially consistent (**Figure 2 and Table 3**).

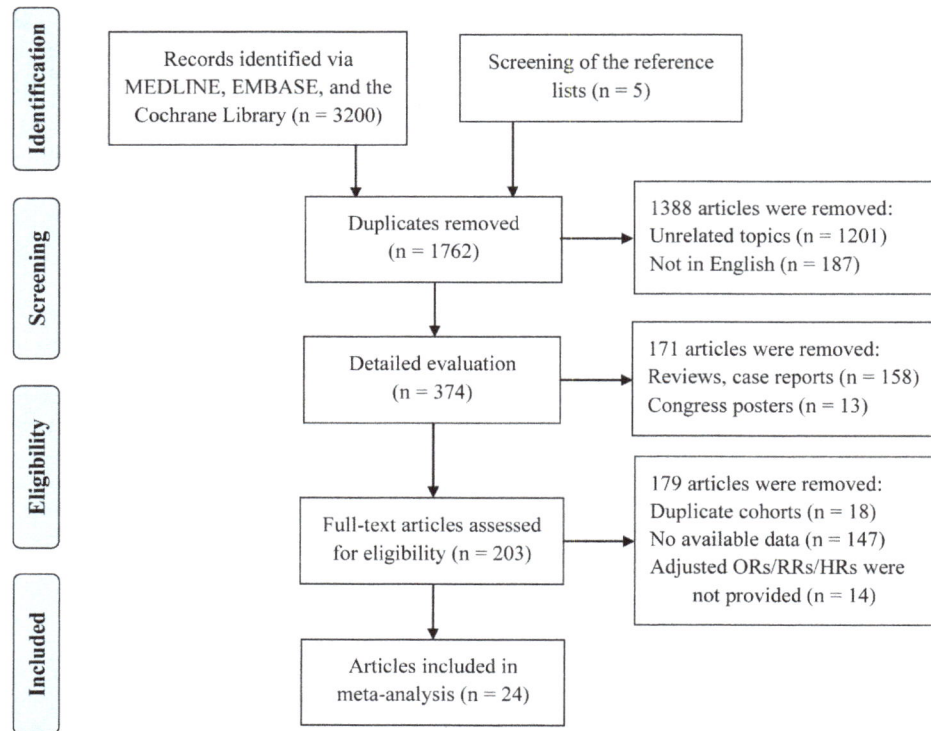

Figure 1. Flow chart depicting the screening process for inclusion in the meta-analysis.

According to the meta-analysis of 7 cohort studies, diabetes was associated with AMD (OR, 1.05; 95% CI, 1.00–1.11). Subgroup analysis based on AMD stages revealed diabetes as a marginal risk factor for late AMD (OR, 1.05; 95% CI, 0.99–1.10), but not for its early form (OR, 0.83; 95% CI, 0.60–1.15). Subgroup analysis by AMD subtypes showed that the pooled OR of diabetes for risk of nAMD was 1.10 (95% CI, 0.96–1.26), for risk of GA was 1.63 (95% CI, 0.51–5.21). In the 9 cross-sectional study populations, diabetes was found increasing AMD risk (OR, 1.21; 95% CI, 1.00–1.45). Subgroup analysis confirmed this effect for late AMD (OR, 1.48; 95% CI, 1.44–1.51), and nAMD (OR, 1.48; 95% CI, 1.44–1.51), but not for early AMD (OR, 0.99; 95% CI, 0.88–1.12) or GA (OR, 1.58; 95% CI, 0.63–3.99). The results kept consistent in the analysis of 11 case-control studies. The pooled OR of diabetes for AMD was 1.29 (95% CI, 1.13–1.49). The pooled OR was 1.16 (95% CI, 1.11–1.21) for late AMD, and 1.15 (95% CI, 1.11–1.21) for nAMD. To reduce the methodological heterogeneity and the potential effect led by other risk factors, we also conducted meta-analysis solely using multivariate-adjusted outcomes. Only 3 cohort studies and 2 cross-sectional were included, and the results varied from the overall data, which was probably due to the limited number of included studies. However, in both groups, diabetes was found as a marginal risk factor for nAMD in cross-sectional studies (OR, 1.04; 95% CI, 0.99–1.10) and a solid risk factor for late AMD in cohort studies (OR, 1.81; 95% CI, 1.10–2.98). No association between diabetes and early AMD or GA was found in both groups (**Table 4**). Subgroup analyses by ethnic group were further performed. The associations of diabetes and overall and early AMD were similar between the Asian and Caucasian populations (**Table 5**), while associations between diabetes and all subtypes of late AMD were suggested only for the Caucasian group, but not for the overall Asian population or any of its subgroups. No indication of any obvious asymmetry was observed according to the shapes of Begg's funnel plots and Egger's test for all groups as detailed in **Tables 3–5**.

Risk of Bias Assessment and Sensitivity Analysis

In our assessment, we found most studies have a robust design and reported in a clear manner, thus have lower risks in introducing bias (**Tables S1–S3**). However, we did identify one cross-sectional study which had relative higher risk to introduce biases when used to evaluate risk-modifying effect of diabetes for AMD [14] (**Tables S2**), thus were subjected to sensitivity analysis. In sensitivity analysis, we sequentially omitted one study at a time and removed studies of higher risk of introducing bias to affirm the associations. Sensitivity analyses revealed that the study conducted by Alexander et al [52] contributed to the heterogeneity in the subgroup analysis of case-control studies, but did not alter the results in each subgroup. When removing the studies conducted by Shalev et al and Hahn et al in the subgroup analysis of cohort studies, respectively, although the *p* values for diabetes and AMD became insignificant, the direction of ORs was kept and associations of marginal significance were revealed (removing study by Shalev et al: OR, 1.04; 95% CI, 0.99–1.10; Hahn et al: OR, 1.12; 95% CI, 0.98–1.29). Similar findings were revealed by subgroup analyses involving cross-sectional and case-control studies. In the analysis of cross-sectional studies, the removal of studies by Vaičaitienė et al [14], Duan et al [45], Xu et al [16], and Choi et al [47] would also lead to borderline results (removing study by Vaičaitienė et al: OR, 1.10; 95% CI, 0.98–1.23; Duan et al: OR, 1.30; 95% CI, 0.97–1.73; Xu et al: OR, 1.21; 95% CI, 0.99–1.47; Choi et al: OR, 1.16; 95% CI, 0.96–1.41). In addition, in the subgroup analysis of case-control studies, an association of borderline significance between diabetes and AMD (OR, 1.23;

Table 1. Characteristics of Included Cohorts.

First Author (Publication Year)	Study	Study Period	Region	Race	Sample Size	Diagnostic Criteria AMD	Diagnostic Criteria Diabetes
Cohort Studies (Prospective & Retrospective)							
Tomany et al (2004)	BDES	1993–1995	US	Caucasian	3562	I & W	PGL & S
	BMES	1997–1999	Australia	Caucasian	2330	I & W	PGL & S
	RS	1997–1999	Netherlands	Caucasian	3631	I & W	PGL & S
Leske et al (2006)	BISED II	1987–1992	Barbados	Mixed	2793	W	M & S
Yasuda et al (2009)	Hisayama Study	2007	Japan	East Asian	1401	I & W	M & PGL
Shalev et al (2011)	MHS	1998–2007	Israel	West Asian	108973	ICD9	M
Hahn et al (2013)	NA	1995–2005	US	Caucasian	16510	ICD9	ICD9
Cross-sectional Studies							
Delcourt et al (2001)	POLA	1995–1997	France	Caucasian	2584	I & W	Interview
Vaičaitienė et al (2003)	NA	1995–1997	Lithuania	Caucasian	438	NA	NA
Duan et al (2007)	NA	2000–2001	US	Caucasian	1519086	ICD9	ICD9
Klein et al (2007)	WHISE	1993–2002	US	Caucasian	4288	W	M
Topouzis et al (2009)	EUREYE study	2000–2003	Europe†	Caucasian	4722	I	S
Xu et al (2009)	Beijing Eye Study	2006	China	East Asian	2960	W	PGL & S
Choi et al (2011)	NA	2006–2008	Korea	East Asian	3008	W	M & PGL
Cheung et al (2013)	SIES	2007–2009	Singapore	Southeast Asian	3337	W	PGL & S
	CIEMS	2006–2008	India	South Asian	3422	W	PGL & S
Case-control Studies							
Blumenkranz et al (1986)	NA	NA	US	Caucasian	49	NA	PGL
Ross et al (1998)	NA	NA	US	Caucasian	94	Detailed in paper.	M
McGwin et al (2003)	NA	1997–2001	US	Caucasian	6050	ICD9	ICD9
Moeini et al (2005)	NA	2001	Iran	West Asian	130	NA	PGL
Alexander et al (2007)	NA	2001–2003	US	Caucasian	62179	ICD9	ICD9
Kim et al (2008)	NA	1998–2003	US	Caucasian	204	W	Questionnaire
Lin et al (2008)	NA	2002–2006	Taiwan	East Asian	280	I	NA
Nitsch et al (2008)	GPRD	1987–2002	UK	Caucasian	104176	Readcodes & OXMIS	Readcodes & OXMIS
Cackett et al (2011)	NA	2007–2008	Singapore	Southeast Asian	1617	W	Questionnaire
Sogut et al (2013)	NA	NA	Turkey	West Asian	280	W	ADA
Torre et al (2013)	NA	2011	Italy	Caucasian	246	NA	Questionnaire

† Europe: Estonia, France, Greece, Italy, Norway, Spain, UK;

Abbreviation: BDES: Beaver Dam Eye Study; BMES: Blue Mountains Eye Study; RS: Rotterdam Study; BISED II: Barbados Incidence Study of Eye Diseases; MHS: Maccabi Healthcare Services; NA: not available; POLA: Pathologies Oculaires Liées àl'Age Study; WHISE: Women's Health Initiative Sight Examination; SIES: Singapore Indian Eye Study; CIEMS: Central India Eye and Medical Study; GPRD: General Practice Research Database; AMD: Age Related Macular Degeneration; &: represents a combination of two diagnostic methods; I: International Classification and Grading System for AMD; W: Wisconsin Age-Related Maculopathy Grading System; ICD9: International Classification of Diseases with Clinical Modifications, Ninth Revision; PGL: Plasma Glucose Level; S: Self-reported diabetic history or medications; M: Medical recorded diabetic history or medications; ADA: American Diabetes Association diagnostic criteria.

Table 2. Detailed Analytical Information for Included Cohorts.

First Author(Publication Year)	OR/RR/HR$^\Lambda$ [95% CI]					Adjusted Variables
	Early AMD	Late AMD			AMD	
		nAMD	GA	Total		
Cohort Studies (Prospective & Retrospective)						
Tomany (2004)	—	0.67 [0.24, 1.86]	2.05 [0.84, 4.99]	1.21 [0.62, 2.36]	1.21 [0.62, 2.36]	Age, Sex
BDES	—	—	0.79 [0.10, 6.31]	—	—	Age, Sex
BMES	—	—	8.31 [2.34, 29.50]	—	—	Age, Sex
RS	—	—	0.79 [0.10, 6.19]	—	—	Age, Sex
Leske (2006)	0.88 [0.60, 1.30]	—	—	2.70 [1.00, 7.30]	1.02 [0.71, 1.47]	Age
Yasuda (2009)	0.70 [0.37, 1.31]	—	—	0.69 [0.16, 2.95]	0.69 [0.39, 1.24]	Multiple Factors#
Shalev (2011)	—	—	—	—	1.18 [1.01, 1.38]	Mutually adjusted
Hahn (2013)	—	1.11 [0.97, 1.27]	1.03 [0.97, 1.09]	1.04 [0.99, 1.10]	1.04 [0.99, 1.10]	Multiple Factors*
Cross-sectional Studies						
Delcourt (2001)	—	—	—	1.22 [0.45, 3.29]	1.22 [0.45, 3.29]	Age, Sex
Vaičaitienė (2003)	—	—	—	—	4.61 [2.45, 8.67]	Age, Sex
Duan (2007)	—	1.48 [1.44, 1.51]	—	1.48 [1.44, 1.51]	1.18 [1.16, 1.19]	Age, Sex, Race
Klein (2007)	0.87 [0.67, 1.12]	2.49 [1.17, 5.31]	2.28 [0.63, 8.28]	2.43 [1.26, 4.70]	0.94 [0.74, 1.20]	Age
Topouzis (2009)	0.98 [0.83, 1.17]	1.81 [1.10, 2.98]	1.06 [0.28, 4.04]	1.38 [0.90, 2.12]	1.01 [0.85, 1.19]	Multiple Factors‡
Xu (2009)	1.30 [0.69, 2.43]	—	—	1.13 [0.14, 9.40]	1.28 [0.70, 2.34]	None
Choi (2011)	1.87 [1.07, 3.28]	—	—	—	1.87 [1.07, 3.28]	Multiple Factors†
Cheung (2013)						
SIES	0.93 [0.68, 1.28]	—	—	—	0.93 [0.68, 1.28]	Age, Sex
CIEMS	1.14 [0.47, 2.77]	—	—	—	1.14 [0.47, 2.77]	Age, Sex
Case-control Studies						
Blumenkranz (1986)	—	—	—	0.53 [0.06, 4.71]	0.53 [0.06, 4.71]	Use siblings
Ross (1998)	—	—	—	—	1.09 [0.21, 5.59]	Age
McGwin Jr (2003)	—	—	—	—	1.78 [1.43, 2.20]	Age, Sex
Moeini (2005)	—	—	—	—	1.29 [0.52, 3.21]	Age, Sex, Risk factors
Alexander (2007)	—	1.16 [1.11, 1.21]	—	1.16 [1.11, 1.21]	1.16 [1.11, 1.21]	Age, Sex, Race, Database length
Kim (2008)	—	0.61 [0.27, 1.39]	—	0.61 [0.27, 1.39]	0.61 [0.27, 1.39]	Use siblings
Lin (2008)	—	1.20 [0.44, 3.26]	0.97 [0.36, 2.63]	1.07 [0.45, 2.57]	1.07 [0.45, 2.57]	Age, Sex
Nitsch (2008)	—	—	—	—	1.36 [1.29, 1.43]	Age, Sex, Practice, Consultation Rate
Cackett (2011)	—	0.92 [0.50, 1.70]	—	0.92 [0.50, 1.70]	0.92 [0.50, 1.70]	Age, Sex
Sogut (2013)	—	—	—	1.68 [0.76, 3.69]	1.68 [0.76, 3.69]	Age, Sex
Torre (2013)	—	—	—	—	0.80 [0.08, 8.07]	Age, Sex, Smoking

$^\Lambda$OR is for cross-sectional and case-control studies, RR is for prospective cohort studies, HR is for retrospective cohort studies;
#Age, Sex, Smoking habit, White blood cells;
*Age, Sex, Race, History of hypertension, Atherosclerosis, Stroke, Coronary heart disease, Hyperlipidemia, Charlson index;
‡Age, Sex, Smoking, Education, BMI, Alcohol consumption, Cardiovascular disease, Aspirin use, Systolic blood pressure, Alpha-tocopherol ratio, Vitamin C, Lutein;
†Age, Sex, Current smoking, Obesity, Hypertension.
Abbreviations: OR: odds ratio; RR: risk ratio; HR: hazard ratio; CI: confidence interval; AMD: Age-related macular degeneration; nAMD: neovascular AMD; GA: geographic atrophy; WBC: white blood cell.

95% CI, 0.97–1.56) was presented if the study by Nitsch et al [13] was excluded.

Discussion

Diabetes is a major concern in ophthalmic care. Whether it contributes to the prevalence of AMD has been an unsolved dilemma targeted by a large number of studies. However, obvious inconsistencies between studies, including a few large cohorts, suggest the necessity to conduct an exhaustive review and quantitative analysis on all the evidences to determine its effect. In the present systemic review and meta-analysis, we reviewed 3205 published reports and completed analysis on 1858350 participants of 27 study populations from 24 original studies. We found that diabetes is a risk factor for AMD, especially for nAMD. To our knowledge, this is the first meta-analysis addressing the

A

Study or Subgroup	Weight	Risk Ratio IV, Fixed, 95% CI
Tomany 2004	0.5%	1.21 [0.62, 2.36]
Leske 2006	1.8%	1.02 [0.71, 1.47]
Yasuda 2009	0.7%	0.70 [0.39, 1.24]
Shalev 2011	9.9%	1.18 [1.01, 1.38]
Hahn 2013	87.0%	1.04 [0.99, 1.10]
Total (95% CI)	100.0%	1.05 [1.00, 1.11]

Heterogeneity: Chi² = 4.34, df = 4 (P = 0.36); I² = 8%
Test for overall effect: Z = 2.09 (P = 0.04)

Risk Ratio IV, Fixed, 95% CI — 0.5 0.7 1 1.5 2 — Non-Diabetes Diabetes

B

Study or Subgroup	Weight	Odds Ratio IV, Random, 95% CI
Delcourt 2001	3.0%	1.22 [0.45, 3.29]
Vaičaitienė 2003	6.3%	4.61 [2.45, 8.67]
Duan 2007	23.2%	1.17 [1.16, 1.19]
Klein 2007	16.6%	0.94 [0.74, 1.20]
Topouzis 2009	19.4%	1.01 [0.85, 1.19]
Xu 2009	6.7%	1.28 [0.70, 2.34]
Choi 2011	7.4%	1.87 [1.07, 3.28]
Cheung 2013 SIES	13.8%	0.93 [0.68, 1.28]
Cheung 2013 CIEMS	3.7%	1.14 [0.47, 2.77]
Total (95% CI)	100.0%	1.21 [1.00, 1.45]

Heterogeneity: Tau² = 0.04; Chi² = 29.20, df = 8 (P = 0.0003); I² = 73%
Test for overall effect: Z = 2.00 (P = 0.05)

Odds Ratio IV, Random, 95% CI — 0.5 0.7 1 1.5 2 — Non-Diabetes Diabetes

C

Study or Subgroup	Weight	Odds Ratio IV, Random, 95% CI
Blumenkranz 1986	0.4%	0.53 [0.06, 4.71]
Ross 1998	0.7%	1.09 [0.21, 5.59]
McGwin Jr 2003	18.7%	1.78 [1.43, 2.20]
Moeini 2005	2.1%	1.29 [0.52, 3.21]
Alexander 2007	33.0%	1.16 [1.11, 1.21]
Kim 2008	2.6%	0.61 [0.27, 1.39]
Lin 2008	2.3%	1.08 [0.45, 2.57]
Nitsch 2008	32.5%	1.36 [1.29, 1.43]
Cackett 2011	4.4%	0.92 [0.50, 1.70]
Torre 2013	0.4%	0.80 [0.08, 8.07]
Sogut 2013	2.8%	1.67 [0.76, 3.69]
Total (95% CI)	100.0%	1.29 [1.13, 1.49]

Heterogeneity: Tau² = 0.01; Chi² = 37.39, df = 10 (P < 0.0001); I² = 73%
Test for overall effect: Z = 3.67 (P = 0.0002)

Odds Ratio IV, Random, 95% CI — 0.05 0.2 1 5 20 — Non-Diabetes Diabetes

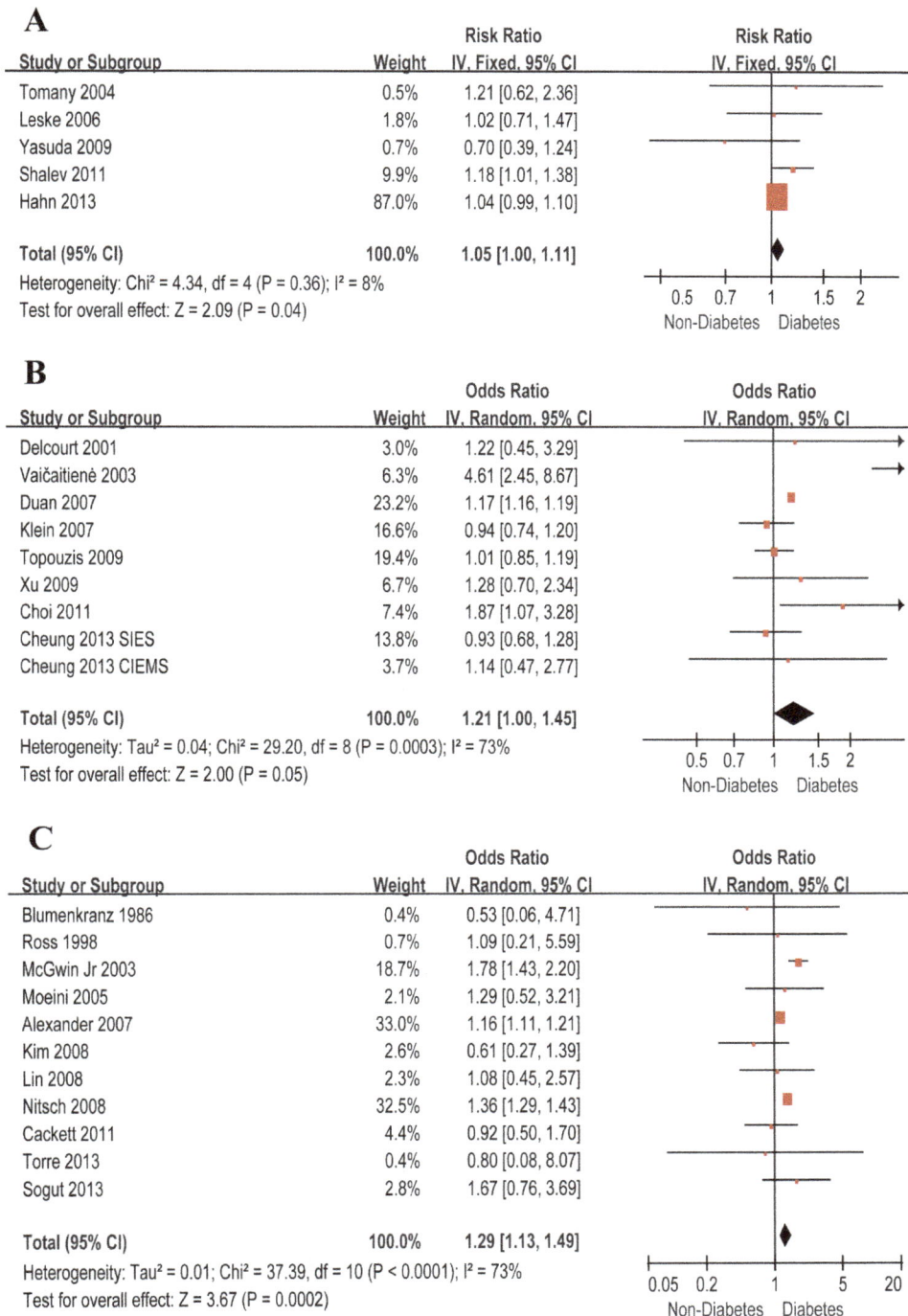

Figure 2. Effects of diabetes on AMD risks. Graphs showing the effects of diabetes on the risk of Age-related Macular Degenerations in longitudinal cohort studies (A), cross-sectional studies (B), and case-control studies (C). IV: inverse variance, CI: confidence interval.

topic for AMD and all its subtypes, and by using data from a comprehensive collection of prospective and retrospective cohort, cross-sectional, and case-control studies.

Clinically, AMD can be classified based on drusen features and retinal pigment epithelial abnormalities, we found most included studies follow the Wisconsin Age-related Maculopathy Grading Scheme, according to 4 levels: level 1 (no AMD), level 2 and 3 (early AMD), and level 4 (late AMD) [57,60]. The contribution of

diabetes to early AMD is inconsistent in studies. Diabetic patients have increased occurrence of early AMD in a cross-sectional study of a Korean cohort of 3008 adults [47]. No similar association has been observed in other studies. An inverse relationship is observed in the Age-Related Eye Disease Study (AREDS) [17]. In the Beaver Dam Eye Study (BDES), diabetes was found to be a protective factor for incident reticular drusen based on a 15-year cumulative incidence [61]. In this meta-analysis, no clear

Table 3. Analysis of Diabetes as a Risk Factor for AMD in Different AMD Types.

Study Design	No. of Cohorts	Sample Size	Overall Effect			Heterogeneity		Egger's Test
			OR/RR* [95% CI]	Z score	p value	I² (%)	Q (p)	
Cohort Studies								
AMD	7	139200	1.05 [1.00, 1.11]	2.09	0.037	8	0.361	0.961
Early AMD	2	4194	0.83 [0.60, 1.15]	1.12	0.261	0	0.529	NA
Late AMD	6	30227	1.05 [0.99, 1.10]	1.70	0.088	25	0.260	0.504
nAMD	4	26033	1.10 [0.96, 1.26]	1.40	0.160	0	0.335	NA
GA	4	26033	1.63 [0.51, 5.21]†	0.83	0.407	72	0.014	0.523
Cross-sectional Studies								
AMD	9	1543845	1.21 [1.00, 1.45]†	2.00	0.045	73	0.000	0.813
Early AMD	6	21737	0.99 [0.88, 1.12]	0.15	0.883	28	0.224	0.205
Late AMD	5	1533640	1.48 [1.44, 1.51]	32.20	0.000	0	0.642	0.774
nAMD	3	1528096	1.48 [1.44, 1.51]	32.23	0.000	20	0.287	0.154
GA	2	9010	1.58 [0.63, 3.99]	0.97	0.333	0	0.419	NA
Case-control Studies								
AMD	11	175305	1.29 [1.13, 1.49]†	3.67	0.000	73	0.000	0.976
Late AMD	6	64609	1.16 [1.11, 1.21]	6.65	0.000	0	0.520	0.334
nAMD	4	62179	1.15 [1.11, 1.21]	6.55	0.000	0	0.416	0.257
GA	1	280	0.97 [0.36, 2.63]	0.06	0.954	NA	NA	NA

* OR is for cross-sectional and case-control studies, RR is for cohort studies.
† Studies using random effect model.
Abbreviations: OR: odds ratio; RR: risk ratio; CI: confidence interval; AMD: age related macular degeneration; nAMD: neovascular AMD; GA: geographic atrophy; NA: not available.

Table 4. Analysis of Diabetes as a Risk Factor for AMD in Different AMD Types with Multivariate-adjusted ORs/RRs/HRs.

Study Design	No. of Cohorts	Sample Size	Overall Effect				Heterogeneity		Egger's Test
			OR/RR* [95% CI]	Z score	p value		I² (%)	Q (p)	
Cohort Studies									
AMD	3	126884	1.07 [0.93, 1.22]†	0.96	0.339		52	0.125	0.904
Early AMD	1	1401	0.70 [0.37, 1.31]	1.12	0.262		NA	NA	NA
Late AMD	2	17911	1.04 [0.99, 1.10]	1.56	0.118		0	0.574	NA
nAMD	1	16510	1.11 [0.97, 1.27]	1.52	0.129		NA	NA	NA
GA	1	16510	1.03 [0.97, 1.09]	0.94	0.349		NA	NA	NA
Cross-sectional Studies									
AMD	2	7730	1.29 [0.71, 2.35]†	0.85	0.397		77	0.038	NA
Early AMD	2	7730	1.28 [0.69, 2.39]†	0.78	0.640		78	0.031	NA
Late AMD	1	4722	1.38 [0.90, 2.12]	1.46	0.145		NA	NA	NA
nAMD	1	4722	1.81 [1.10, 2.98]	2.34	0.020		NA	NA	NA
GA	1	4722	1.06 [0.28, 4.04]	0.09	0.928		NA	NA	NA

* OR is for cross-sectional and case-control studies, RR is for cohort studies.
† Studies using random effect model.
Abbreviations: OR: odds ratio; RR: risk ratio; CI: confidence interval; AMD: age related macular degeneration; nAMD: neovascular AMD; GA: geographic atrophy; NA: not available.

Table 5. Analysis of Diabetes as a Risk Factor for AMD in Different Ethnic Groups.

Ethnic Group	No. of cohorts	Sample Size	Overall Effect OR/RR* [95% CI]	Z score	p value	Heterogeneity I² (%)	Heterogeneity Q (p)	Egger's Test
AMD								
Caucasian	16	1730149	1.20 [1.12, 1.29]†	4.86	0.000	84	0.000	0.733
Asian	10	125408	1.14 [1.01, 1.29]	2.11	0.035	2	0.423	0.978
East Asian	4	7649	1.18 [0.86, 1.61]	1.03	0.301	49	0.115	0.856
West Asian	3	109383	1.20 [1.03, 1.39]	2.35	0.019	0	0.688	0.385
Southeast Asian	2	4954	0.93 [0.70, 1.23]	0.50	0.616	0	0.973	NA
South Asian	1	3422	1.14 [0.47, 2.77]	0.29	0.771	NA	NA	NA
Total	27	1858350	1.18 [1.11, 1.26]†	5.11	0.000	74	0.000	0.909
Early AMD								
Caucasian	2	9010	0.95 [0.82, 1.09]	0.77	0.442	0	0.422	NA
Asian	5	14128	1.06 [0.85, 1.34]	0.54	0.588	40	0.152	0.626
East Asian	3	7369	1.21 [0.68, 2.14]†	0.65	0.517	62	0.070	0.385
Southeast Asian	1	3337	0.93 [0.68, 1.28]	0.43	0.667	NA	NA	NA
South Asian	1	3422	1.14 [0.47, 2.77]	0.29	0.771	NA	NA	NA
Total	8	25931	0.97 [0.86, 1.09]	0.53	0.595	16	0.303	0.478
Late AMD								
Caucasian	11	1619145	1.25 [1.05, 1.49]†	2.50	0.013	96	0.000	0.479
Asian	5	6538	1.09 [0.73, 1.63]	0.44	0.663	0	0.770	0.882
East Asian	3	4641	0.97 [0.48, 1.97]	0.07	0.941	0	0.865	0.800
Southeast Asian	1	1617	0.92 [0.50, 1.70]	0.26	0.795	NA	NA	NA
West Asian	1	280	1.68 [0.76, 3.69]	1.28	0.200	NA	NA	NA
Total	17	1628476	1.25 [1.07, 1.46]†	2.74	0.006	92	0.000	0.454
Neovascular AMD								
Caucasian	9	1616512	1.29 [1.09, 1.54]†	2.92	0.003	94	<0.001	0.524
Asian	2	1897	0.99 [0.59, 1.67]	0.04	0.970	0	0.662	NA
East Asian	1	280	1.20 [0.44, 3.26]	0.35	0.724	NA	NA	NA
Southeast Asian	1	1617	0.92 [0.50, 1.70]	0.26	0.795	NA	NA	NA
Total	11	1618409	1.27 [1.07, 1.50]†	2.81	0.005	93	<0.001	0.429
Geographic Atrophy								
Caucasian	6	24408	1.97 [1.07, 3.64]	2.17	0.030	35	0.172	0.178
Asian	1	280	0.97 [0.36, 2.63]	0.06	0.954	NA	NA	NA
East Asian	1	280	0.97 [0.36, 2.63]	0.06	0.954	NA	NA	NA
Total	7	24688	1.62 [0.96, 2.74]	1.82	0.069	34	0.166	0.687

* OR is for cross-sectional and case-control studies, RR is for prospective cohort studies.
† Studies using random effect model.
Abbreviations: OR: odds ratio; RR: relative risk; CI: confidence interval; AMD: age related macular degeneration.

association was detected between diabetes and early AMD based on 16 relevant cohorts.

The associations of diabetes with late AMD are also inconsistent among previous reports. According to analysis from 5 cross-sectional and 6 case-control studies, diabetes is significantly correlated with late AMD, especially with nAMD, but not for GA. Temporal relationships revealed by 7 cohort studies further supports diabetes as a potential risk factor for late AMD, only for nAMD but not for GA. However, an association between diabetes and GA was identified in Caucasians. Also, the Blue Mountains Eye Study (BMES) has revealed diabetes as a predictor of incident GA, but not incident nAMD. This is consistent with a cross-sectional baseline report [62,63], to 5-year [42] and 10-year [59] incident reports, providing evidence for a diabetes and GA association.

In the current meta-analysis, we found no obvious ethnic divergence regarding the association between the diabetes and risk of overall AMD and its early form. The results obtained from different Asian groups are consistent in all types of AMD. However, the association between diabetes and late AMD in the Caucasian population differs from that in the Asian population, which is probably due to the large variation of genetic factors among different ethnic groups [64], and the differences in dietary habits and lifestyles.

The biological interplay between diabetes and AMD is complicated and has not been fully elucidated. First, diabetic conditions may lead to the accumulation of the highly stable advanced glycation end products (AGEs) in multiple tissues, including the retinal pigment epithelium (RPE) cell layers and photoreceptors [51,65]. These AGEs would first contribute to the modification of molecules, leading to the activation of NFκB, NFκB nuclear translocation, and up-regulation in the expression of the receptor for AGEs (RAGE) [66]. Further, the up-regulated RAGE, which usually localized to the neuroglia in the inner retina [67], would integrate with AGE, thus leading to high levels of the nondegradable aggregates AGE-RAGE ligands in retina [65]. Therefore, accumulated AGEs would reduce the dosage dependent RAGE-mediated activation of RPE/photoreceptor cells [68]. AGEs and RAGE were found in the RPE or both RPE and photoreceptors in the maculas of human donor retina from patients with AMD, but not in normal eyes [66,68], indicating that AGE deposition and RAGE up-regulation in diabetic conditions are implicated in the pathogenesis of AMD.

Second, hyperglycemia and dyslipidemia in diabetic patients will disturb homeostasis of the retina by inducing inflammatory responses in tissue cells, including oxidative stress [69]. Significantly elevated oxidative stress markers and total oxidative stress (TOS), as well as decreased total anti-oxidant capacity (TAC), are found in the serum of AMD patients when compared with age-matched controls free of AMD [70,71]. Meanwhile, anti-oxidants and omega-3 fatty acids have been shown to help with the preservation of RPE health and prevent retinal degeneration in animal models [72,73]. Therefore, oxidative stress is recognized as one of the principle pathogenic elements in AMD [74]. Oxidative stress may further activate NF-κB regulated inflammatory genes and lead to inflammation, which would in turn generate reactive oxygen species and aggregate oxidative stress. Inflammation disrupts the NF-κB, JUN N-terminal kinase (JNK), and the NADPH oxidase pathways, consequently dysregulations of many inflammatory cytokines and chemokines, involving the tumor necrosis factor (TNF), interleukin-6 (IL-6), IL-1β, C-reactive protein (CRP), CC-chemokine ligand 2 (CCL2), and adipokines [75]. These inflammatory activations would lead to the dysfunction and even death of the RPE/photoreceptor cells [69]. Thus,

oxidative stress and inflammations in the retina are pre-requites for development of AMD [74].

Meanwhile, diabetic microangiopathy shares common pathogenic pathways with AMD. Hyperglycemia and dyslipidemia in diabetic patients will lead to multiple microvascular complications, including diabetic retinopathy (DR). AMD and DR share some common features in pathogenesis and treatment. In a longitudinal study over 10 years, individuals with DR, including both the nonproliferative and proliferative form, were at higher risk for nAMD when compared to diabetic patients without DR or normal controls [39]. Vascular endothelial growth factor (VEGF) seems to play an important role in both DR and AMD, and anti-VEGF treatment are useful for both [76,77]. Apolipoproteins are also involved. Lower apoAI and higher apoB and apoB/AI levels, biomarkers for diabetic retinopathy [78], are involved in the pathogenesis of cardiovascular diseases [79], which is a risk factor for AMD [8,59]. Meanwhile, mitochondrial dysfunctions have been reported to contribute to metabolic disorders as well as AMD [74,80,81]. All these suggested that hyperglycemia probably affects the function and structure of the retinal pigment epithelium, Bruch membrane, and the choroidal circulation [47], thus increase the risk of AMD. Our study indicates a potential relationship between diabetes and late AMD, but further evidences from more epidemiological and biological investigations are required.

To enhance the reliability of our results, we adopted quality assessment tools recommended by the AHRQ and NOS for observational studies. Only studies discussing diabetes as the main exposure or providing adjusted ORs/HRs/RRs were included in the present meta-analysis for a more precise association of diabetes as a relatively independent risk factor for AMD. In addition, for studies reporting duplicated cohorts, only those with the latest follow-up information or provides better adjusted results were included. Subgroup analysis was performed to affirm the association and to explorer the sources of the heterogeneity. Meanwhile, our study entailed some limitations. Data obtained from prospective cohort studies would be more convincing. But the number of prospective cohort studies was quite limited. Retrospective cohort, cross-sectional, and case-control studies were also included in the present study, which may partly help to reflect the association between diabetes and AMD. However, these studies have limitation. Retrospective cohort studies use healthcare databases and have inherent methodological limitations, which may obscure the association between diabetes and AMD [82]. Cross-sectional does not establish temporality and case-control studies may introduce selection bias and established temporality [82]. Early AMD can be further classified into more specific categories. Herein, we could only judge the relationship between diabetes and early AMD. Other than diabetic status, plenty of other risk factors have been suggested for AMD. Although we have tried to narrow down the influence of other risk factors by selecting studies with adjusted data, some included studies only reported data adjusted for age and sex, and the number of studies providing multivariate-adjusted data was quite limited. With the limited information provided by each individual study, therefore, this present meta-analysis only deals with the relationship between diabetic disease status and risk of AMD, but not the specific type of diabetes, the disease course, and blood glucose levels.

In conclusion, results of this meta-analysis indicate diabetes as a potential risk factor for AMD, especially for its late form. No clear association between diabetes and early AMD is identified. More longitudinal studies are needed to ascertain the association between diabetes and AMD. And biological studies involving the inflammatory pathways might help understand the molecular basis behind this association.

Author Contributions

Conceived and designed the experiments: CP CZ. Performed the experiments: XC SR. Analyzed the data: XC SR QX FT YL HG. Contributed reagents/materials/analysis tools: PT LC MB. Wrote the paper: XC SR CP CZ.

References

1. Bressler NM (2004) Age-related macular degeneration is the leading cause of blindness. JAMA 291: 1900–1901.
2. Jager RD, Mieler WF, Miller JW (2008) Age-related macular degeneration. N Engl J Med 358: 2606–2617.
3. Lim LS, Mitchell P, Seddon JM, Holz FG, Wong TY (2012) Age-related macular degeneration. Lancet 379: 1728–1738.
4. Cheung N, Shankar A, Klein R, Folsom AR, Couper DJ, et al. (2007) Age-related macular degeneration and cancer mortality in the atherosclerosis risk in communities study. Arch Ophthalmol 125: 1241–1247.
5. Mitchell P, Wang JJ, Foran S, Smith W (2002) Five-year incidence of age-related maculopathy lesions: the Blue Mountains Eye Study. Ophthalmology 109: 1092–1097.
6. Kawasaki R, Yasuda M, Song SJ, Chen SJ, Jonas JB, et al. (2010) The prevalence of age-related macular degeneration in Asians: a systematic review and meta-analysis. Ophthalmology 117: 921–927.
7. Friedman DS, Katz J, Bressler NM, Rahmani B, Tielsch JM (1999) Racial differences in the prevalence of age-related macular degeneration: the Baltimore Eye Survey. Ophthalmology 106: 1049–1055.
8. Chakravarthy U, Wong TY, Fletcher A, Piault E, Evans C, et al. (2010) Clinical risk factors for age-related macular degeneration: a systematic review and meta-analysis. BMC Ophthalmol 10: 31.
9. Topouzis F, Anastasopoulos E, Augood C, Bentham GC, Chakravarthy U, et al. (2009) Association of diabetes with age-related macular degeneration in the EUREYE study. Br J Ophthalmol 93: 1037–1041.
10. Borger PH, van Leeuwen R, Hulsman CA, Wolfs RC, van der Kuip DA, et al. (2003) Is there a direct association between age-related eye diseases and mortality? The Rotterdam Study. Ophthalmology 110: 1292–1296.
11. Karesvuo P, Gursoy UK, Pussinen PJ, Suominen AL, Huumonen S, et al. (2013) Alveolar bone loss associated with age-related macular degeneration in males. J Periodontol 84: 58–67.
12. McGwin G Jr, Owsley C, Curcio CA, Crain RJ (2003) The association between statin use and age related maculopathy. Br J Ophthalmol 87: 1121–1125.
13. Nitsch D, Douglas I, Smeeth L, Fletcher A (2008) Age-related macular degeneration and complement activation-related diseases: a population-based case-control study. Ophthalmology 115: 1904–1910.
14. Vaicaitiene R, Luksiene DK, Paunksnis A, Cerniauskiene LR, Domarkiene S, et al. (2003) Age-related maculopathy and consumption of fresh vegetables and fruits in urban elderly. Medicina (Kaunas) 39: 1231–1236.
15. Fraser-Bell S, Wu J, Klein R, Azen SP, Hooper C, et al. (2008) Cardiovascular risk factors and age-related macular degeneration: the Los Angeles Latino Eye Study. Am J Ophthalmol 145: 308–316.
16. Xu L, Xie XW, Wang YX, Jonas JB (2009) Ocular and systemic factors associated with diabetes mellitus in the adult population in rural and urban China. The Beijing Eye Study. Eye (Lond) 23: 676–682.
17. Clemons TE, Rankin MW, McBee WL (2006) Cognitive impairment in the Age-Related Eye Disease Study: AREDS report no. 16. Arch Ophthalmol 124: 537–543.
18. (2011) Cochrane Handbook for Systematic Reviews of Interventions. In: Julian PT Higgins, Green S, editors: The Cochrane Collaboration.
19. Stroup DF, Berlin JA, Morton SC, Olkin I, Williamson GD, et al. (2000) Meta-analysis of observational studies in epidemiology: a proposal for reporting. Meta-analysis Of Observational Studies in Epidemiology (MOOSE) group. JAMA 283: 2008–2012.
20. Yuan D, Yuan S, Liu Q (2013) The age-related maculopathy susceptibility 2 polymorphism and polypoidal choroidal vasculopathy in Asian populations: a meta-analysis. Ophthalmology 120: 2051–2057.
21. Rostom A, Dubé C, Cranney A, Saloojee N, Sy R, et al. (2004) Evidence Reports/Technology Assessments, No. 104.Celiac Disease: Rockville (MD): Agency for Healthcare Research and Quality (US).
22. DerSimonian R, Laird N (1986) Meta-analysis in clinical trials. Control Clin Trials 7: 177–188.
23. Kuritz SJ, Landis JR, Koch GG (1988) A general overview of Mantel-Haenszel methods: applications and recent developments. Annu Rev Public Health 9: 123–160.
24. Davis MD, Gangnon RE, Lee LY, Hubbard LD, Klein BE, et al. (2005) The Age-Related Eye Disease Study severity scale for age-related macular degeneration: AREDS Report No. 17. Arch Ophthalmol 123: 1484–1498.
25. Ferris FL, Davis MD, Clemons TE, Lee LY, Chew EY, et al. (2005) A simplified severity scale for age-related macular degeneration: AREDS Report No. 18. Arch Ophthalmol 123: 1570–1574.
26. Begg CB, Mazumdar M (1994) Operating characteristics of a rank correlation test for publication bias. Biometrics 50: 1088–1101.
27. Egger M, Davey Smith G, Schneider M, Minder C (1997) Bias in meta-analysis detected by a simple, graphical test. BMJ 315: 629–634.
28. Wong TY, Klein R, Sun C, Mitchell P, Couper DJ, et al. (2006) Age-related macular degeneration and risk for stroke. Ann Intern Med 145: 98–106.
29. Jeganathan VS, Kawasaki R, Wang JJ, Aung T, Mitchell P, et al. (2008) Retinal vascular caliber and age-related macular degeneration: the Singapore Malay Eye Study. Am J Ophthalmol 146: 954–959 e951.
30. Baker ML, Wang JJ, Rogers S, Klein R, Kuller LH, et al. (2009) Early age-related macular degeneration, cognitive function, and dementia: the Cardio-vascular Health Study. Arch Ophthalmol 127: 667–673.
31. Pokharel S, Malla OK, Pradhananga CL, Joshi SN (2009) A pattern of age-related macular degeneration. JNMA J Nepal Med Assoc 48: 217–220.
32. Hu CC, Ho JD, Lin HC (2010) Neovascular age-related macular degeneration and the risk of stroke: a 5-year population-based follow-up study. Stroke 41: 613–617.
33. Weiner DE, Tighiouart H, Reynolds R, Seddon JM (2011) Kidney function, albuminuria and age-related macular degeneration in NHANES III. Nephrol Dial Transplant 26: 3159–3165.
34. Cheung CM, Tai ES, Kawasaki R, Tay WT, Lee JL, et al. (2012) Prevalence of and risk factors for age-related macular degeneration in a multiethnic Asian cohort. Arch Ophthalmol 130: 480–486.
35. Yang K, Zhan SY, Liang YB, Duan X, Wang F, et al. (2012) Association of dilated retinal arteriolar caliber with early age-related macular degeneration: the Handan Eye Study. Graefes Arch Clin Exp Ophthalmol 250: 741–749.
36. La Torre G, Pacella E, Saulle R, Giraldi G, Pacella F, et al. (2013) The synergistic effect of exposure to alcohol, tobacco smoke and other risk factors for age-related macular degeneration. Eur J Epidemiol 28: 445–446.
37. Mattes D, Haas A, Renner W, Steinbrugger I, El-Shabrawi Y, et al. (2009) Analysis of three pigment epithelium-derived factor gene polymorphisms in patients with exudative age-related macular degeneration. Mol Vis 15: 343–348.
38. Vine AK, Stader J, Branham K, Musch DC, Swaroop A (2005) Biomarkers of cardiovascular disease as risk factors for age-related macular degeneration. Ophthalmology 112: 2076–2080.
39. Hahn P, Acquah K, Cousins SW, Lee PP, Sloan FA (2013) Ten-year incidence of age-related macular degeneration according to diabetic retinopathy classification among medicare beneficiaries. Retina 33: 911–919.
40. Shalev V, Sror M, Goldshtein I, Kokia E, Chodick G (2011) Statin use and the risk of age related macular degeneration in a large health organization in Israel. Ophthalmic Epidemiol 18: 83–90.
41. Leske MC, Wu SY, Hennis A, Nemesure B, Yang L, et al. (2006) Nine-year incidence of age-related macular degeneration in the Barbados Eye Studies. Ophthalmology 113: 29–35.
42. Tomany SC, Wang JJ, Van Leeuwen R, Klein R, Mitchell P, et al. (2004) Risk factors for incident age-related macular degeneration: pooled findings from 3 continents. Ophthalmology 111: 1280–1287.
43. Yasuda M, Kiyohara Y, Hata Y, Arakawa S, Yonemoto K, et al. (2009) Nine-year incidence and risk factors for age-related macular degeneration in a defined Japanese population the Hisayama study. Ophthalmology 116: 2135–2140.
44. Delcourt C, Michel F, Colvez A, Lacroux A, Delage M, et al. (2001) Associations of cardiovascular disease and its risk factors with age-related macular degeneration: the POLA study. Ophthalmic Epidemiol 8: 237–249.
45. Duan Y, Mo J, Klein R, Scott IU, Lin HM, et al. (2007) Age-related macular degeneration is associated with incident myocardial infarction among elderly Americans. Ophthalmology 114: 732–737.
46. Klein R, Deng Y, Klein BE, Hyman L, Seddon J, et al. (2007) Cardiovascular disease, its risk factors and treatment, and age-related macular degeneration: Women's Health Initiative Sight Exam ancillary study. Am J Ophthalmol 143: 473–483.
47. Choi JK, Lym YL, Moon JW, Shin HJ, Cho B (2011) Diabetes mellitus and early age-related macular degeneration. Arch Ophthalmol 129: 196–199.
48. Gemmy Cheung CM, Li X, Cheng CY, Zheng Y, Mitchell P, et al. (2013) Prevalence and risk factors for age-related macular degeneration in Indians: a comparative study in Singapore and India. Am J Ophthalmol 155: 764–773, 773 e761–763.
49. Blumenkranz MS, Russell SR, Robey MG, Kott-Blumenkranz R, Penneys N (1986) Risk factors in age-related maculopathy complicated by choroidal neovascularization. Ophthalmology 93: 552–558.
50. Ross RD, Barofsky JM, Cohen G, Baber WB, Palao SW, et al. (1998) Presumed macular choroidal watershed vascular filling, choroidal neovascularization, and systemic vascular disease in patients with age-related macular degeneration. Am J Ophthalmol 125: 71–80.

51. Monnier VM, Sell DR, Genuth S (2005) Glycation products as markers and predictors of the progression of diabetic complications. Ann N Y Acad Sci 1043: 567–581.

52. Alexander SL, Linde-Zwirble WT, Werther W, Depperschmidt EE, Wilson LJ, et al. (2007) Annual rates of arterial thromboembolic events in medicare neovascular age-related macular degeneration patients. Ophthalmology 114: 2174–2178.

53. Kim IK, Ji F, Morrison MA, Adams S, Zhang Q, et al. (2008) Comprehensive analysis of CRP, CFH Y402H and environmental risk factors on risk of neovascular age-related macular degeneration. Mol Vis 14: 1487–1495.

54. Lin JM, Wan L, Tsai YY, Lin HJ, Tsai Y, et al. (2008) Pigment epithelium-derived factor gene Met72Thr polymorphism is associated with increased risk of wet age-related macular degeneration. Am J Ophthalmol 145: 716–721.

55. Cackett P, Yeo I, Cheung CM, Vithana EN, Wong D, et al. (2011) Relationship of smoking and cardiovascular risk factors with polypoidal choroidal vasculopathy and age-related macular degeneration in Chinese persons. Ophthalmology 118: 846–852.

56. Sogut E, Ortak H, Aydogan L, Benli I (2013) Association of Paraoxonase 1 L55m and Q192r Single-Nucleotide Polymorphisms with Age-Related Macular Degeneration. Retina.

57. Klein R, Davis MD, Magli YL, Segal P, Klein BE, et al. (1991) The Wisconsin age-related maculopathy grading system. Ophthalmology 98: 1128–1134.

58. Bird AC, Bressler NM, Bressler SB, Chisholm IH, Coscas G, et al. (1995) An international classification and grading system for age-related maculopathy and age-related macular degeneration. The International ARM Epidemiological Study Group. Surv Ophthalmol 39: 367–374.

59. Tan JS, Mitchell P, Smith W, Wang JJ (2007) Cardiovascular risk factors and the long-term incidence of age-related macular degeneration: the Blue Mountains Eye Study. Ophthalmology 114: 1143–1150.

60. (2001) The Age-Related Eye Disease Study system for classifying age-related macular degeneration from stereoscopic color fundus photographs: the Age-Related Eye Disease Study Report Number 6. Am J Ophthalmol 132: 668–681.

61. Klein R, Meuer SM, Knudtson MD, Iyengar SK, Klein BE (2008) The epidemiology of retinal reticular drusen. Am J Ophthalmol 145: 317–326.

62. Mitchell P, Wang JJ (1999) Diabetes, fasting blood glucose and age-related maculopathy: The Blue Mountains Eye Study. Aust N Z J Ophthalmol 27: 197–199.

63. Smith W, Mitchell P, Leeder SR, Wang JJ (1998) Plasma fibrinogen levels, other cardiovascular risk factors, and age-related maculopathy: the Blue Mountains Eye Study. Arch Ophthalmol 116: 583–587.

64. Klein R, Li X, Kuo JZ, Klein BE, Cotch MF, et al. (2013) Associations of Candidate Genes to Age-Related Macular Degeneration Among Racial/Ethnic Groups in the Multi-Ethnic Study of Atherosclerosis. Am J Ophthalmol.

65. Stitt AW (2010) AGEs and diabetic retinopathy. Invest Ophthalmol Vis Sci 51: 4867–4874.

66. Hammes HP, Hoerauf H, Alt A, Schleicher E, Clausen JT, et al. (1999) N(epsilon)(carboxymethyl)lysin and the AGE receptor RAGE colocalize in age-related macular degeneration. Invest Ophthalmol Vis Sci 40: 1855–1859.

67. Soulis T, Thallas V, Youssef S, Gilbert RE, McWilliam BG, et al. (1997) Advanced glycation end products and their receptors co-localise in rat organs susceptible to diabetic microvascular injury. Diabetologia 40: 619–628.

68. Howes KA, Liu Y, Dunaief JL, Milam A, Frederick JM, et al. (2004) Receptor for advanced glycation end products and age-related macular degeneration. Invest Ophthalmol Vis Sci 45: 3713–3720.

69. Zhang W, Liu H, Al-Shabrawey M, Caldwell RW, Caldwell RB (2011) Inflammation and diabetic retinal microvascular complications. J Cardiovasc Dis Res 2: 96–103.

70. Totan Y, Yagci R, Bardak Y, Ozyurt H, Kendir F, et al. (2009) Oxidative macromolecular damage in age-related macular degeneration. Curr Eye Res 34: 1089–1093.

71. Venza I, Visalli M, Cucinotta M, Teti D, Venza M (2012) Association between oxidative stress and macromolecular damage in elderly patients with age-related macular degeneration. Aging Clin Exp Res 24: 21–27.

72. Cao X, Liu M, Tuo J, Shen D, Chan CC (2010) The effects of quercetin in cultured human RPE cells under oxidative stress and in Ccl2/Cx3cr1 double deficient mice. Exp Eye Res 91: 15–25.

73. Tuo J, Ross RJ, Herzlich AA, Shen D, Ding X, et al. (2009) A high omega-3 fatty acid diet reduces retinal lesions in a murine model of macular degeneration. Am J Pathol 175: 799–807.

74. Ardeljan D, Chan CC (2013) Aging is not a disease: distinguishing age-related macular degeneration from aging. Prog Retin Eye Res 37: 68–89.

75. Donath MY, Shoelson SE (2011) Type 2 diabetes as an inflammatory disease. Nat Rev Immunol 11: 98–107.

76. Ho AC, Scott IU, Kim SJ, Brown GC, Brown MM, et al. (2012) Anti-vascular endothelial growth factor pharmacotherapy for diabetic macular edema: a report by the American Academy of Ophthalmology. Ophthalmology 119: 2179–2188.

77. Rofagha S, Bhisitkul RB, Boyer DS, Sadda SR, Zhang K (2013) Seven-Year Outcomes in Ranibizumab-Treated Patients in ANCHOR, MARINA, and HORIZON: A Multicenter Cohort Study (SEVEN-UP). Ophthalmology 120: 2292–2299.

78. Sasongko MB, Wong TY, Nguyen TT, Kawasaki R, Jenkins AJ, et al. (2012) Serum apolipoproteins are associated with systemic and retinal microvascular function in people with diabetes. Diabetes 61: 1785–1792.

79. Di Angelantonio E, Sarwar N, Perry P, Kaptoge S, Ray KK, et al. (2009) Major lipids, apolipoproteins, and risk of vascular disease. JAMA 302: 1993–2000.

80. Turner N, Robker RL (2014) Developmental programming of obesity and insulin resistance: does mitochondrial dysfunction in oocytes play a role? Mol Hum Reprod.

81. Sorriento D, Pascale AV, Finelli R, Carillo AL, Annunziata R, et al. (2014) Targeting mitochondria as therapeutic strategy for metabolic disorders. ScientificWorldJournal 2014: 604685.

82. Wu J, Uchino M, Sastry SM, Schaumberg DA (2014) Age-related macular degeneration and the incidence of cardiovascular disease: a systematic review and meta-analysis. PLoS One 9: e89600.

22

Quantitative Analysis of Cone Photoreceptor Distribution and Its Relationship with Axial Length, Age, and Early Age-Related Macular Degeneration

Ryo Obata*, Yasuo Yanagi

Department of Ophthalmology, University of Tokyo School of Medicine, Bunkyo-ku, Tokyo, Japan

Abstract

Purpose: It has not been clarified whether early age-related macular degeneration (AMD) is associated with cone photoreceptor distribution. We used adaptive optics fundus camera to examine cone photoreceptors in the macular area of aged patients and quantitatively analyzed its relationship between the presence of early AMD and cone distribution.

Methods: Sixty cases aged 50 or older were studied. The eyes were examined with funduscopy and spectral-domain optical coherence tomography to exclude the eyes with any abnormalities at two sites of measurement, $2°$ superior and $5°$ temporal to the fovea. High-resolution retinal images with cone photoreceptor mosaic were obtained with adaptive optics fundus camera (rtx1, Imagine Eyes, France). After adjusting for axial length, cone packing density was calculated and the relationship with age, axial length, or severity of early AMD based on the age-related eye disease study (AREDS) classification was analyzed.

Results: Patient's age ranged from 50 to 77, and axial length from 21.7 to 27.5 mm. Mean density in metric units and that in angular units were 24,900 cells/mm^2, 2,170 cells/deg^2 at $2°$ superior, and 18,500 cells/mm^2, 1,570 cels/deg^2 at $5°$ temporal, respectively. Axial length was significantly correlated with the density calculated in metric units, but not with that in angular units. Age was significantly correlated with the density both in metric and angular units at $2°$ superior. There was no significant difference in the density in metric and angular units between the eyes with AREDS category one and those with categories two or three.

Conclusion: Axial length and age were significantly correlated with parafoveal cone photoreceptor distribution. The results do not support that early AMD might influence cone photoreceptor density in the area without drusen or pigment abnormalities.

Editor: Steven Barnes, Dalhousie University, Canada

Funding: This study was supported in part by a Grant in Aid for scientific research (B) number 24791837 from the Ministry of Education, Culture, Sports, Science and Technology of Japan. The funder had no role in study design, data collection and analysis, decision to publish, or preparation of the manuscript. No additional external funding was received for this study.

Competing Interests: The authors have declared that no competing interests exist.

* E-mail: robata-tky@umin.ac.jp

Introduction

Age-related macular degeneration (AMD) is a leading cause of blindness in developed countries. [1] AMD has two stages; i.e., early AMD and late AMD. Drusen and pigment abnormalities are the hallmarks of early AMD. [2,3] They are usually recognized in focal areas, but the pathological investigation proved diffusely distributed membranous deposits on the basement membrane of the retinal pigment epithelium throughout the macula. [4–6] Early AMD is predisposed to late AMD, which is characterized by development of choroidal neovascularization or progressive retinochoroidal atrophy resulting in severe vision loss. Susceptible genes and environmental risk factors have been reported, [7] which suggest that RPE damage is critical in AMD pathogenesis.

Photoreceptor loss is also documented in early AMD, disorganization of rod photoreceptor has been well demonstrated both pathologically [8,9] and physiologically. [10] Meanwhile, alter-

ation in cone photoreceptors has not been fully understood. Some previous studies pathologically demonstrated that cone photoreceptors were disorganized at the fovea or parafovea in early AMD patients. [9,11] Other studies reported that central visual field, [12] cone adaptation, [13] blue cone sensitivity, [14] focal ERG, [15] and multifocal ERG [16] showed impaired cone function even in the early stage of the disease. It has also been demonstrated pathologically that cone photoreceptor density was decreased in the parafovea of three eyes with early AMD. [5] However, another study reported the photoreceptor damage was confined to areas directly overlying drusen. [17].

High-resolution retinal images using adaptive optics (AO) has been introduced recently,[18–21] making it possible to analyze photoreceptor distribution in areas of interest in living normal [22–24] or affected eyes [25–29] non-invasively. Regarding the influence of AMD, a pilot study described slight disruption in the cone photoreceptor mosaic in early AMD. [30] However, large number of subjects and adjustment for potentially confounding factors such as eccentricity to the fovea, axial length, or age are essential to clarify the influence of AMD on cone photoreceptor distribution.

Here we used AO fundus camera to examine cone photoreceptor distribution in the macular area of a relatively large number of aged patients and quantitatively analyzed the relationship between cone photoreceptor distribution and axial length, age, or the presence of early AMD.

Materials and Methods

This observational case series study was approved by the institutional review board of University of Tokyo Graduate School of Medicine. Written consent was given by the patients for their information to be stored in the hospital and used for research. The study adhered to the tenets of the Declaration of Helsinki.

Patients

Sixty-nine patients (37 men and 32 women; mean age 65.0 years, range 50–80 years) who visited Macular Clinic, University of Tokyo Hospital between September 2012 and October 2012 with unilaterally affected macular diseases were included. The unaffected eye was used for study. If the patients had any ocular diseases other than early AMD in the unaffected eye or the best-corrected decimal visual acuity (BCVA) in the unaffected eye was worse than 0.8, they were excluded from the study.

Examination

Each patient underwent complete examination, including axial length measurement, anterior segment and fundus examination by slit-lamp biomicroscopy after pupil dialation. Fundus autofluorescence images were also acquired with HRAII (Heidelberg Engineering, Heidelberg, Germany), if possible. Axial length was measured with IOL master (Carl Zeiss Meditec, Jena, Germany). The study eye was classified into AMD category 1, 2, or 3 according to the criteria reported by age-related eye disease study group [31,32] based on the fundoscopic findings within two disc diameters of the center of the macula. Briefly, category 1 included eyes with no or small (<63 μm) drusen, category 2 included eyes with intermediate (≥63, <125 μm) drusen or pigment abnormalities, and category 3 with large (≥125 μm) drusen.

Spectral-domain optical coherence tomography (SD-OCT) images were obtained with SpectralisOCT (Heidelberg Engineering, Heidelberg, Germany). Thirty-degree horizontally or vertically scanned images centered on the fovea were taken. Using eye-tracking system, at most 100 tomographs captured at the same location were overlaid to decrease random speckle noise. Infrared (IR, 815 nm) reflectance images 30° by 30° were simultaneously obtained with OCT scan (**Figure 1**). By referring to the OCT images, the center of the fovea was located on the IR image. Then the IR image was imported into an open-source imaging program (GIMP, version 2.8.2). The points at 2° superior and 5° temporal to the fovea were located on the IR image, using the corresponding distance in pixel units calculated by dividing the pixel length of the whole IR image (30°) by 15 or 6. After the sites at 2° superior and 5° temporal to the fovea were located, funduscopy and the OCT scan were reviewed. If any drusen or RPE disturbance were detected at any of these points, it was excluded from the analysis.

Adaptive Optics Fundus Camera

High-resolution retinal images with cone photoreceptor mosaic were obtained with flood-illuminated adaptive optics fundus camera (rtx1, Imagine Eyes, Orsey, France).[33–36] The rtx1 has a resolution of 1.6 μm with a 4.2° by 4.2° imaging field of view and an illumination wavelength of 850 nm. Patients were instructed to gaze a built-in fixation target that could be moved within $\pm10°$ horizontally and $\pm8°$ vertically. After checking whether the patient was properly fixating, 40 images were acquired during approximately four seconds. These images are processed and overlaid to yield a 4° by 4° highly contrasted image.

Measurement of Cone Distribution

The processed AO image was imported into the imaging program (GIMP). It was manually overlaid with the IR image using the functions of resizing, parallel translation, or rotation by referring to retinal vessels. Thereby the locations at 2° superior and 5° temporal to the fovea were identified on the AO images. Cone distribution was measured at each site firstly using the software provided by the manufacturer (AOdetect Ver. 0.1. Imagine Eyes). [35] A 60 pixel by 60 pixel square was placed at 2° superior and 5° temporal to the fovea. The area was chosen not to include defects. The size of the square in each image was also expressed in the metric unit after it was calibrated with the axial length according to the formula by Bennett et al. [37]. In eyes with axial length of 24 mm, 60 pixel of the image corresponds approximately to 50 μm. Within the square, cone photoreceptor density and spacing were automatically calculated by cells/mm^2 and by μm. Furthermore, Voronoi diagram was automatically constructed from each cone mosaic to calculate the proportion of hexagonal Voronoi domains, that indicates regularity of cone packing arrangement. [28,38,39] We also calculated cone angular density (cells/deg^2). [23,24] It was provided by dividing the absolute number of cones (cells) within this square by the area of the square (deg^2). The area of the square (deg^2) was obtained by multiplying the area of the AO image (equal to 16 deg^2) by the proportion of the area of the square (pixel^2) to that of the whole AO image (equal to 140,625 pixel^2).

In all images, automatically detected cones were inspected and modified manually by two independent observers without knowledge of the backgrounds or the fundus image of each case. The inter-observer variability was calculated as the absolute difference in cone numbers between observers divided by the average cone number. If the variability was less than 5%, the average cone number was used as the final count to calculate the cone density. When the variability was 5% or more, two observers re-examined the image together and performed a third count as the final one.

Statistical Analysis

Student t test was used for comparison of the background characteristics between eyes with AMD category 1 and those with AMD categories 2 or 3. Relationship between parameters of cone distribution and axial length, age, and AMD category was analyzed by multiple linear regression analysis. P value less than 0.05 was considered to be statistically significant. The software package JMP (SAS Institute, Cary, NC) was used for the analyses.

Results

Patient Demography

Of all 69 enrolled patients, nine patients were excluded because of blurred images which resulted from media opacity such as cataract or dry eye. Of the remaining 60 patients, the site at 2° superior to the fovea in 9 patients and that at 5° temporal in 12 patients were excluded from the measurement since drusen or RPE abnormality was detected by funduscopy or OCT scan.

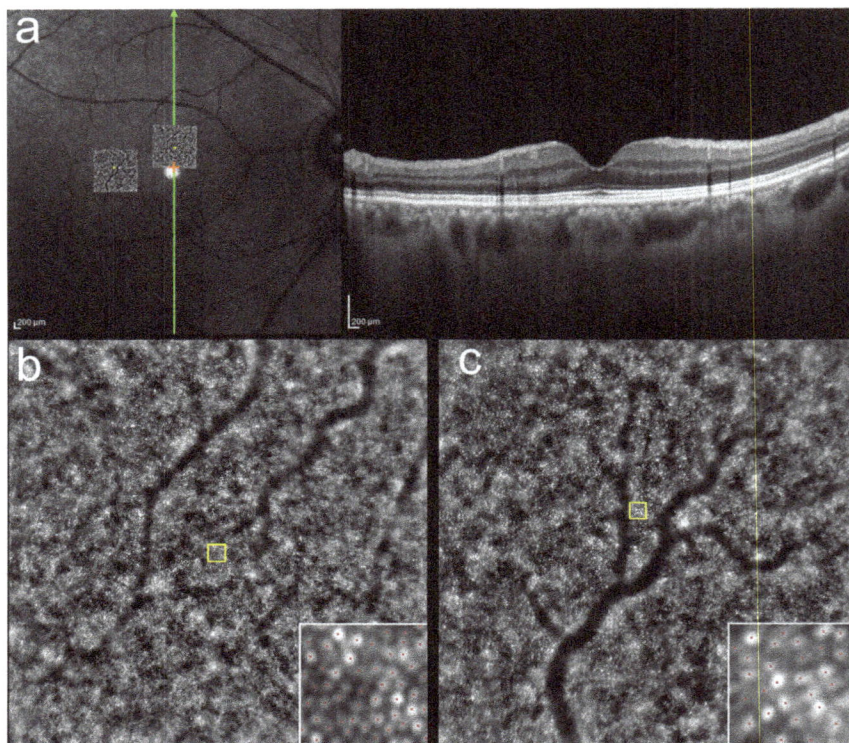

Figure 1. Identification of the sites for measurement in the images taken by adaptive optics fundus camera. Identification and measurement of cone distribution at $2°$ superior and $5°$ temporal to the fovea. Figures of a representative case are shown. Horizontal and vertical SD-OCT scan images centered on the fovea were obtained simultaneously with IR images using Spectralis (a). After the site corresponding to the fovea was identified on the IR image (orange cross in a) by referring to the OCT images, the sites at $2°$ superior and $5°$ temporal to the fovea on the IR image were located (yellow squares in a). Processed images from the adaptive optics (AO) fundus camera were overlaid with IR images by referring to retinal vessels in order to identify the sites of interest on AO images. A 60 pixel by 60 pixel square was placed at these sites (yellow square in b and c). Cone mosaic within the square was identified (red dots in the insets of 1b and 1c) and its distribution was assessed.

Therefore, the data at $2°$ superior of 51 eyes and that at $5°$ temporal of 48 eyes in 60 patients were used for analysis. The demography of the 60 patients was shown in **Table 1**. Mean age was 64.2 (range: 50–77). Thirty-two (53%) patients were unilaterally affected by neovascular AMD, and 28 (47%) by other diseases such as branch retinal vein occlusion (16 eyes), central retinal vein occlusion (5 eyes), idiopathic epiretinal membrane (4 eyes), and idiopathic full-thickness macular hole (3 eyes). Best-corrected decimal visual acuity ranged 0.8 to 1.2 (median, 1.0). Thirty (50%), 18 (30%), and 12 (20%) eyes were classified as AMD category 1, 2, and 3, respectively. Sex predominance, age, axial length, and proportion of neovascular AMD in the contralateral eye were not significantly different between the eyes in AMD category 1 and those in categories 2 or 3.

Parameters of Cone Distribution

Out of 60 patients, parameters of cone distribution at $2°$ in 51 patients and those at $5°$ in 48 patients were measured. Mean cone density in metric units and angular units, after manual modification were $24,900 \pm 3,400$ cells/mm^2, $2,170 \pm 400$ cells/deg^2, respectively, at $2°$ superior, and $18,500 \pm 2,600$ cells/mm^2, $1,570 \pm 140$ cells/deg^2, respectively, at $5°$ temporal(**Table 2**). Cone spacing in metric and angular units, and proportion of hexagonal Voronoi domains were automatically calculated and shown in Table S1. During manual modification, the inter-observer variability were $1.4 \pm 3.5\%$ and $0.4 \pm 5.1\%$ (mean $\pm$ SD) at $2°$ and $5°$, respectively.

Correlation with Axial Length, Age, and AMD Category

Multiple linear regression coefficients analyzing effect of patient's demography on cone densities are shown in **Table 3** and **Table 4**. Cone density in metric units was significantly correlated negatively both with axial length and age, but not with AMD category at $2°$ (**Table 3**) and with axial length but not with AMD category at $5°$ (**Table 4**). In contrast, cone density in angular units was significantly correlated only with age at $2°$ (**Table 3**). Additionally, cone density in metric and angular units were not significantly different between the patients with neovascular AMD and those with other diseases in the affected eye (data not shown). Representative cases with various AMD categories are shown in **Figure 2, 3, and 4**.

Discussion

In the present study, we used adaptive optics (AO) fundus camera to examine cone photoreceptor distribution in the macular area of aged patients and, quantitatively analyzed its relationship with age, axial length, and early age-related macular degeneration (AMD). Since previous reports suggested that cone distribution might vary according to eccentricity to the fovea, axial length, or age, quantitative analyses investigating any difference between patients and controls should take these confounding factors into consideration. Therefore we examined cone distribution at the specific eccentricities with adjustment for these confounding factors.

Table 1. Patient demographics.

	Total	AMD category	AMD categories
		1	2 or 3
No. of eyes	60	30	30
Male (%)	31 (52)	15 (50)	16 (53)
Mean axial length (mm)	23.9	24	23.8
[95% CI]	[23.6:24.2]	[23.6:24.5]	[23.2:24.3]
(range)	(21.7–27.5)	(22.3–26.5)	(21.7–27.5)
Mean age	64.2	63.6	64.9
[95% CI]	[62.5:65.9]	[60.9:66.3]	[62.7:67.0]
(range)	(50–77)	(50–77)	(53–77)
Neovascular AMD	32 (53)	14 (47)	18 (60)
in the affected eye (%)			

There was no statistically significant difference in background characteristics between eyes with AMD category 1 and those with categories 2 or 3.

As previously discussed, acquisition of fundus images of aged patients is technically challenging. [30] The difficulty derives from various factors such as unstable fixation or opaque media. In the present study, we selected patients with good visual acuity to address this problem. Although part of the examined eyes was still excluded from the study because of blurred images by cataract or dry eye, we were able to obtain the AO images from a number of the aged patients with good to excellent repeatability.

In cone counting, automatic counting software is useful and will be essential when large quantity of data is to be analyzed. However, currently, manually modified count is more reliable. [38,40,41] In the present study automatic counting was manually edited by two observers. Inter-observer differences were 0.4 to 1.4%, and in the cases with variability 5% or higher, recount was performed to enhance the reliability of manual modification.

Axial length negatively influenced on cone density calculated in metric units both at $2°$ and $5°$, while it did not if calculated in angular units. As previously discussed,[22–24,39] axial length is a major variable to be taken care of in calculating cone distribution outside the fovea. There may be two reasons; Firstly, a particular angular eccentricity corresponds to different distances from the fovea in metric units with different axial lengths. For example, $2°$ and $5°$ eccentricity corresponds approximately to 0.53 to 0.64 and 1.3 to 1.6 mm with axial length of 22 to 26 mm, respectively. Secondly, as axial length increases, retinal size in metric units of a particular angular area increases, leading cone density to less value when calculated in metric units. Therefore we measured at the same eccentricities from the fovea described in angular units and calculated cone density both in metric units and angular units. In a previous report [22] studying 19 normal subjects aged 20 to 52 with AO imaging, eyes with moderate to high myopia showed significantly longer cone spacing in metric units than those with normal to low myopia. Other studies [23,24] investigated cone distribution in young healthy eyes and reported that cone density in metric units negatively correlated with axial length while angular density shows no significant correlation. The results of the present study indicate that this relationship also applies to aged patients. Recently another study showed that axial length was significantly correlated with cone density in metric units at 0.5 mm eccentricity from the fovea, while not at 1.0 mm and 1.5 mm eccentricities. 1.5 mm eccentricity corresponds to approximately $5°$. [39] Discrepancy with the result of the present study may be partly because, as discussed in the previous report, [24] when eccentricity was set in metric units, the eccentricity calculated in angular units becomes narrower with longer axial length, and it may tend to attenuate the negative relationship between cone density in metric units and axial length.

Additionally age was negatively correlated with cone density after adjustment for axial length at 2 degrees eccentric to the fovea. Decrease in cone function with age was reported in a physiological study. [42] Transfer of metabolic products across the RPE layer is impaired with the accumulation of age-related deposits in Bruch's membrane and retinal pigment epithelium, and the resultant insufficiency of the nutrients and ischemia is indicated to lead to dysfunction of cone photoreceptors. [8] Histologically cone photoreceptor decreases at the parafoveal

Table 2. Cone photoreceptor density in metric and angular units at $2°$ and $5°$ to the fovea.

	2° superior	5° temporal
Cone density (mean±SD)		
(cells/mm2)	24,900±3,400	18,500±2,600
[95%CI]	[24,000:25,900]	[17,700:19,200]
(cells/deg2)	2,170±400	1,570±140
[95%CI]	[2,060:2,290]	[1,530:1,610]

It was firstly automatically counted and then manually edited.

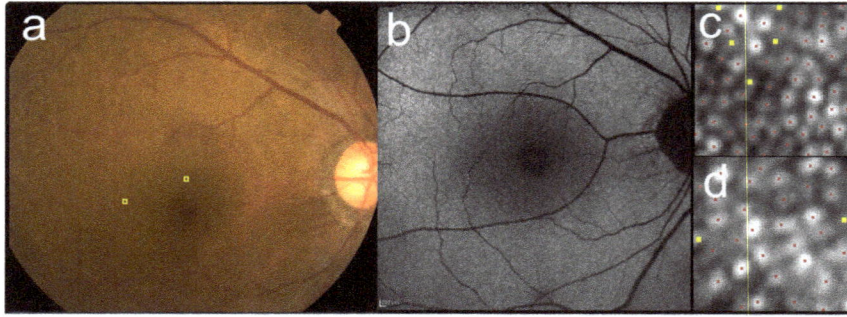

Figure 2. Cone mosaic images of the case with AREDS category 1 (no drusen). The right eye of 69-year-old male (the same eye as Figure 1) as a representative case with AREDS category 1 (no drusen). The fundus photo (**a**) did not show any sign of drusen or pigmentary abnormalities. The fundus autofluorescence (FAF) (**b**) was also unremarkable. After AO image was taken, the 60 pixel by 60 pixel square image was cropped at 2° superior (**c**) and 5° temporal (**d**) to the fovea (also shown as yellow squares in **a**). Cone mosaic was identified automatically at first (red dots in **c** and **d**), then added (yellow dots) in manual modification. Cone density were 25,500 cells/mm^2 (2,340 cells/deg^2) at 2° and 14,030 cells/mm^2 (1,290 cells/deg^2) at 5°.

lesion [43] and appreciable number of nuclei was displaced from the outer nuclear layer to the photoreceptor layer over the age of 40, causing disarray of photoreceptor inner or outer segment. [44] Inner segments also showed deposition of lipofuscin with aging [45,46] and outer segment revealed accumulation of amyloid beta, [47] indicating disorganization within inner or outer segments with aging. Since AO imaging detects the reflected light guided through the inner and outer segment, [20] the loss, disarray, and/or disorganization with aging should influence in the number of cones detected by AO imaging. Indeed, age-related decline in the cone density in the parafoveal area was previously suggested. [48,49] Another recent study also reported that cone density in the parafovea showed a trend towards negative correlation to age. [39]

The result in the present study, with large number of patients, was compatible with these report.

Several reports investigated cone density in normal subjects histologically or using AO imaging. They showed that cone density rapidly decreases with increasing eccentricity, with the value between approximately 35,000 and 15,000 cells/mm^2 at 0.5 mm to 1.0 mm to the fovea. [27,39,48] In contrast, cone density decreases more slowly at the more eccentric area, with the value from approximately 19,000 to 11,000 cells/mm^2 at 1.0 mm to 1.9 mm to the fovea. [27,39,48] However, these values were not fully adjusted for axial length, the unit used for indicating eccentricity, and horizontal or vertical meridian, all of which were reported to influence cone density. [39,48,50] Even after adjusting them, considerable individual variation have been

Table 3. Multiple linear regression coefficients analyzing effects of demographic valuables on cone photoreceptor distribution at 2°.

	Retinal density	Angular density
(Constant)		
P	<0.0001	0.022
b coefficient	67,500	3,160
[95%CI]	[45,400:89,600]	[480:5,850]
Axial length		
P	0.0002	0.56
b coefficient	−1,390	
[95%CI]	[−2,090:−683]	
Age		
P	0.042	0.0054
b coefficient	−147	−24.8
[95%CI]	[−287:−6]	[−41.9:−7.7]
AMD category (1 or 2–3)		
P	0.96	0.44
b coefficient		
[95%CI]		

Coefficients that were not statistically significant are not shown.

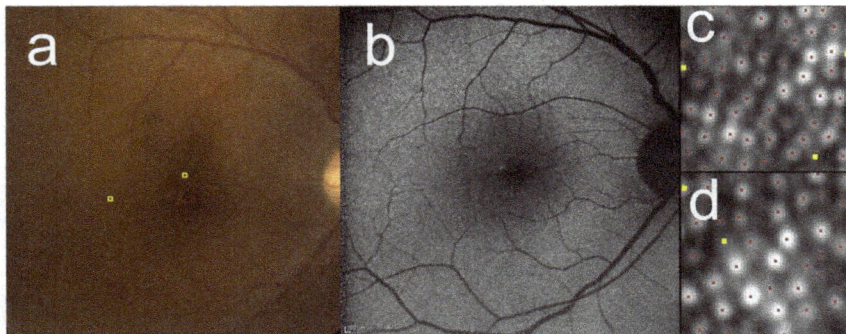

Figure 3. Cone mosaic images of the case with AREDS category 2 (pigmentary abnormality). The right eye of 59-year-old male with AREDS category 2. The fundus photo (**a**) showed hypopigmentation temporal to the fovea. FAF (**b**) showed irregular hyper- and hypofluorescence corresponding to the area. After AO image was taken, the 60 pixel by 60 pixel square image was cropped at 2° superior (**c**) and 5° temporal (**d**) to the fovea (also shown as yellow squares in **a**). Cone mosaic was identified automatically at first (red dots in **c** and **d**), then added (yellow dots) in manual modification. Cone density were 22,600 cells/mm^2 (2,190 cells/deg^2) at 2° and 14,900 cells/mm^2 (1,450 cells/deg^2) at 5°.

observed. [23,48,51] Therefore it is difficult to directly compare the cone density from different studies. However, it should be noted that the mean cone density at 2° in the present study seems slightly lower than a previous report [48] in that 10 normal eyes aged 50 to 65 showed 29,400 cells/mm^2 at 0.54 mm and 23,200 cells/mm^2 at 0.72 mm to the fovea. Since the slight decrease was observed only at 2° but not at 5°,it is unlikely to be explained by impaired image quality from media opacity or increased aberration in the aged patients. The previous study [48] reported that, comparing normal subjects aged 50 to 65 with those aged 22 to 35, there was significant decrease in cone density only within 0.5 mm to the fovea. Although the mechanism remains unclear, the current findings, together with previous studies, seems to suggest that as the subjects become older, cone density decreases at the parafovea.

In the present study, cone distribution was not significantly different between eyes with low and high severity of early AMD or between patients affected with neovascular AMD and other macular diseases in the contralateral eye. Although cone dysfunction has been demonstrated in eyes with early AMD, alteration in cone distribution in the area without drusen or pigmentary abnormalities has not been clarified. Therefore, we examined the region where drusen or pigmentary abnormalities were not detected. The results of this study do not support that severity of early AMD might be associated with cone photoreceptor distribution in the area without drusen or pigment abnormalities. For future analysis, it will be of much interest to

Table 4. Multiple linear regression coefficients analyzing effects of demographic valuables on cone photoreceptor distribution at 5°.

	Retinal density	Angular density
(Constant)		
P	<0.0001	0.0009
b coefficient	56,800	1,840
[95%CI]	[43,000:70,600]	[800:2,880]
Axial length		
P	<0.0001	0.77
b coefficient	−1,510	
[95%CI]	[−1,970:−1,060]	
Age		
P	0.43	0.47
b coefficient		
[95%CI]		
AMD category (1 or 2–3)		
P	0.72	0.95
b coefficient		
[95%CI]		

Coefficients that were not statistically significant are not shown.

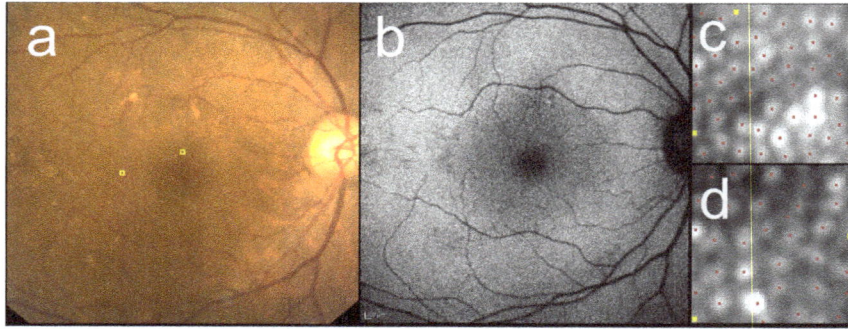

Figure 4. Cone mosaic images of the case with AREDS category 3 (large drusen). The right eye of 68-year-old female with AREDS category 3. The fundus photo (**a**) showed large drusen superior and temporal to the fovea. FAF (**b**) revealed hyper- and hypopigmentation corresponding to the drusen. After AO image was taken, the 60 pixel by 60 pixel square image was cropped at 2° superior (**c**) and 5° temporal (**d**) to the fovea (also shown as yellow squares in **a**). Cone mosaic was identified automatically at first (red dots in **c** and **d**), then added (yellow dots) in manual modification. Cone density were 25,700 cells/mm^2 (1,990 cells/deg^2) at 2° and 14,900 cells/mm^2 (1,450 cells/deg^2) at 5°.

analyze the cone distribution overlying drusen or pigmentary abnormalities by taking images with sufficient quality and adjusting several aforementioned confounding factors.

However, there are some limitations in the study such as retrospective nature of the study design. Additionally the sites of measurement were restricted to small area. Nevertheless, these results indicate that AO imaging technique can be used to evaluate cone distribution of aged patients with good visual acuity and transparent media, and might contribute to understanding in the relationship between cone distribution and confounding factors in aged patients or AMD.

In conclusion, we used AO fundus camera to examine cone photoreceptor distribution in the macular area of aged patients and quantitatively analyzed its relationship with age, axial length, and early age-related macular degeneration (AMD). Axial length and age showed significant correlation with parafoveal cone photoreceptor distribution. Severity of early AMD may not be associated with cone distribution in the area without apparent drusen or pigment abnormalities. AO imaging can be used to assess cone photoreceptor distribution of aged patients and might

be helpful to clarify the relationship between cone photoreceptor distribution, aging, and AMD.

Acknowledgments

The authors thank Mako Ogawa for data acquisition, Nicolas Chateau, Erika Boyenga Odlund, Frida Rosander and Fanny Poulon for technical assistance, and Kiyoko Gocho-Nakashima for valuable advices.

Author Contributions

Conceived and designed the experiments: RO YY. Performed the experiments: RO. Analyzed the data: RO. Contributed reagents/materials/analysis tools: RO. Wrote the paper: RO YY.

References

1. Klein R, Wang Q, Klein BE, Moss SE, Meuer SM (1995) The relationship of age-related maculopathy, cataract, and glaucoma to visual acuity. Invest Ophthalmol Vis Sci 36: 182–191.
2. Klein R, Davis MD, Magli YL, Segal P, Klein BE, et al. (1991) The Wisconsin age-related maculopathy grading system. Ophthalmology 98: 1128–1134.
3. Bird AC, Bressler NM, Bressler SB, Chisholm IH, Coscas G, et al. (1995) An international classification and grading system for age-related maculopathy and age-related macular degeneration. Surv Ophthalmol 39: 367–374.
4. Sarks SH (1976) Ageing and degeneration in the macular region: a clinico-pathological study. Br J Ophthalmol 60: 324–341.
5. Curcio CA, Medeiros NE, Millican CL (1996) Photoreceptor loss in age-related macular degeneration. Invest Ophthalmol Vis Sci 37: 1236–1249.
6. Curcio CA (2001) Photoreceptor topography in ageing and age-related maculopathy. Eye 15: 376–383.
7. Lim LS, Mitchell P, Seddon JM, Holz FG, Wong TY (2012) Age-related macular degeneration. Lancet 379: 1728–1738.
8. Curcio CA, Owsley C, Jackson GR (2000) Spare the Rods, Save the Cones in Aging and Age-related Maculopathy. Invest Ophthalmol Vis Sci 41: 2015–2018.
9. Jackson GR, Owsley C, Curcio CA (2002) Photoreceptor degeneration and dysfunction in aging and age-related maculopathy. Ageing Res Rev 1: 381–396.
10. Eisner A, Stoumbos VD, Klein ML, Fleming SA (1991) Relations between fundus appearance and function. Eyes whose fellow eye has exudative age-related macular degeneration. Invest Ophthalmol Vis Sci 32: 8–20.
11. Kanis MJ, Wisse RPL, Berendschot TTJM, van de Kraats J, van Norren D (2008) Foveal Cone-Photoreceptor Integrity in Aging Macula Disorder. Invest Ophthalmol Vis Sci 49: 2077–2081.
12. Swann PG, Lovie-Kitchin JE (1991) Age-related maculopathy. II: The nature of the central visual field loss. Ophthalmic Physiol Opt J Br Coll Ophthalmic Opt Optom 11: 59–70.
13. Brown B, Tobin C, Roche N, Wolanowski A (1986) Cone adaptation in age-related maculopathy. Am J Optom Physiol Opt 63: 450–454.
14. Eisner A, Fleming SA, Klein ML, Mauldin WM (1987) Sensitivities in older eyes with good acuity: eyes whose fellow eye has exudative AMD. Invest Ophthalmol Vis Sci 28: 1832–1837.
15. Sandberg MA, Miller S, Gaudio AR (1993) Foveal cone ERGs in fellow eyes of patients with unilateral neovascular age-related macular degeneration. Invest Ophthalmol Vis Sci 34: 3477–3480.
16. Wu Z, Ayton LN, Guymer RH, Luu CD (2013) Relationship Between the Second Reflective Band on Optical Coherence Tomography and Multifocal Electroretinography in Age-Related Macular Degeneration. Invest Ophthalmol Vis Sci 54: 2800–2806.
17. Johnson PT, Lewis GP, Talaga KC, Brown MN, Kappel PJ, et al. (2003) Drusen-Associated Degeneration in the Retina. Invest Ophthalmol Vis Sci 44: 4481–4488.
18. Miller DT, Williams DR, Morris GM, Liang J (1996) Images of cone photoreceptors in the living human eye. Vision Res 36: 1067–1079.
19. Roorda A, Williams DR (1999) The arrangement of the three cone classes in the living human eye. Nature 397: 520–522.
20. Godara P, Dubis AM, Roorda A, Duncan JL, Carroll J (2010) Adaptive Optics Retinal Imaging: Emerging Clinical Applications. Optom Vis Sci Off Publ Am Acad Optom 87: 930–941.
21. Lombardo M, Serrao S, Devaney N, Parravano M, Lombardo G (2012) Adaptive Optics Technology for High-Resolution Retinal Imaging. Sensors 13: 334–366.

22. Kitaguchi Y, Bessho K, Yamaguchi T, Nakazawa N, Mihashi T, et al. (2007) In Vivo Measurements of Cone Photoreceptor Spacing in Myopic Eyes from Images Obtained by an Adaptive Optics Fundus Camera. Jpn J Ophthalmol 51: 456–461.

23. Chui TYP, Song H, Burns SA (2008) Individual variations in human cone photoreceptor packing density. Invest Ophthalmol Vis Sci 49: 4679–4687.

24. Li KY, Tiruveedhula P, Roorda A (2010) Intersubject Variability of Foveal Cone Photoreceptor Density in Relation to Eye Length. Invest Ophthalmol Vis Sci 51: 6858–6867.

25. Wolfing JI, Chung M, Carroll J, Roorda A, Williams DR (2006) High-Resolution Retinal Imaging of Cone–Rod Dystrophy. Ophthalmology 113: 1014–1019.

26. Duncan JL, Zhang Y, Gandhi J, Nakanishi C, Othman M, et al. (2007) High-Resolution Imaging with Adaptive Optics in Patients with Inherited Retinal Degeneration. Invest Ophthalmol Vis Sci 48: 3283–3291.

27. Ooto S, Hangai M, Sakamoto A, Tsujikawa A, Yamashiro K, et al. (2010) High-Resolution Imaging of Resolved Central Serous Chorioretinopathy Using Adaptive Optics Scanning Laser Ophthalmoscopy. Ophthalmology 117: 1800–1809.

28. Ooto S, Hangai M, Takayama K, Sakamoto A, Tsujikawa A, et al. (2011) High-Resolution Imaging of the Photoreceptor Layer in Epiretinal Membrane Using Adaptive Optics Scanning Laser Ophthalmoscopy. Ophthalmology 118: 873–881.

29. Hayashi A, Tojo Nakamura, Fuchizawa Oiwake (2013) Adaptive optics fundus images of cone photoreceptors in the macula of patients with retinitis pigmentosa. Clin Ophthalmol: 203.

30. Boretsky A, Khan F, Burnett G, Hammer DX, Ferguson RD, et al. (2012) In vivo imaging of photoreceptor disruption associated with age-related macular degeneration: A pilot study. Lasers Surg Med 44: 603–610.

31. (1999) The Age-Related Eye Disease Study (AREDS): design implications. AREDS report no. 1 Control Clin Trials 20: 573–600.

32. (2001) A randomized, placebo-controlled, clinical trial of high-dose supplementation with vitamins C and E, beta carotene, and zinc for age-related macular degeneration and vision loss: AREDS report no. 8 Arch Ophthalmol 119: 1417–1436.

33. Lombardo M, Lombardo G, Ducoli P, Serrao S (2012) Adaptive Optics Photoreceptor Imaging. Ophthalmology 119: 1498–1498.

34. Lombardo M, Parravano M, Lombardo G, Varano M, Boccassini B, et al. (2013) Adaptive optics imaging of parafoveal cones in type 1 diabetes. Retina. Published ahead of print August 7,2013, doi:10.1097/IAE.0b013e3182a10850.

35. Mrejen S, Sato T, Curcio CA, Spaide RF (2013) Assessing the Cone Photoreceptor Mosaic in Eyes with Pseudodrusen and Soft Drusen In Vivo Using Adaptive Optics Imaging. Ophthalmology. Published ahead of print October 30,2013, doi:10.1016/j.ophtha.2013.09.026.

36. Tojo N, Nakamura T, Fuchizawa C, Oiwake T, Hayashi A (2013) Adaptive optics fundus images of cone photoreceptors in the macula of patients with retinitis pigmentosa. Clin Ophthalmol Auckl NZ 7: 203–210.

37. Bennett AG, Rudnicka AR, Edgar DF (1994) Improvements on Littmann's method of determining the size of retinal features by fundus photography. Graefes Arch Clin Exp Ophthalmol 232: 361–367.

38. Li KY, Roorda A (2007) Automated identification of cone photoreceptors in adaptive optics retinal images. J Opt Soc Am A 24: 1358–1363.

39. Park SP, Chung JK, Greenstein V, Tsang SH, Chang S (2013) A study of factors affecting the human cone photoreceptor density measured by adaptive optics scanning laser ophthalmoscope. Exp Eye Res 108: 1–9.

40. Garrioch R, Langlo C, Dubis AM, Cooper RF, Dubra A, et al. (2012) The Repeatability of In Vivo Parafoveal Cone Density and Spacing Measurements. Optom Vis Sci 89: 632–643.

41. Cooper RF, Langlo CS, Dubra A, Carroll J (2013) Automatic detection of modal spacing (Yellott's ring) in adaptive optics scanning light ophthalmoscope images. Ophthalmic Physiol Opt 33: 540–549.

42. Jackson GR, Owsley C (2000) Scotopic sensitivity during adulthood. Vision Res 40: 2467–2473.

43. Panda-Jonas S, Jonas JB, Jakobczyk-Zmija M (1995) Retinal photoreceptor density decreases with age. Ophthalmology 102: 1853–1859.

44. Gartner S, Henkind P (1981) Aging and degeneration of the human macula. 1. Outer nuclear layer and photoreceptors. Br J Ophthalmol 65: 23–28.

45. Tucker GS (1986) Refractile bodies in the inner segments of cones in the aging human retina. Invest Ophthalmol Vis Sci 27: 708–715.

46. Iwasaki M, Inomata H (1988) Lipofuscin granules in human photoreceptor cells. Invest Ophthalmol Vis Sci 29: 671–679.

47. Hoh Kam J, Lenassi E, Jeffery G (2010) Viewing Ageing Eyes: Diverse Sites of Amyloid Beta Accumulation in the Ageing Mouse Retina and the Up-Regulation of Macrophages. PLoS ONE 5: e13127.

48. Song H, Chui TYP, Zhong Z, Elsner AE, Burns SA (2011) Variation of Cone Photoreceptor Packing Density with Retinal Eccentricity and Age. Invest Ophthalmol Vis Sci 52: 7376–7384.

49. Chui TYP, Song H, Clark CA, Papay JA, Burns SA, et al. (2012) Cone Photoreceptor Packing Density and the Outer Nuclear Layer Thickness in Healthy Subjects. Invest Ophthalmol Vis Sci 53: 3545–3553.

50. Curcio CA, Sloan KR, Kalina RE, Hendrickson AE (1990) Human photoreceptor topography. J Comp Neurol 292: 497–523.

51. Curcio CA, Sloan KR (1992) Packing geometry of human cone photoreceptors: variation with eccentricity and evidence for local anisotropy. Vis Neurosci 9: 169–180.

23

Systemic Adverse Events after Intravitreal Bevacizumab versus Ranibizumab for Age-Related Macular Degeneration: A Meta-Analysis

Wei Wang, Xiulan Zhang*

Zhongshan Ophthalmic Center, State Key Laboratory of Ophthalmology, Sun Yat-Sen University, Guangzhou, People's Republic of China

Abstract

Objective: To assess whether the incidence of systemic adverse events differs between those who used bevacizumab and those who used ranibizumab in the treatment of age-related macular degeneration (AMD).

Methods: A systematic literature search was conducted to identify randomised controlled trials (RCTs) comparing the use of intravitreal bevacizumab with the use of ranibizumab in AMD patients. Results were expressed as risk ratios (RRs) with accompanying 95% confidence intervals (CIs). The data were pooled using the fixed-effect or random-effect model according to the heterogeneity present.

Results: Four RCTs were included in the final meta-analysis. Overall, the quality of the evidence was high. There were 2,613 treated patients: 1,291 treated with bevacizumab and 1,322 treated with ranibicizumab. No significant differences between bevacizumab use and ranizumab use were found in terms of the incidence of death from all causes, arteriothrombotic events, stroke, nonfatal myocardial infarction, vascular death, venous thrombotic events, and hypertension, with the pooled RRs being 1.11 (0.77, 1.61), 1.03 (0.69,1.55), 0.84 (0.39,1.80), 0.97 (0.48, 1.96), 1.24 (0.63, 2.44), 2.38 (0.94, 6.04), and 1.02 (0.29, 3.62), respectively.

Conclusions: The meta-analysis shows that both treatments are comparably safe. However, the findings from our study must be confirmed in future research via well-designed cohort or intervention studies because of the limited number of studies.

Editor: Andreas Wedrich, Medical University Graz, Austria

Funding: This research was supported by the National Natural Science Foundation of China (81371008). No additional external funding was received. The funders had no role in study design, data collection and analysis, decision to publish, or preparation of the manuscript.

Competing Interests: The authors have declared that no competing interests exist.

* Email: zhangxl2@mail.sysu.edu.cn

Introduction

Age-related macular degeneration (AMD) is the most common cause of blindness in individuals over 50 years of age [1–3]. Although an estimated 80% of patients with AMD have the non-neovascular (dry) form, the neovascular (wet) form is responsible for almost 90% of severe visual losses resulting from AMD [4–6]. Vascular endothelial growth factor-A (VEGF-A) has been proven to play a major role in the pathogenesis of wet AMD [7,8]. Since the mid-2000s, antivascular endothelial growth factor (anti-VEGF) therapy has become the mainstay of treatment for wet AMD [9].

Ranibizumab (Lucentis, Genentech, Inc., South San Francisco, CA, USA) is a recombinant humanized immunoglobulin G1κ isotype monoclonal antibody fragment directed toward all isoforms of VEGF-A [7]. It has been approved for the treatment of wet AMD by the food and drug administration (FDA) in the US (2006), Europe (2007), Japan (2009), and many other countries. However, the cost of ranibizumab is immense: monthly injections

at a dose of 0.5 mg result in an annual cost greater than US $23,000 per patient [10].

Similar to ranibizumab, bevacizumab (Avastin, Genentech, Inc., South San Francisco, CA, USA) is a recombinant humanized full-length antibody that can inhibit all isoforms of VEGF-A [11]. In 2004, it was approved for the treatment of metastatic cancer of the colon or rectum, but it has not gained FDA approval for intravitreal use. Therefore, it can be utilized only in an off-label setting. For the past several years, it has been used off-label to treat wet AMD with very encouraging results. Bevacizumab has attracted more and more interest because of its low cost, which is especially important considering the number of injections that are necessary at 4- to 6-week intervals. A report suggested that the US medicare system could save more than US$1 billion within 2 years if bevacizumab replaced ranibizumab [7,10].

Although anti-VEGF agents are injected in small quantities into the eye, concerns about systemic safety have been raised, especially for the off-label use of bevacizumab. Research has shown that the systemic administration of bevacizumab, along with chemotherapeutic agents, can increase the risk of thromboembolic events two-fold over chemotherapy alone [12]. Many recently published randomized clinical trials (RCTs) have evaluated intravitreal bevacizumab and ranibizumab for the treatment of wet AMD. The results of the comparison of the AMD Treatments Trial (CATT) and the Age-related Choroidal Neovascularization Trial (IVAN) demonstrated that bevacizumab was not inferior to ranibizumab in the treatment of wet AMD [13,14]. However, these studies were not sufficiently powerful to detect drug-specific differences in the rates of systemic adverse events. Hence, the crucial question of whether adverse effects differ between off-label bevacizumab and licensed ranibizumab has not yet been answered [15].

To determine whether the intravitreal injection of bevacizumab creates a higher risk of systemic adverse events than ranibizumab injection does, we undertook a systematic review and meta-analysis of all relevant head-to-head RCTs.

Methods

This study was reported in accordance with the Preferred Reporting Items for Systematic Reviews and Meta-Analyses (PRISMA) statement (Checklist S1) [16]. All stages of study selection, data extraction, and quality assessment were performed independently by two reviewers (W.W. and X.Z.). Any disagreement was resolved via discussion and consensus.

1. Literature Search

Studies were identified through a systematic search of Pubmed, Embase, the Chinese Biomedicine Database, and the Cochrane library from inception up to December 2013. The initial search terms were (Ranibizumab or Lucentis) AND (Bevacizumab or Avastin) AND ("Macular degeneration" or AMD), which were filtered by "Humans" and "Randomized Controlled Trial." In addition, the reference lists of identified studies were manually checked to include other potentially eligible trials. This process was performed iteratively until no additional articles could be identified.

2. Study Selection

Studies were considered acceptable for inclusion in the meta-analysis if they met the following criteria: (1) the study design included randomized clinical trials; (2) the population was patients with wet AMD; (3) the interventions were intravitreal bevacizumab and intravitreal ranibizumab, which were directly compared in head-to-head design; (4) the incidence of systemic adverse events was reported; (5) there was a follow-up time of at least 1 year; and (6) there were at least ten patients in each arm. If there were multiple reports for a particular study, the most recent publication was included. Trials were excluded if they (1) were abstracts, letters, or meeting proceedings; (2) had repeated data or did not report outcomes of interest; or (3) included patients with other indications than wet AMD, patients previously treated with VEGF inhibitors, or patients receiving systemic anti-VEGF therapy.

3. Data Extraction

The following information was extracted from each study: first author; year of publication; study design; inclusion and exclusion criteria; number of patients in each group; characteristics of the study population; adverse events; the period, and number of injections preceding an adverse event. A Thromboembolic Event (TEE) was defined as any arteriothrombotic or venous thrombotic event [17].

4. Quality Assessment

The methodological quality of each trial was evaluated using the Jadad scale [18]. The scale consists of three items describing randomization (0–2 points), blinding (0–2 points), and dropouts and withdrawals (0–1 points) in the reporting of a randomized controlled trial. A score of 1 is given for each of the points described. A further point is awarded when the method of randomization and/or blinding is given and is appropriate, whereas when it is inappropriate, a point is deducted. The quality scale ranges from 0 to 5 points. Higher scores indicate better reporting. The studies are said to be of low quality if the Jadad score is ≤ 2 and of high quality if the score is ≥ 3.

5. Statistical Analysis

All outcomes were expressed as risk ratios (RRs) with accompanying 95% confidence intervals (CIs). Outcome measure was assessed on an intent-to-treat (ITT) basis, the ITT population being comprised of all randomized patients who received the study medication and provided a valid baseline measurement. The cochrane Q test was used to detect the heterogeneity of the effects. Significant heterogeneity was defined as a P value of <0.05. A fixed-effects model or random-effects model was used, depending on the presence or absence of heterogeneity. The I^2 value was used to demonstrate the percentage of the variability attributable to heterogeneity rather than to sampling error. Studies with an I^2 statistic of <25% are considered to have no heterogeneity, those with an I^2 statistic of 25% to 50% are considered to have low heterogeneity, those with an I^2 statistic of 50% to 75% are considered to have moderate heterogeneity, and those with an I^2 statistic of >75% are considered to have high heterogeneity [19]. Sensitivity analyses were performed by investigating the influence of a single study on the overall pooled estimate via omitting one study at a time. Potential publication bias was assessed by using Begg's and Egger's tests [20,21]. A P value <0.05 was judged to be statistically significant, except when otherwise specified. All statistical analyses were performed using Stata version 12.0 (Stata Corp, College Station, TX).

Results

1. Literature Search

The selection process and reasons for exclusion are detailed in Figure 1. The initial search identified 125 potentially relevant articles, of which 71 were excluded based on the titles and abstracts. The remaining 54 were retrieved for a full-text review, and 40 of them were excluded because 38 included unqualified patients, two involved unqualified interventions, eight contained duplicated data [22–29], one did not report outcomes of interest [30], and one contained only one patients (<10) in the ranibizumab arm [31]. Thus, four RCTs [13,14,32,33] were included in the final meta-analysis.

2. Study Characteristics and Quality

The main characteristics of the four RCTs included in the meta-analysis are presented in Table 1, and the outcome data of each included trial are described in Table 2. These studies were published between 2012 and 2013. The sizes of the RCTs ranged from 317 to 1,185 patients (a total of 2,613; 1,291 with bevacizumab and 1,322 with ranibicizumab). Of the four trials, one was done in the USA [14], one in the UK [13], one in France [33], and one in Australia [32]. The trials included in this

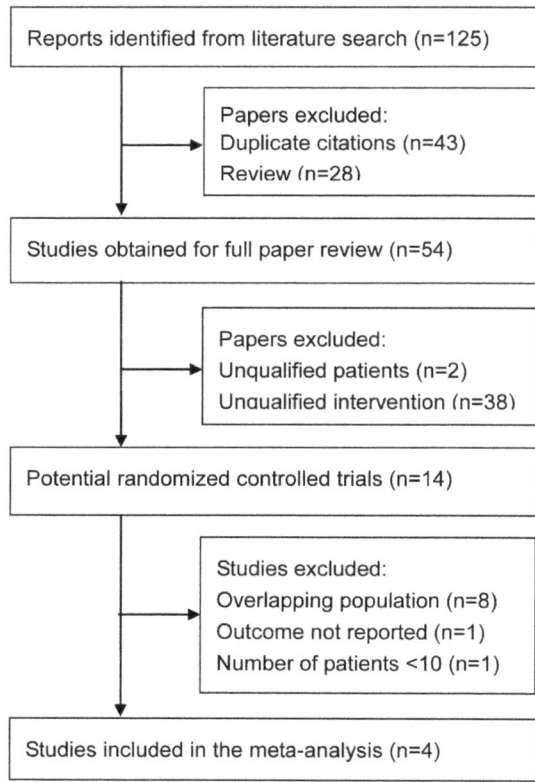

Figure 1. Flowchart of studies included in meta-analysis. RCT, randomized controlled trial.

meta-analysis appeared to have been reasonably designed and conducted. All studies had a statement regarding randomization and double-blindness. Four trials described the methods of randomization. Four trials reported withdrawals and dropouts. All trials described the main outcome, and no missing data seemed to influence the results. The Jadad score of the studies included was 5.

3. Risk of Systemic Adverse Events

The risk estimates for systemic adverse events associated with intravitreal bevacizumab, as compared with ranibizumab, were summarized in Table 3. No significant differences between bevacizumab and ranizumab were found in terms of the incidence of death from all causes, arteriothrombotic events, stroke, nonfatal myocardial infarction, vascular death, venous thrombotic events, and hypertension, with the pooled RRs being 1.11 (0.77, 1.61), 1.03 (0.69,1.55), 0.84 (0.39,1.80), 0.97 (0.48, 1.96), 1.24 (0.63, 2.44), 2.38 (0.94, 6.04), and 1.02 (0.29, 3.62), respectively. When any arteriothrombotic or venous thrombotic events, such as TEE, were combined, no significant difference was detected (RR, 1.22; 95% CI: 0.85 to 1.75; P = 0.292) (Figure 2). Furthermore, when adverse events were divided by MedDRA system organ class, there was also no significant difference between bevacizumab and ranibizumab injections. The tests for heterogeneity were all non-significant (all P>0.1). We tested the robustness of our analyses by performing sensitivity analyses excluding the CATT study (largest trial). Excluding this study did not change our final results.

Table 1. Baseline characteristics of the head-to-head studies comparing ranibizumab with bevacizumab.

Study	Location	Center	Blind	Duration	Intervention	No. of eyes	Age (years)	Male (%)	Visual acuity (letters)	Foveal thickness (mm)
CATT	USA	44	double	2 years	Ranibizumab Monthly	301	79.2±7.4	39.2%	60.1±14.3	458±184
					Bevacizumab Monthly	286	80.1±7.3	37.1%	60.2±13.1	463±196
					Ranibizumab as Needed	298	78.4±7.8	37.9%	61.5±13.2	458±193
					Bevacizumab as Needed	300	79.3±7.6	38.7%	60.4±13.4	461±175
IVAN	UK	23	double	2 years	Ranibizumab	314	77.8±7.6	41%	67.8±17.0	471.6±192.5
					Bevacizumab	296	77.7±7.3	39%	66.1±18.4	465.6±183.1
GEFAL	France	38	double	1 year	Ranibizumab	129	78.68±7.27	31.21%	55.78±13.99	354.75±109.90
					Bevacizumab	119	79.62±6.90	35.82%	54.62±14.07	359.21±120.72
MANTA	Austria	10	double	1 year	Ranibizumab	163	77.6±8.1	36.20%	56.4±13.5	365.0±8.1
					Bevacizumab	154	76.7±7.8	36.36%	57.0±13.0	374.6±8.4

CATT = The Comparison of Age-related macular degeneration Treatments Trials; IVAN = The Alternative treatments to Inhibit VEGF in Age-related choroidal Neovascularization study; MANTA = The Multicenter Anti-VEGF Trial; GEFAL = The Groupe d'Etude Français Avastin versus Lucentis dans la DMLA néovasculaire (The French Study Group Avastin versus Lucentis for neovascular AMD).

Table 2. Outcome data of randomized controlled trials included in the meta-analysis.

Adverse events	CAAT Ranibizumab (N = 599)	CAAT Bevacizumab (N = 586)	IVAN Ranibizumab (N = 314)	IVAN Bevacizumab (N = 296)	GEFAL Ranibizumab (N = 246)	GEFAL Bevacizumab (N = 255)	MANTA Ranibizumab (N = 163)	MANTA Bevacizumab (N = 154)
Systemic adverse event								
Death-all causes	32	36	15	15	3	2	2	3
Arteriothrombotic events	28*	29	13	10	1	1	3	5
Stroke	8	8	6	3	0	0	1	1
Nonfatal myocardial infarction	9	7	4	4	1	1	2	3
Vascular death	12	14	3	4	0	0	0	0
Venous thrombotic events	3	10	3	4	0	1	0	0
Hypertension	3	4	0	0	2	1	0	0
MedDRA system organ class								
Cardiac disorders	47	62	20	19	5	2	1	1
Infections	41	54	9	12	2	4	3	3
Nervous system disorders	34	36	9	8	0	3	1	2
Injury and procedural complications	23	35	12	10	2	4	3	2
Neoplasms benign and malignant	27	22	11	14	1	1	2	1
Surgical and medical procedures	0	0	16	14	0	5	0	1
Gastrointestinal disorders	11	28	3	9	5	3	0	0
Any other system organ class	81	104	25	27	11	10	2	3

Table 3. Risk ratio of systemic adverse events associated with intravitreal bevacizumab compared with ranibizumab.

Avastin vs Lucentis	Study(n)	RR (95%CI)			Heterogeneity		Overall Effect	
		Estimate	Lower	Up	P	I²(%)	Z	P
Death-all causes	4	1.11	0.77	1.61	0.907	0.00%	0.56	0.572
Arteriothrombotic events	4	1.03	0.69	1.55	0.828	0.00%	0.15	0.879
Stroke	3	0.84	0.39	1.80	0.737	0.00%	0.46	0.649
Nonfatal myocardial infarction	4	0.97	0.48	1.96	0.925	0.00%	0.09	0.928
Vascular death	2	1.24	0.63	2.44	0.842	0.00%	0.61	0.541
Venous thrombotic events	3	2.38	0.94	6.04	0.676	0.00%	1.83	0.067
Hypertension	2	1.02	0.29	3.62	0.471	0.00%	0.03	0.977
MedDRA system organ class								
Cardiac disorders	4	1.20	0.88	1.62	0.460	0.00%	1.16	0.245
Infections	4	1.36	0.97	1.91	0.965	0.00%	1.79	0.074
Nervous system disorders	4	1.11	0.75	1.66	0.606	0.00%	0.52	0.602
Injury and procedural complications	4	1.31	0.87	1.98	0.578	0.00%	1.30	0.194
Neoplasms benign and malignant	4	0.96	0.62	1.48	0.743	0.00%	0.18	0.854
Surgical and medical procedures	3	1.75	0.43	7.16	0.222	33.60%	0.78	0.434
Gastrointestinal disorders	3	1.90	0.78	4.62	0.141	49.00%	1.41	0.158
Any other system organ class	4	1.25	0.99	1.56	0.803	0.00%	1.90	0.058

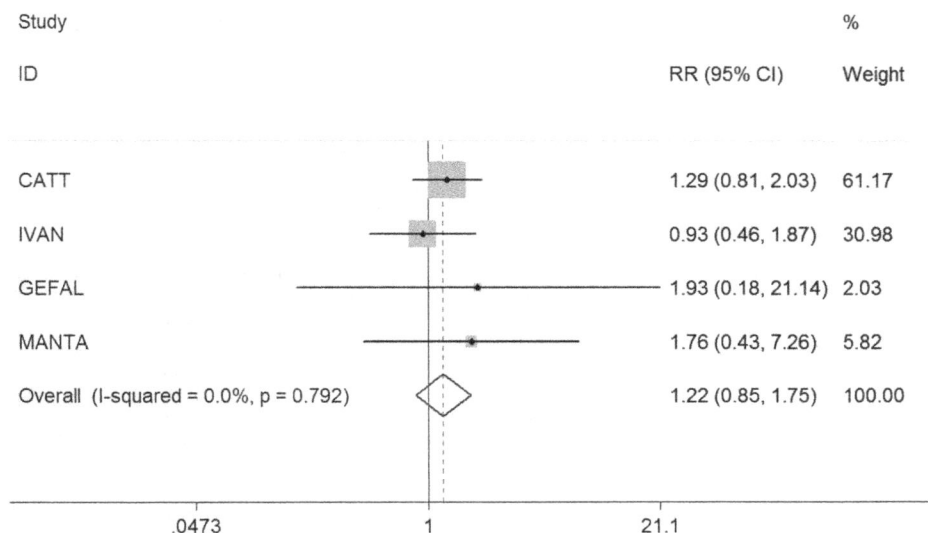

Figure 2. Risk ratio of thromboembolic events associated with intravitreal bevacizumab compared with ranibizumab. Each study is shown by the point estimate of relative risk "risk ratio" (RR) - the size of the square is proportional to the weight of the study - and 95%confidence interval for the RR (lines extending from the squares); the pooled RR and 95%confidence interval are shown as a diamond.

4. Publication Bias

Due to the limited number (<10) of studies included in each analysis, publication bias was not assessed.

Discussion

The development of VEGF inhibitors has revolutionized the treatment of AMD. Bevacizumab and ranibizumab are the two most common VEGF inhibitors in ophthalmic practice [34]. Although anti-VEGF agents are injected into the eye in small quantities, concerns about systemic safety have been raised [35]. Until relatively recently, high-quality data comparing the efficacy and safety of ranibizumab and bevacizumab in AMD were lacking. Because many adverse events are relatively uncommon, clinical trials often lack the power to detect small but clinically important risk differences. Hence, meta-analyses pooling data from multiple studies provide important insights [15,36]. The main aim of this study is to provide an evidence-based analysis of the safety profile for bevacizumab versus that of intravitreal ranibizumab injections in patients with AMD. In the present meta-analysis, we have reviewed the literature regarding the safety of intravitreal bevacizumab as compared with that of ranibizumab. The pooled results suggest that the incidence of specific systemic complications did not differ significant between bevacizumab and ranibizumab. Also, no heterogeneity was observed across the studies.

Several high-quality non-randomized studies [37–40] focusing on adverse effects for bevacizumab versus ranibizumab are summarized in Table 4. All of them reported that the rates of specific systemic adverse events, such as all-cause mortality, stroke, acute myocardial infarction, and venous thromboembolism during the bevacizumab and ranibizumab periods were not different. However, the limitation of these studies was that a non-randomized study design was used (case control or cohort study). The principal finding of our meta-analysis is consistent with the aforementioned studies on the topic.

Thus far, ranibizumab and bevacizumab have been evaluated in several systematic reviews [11,17,34,41]. However, the published reviews focused on the beneficial effects and clinical effectiveness of VEGF inhibitors, without adequately addressing their adverse effects. Furthermore, they are mainly based on indirect comparative studies; this may lower the evidence level. In Schmucker and colleagues' report [41], only one multiple-center, head-to-head RCT (CATT) was included; it had relatively modest sample sizes. In another meta-analysis by Chakravarthy et al. [13], no difference in the frequency of death, arterial thrombotic events, or hospital admission for heart failure was recorded between the drugs. Their study is limited by the fact that only 1-year CATT data were included. In our study, we incorporated the 2-year CATT data and two other well-designed RCTs. We found a similar risk of specific adverse events between the bevacizumab and ranibizumab groups. From a theoretical viewpoint, the risk of the development of systemic adverse events may be higher with bevacizumab than with ranibizumab [10]. Bevacizumab is more likely to induce immunologic activation and will remain in systemic circulation than ranibizumab. Thus, bevacizumab administration may create a higher risk of systemic adverse events. These highlight the need for ongoing surveillance and large population-based studies to investigate these outcomes [15].

The results of this meta-analysis must be interpreted cautiously in light of the strengths and limitations of the included trials. A key strength of this study is the fact that all the studies included in this meta-analysis were published by established centers of excellence using a randomized controlled design and all of them were well-performed and of high quality. In addition, with the enlarged sample size, we have enhanced statistical power to provide more precise and reliable effect estimates. Despite our rigorous methodology, some limitations of the current study should not be ignored. First, we cannot fully exclude publication bias. The number of included studies is insufficient to carry out further statistical testing to detect publication bias through an asymmetry plot. In addition, we did not attempt to gain access to unpublished results. More RCTs are warranted to confirm or refute our finding in the future update meta-analysis. Second, all studies have come from western populations with predominately Caucasian participants. The relatively good distribution of the study population makes findings from this meta-analysis a fair representation of the general population. The safety of these drugs for other ethnicities,

Table 4. Summary of high-quality non-randomized studies comparing ranibizumab with bevacizumab.

Author, country	Design	Population	Method	Results
Campbell et al., 2012, Canada	Population based nested case-control study	Older adults with a history of physician diagnosed retinal disease identified between 1 April 2006 and 31 March 2011.	Cases were patients admitted to hospital for ischaemic stroke, acute myocardial infarction, venous thromboembolism, for congestive heart failure. Event-free controls were matched to cases on the basis of year of birth, sex, history of the outcome in the previous 5 years, and diabetes	Adjusted odds ratios for bevacizumab relative to ranibizumab were 1.03 (0.67 to 1.60) for ischaemic stroke, 1.23 (0.85 to 1.77) for acute myocardial infarction, 0.92 (0.51 to 1.69) for venous thromboembolism, and 1.35 (0.93 to 1.95) for congestive heart failure. Results showed these risks did not differ significantly between bevacizumab and ranibizumab injections.
Campbell et al., 2012, Canada	Population-based, time series analysis	All patients aged 66 years or older with physician-diagnosed retinal disease between 2002 and 2010 (N = 116 388).	Segmented regression analysis was used to evaluate changes in the rate of hospitalization for ischemic stroke associated with the introduction of bevacizumab and ranibizumab.	Bevacizumab trend change coefficient: -0.0026 stroke hospitalizations/1000 subjects/month (P = 0.20); Ranibizumab trend change coefficient: -0.0011 stroke hospitalizations/1000 subjects/month (P = 0.78). Results showed that stroke rates in the bevacizumab and ranibizumab periods were not different.
French et al., 2011, USA	Cohort study	Beneficiaries of the Veterans Health Administration aged ≥55 years with AMD in fiscal years 2007-2009 were included.	Anti-vascular endothelial growth factor exposure was identified through pharmacy records. Cox proportional hazard model was adjusted for age, gender, number of injections, and ocular and medical comorbidities.	The adjusted HR for all-cause mortality were 0.94 (95%CI: 0.72 to 1.22) for bevacizumab and 0.85 (95%CI: 0.67 to1.08) for ranibizumab. Results showed lack an association between the use of either ranibizumab or bevacizumab and mortality.
Curtis et al., 2010, USA	Cohort study	Medicare beneficiaries 65 years or older with a claim for AMD in fiscal years 2005-2006 were included.	When the patients received a therapy different from the initial therapy, the data were censored. The associations between anti-VEGF therapies and the risks of all-cause mortality, incident myocardial infarction, bleeding, and incident stroke were calculated.	Adjusted HRs for ranibizumab relative to bevacizumab were 0.90 (0.79-1.02) for all-cause mortality, 0.84 (0.66-1.06) for myocardial infarction, 1.03 (0.93-1.15) for bleeding, 0.81 (0.68-0.98) for stroke. Results showed these risks did not differ significantly between bevacizumab and ranibizumab injections.

such as Asians, must be tested. Furthermore, patients enrolled in RCTs meet strict eligibility criteria, which may exclude many patients at a higher risk for systemic adverse events. These limitations likely resulted in an underestimation of the incidence of systemic adverse events. However, the determination of the risk of systemic adverse events associated with bevacizumab versus ranibizumab was not likely affected, because this underestimation should have had similar impacts on both arms. Finally, given that the treatment of wet AMD is not limited to 2 years, more data from studies of longer durations are needed to determine the relative safety of each anti-VEGF agent over the long term.

In conclusion, there is no difference between bevacizumab and ranibizumab in terms of the risk of specific systemic adverse events. However, the results should be interpreted cautiously because the relevant evidence remains limited, and the findings must be confirmed through future research involving well-designed cohort studies or RCTs.

Author Contributions

Conceived and designed the experiments: WW XZ. Performed the experiments: WW XZ. Analyzed the data: WW XZ. Contributed reagents/materials/analysis tools: WW XZ. Wrote the paper: WW XZ.

References

1. Owen CG, Jarrar Z, Wormald R, Cook DG, Fletcher AE, et al. (2012) The estimated prevalence and incidence of late stage age related macular degeneration in the UK. Br J Ophthalmol 96: 752–756.
2. Rudnicka AR, Jarrar Z, Wormald R, Cook DG, Fletcher A, et al. (2012) Age and gender variations in age-related macular degeneration prevalence in populations of European ancestry: a meta-analysis. Ophthalmology 119: 571–580.
3. Kawasaki R, Yasuda M, Song SJ, Chen SJ, Jonas JB, et al. (2010) The prevalence of age-related macular degeneration in Asians: a systematic review and meta-analysis. Ophthalmology 117: 921–927.
4. Schmier JK, Jones ML, Halpern MT (2006) The burden of age-related macular degeneration. Pharmacoeconomics 24: 319–334.
5. Brown MM, Brown GC, Sharma S, Stein JD, Roth Z, et al. (2006) The burden of age-related macular degeneration: a value-based analysis. Curr Opin Ophthalmol 17: 257–266.
6. Ferris FR, Wilkinson CP, Bird A, Chakravarthy U, Chew E, et al. (2013) Clinical classification of age-related macular degeneration. Ophthalmology 120: 844–851.
7. Frampton JE (2013) Ranibizumab: a review of its use in the treatment of neovascular age-related macular degeneration. Drugs Aging 30: 331–358.

8. Ambati J, Fowler BJ (2012) Mechanisms of age-related macular degeneration. Neuron 75: 26–39.
9. Lally DR, Gerstenblith AT, Regillo CD (2012) Preferred therapies for neovascular age-related macular degeneration. Curr Opin Ophthalmol 23: 182–188.
10. Campbell RJ, Bell CM, Campbell EL, Gill SS (2013) Systemic effects of intravitreal vascular endothelial growth factor inhibitors. Curr Opin Ophthalmol 24: 197–204.
11. Schmucker C, Ehlken C, Hansen LL, Antes G, Agostini HT, et al. (2010) Intravitreal bevacizumab (Avastin) vs. ranibizumab (Lucentis) for the treatment of age-related macular degeneration: a systematic review. Curr Opin Ophthalmol 21: 218–226.
12. Hurwitz HI, Tebbutt NC, Kabbinavar F, Giantonio BJ, Guan ZZ, et al. (2013) Efficacy and safety of bevacizumab in metastatic colorectal cancer: pooled analysis from seven randomized controlled trials. Oncologist 18: 1004–1012.
13. Chakravarthy U, Harding SP, Rogers CA, Downes SM, Lotery AJ, et al. (2013) Alternative treatments to inhibit VEGF in age-related choroidal neovascularisation: 2-year findings of the IVAN randomised controlled trial. Lancet 382: 1258–1267.

14. Martin DF, Maguire MG, Fine SL, Ying GS, Jaffe GJ, et al. (2012) Ranibizumab and bevacizumab for treatment of neovascular age-related macular degeneration: two-year results. Ophthalmology 119: 1388–1398.

15. Cheung CM, Wong TY (2013) Treatment of age-related macular degeneration. Lancet 382: 1230–1232.

16. Moher D, Liberati A, Tetzlaff J, Altman DG (2009) Preferred reporting items for systematic reviews and meta-analyses: the PRISMA statement. J Clin Epidemiol 62: 1006–1012.

17. Abouammoh MA (2013) Ranibizumab injection for diabetic macular edema: meta-analysis of systemic safety and systematic review. Can J Ophthalmol 48: 317–323.

18. Jadad AR, Moore RA, Carroll D, Jenkinson C, Reynolds DJ, et al. (1996) Assessing the quality of reports of randomized clinical trials: is blinding necessary? Control Clin Trials 17: 1–12.

19. Higgins JP, Thompson SG, Deeks JJ, Altman DG (2003) Measuring inconsistency in meta-analyses. BMJ 327: 557–560.

20. Egger M, Davey SG, Schneider M, Minder C (1997) Bias in meta-analysis detected by a simple, graphical test. BMJ 315: 629–634.

21. Begg CB, Mazumdar M (1994) Operating characteristics of a rank correlation test for publication bias. Biometrics 50: 1088–1101.

22. Ying GS, Huang J, Maguire MG, Jaffe GJ, Grunwald JE, et al. (2013) Baseline predictors for one-year visual outcomes with ranibizumab or bevacizumab for neovascular age-related macular degeneration. Ophthalmology 120: 122–129.

23. Jaffe GJ, Martin DF, Toth CA, Daniel E, Maguire MG, et al. (2013) Macular morphology and visual acuity in the comparison of age-related macular degeneration treatments trials. Ophthalmology 120: 1860–1870.

24. DeCroos FC, Toth CA, Stinnett SS, Heydary CS, Burns R, et al. (2012) Optical coherence tomography grading reproducibility during the Comparison of Age-related Macular Degeneration Treatments Trials. Ophthalmology 119: 2549–2557.

25. Chakravarthy U, Harding SP, Rogers CA, Downes SM, Lotery AJ, et al. (2012) Ranibizumab versus bevacizumab to treat neovascular age-related macular degeneration: one-year findings from the IVAN randomized trial. Ophthalmology 119: 1399–1411.

26. Grunwald JE, Daniel E, Ying GS, Pistilli M, Maguire MG, et al. (2012) Photographic assessment of baseline fundus morphologic features in the Comparison of Age-Related Macular Degeneration Treatments Trials. Ophthalmology 119: 1634–1641.

27. Martin DF, Maguire MG, Ying GS, Grunwald JE, Fine SL, et al. (2011) Ranibizumab and bevacizumab for neovascular age-related macular degeneration. N Engl J Med 364: 1897–1908.

28. Donahue SP, Recchia F, Sternberg PJ (2010) Bevacizumab vs ranibizumab for age-related macular degeneration: early results of a prospective double-masked, randomized clinical trial. Am J Ophthalmol 150: 287, 287.

29. Subramanian ML, Ness S, Abedi G, Ahmed E, Daly M, et al. (2009) Bevacizumab vs ranibizumab for age-related macular degeneration: early results of a prospective double-masked, randomized clinical trial. Am J Ophthalmol 148: 875–882.

30. Biswas P, Sengupta S, Choudhary R, Home S, Paul A, et al. (2011) Comparative role of intravitreal ranibizumab versus bevacizumab in choroidal neovascular membrane in age-related macular degeneration. Indian J Ophthalmol 59: 191–196.

31. Subramanian ML, Abedi G, Ness S, Ahmed E, Fenberg M, et al. (2010) Bevacizumab vs ranibizumab for age-related macular degeneration: 1-year outcomes of a prospective, double-masked randomised clinical trial. Eye (Lond) 24: 1708–1715.

32. Krebs I, Schmetterer L, Boltz A, Told R, Vecsei-Marlovits V, et al. (2013) A randomised double-masked trial comparing the visual outcome after treatment with ranibizumab or bevacizumab in patients with neovascular age-related macular degeneration. Br J Ophthalmol 97: 266–271.

33. Kodjikian L, Souied EH, Mimoun G, Mauget-Faysse M, Behar-Cohen F, et al. (2013) Ranibizumab versus Bevacizumab for Neovascular Age-related Macular Degeneration: Results from the GEFAL Noninferiority Randomized Trial. Ophthalmology.

34. Mitchell P (2011) A systematic review of the efficacy and safety outcomes of anti-VEGF agents used for treating neovascular age-related macular degeneration: comparison of ranibizumab and bevacizumab. Curr Med Res Opin 27: 1465–1475.

35. Aujla JS (2012) Replacing ranibizumab with bevacizumab on the Pharmaceutical Benefits Scheme: where does the current evidence leave us? Clin Exp Optom 95: 538–540.

36. Torjesen I (2013) Avastin is as effective as Lucentis in treating wet age related macular degeneration, study finds. BMJ 347: f4678.

37. Campbell RJ, Gill SS, Bronskill SE, Paterson JM, Whitehead M, et al. (2012) Adverse events with intravitreal injection of vascular endothelial growth factor inhibitors: nested case-control study. BMJ 345: e4203.

38. Campbell RJ, Bell CM, Paterson JM, Bronskill SE, Moineddin R, et al. (2012) Stroke rates after introduction of vascular endothelial growth factor inhibitors for macular degeneration: a time series analysis. Ophthalmology 119: 1604–1608.

39. French DD, Margo CE (2011) Age-related macular degeneration, anti-vascular endothelial growth factor agents, and short-term mortality: a postmarketing medication safety and surveillance study. Retina 31: 1036–1042.

40. Curtis LH, Hammill BG, Schulman KA, Cousins SW (2010) Risks of mortality, myocardial infarction, bleeding, and stroke associated with therapies for age-related macular degeneration. Arch Ophthalmol 128: 1273–1279.

41. Schmucker C, Ehlken C, Agostini HT, Antes G, Ruecker G, et al. (2012) A safety review and meta-analyses of bevacizumab and ranibizumab: off-label versus goldstandard. PLoS One 7: e42701.

Permissions

All chapters in this book were first published in PLOS ONE, by The Public Library of Science; hereby published with permission under the Creative Commons Attribution License or equivalent. Every chapter published in this book has been scrutinized by our experts. Their significance has been extensively debated. The topics covered herein carry significant findings which will fuel the growth of the discipline. They may even be implemented as practical applications or may be referred to as a beginning point for another development.

The contributors of this book come from diverse backgrounds, making this book a truly international effort. This book will bring forth new frontiers with its revolutionizing research information and detailed analysis of the nascent developments around the world.

We would like to thank all the contributing authors for lending their expertise to make the book truly unique. They have played a crucial role in the development of this book. Without their invaluable contributions this book wouldn't have been possible. They have made vital efforts to compile up to date information on the varied aspects of this subject to make this book a valuable addition to the collection of many professionals and students.

This book was conceptualized with the vision of imparting up-to-date information and advanced data in this field. To ensure the same, a matchless editorial board was set up. Every individual on the board went through rigorous rounds of assessment to prove their worth. After which they invested a large part of their time researching and compiling the most relevant data for our readers.

The editorial board has been involved in producing this book since its inception. They have spent rigorous hours researching and exploring the diverse topics which have resulted in the successful publishing of this book. They have passed on their knowledge of decades through this book. To expedite this challenging task, the publisher supported the team at every step. A small team of assistant editors was also appointed to further simplify the editing procedure and attain best results for the readers.

Apart from the editorial board, the designing team has also invested a significant amount of their time in understanding the subject and creating the most relevant covers. They scrutinized every image to scout for the most suitable representation of the subject and create an appropriate cover for the book.

The publishing team has been an ardent support to the editorial, designing and production team. Their endless efforts to recruit the best for this project, has resulted in the accomplishment of this book. They are a veteran in the field of academics and their pool of knowledge is as vast as their experience in printing. Their expertise and guidance has proved useful at every step. Their uncompromising quality standards have made this book an exceptional effort. Their encouragement from time to time has been an inspiration for everyone.

The publisher and the editorial board hope that this book will prove to be a valuable piece of knowledge for researchers, students, practitioners and scholars across the globe.

List of Contributors

Paul Mitchell and Elena Rochtchina
Department of Ophthalmology and Westmead Millennium Institute, University of Sydney, Westmead, New South Wales, Australia

Neil Bressler
Wilmer Eye Institute, Johns Hopkins University, Baltimore, Maryland, United States of America

Quan V. Doan and Mark Danese
Outcomes Insights, Inc., Westlake Village, California, United States of America

Chantal Dolan
CMD Consulting, Inc., Sandy, Utah, United States of America

Alberto Ferreira and Aaron Osborne
Novartis, Basel, Switzerland

Shoshana Colman
Genentech, Inc., South San Francisco, California, United States of America

Tien Y. Wong
Singapore Eye Research Institute, National University of Singapore, Singapore, Singapore
Centre for Eye Research Australia, University of Melbourne, Parkville, Victoria, Australia

M. Cristina Kenney, Marilyn Chwa, Shari R. Atilano, Janelle M. Pavlis, Payam Falatoonzadeh, Claudio Ramirez, Deepika Malik, Tiffany Hsu, Grace Woo, Kyaw Soe, Baruch D. Kuppermann and Nitin Udar
Gavin Herbert Eye Institute, University of California Irvine, Irvine, California, United States of America

Anthony B. Nesburn
Gavin Herbert Eye Institute, University of California Irvine, Irvine, California, United States of America
Cedars-Sinai Medical Center, Los Angeles, California, United States of America

David S. Boyer
Retina-Vitreous Associates Medical Group, Beverly Hills, California, United States of America

S. Michal Jazwinski and Michael V. Miceli
Tulane Center for Aging and Department of Medicine, Tulane University, New Orleans, Louisiana, United States of America

Douglas C. Wallace
Children's Hospital of Pittsburgh, Pittsburgh, Pennsylvania, United States of America

Peng Zhou, Hong-Fei Ye, Yong-Xiang Jiang, Jin Yang, Xiang-Jia Zhu, Xing-Huai Sun, Yi Luo and Yi Lu
Department of Ophthalmology, Eye and ENT Hospital of Fudan University, Shanghai, People's Republic of China

Guo-Rui Dou and Yu-Sheng Wang
Department of Ophthalmology, Xijing Hospital, Fourth Military Medical University, Xi'an, People's Republic of China

Mahsa Sohrab, Katherine Wu and Amani A. Fawzi
Department of Ophthalmology, Northwestern University, Feinberg School of Medicine, Chicago, Illinois, United States of America

John Paul SanGiovanni and Emily Y. Chew
Clinical Trials Branch, National Eye Institute, National Institutes of Health, Bethesda, Maryland, United States of America

Jing Chen, Christopher M. Aderman and Lois E. H. Smith
Department of Ophthalmology, Harvard Medical School, The Children's Hospital, Boston, Massachusetts, United States of America

Przemyslaw Sapieha
Department of Ophthalmology, Maisonneuve-Rosemont Hospital Research Centre, University of Montreal, Montreal, Quebec, Canada

Andreas Stahl
Department of Ophthalmology, University Eye Hospital Freiburg, Freiburg, Germany

Traci E. Clemons
The EMMES Corp., Rockville, Maryland, United States of America

Stuart Cantsilieris
Centre for Eye Research Australia, University of Melbourne, Royal Victorian Eye and Ear Hospital, East Melbourne, Victoria, Australia
Centre for Reproduction and Development, Monash Institute of Medical Research, Melbourne, Victoria, Australia

Stefan J. White
Centre for Reproduction and Development, Monash Institute of Medical Research, Melbourne, Victoria, Australia

Andrea J. Richardson, Robyn H. Guymer and Paul N. Baird
Centre for Eye Research Australia, University of Melbourne, Royal Victorian Eye and Ear Hospital, East Melbourne, Victoria, Australia

Johanna M. Seddon
Ophthalmic Epidemiology and Genetics Service, Tufts University School of Medicine and Tufts Medical Center, New England Eye Center, Boston, Massachusetts, United States of America
Department of Ophthalmology, Tufts University School of Medicine, Boston, Massachusetts, United States of America

Robyn Reynolds and Yi Yu
Ophthalmic Epidemiology and Genetics Service, Tufts University School of Medicine and Tufts Medical Center, New England Eye Center, Boston, Massachusetts, United States of America

Bernard Rosner
Channing Laboratory, Brigham and Women's Hospital and Harvard School of Public Health, Harvard University, Boston, Massachusetts, United States of America

Akshay Anand, Neel Kamal Sharma, Sudesh Prabhakar and Pawan Kumar Gupta
Department of Neurology, Post Graduate Institute of Medical Education and Research (PGIMER), Chandigarh, India

Amod Gupta and Ramandeep Singh
Department of Ophthalmology, Post Graduate Institute of Medical Education and Research (PGIMER), Chandigarh, India

Suresh Kumar Sharma
Department of Statistics, Panjab University, Chandigarh, India

Michal Lederman and Alexey Obolensky
Department of Ophthalmology, Hadassah-Hebrew University Medical Center, and the Hebrew University-Hadassah School of Medicine, Jerusalem, Israel
Department of Cellular Biochemistry and Human Genetics, Hadassah-Hebrew University Medical Center, and the Hebrew University-Hadassah School of Medicine, Jerusalem, Israel

Shira Hagbi-Levi, Michelle Grunin, Eyal Banin and Itay Chowers
Department of Ophthalmology, Hadassah-Hebrew University Medical Center, and the Hebrew University-Hadassah School of Medicine, Jerusalem, Israel

Eduard Berenshtein and Mordechai Chevion
Department of Cellular Biochemistry and Human Genetics, Hadassah-Hebrew University Medical Center, and the Hebrew University-Hadassah School of Medicine, Jerusalem, Israel

Xia Li, Yan Cai, Yu-Sheng Wang, Yuan-Yuan Shi, Hai-Yan Wang and Zi Ye
Department of Ophthalmology, Xijing Hospital, Fourth Military Medical University, Xi'an, Shaanxi Province, People's Republic of China

Wei Hou
Department of Orthopedics, Xijing Hospital, Fourth Military Medical University, Xi'an, Shaanxi Province, People's Republic of China

Chun-Sheng Xu
State Key Laboratory of Cancer Biology, Department of Gastrointestinal Surgery, Xijing Hospital, Fourth Military Medical University, Xi'an, Shaanxi Province, People's Republic of China

Li-Bo Yao and Jian Zhang
State Key Laboratory of Cancer Biology, Department of Biochemistry and Molecular Biology, Fourth Military Medical University, Xi'an, Shaanxi Province, People's Republic of China

Bum-Joo Cho, Jang Won Heo and Hum Chung
Department of Ophthalmology, Seoul National University College of Medicine, Seoul, Korea
Department of Ophthalmology, Seoul National University Hospital, Seoul, Korea

Jae Pil Shin
Department of Ophthalmology, Kyungpook National University School of Medicine, Daegu, Korea

Jeeyun Ahn and Tae Wan Kim
Department of Ophthalmology, Seoul National University College of Medicine, Seoul, Korea
Department of Ophthalmology, Seoul Metropolitan Government Seoul National University Boramae Medical Center, Seoul, Korea

Fernando Cruz-Guilloty and Victor L. Perez
Bascom Palmer Eye Institute, Department of Ophthalmology, University of Miami Miller School of Medicine, Miami, Florida, United States of America

Department of Microbiology and Immunology, University of Miami Miller School of Medicine, Miami, Florida, United States of America

Ali M. Saeed, Stephanie Duffort, Asha Ballmick and Yaohong Tan
Bascom Palmer Eye Institute, Department of Ophthalmology, University of Miami Miller School of Medicine, Miami, Florida, United States of America

Marisol Cano, Katayoon B. Ebrahimi and James T. Handa
Wilmer Eye Institute, Department of Ophthalmology, Johns Hopkins University School of Medicine, Baltimore, Maryland, United States of America

Hua Wang, James M. Laird and Robert G. Salomon
Department of Chemistry, Case Western Reserve University, Cleveland, Ohio, United States of America

Alice L. Yu and Johannes Burger
Department of Ophthalmology, Ludwig-Maximilians-University, Muenchen, Germany

Kerstin Birke and Ulrich Welge-Lussen
Department of Ophthalmology, Friedrich-Alexander-University, Erlangen, Germany

Felix Grassmann, Lars G. Fritsche and Bernhard H. F. Weber
Institute of Human Genetics, University of Regensburg, Regensburg, Germany

Claudia N. Keilhauer
University Eye Hospital Würzburg, Würzburg, Germany

Iris M. Heid
Institute of Epidemiology and Preventive Medicine, University Hospital Regensburg, Regensburg, Germany Institute of Genetic Epidemiology, Helmholtz Zentrum München, German Research Center for Environmental Health, Neuherberg, Germany

Yong Cheng, Lv Zhen Huang and Xiaoxin Li
Department of Ophthalmology, People's Hospital, Peking University, Beijing, China Key Laboratory of Vision Loss and Restoration, Ministry of Education, Beijing, China

Peng Zhou
Department of Ophthalmology, Eye and ENT Hospital of Fudan University, Shanghai, China

Wotan Zeng
Chinese National Human Genome Center, Beijing, China

ChunFang Zhang
Department of Clinical Epidemiology, People's Hospital, Peking University, Beijing, China

Kee Dong Yoon, Kazunori Yamamoto, Keiko Ueda and Jilin Zhou
Department of Ophthalmology, Columbia University, New York, New York, United States of America

Janet R. Sparrow
Department of Ophthalmology, Columbia University, New York, New York, United States of America Department of Pathology and Cell Biology, Columbia University, New York, New York, United States of America

Michaela Dithmer, Elisabeth Richert, Johann Roider and Alexa Klettner
University of Kiel, University Medical Center, Department of Ophthalmology, Kiel, Germany

Sabine Fuchs and Yang Shi
University of Kiel, University Medical Center, Experimental Trauma Surgery, Kiel, Germany

Harald Schmidt
MetaPhysiol, Essenheim, Germany

Ian J. Saldanha, Kay Dickersin, Xue Wang, Tianjing Li
Department of Epidemiology, Johns Hopkins Bloomberg School of Public Health, Baltimore, Maryland, United States of America

Elton R. Kelly, Aize Kijlstra and Tos T. J. M. Berendschot
University Eye Clinic Maastricht, Maastricht University, Maastricht, the Netherlands

Jogchum Plat
Department of Human Biology, Maastricht University, Maastricht, the Netherlands

Guido R. M. M. Haenen
Department of Pharmacology and Toxicology, Maastricht University, Maastricht, the Netherlands

Michael Janusz Koss
Department of Ophthalmology, Goethe University, Frankfurt am Main, Germany Doheny Eye Institute, Los Angeles, California, United States of America Department of Ophthalmology, Ruprecht Karls University, Heidelberg, Germany

Janosch Hoffmann and Julie Klein
Mosaiques Diagnostics, Hannover, Germany

Nauke Nguyen and Frank Koch
Department of Ophthalmology, Goethe University, Frankfurt am Main, Germany

Marcel Pfister
Doheny Eye Institute, Los Angeles, California, United States of America

Harald Mischak
Mosaiques Diagnostics, Hannover, Germany
BHF Glasgow Cardiovascular Research Centre, University of Glasgow, Glasgow, United Kingdom

William Mullen and Holger Husi
BHF Glasgow Cardiovascular Research Centre, University of Glasgow, Glasgow, United Kingdom

Robert Rejdak
Department of General Ophthalmology, Lublin University, Poland

Joachim Jankowski and Katharina Krueger
Department of Nephrology, Endocrinology, and Transplantation Medicine Charité-Universitaetsmedizin, Berlin, Germany

Thomas Bertelmann
Department of Ophthalmology, Philipps University, Marburg, Germany

Joost P. Schanstra
Mosaiques Diagnostics, Hannover, Germany
Institut National de la Santé et de la Recherche Me´dicale (INSERM), U1048, Institut of Cardiovascular and Metabolic Disease, Toulouse, France
Universite´ Toulouse III Paul-Sabatier, Toulouse, France

Justyna Siwy
Mosaiques Diagnostics, Hannover, Germany
Department of Nephrology, Endocrinology, and Transplantation Medicine Charite´-Universitaetsmedizin, Berlin, Germany

Xue Chen
Department of Ophthalmology, The First Affiliated Hospital of Nanjing Medical University and State Key Laboratory of Reproductive Medicine, Nanjing Medical University, Nanjing, China
Department of Ophthalmology and Visual Sciences, The Chinese University of Hong Kong, Hong Kong, China

Shi Song Rong, Fang Yao Tang, Pancy O. S. Tam, Li Jia Chen, Mårten E. Brelén and Chi Pui Pang
Department of Ophthalmology and Visual Sciences, The Chinese University of Hong Kong, Hong Kong, China

Qihua Xu
Department of Ophthalmology, The First Affiliated Hospital of Nanjing Medical University and State Key Laboratory of Reproductive Medicine, Nanjing Medical University, Nanjing, China
Department of Ophthalmology, The Affiliated Jiangyin Hospital of Southeast University Medical College, Jiangyin, China

Yuan Liu and Chen Zhao
Department of Ophthalmology, The First Affiliated Hospital of Nanjing Medical University and State Key Laboratory of Reproductive Medicine, Nanjing Medical University, Nanjing, China

Hong Gu
Department of Ophthalmology and Visual Sciences, The Chinese University of Hong Kong, Hong Kong, China
Department of Ophthalmology, Ningbo Medical Treatment Center Lihuili Hospital, Ningbo, China

Ryo Obata and Yasuo Yanagi
Department of Ophthalmology, University of Tokyo School of Medicine, Bunkyo-ku, Tokyo, Japan

Wei Wang and Xiulan Zhang
Zhongshan Ophthalmic Center, State Key Laboratory of Ophthalmology, Sun Yat-Sen University, Guangzhou, People's Republic of China

Index

www.ingramcontent.com/pod-product-compliance
Lightning Source LLC
Chambersburg PA
CBHW080512200326
41458CB00012B/4180